Basic Principles of Pharmacology with Dental Hygiene Applications

Basic Principles of Pharmacology with Dental Hygiene Applications

Frieda Atherton Pickett, RDH, MS
Dental Hygiene Educator, Author, Lecturer
Former Associate Professor, Caruth School of Dental Hygiene
Texas A&M Baylor College of Dentistry
Dallas, Texas

Géza T. Terézhalmy, DDS, MA
Endowed Professor in Clinical Dentistry
Dental School Professor, Department of Pharmacology
Graduate School of Biomedical Sciences
The University of Texas Health Science Center at San Antonio
San Antonio, Texas

Professor and Dean Emeritus
School of Dental Medicine
Case Western Reserve University
Cleveland, Ohio

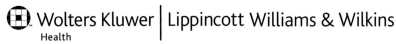

Wolters Kluwer | Lippincott Williams & Wilkins
Health
Philadelphia · Baltimore · New York · London
Buenos Aires · Hong Kong · Sydney · Tokyo

Acquisitions Editor: John Goucher
Managing Editor: Jennifer Walsh and Jessica Schultheis
Marketing Manager: Zhan Caplan
Production Editor: Paula C. Williams
Designer: Stephen Druding
Production Services: Aptara®

9 8 7 6 5 4 3 2 1

Library of Congress Cataloging-in-Publication Data

Pickett, Frieda Atherton.
  Basic principles of pharmacology with dental hygiene applications / Frieda Atherton Pickett, Géza T. Terézhalmy.—1st ed.
    p. ; cm.
  Includes bibliographical references and index.
  ISBN 978-0-7817-6536-7
1. Dental pharmacology.   2. Pharmacology.   3. Dental hygiene.   I. Terézhalmy, G. T. (Géza T.)
II. Title.
  [DNLM: 1. Pharmaceutical Preparations.   2. Dental Hygiene.   3. Drug Therapy.   QV 55
P597b 2009]
  RK701.P62 2009
  617.6′01–dc22

                                                                  2008024240

To purchase additional copies of this book, call our customer service department at **(800) 638-3030** or fax orders to **(301) 223-2320**. International customers should call **(301) 223-2300**.

Visit Lippincott Williams & Wilkins on the Internet: http://www.lww.com. Lippincott Williams & Wilkins customer service representatives are available from 8:30 am to 6:00 pm, EST.

To dental hygiene students who require textbook information to be clinically relevant.
For dental hygiene faculty who appreciate a clearly worded presentation of basic
information and materials to assist in the educational process.

F. A. P.
G. T. T.

PREFACE

The primary goals of this textbook are to present up-to-date pharmacologic principles in an easy-to-read language while identifying applications of the information to everyday life of dental hygiene practice. The unique author team of Frieda Pickett, RDH, MS, a dental hygiene educator, and Géza Terézhalmy, DDS, MA, Professor of Oral Medicine and Pharmacology, have developed a text that coordinates principles of pharmacology with pathophysiology and identifies applications to the oral health treatment plan and treatment record information.

Previous texts on this topic have not been directly relevant to clinical uses of pharmacologic information in dental hygiene practice, whereas this textbook includes several useful subjects that are not found in other pharmacology textbooks for dental hygiene students. This information includes:

- a chapter dealing specifically with adverse drug effects (Chapter 5)
- a chapter dealing with substance abuse, which includes sources for assisting the oral health professional with a substance abuse problem (Chapter 23)
- a chapter discussing herbal products used in oral care (Chapter 20)
- an eight-page color insert containing clinical images of adverse drug effects
- information on Canadian regulatory agencies

The text emphasis is on drug products that are likely to be administered by dental hygienists or taken by dental patients. Detailed information on product selection is discussed in the chapters dealing with local and topical anesthetics, fluorides, and desensitizing agents. Attention is paid to the use of dental drugs in special populations, such as during pregnancy and lactation, or in clients taking medications to control the effects of common chronic diseases. Because dental hygienists do not write prescriptions (other than in one province of Canada), less emphasis is given to pharmacokinetics of various drug classifications than is found in other textbooks.

This textbook can be used in conjunction with the same author team's *Dental Drug Reference with Clinical Implications*, published in 2008, which includes detailed information on clinical considerations for the dental professional.

ORGANIZATIONAL PHILOSOPHY

The text is organized into four parts:

- **General Principles of Pharmacology** includes general information about drugs, how drugs work and what happens to them after administration, rules for prescribing drugs and information on prescription labels relevant to the dental hygienist, autonomic pharmacology, and adverse drug effects.
- **Drugs Used in the Provision of Oral Healthcare** includes pharmacologic properties of local anesthetics, various topical products used or recommended by the dental hygienist, analgesic agents recommended or prescribed for oral pain, antibacterial agents and the relevance to dentistry, antifungal and antiviral drugs and the relevance to dentistry, drugs used for conscious sedation and general anesthesia, emergency drugs, and pharmacologic management of common oral conditions. Clinical application activities in these chapters focus on product selection and uses for dental hygiene procedures.
- **Drugs Used to Control Systemic Disorders** describes the disease condition and agents used to manage signs and symptoms. Clinical implications are highlighted as each chapter ends with a discussion of dental hygiene applications relevant to the medical condition or drug effects.
- **Drugs Used by Special Populations** includes significant information relevant to clinical considerations of clients in these categories when they present for oral health care. Agents used in dentistry are highlighted in the chapter on herbal supplements, and sources for helping individuals seek treatment for substance abuse is discussed in Chapter 23. Special considerations for the pregnant client are highlighted in this section.

FEATURES

Basic Pharmacology with Dental Hygiene Applications contains the following elements that are geared toward practicing dental hygienists and the dental hygiene student:

- **Key terms** are bolded throughout the textbook, and the definitions of these terms are summarized on each chapter's opening page and in the **glossary**.
- **Self-study review questions** follow each major division within the chapters to identify and reinforce main concepts before continuing with the reading. This section also provides a guideline for test preparation as faculty test items are developed from the self-study items.
- **Boxes** summarize dental hygiene applications of the chapter information.
- **Clinical application exercises** at the end of each chapter are related to dental hygiene services, including issues that would be addressed by the dental hygienist as part of the drug history review and determination of treatment

plan modifications. These exercises link what the student is learning to what actually happens in practice. When appropriate, Web-based activities are included. For drug card information, authors direct the reader to use a dental drug reference text for drug investigation.

ART

- **Figures** assist in understanding of concepts are included.
- **Colored clinical images** are provided to illustrate the appearance of adverse drug effects within the oral cavity.

STUDENT AND INSTRUCTOR RESOURCES

Student Resources

A Student Resource Center at http://thePoint.lww.com/pickett includes the following materials from the text:

- A **glossary** of key terms found throughout the text and their definitions.
- An appendix with **answers** to the clinical application exercises

Instructor Resources

In addition to the student resources, an Instructor's Resource Center at http://thePoint.lww.com/pickett includes the following:

- A Test Generator with 770 multiple-choice questions
- PowerPoint presentations in the form of lecture outlines
- An Image Bank containing all figures and tables found in the textbook

REVIEWERS

Darlene A. Armstrong, RDHAP, RDH, MA
Assistant Professor
Dental Hygiene Department
Loma Linda University, School of Dentistry
Loma Linda, California

Cynthia Baker, DDS
Department Head for Dental Assisting
Greenville Technical College
Greenville, South Carolina

Barbara Bennett, CDA, RDH, MS
Division Director
Allied Health Division
Texas State Technical College
Harlingen, Texas

Stephanie Bossenberger, RDH, MS
Professor and Department Chair
Dental Hygiene Department
Weber State University
Ogden, Utah

Elvir Dincer, DDS
Assistant Professor
Dental Hygiene Program
Eugenio Maria de Hostos Community College of the
   City of New York
Bronx, New York

Juli Kagan, RDH, MEd
Clinical Instructor
Department of Dental Hygiene
Broward Community College
Davie, Florida

Rachel Leo, RDH, MA
Assistant Professor
Allied Dental Health Department
New Hampshire Institute of Technology
Londonderry, New Hampshire

Donal Scheidel, DDS
Associate Professor
Department of Dental Hygiene
University of South Dakota
Vermillion, South Dakota

Jane Weiner, RDH
Instructor
PreDoctoral Periodontics Department
Nova Southeastern College of Dental Medicine
Fort Lauderdale, Florida

ACKNOWLEDGMENTS

The preparation of this book could not have been completed without the generous help and support of many individuals. Ruth Tornwall, Lamar University, Dental Hygiene Program assisted in the development of PowerPoint slides. We have incorporated the suggestions volunteered by the faculties of several universities. This includes review of the chapter on drugs used by the dental hygienist by Ruth Tornwall, Lamar University and Kathy Muzzin, Caruth School of Dental Hygiene, Texas A&M Baylor College of Dentistry. Our managing editor, Jessica Schultheis, provided excellent guidance and assistance in manuscript preparation, acquiring permissions and ancillary products.

Finally, we appreciate the support and encouragement of our spouses whom we may have neglected during this lengthy manuscript preparation.

Frieda Pickett, RDH, MS and
Géza T. Terézhalmy, DDS, MA

CONTENTS

Part 1

General Principles of Pharmacology

1

Introduction to Pharmacology: Role of Dental Hygienist, Regulations, and Sources of Information

Pharmacology is the study of **drugs** and their interactions with living cells or systems. It deals with legal and illegal drugs, prescription and nonprescription medications, and herbal and nonherbal supplements. *Drugs are chemical substances that affect living tissue and are used in the diagnosis, treatment, or prevention of a disease or medical condition.* This definition includes mineral and vitamin supplements. Food is not included in this definition, although the distinction is becoming less clear with the recent advent of adding chemical substances from plants into foods for a variety of medical effects. One example is the addition of plant stanol esters into a margarine product to lower cholesterol levels. Normally one considers drugs to be helpful and necessary; however, drugs also have the potential to cause harm. This result can occur from adverse side effects (ADEs) that are possible with almost all drugs. Therefore, the health care professional (HCP) must be thoroughly informed about each

drug likely to be administered to a client. To safely administer a drug, one must know:

- the appropriate dose to use (given the client's weight, age, and physiological status—i.e., children and elderly often require lower doses of drugs);
- the route of administration;
- the indication or reason for using the drug;
- significant side effects and potential adverse reactions;
- relevant drug interactions;
- contraindications for using the drug in a particular client;
- appropriate monitoring techniques and interventions in case of a medical emergency.

Pharmacology courses for dental hygienists in the past have been general in nature, with an emphasis on implications in dentistry. However, if pharmacology is important, then greater emphasis on its relationship to dental hygiene procedures should be included in these courses, and applications to the typical dental hygiene clinical treatment plan should be highlighted. That is the goal of this pharmacology textbook. In addition, the text should include information relevant to potential users. Therefore, in order to include dental hygiene students in Canada, this chapter includes both U.S. and Canadian governmental divisions and laws in the section that deals with drug regulation.

■ Self-Study Review

1. What is *not* included in the definition of a drug product?
2. What is a substance used in the diagnosis, prevention, or treatment of a disease or a medical condition?
3. What information is essential to know for safe administration of a drug?

HISTORY OF DRUGS

The search for substances to treat and cure disease has existed since the beginning of time. The oldest prescriptions known to exist were found on a clay tablet written by a Sumerian physician around 3000 B.C. Hippocrates (5th century B.C.), the "father of medicine," promoted the idea that disease resulted from natural causes rather than evil spirits. He believed the body had the ability to recuperate from disease and that the role of the HCP was to assist in that recuperative process. History reveals that herbs and medicinal plants grown in monastery gardens were used by religious orders to treat the sick. In the 16th century, the first pharmacopeia was written as an authoritative set of drug standards. A **pharmacopeia** is a collection of drug information in a specific geographic area. It contains all of the authorized drugs available within a country, including their descriptions, formulas, strengths, standards of purity, and doseforms. The first British pharmacopeia appeared in 1618, and many preparations included in that document are still in use today. The French produced their document in 1818, followed by the United States' pharmacopeia in 1820. Drugs and dosages were used *empirically*, which means "by best guess or statistical probabilities, using experience." In the 19th century, much research was directed at determining accurate drug dosages. As a result, drug dosages and knowledge of their expected effects became more precise. This led to the building of large manufacturing plants to produce more uniform drug products. Scientific pharmacologic practices have begun to replace **empirical** drug use.

SOURCES OF DRUGS

Drugs originally were derived from plants. As science developed, animal substances were used (insulin, estrogens),

as were mineral products (iron, calcium). Today most drugs are produced synthetically in laboratories. However, some leaves, roots, seeds, or other plant parts still are processed in laboratories for medicinal use. In this event, the pharmacologically active constituent of the plant part is separated from the plant. The resulting substance is usually more potent than that derived from chewing the plant or drinking a tea from the plant parts. Essential oils—active ingredients in some mouth rinse formulations (e.g., Listerine mouth rinse)—are secured in this way.

DRUG NOMENCLATURE

As a drug passes through the phases of drug trials before it is approved and sold, it collects three different names: (a) a chemical name, (b) a **generic** or "official" name, and (c) a trade or brand name (also called the **proprietary** name). The chemical name is a description of the chemical composition and molecular structure (such as N-acetyl-P-aminophenol). The generic name is a shorter name derived from the chemical name (such as acetaminophen). The brand name is the name a manufacturer copyrights and gives to its approved drug product (such as Tylenol). This copyright restricts the name for use only by the drug's manufacturer. To get a legitimate return for the costs of research, drug companies need to patent their products, giving them exclusive rights to the manufacture and sale for a specified period. The patent for exclusive manufacture and marketing of a drug lasts for approximately 17 years. Following this period's expiration, other drug companies can manufacture the drug under the generic name or a different brand name. Occasionally the generic name is used as the brand name. Different doseforms (tablet, patch, gel, etc.) may have different brand names. For example, lidocaine is an anesthetic agent used in dentistry. It has both topical and injectable doseforms. Topical doseforms of lidocaine are supplied as gels, sprays, ointments, liquids, or patches. Table 1-1 illustrates generic and brand names for several drugs used in dentistry.

Before the FDA approves a drug, the generic name is assigned by the manufacturer with the approval of the United States Adopted Names (USAN) Council. The generic name of the drug is listed in an official pharmacopeia and often is referred to as the "official" name of the drug. All drugs have one generic name, but they can have numerous brand names.

Table 1-1 Generic Name and Brand Names of Drugs	
Generic Name	**Brand Name**
ibuprofen	Advil, Motrin IB, Motrin, Ibutab, Midol, Menadol, PediaCare
lidocaine	**Topical:** Xylocaine Viscous, Xylocaine Liquid, Xylocaine Spray, Xylocaine Ointment, Xylocaine Solution, Xylocaine Jelly, Anestacon Jelly **Patch:** DentiPatch **Injection:** Octocaine, Xylocaine, Xylocaine-MPF, Lidocaine HCl

To avoid confusion, the generic name for a drug is usually identified in the lower case, and the brand name is capitalized.

A drug can be a prescription, or **legend**, drug—which means it can only be secured with a prescription—or a drug can be a nonprescription drug and sold over-the-counter (OTC). When multiple drugs are included into a single dose-form, they create a *combination product*. Combination products have unique brand names, but when these drugs are investigated in a drug reference, all drugs in the combination products must be examined for pertinent drug effects and clinical implications. Occasionally the Food and Drug Administration (FDA) allows drugs that formerly were sold by "prescription only" to be sold OTC. When prescription drugs are approved for OTC sale, they usually are sold in low doses considered safe for consumer purchase. An example is ibuprofen, which is sold in a 200-mg tablet OTC (Advil, Motrin IB) but can be secured as a prescription product for the 400-, 600-, or 800-mg tablet.

Each year a list of the top 200 drugs prescribed the previous year is published. This list can be found by searching the Internet. One Web site that often contains the information is www.pharmacytimes.com. A rank of one indicates this drug was the most commonly prescribed drug in the prior year. It should be noted that both generic drug names (e.g., hydrocodone with acetaminophen) and brand names (e.g., Lipitor) are included in the listing. When the generic name appears, it means that the generic drug was prescribed more often than a brand-name product. All drugs included in the top-200 list are included in this textbook so the student will become familiar with drugs likely to be reported on a client's health history. Often the client will report drugs by their brand names. Knowing the generic names for all brand-name products is important because if the client reports an allergy to Xylocaine (the brand name for lidocaine), then any brand of lidocaine would be expected to produce an allergic reaction.

DRUG EQUIVALENCY

There is a trend to encourage clinicians to write prescriptions for generic drug products due to the lower cost of the generic drug when compared to the brand-name drug. Although there are exceptions, most generic drug formulations are considered to be therapeutically equivalent to the brand-name product. The FDA requires that the active ingredient of the generic product achieve the same therapeutic blood level as the brand-name product. This should ensure equivalent therapeutic results. When two formulations of a drug meet the same chemical and physical standards required by the FDA, they are described as chemically equivalent. Those products that produce similar concentrations of the drug in the blood and tissues are **biologically equivalent**. If clinical trials show the generic drug to have an equal therapeutic effect, it is described as therapeutically equivalent. A drug product may be chemically equivalent, but not therapeutically equivalent. Only generic drugs that are biologically equivalent can be marketed. Biologic and therapeutic equivalence are the same because the amount of a drug in the blood or tissue is a requirement for a therapeutic effect.

DRUG CLASSIFICATION

Drugs are classified by (a) their intended use, or **indication**, (b) by the effect produced in the body, or (c) by their chemical categories. Drugs used to control diabetes are a good example. They may be called antidiabetic drugs (indication), oral hypoglycemic agents (effect produced), or sulfonylureas, alpha-glucosidase inhibitors, biguanides, meglitinides, or thiazolidinediones (chemical classifications). Most drugs in this text will be classified by their indications. There are other classifications for individual drugs, such as the FDA pregnancy-safety category. This classification indicates documented problems have occurred in animals or humans when the drug is used during pregnancy. Pregnancy categories will be discussed further in Chapter 21.

■ Self-Study Review

4. Define the terms pharmacopeia, empirical, legend drug, and biologic equivalence.
5. How is a legend drug obtained?
6. What is the original source for drugs?
7. All drugs have an official name, called the _____ name.
8. The proprietary name for a drug is the _____ name.
9. Biologic equivalence is equal to _____ equivalence.
10. What is the time period of patent protection for the manufacture and marketing of a drug?

REGULATORY AGENCIES IN THE UNITED STATES AND CANADA

Drugs sold in the United States are regulated by various agencies in the federal government. Each agency has a different responsibility.

- FDA: The FDA is an agency within the Department of Health and Human Services charged with the responsibility to approve drugs that have been shown to be safe and effective.[1] The FDA also tests food products to ensure they are safe to consume.[2,3] It enforces the Food, Drug, and Cosmetic Act (1938), which gives the agency the authority to regulate labeling and packaging of drug products, and to establish standards for purity and strength. It oversees quality control in drug manufacturing facilities and takes pharmacologic products off the market when manufacturing standards are not met. To improve the drug approval process, this act was updated as the FDA Modernization Act of 1997 (www.fda.gov/opacom/backgrounders/modact.htm). The main changes allowed drug manufacturers to discuss unapproved, or "off label," indications for drug products with practitioners; provided for accelerated drug approvals for life-threatening medical disorders; made

| Table 1-2 | Selected FDA Drug Safety Summaries in 2005 |

Product	Safety Issue
pamidronate (Aredia) zolendronic acid (Zometa)	May 2005: The manufacturer alerted health care professionals to the possibility of osteonecrosis of the jaw associated with the use of IV bisphosphonates in cancer patients. Based on reports, the manufacturer recommended that cancer patients receiving these drugs receive a dental examination prior to the initiation of therapy and avoid invasive dental procedures during therapy (www.fda.gov/medwatch/SAFETY/2005/zometa_deardentite_5-5-05.pdf)
Able Laboratories	May, June 2005: In May, the FDA notified patients regarding the recall of drugs manufactured by Able Laboratories because of serious concerns that they were not produced according to quality assurance standards. In June, the recall was expanded to include Quality Care Products, a federally licensed drug repackager that repackaged Able Laboratories' medications (www.fda.gov/bbs/topics/NEWS/2005/NEW01182.html).
acetaminophen (Tylenol)	June 2005: McNeil Consumer & Specialty Pharmaceuticals recalled all lots and flavors of Children's Tylenol Meltaways and SoftChews (80 mg) because of confusing labeling regarding dosing, which could lead to improper administration (www.fda.gov/oc/po/firmrecalls/mcneil05_05.html)

Adapted from the Food and Drug Administration Web site.

provisions for pediatric drug research; and revised the communication between the FDA and individuals conducting clinical trials for drugs (www.fda.gov/cder/guidance/105-115.htm). The FDA decides which drugs are sold by prescription and which drugs can be sold OTC. It regulates claims on labels and advertisements of prescription drugs. The FDA maintains a Web site summarizing new safety information about drugs, dietary supplements, biologics, medical devices, and other topics of interest (www.fda.gov/medwatch/safety/2005/safety05.htm). An example of a recent safety report from the FDA is included in Table 1-2. The FDA runs an adverse reaction reporting program that requests HCPs to report unusual occurrences or increased numbers of known adverse events associated with a drug. Reporting of adverse drug reactions can be made by telephone to the FDA or by completing an adverse event form found on the Web site. These reports may result in changes in the drug's package insert information, or it may result in a drug being removed from the market, as was the case with the analgesic Vioxx, which was shown to be associated with an increased number of adverse cardiovascular events.

- Federal Trade Commission (FTC): The FTC enforces federal consumer protection laws (www.ftc.gov) and regulates marketing practices and advertising on foods, nonprescription drugs, dietary supplements, and products promising health benefits. For example, in the 1980s, advertisements for Listerine mouth rinse used the slogan "Kills the germs that cause bad breath." The FTC banned use of the slogan because there was no scientific evidence to support the claim. The old slogan was replaced with a new one—"Kills the germs that cause gingivitis"—following the completion of properly designed studies. The FTC protects rights of competition and fair-pricing practices, including pricing for prescription drugs and health care. It prohibits false advertising of foods, nonprescription drugs, and cosmetics. People also can visit the FTC Web site for consumer services, such as ordering a free credit report or reporting fraudulent spam e-mail (spam@uce.gov).
- Drug Enforcement Administration (DEA): The DEA is an agency within the Department of Justice that administers the requirements outlined in the Controlled Substances Act

(1970). This act identifies drugs capable of causing addiction and sets requirements for prescribing drugs with potential for abuse, such as narcotics, barbiturates, and benzodiazepines.

FDA Approval Process for New Drugs

Table 1-3 gives the success rate and the length of time each step takes in the FDA drug-approval process. Here is an overview of how a drug becomes FDA approved.

- Preclinical trials: A new drug is tested in animals to prove its safety.
- Phase I clinical trial: Low doses of the drug are tested in a group of 20 to 80 healthy volunteers to study safety profiles and determine pharmacokinetic characteristics.
- Phase II clinical trials: Controlled studies involving 100 to 300 volunteers assess the drug's effectiveness.
- Phase III clinical trials: Controlled studies involving 1,000 to 3,000 volunteers to confirm the drug's safety and efficacy, and identify adverse drug effects (ADEs).
- Postmarketing surveillance: Determine the true risk–benefit profile of the new drug.

Drug Trials

Premarketing drug trial groups generally include only 3,000 to 4,000 subjects. From a statistical perspective, a population of 30,000 would have to be exposed to the drug to have a 95% chance of detecting an ADE with an incidence of 1 in 10,000 subjects. Therefore, ADEs that occur at low frequencies easily can be missed. In addition, premarketing clinical trials are of relatively short duration. ADEs that develop when a drug is taken on a regular basis or those that have long latency periods also may escape detection. Study groups often exclude children, women, and the elderly, making ADEs in this population unlikely to be identified in data supplied to the FDA for drug approval. Finally, the efficacy of a drug is evaluated for only a narrow set of indications and may not include the actual evolving use of a drug. Consequently, premarketing clinical trials are designed to detect only the most common ADEs, including those occurring more frequently than 1 in

Table 1-3	The Chronology of Testing and Introducing New Drugs

Preclinical Testing (3.5 y)	Clinical Trials (8.5 y)	Postmarketing Surveillance

Laboratory studies
• Isolation or synthesis of a new chemical
Animal studies
• Assess safety and biological activity
Pharmaceutical company files an Investigational New Drug (IND) application with the FDA
• FDA approval
IND reviewed and approved by the Institutional Review Board where the studies will be conducted
• Progress reports on clinical trials submitted to FDA annually
	Phase I (1 y):
	• 20 to 80 healthy volunteers
	    Dosage range
	    Safety profile
	Phase II (2 y):
	• 100 to 300 volunteers with a specific disease
	    Short-term effectiveness
	    Adverse drug events
	Phase III (3 y):
	• 1,000 to 3,000 volunteers with a specific disease
	    Long-term effectiveness
	    Adverse drug events
	Pharmaceutical company files a New Drug Application (NDA) with the FDA
	• FDA approval
		Monitoring for safety during postmarketing clinical use to determine the true risk–benefit profile of the new drug
		• Pharmaceutical company must continue to submit periodic reports to the FDA
		    Case reports of adverse drug reactions
		    Quality control records
		• FDA may require additional clinical trials (Phase IV studies)

5,000 potential drugs evaluated	5 drugs are approved for clinical trials	1 drug approved for marketing

y = years

1,000; these are listed in the product's official labeling at the time of approval.

U.S. Legislation That Affects Narcotics

• Harrison Narcotics Act (HNA): This was the first federal law (1914) intended to reduce drug addiction or substance abuse. The HNA established regulations governing the use of opium products, cocaine, and their derivatives. It was amended in 1937 to add marijuana. This act provided federal control over the prescription of narcotics and required registration of practitioners who prescribed narcotics. Prior to the HNA, both opium mixtures and cocaine products could be purchased OTC. This practice was responsible for many cases of drug addiction and ended with the passage of this legislation.

• Comprehensive Drug Abuse Prevention and Control Act of 1970: This act is usually referred to as the Controlled Substances Act (CSA). The HNA was replaced by the CSA and other legislation related to narcotic drug prescription. It was designed to prevent drug abuse and dependence and to include recommendations for treatment and rehabilitation of drug-dependent persons. It also includes regulations for the manufacturing, distribution, and dispensing of controlled substances. The CSA identifies drugs that have the potential to cause dependence or abuse and classifies them according to their abuse potential. It also identifies drugs within each of five schedules (Schedule I, II, III, IV, V) and sets requirements for writing prescriptions for these scheduled drugs. Some of these agents frequently are prescribed by dentists for relief of dental pain and to reduce anxiety. The schedules are discussed in Chapter 3. Other countries have similar legislation; for example, Canada has a controlled substance schedule similar to the U.S. schedule, but there are some differences in how drugs are classified in the Canadian schedules when compared to U.S. regulations.

Canadian Regulatory Agencies

The Health Protection Branch of the Department of National Health and Welfare in Canada is responsible for the administration and enforcement of the laws governing drug prescriptions in Canada. It oversees the Food and Drugs Act, the Proprietary or Patent Medicine Act, and the Narcotic Control Act. These acts are designed to protect the consumer from fraud, deception, and health hazards due to the use of foods, drugs, cosmetics, and medical devices. The Department of National Health and Welfare also authorizes substance abuse treatment, including the use of methadone for narcotic addicts.

Canadian Legislation That Affects Narcotics

The following acts regulate narcotics in Canada.

• The Canadian Food and Drugs Act (1953): This act requires that drugs comply with prescribed standards stated in recognized pharmacopeias and formularies or with the professed standards under which the drugs are sold. Drug labels must include the legend "Canadian standard drug" or the abbreviation "CSD" to signify these standards have been met. It specifies rules regarding advertising or marketing to the general public. Drugs used as treatments (preventive or curative) for alcoholism, arteriosclerosis, or cancer have special rules for advertisement. When it is necessary to provide adequate directions for the safe use of a drug in the treatment of these diseases, that disease or disorder may be mentioned only on or within package inserts that accompany the drug. The act also prohibits the sale of drugs that are contaminated, adulterated, or unsafe, and those whose labels are false, misleading, or deceptive. Controlled substances are included in Part G within the act. Those requirements are discussed in Chapter 3.

• Controlled Drugs and Substance Act: This Act with amendments governs the possession, sale, manufacture, production, and distribution of narcotics. It requires that only authorized persons possess narcotic substances. These include licensed manufacturers or distributors, pharmacists, practitioners, persons in charge of a hospital, or persons acting as agents for practitioners. Members of the Royal Canadian Mounted Police (RCMP) and various governmental or university departments may possess narcotics in connection with their employment. Of course, a person who has secured narcotics after filling a legal prescription is included in the approved category. The Act identifies drugs and derivatives that are subject to provisions and places them into schedules similar to those in the United States. A prescription from a physician is required to secure the drugs in the schedules.

DRUG INFORMATION SOURCES

Another purpose of pharmacology in dental hygiene practice is to guide the practitioner toward using reliable sources of drug information for drug investigation. Both the dentist and dental hygienist consult resources containing pharmacologic information. When drugs are prescribed or used by dental professionals, more than cursory information is needed. Detailed and complete drug information can be found in a variety of publications. Some examples include:

- Facts & Comparisons
- *Physicians' Drug Reference* (PDR)
- The U.S. Pharmacopeia Drug Information
- American Hospital Formulary Service® Drug Information
- Mosby's Dental Drug Reference

These references are updated annually or, in the case of Facts & Comparisons, monthly. Drug information also can be found on the Internet. Several sources include the Hippocrates Web site, the PDR Web site, and MedlinePlus, a governmental drug information site. The PDRhealth Web site provides drug information for consumers. These sites contain information on prescription drugs, OTCs, herbal medicines, and nutritional supplements. There are several concise, but less complete, drug references published each year or every other year, some of which are designed specifically for dental use:

- *Dental Drug Reference with Clinical Implications* (Lippincott Williams & Wilkins)
- *Dental Drug Reference* (Mosby-Elsevier)
- *Drug Information Handbook for Dentistry* (Lexicomp)

Publications that are specific for identifying drug interactions include the following:

- *Drug Interaction Facts* (Facts & Comparisons)
- *Handbook of Adverse Drug Interactions* (The Medical Letter)

Each type of publication is selected based on how it is used. For example, complete and up-to-date references are recommended for drug investigation before drugs are prescribed, whereas a concise, but less complete, reference might be used to investigate drugs that were prescribed by another provider and reported on the health history. Every dental office should have up-to-date drug references to use for drug investigation. Each year new drugs are approved by the FDA. This requires purchasing new, updated references on a regular basis.

■ Self-Study Review

11. What are the functions of the FDA?
12. Which agency oversees nonprescription drug products?
13. Describe the differences between drug trial phases. What is the chance that all ADEs are identified when all the phases are completed?
14. Briefly describe the steps required for a drug to get FDA approval. What groups are often excluded in drug trials? What is the purpose of postmarket surveillance?
15. The CSA is administered by which U.S. governmental agency?
16. Which act identifies rules for writing prescriptions for narcotics in the United States? Which governmental agency enforces this act?
17. Which governmental agency enforces rules for prescribing narcotic drugs in Canada?
18. Identify sources for dentally related drug information that provide fast retrieval of drug information relevant to dental hygiene practice.
19. Define the acronym *FDA*.

ROLES OF THE DENTAL HYGIENIST

Dental hygienists use a variety of drugs in the provision of dental hygiene services. Examples include topical anesthetics, fluorides, and desensitizing agents. Some states permit dental hygienists to administer local anesthetic agents by injection and nitrous oxide gas by inhalation. Dental hygienists may be asked by clients to recommend OTC products for postoperative pain control, antiviral or antifungal treatments, or any other number of reasons. Most agents administered in the dental office should be entered into the treatment record identifying the drug used, the dose or amount applied, and the route of administration. Drug recommendations made to a client also must be recorded in the treatment record, with specific instructions to the client described. During health history review, any medications, herbs, or supplements listed should be investigated to determine drug effects that may warrant treatment plan modifications (Box 1-1).

For the reasons described above, dental hygienists must understand the pertinent pharmacological properties of those drugs used as adjuncts to dental hygiene procedures or those administered by the dental hygienists. This understanding includes identifying specific drugs most appropriate to use in a given situation, plus knowing the proper dose to use, the method of application or administration, and precautions or contraindications in using any given product.

Dental hygienists also have an obligation to understand the **pharmacologic effects** of agents reported on the health history. During the health history drug review, dental hygienists should investigate all drugs, supplements, and herbal products reported by clients. This pretreatment evaluation should, at a minimum, include the name of the product, why

BOX 1-1. Role of the Dental Hygienist in Pharmacology

- Drugs used should be entered into the treatment record, including drug, dose, and route of administration.
- Any drug recommended or given as a sample to a client should be recorded in the treatment record, with the client's instructions.
- Drug or herbal supplement history review should include investigation of potential drug effects and modifications of the treatment plan.

it is being taken, and if it was taken prior to the appointment (Box 1-2). All pharmacologic products should be investigated in a medical or dental drug reference, with attention given to the action of the product and potential ADEs, often referred to as "side effects." The client may or may not experience ADEs identified for a particular drug. For those ADEs which may require modification of the dental hygiene treatment plan, investigation should include evaluation of vital-sign values to identify alterations from normal levels and questioning the client (or examining the oral cavity) to determine if the side effect has occurred. This text identifies treatment plan modifications for common ADEs of various drugs. If a drug will be used by the HCP during the appointment, the investigation should include whether the agent could interact with any drugs reported on the health history. It is clear, then, that the dental hygienist must learn appropriate and selective information on principles of drug effects, both those agents being taken by the client and those drugs used by the dental hygienist. Furthermore, the clinical implications for those effects must be considered. For example, the health history includes medical information that must be evaluated for indications for antibiotic prophylaxis prior to continuing with various dental hygiene procedures. The dentist is responsible for prescribing the indicated antibiotic, but the dental hygienist plays a role as part of the pretreatment evaluation to ensure that the client takes the proper dose and knows when it should

be taken. This information should be recorded in the client's treatment record to verify that this follow-up procedure is done.

DRUG CARD PREPARATION

Most dental hygiene standards of practice require that practitioners investigate drugs reported on the health history and prepare appropriate information regarding clinical implications in a written format. Each chapter of this textbook illustrates significant information to consider and the indicated modifications to the dental hygiene treatment plan. Drug cards should include the following information:

- Drug name (generic name, brand name)
- Indication (why the drug was taken)
- Side effects relevant to dental hygiene care:
  - Xerostomia/dry mouth, oral ulcerations, taste disturbances
  - Effect on blood pressure or pulse
  - Immune response changes
  - Increased bleeding risk
  - Nausea, abdominal pain
  - Respiratory effects
  - Central nervous system effects (tremors, facial tics, etc.)
  - Other side effects relevant to oral health care
- Clinical implications for each drug effect experienced by the client and treatment implications for the indication of the drug
- Oral health information topics related to drug effects, drug warnings, or the condition for which the drug was indicated

An example of a comprehensive drug card is illustrated in Figure 1-1.

■ Self-Study Review

20. Describe three ways the RDH applies knowledge of pharmacology.
21. Which three types of information should be placed in the treatment record?
22. When preparing a drug card, which four items of information should be included?
23. List four to six ADEs that can modify the dental hygiene treatment plan.
24. What information should be considered when investigating drugs reported on the medical history?

BOX 1-2. Follow-up Information for Drug Products Reported on the Health History

- "I see you are taking [drug name]."
- "Why are you taking this drug?"
- "Did you take it today?"

Side Effects Profile
- "Have you noticed a problem with [side effect]?"
- Evaluate values of vital sign information for relationships.
- Examine oral cavity for evidence of drug effects.

CONCLUSION

The dental hygienist has a significant role in understanding drug information and names associated with pharmacology. Principles for safe administration of drugs provide a reliable

---

AMOXICILLIN (Trimox, Amoxil)

Indication:	Antibiotic prophylaxis, hip joint replacement 1 year prior
Adverse/Side Effects:	Discolored tongue, candidiasis, glossitis, stomatitis, thirst, nausea, vomiting, diarrhea, bone marrow depression, immediate (anaphylaxis) or delayed (rash) hypersensitivity reactions
Clinical Consideration:	(1) Check dose taken, timing of dose related to appointment time. (2) Use semisupine chair position if GI side effects are present. (3) Monitor for oral side effect manifestation and opportunistic infection [unlikely in one dose regimen] and (4) monitor for signs of allergy (rash, itching, inability to breathe, hypotension). (5) Examine for oral manifestations of adverse drug effects and discuss potential management issues (i.e., antifungal therapy). (6) Review physician orders for dental treatment.
Oral Health Information:	Inform client that antibiotic prophylaxis following prosthetic hip replacement is recommended during initial two years, following successful surgery and no post-operative infection, but may be discontinued after that time in most cases.

Figure 1-1 Illustration of a Drug Card.

---

system of pharmacology. The regulatory agencies that make and administer laws related to drug function also provide safety in drug use. Drug trials include several phases to identify potential ADEs before marketing the drugs to the public. Reference sources are available to provide information for effective investigation of pharmacologic agents. The information in this chapter is used and applied throughout this textbook.

References

1. Hilts PJ. The FDA at work: Cutting-edge science promoting public health. *FDA Consum.* 2006;40(1):28–39.
2. Meadows M. A century of ensuring safe foods and cosmetics. *FDA Consum.* 2006;40(1):7–13.
3. Meadows M. Promoting safe and effective drugs for 100 years. *FDA Consum.* 2006;40(1):15–20.

CLINICAL APPLICATION EXERCISES (CAE)

☐ Exercise 1. A 62-year-old woman presents for her semiannual dental exam and maintenance care. She reports no changes in her health history, but she is taking a medication for the management of osteoporosis (raloxifene hydrochloride [Evista]). She is unaware of the dose of the medication, but she takes it once daily and reports no associated ADEs. Vital signs are all within normal limits. Prepare a drug card for the medication according to the example in this chapter. You may need to use a dental drug reference to complete this exercise.

☐ Exercise 2. Use a dental drug reference to find the generic drug *metformin*. Why would this drug be taken? What disease or condition would the person have? What brand name(s) might the client report on the health history? What treatment plan modifications would be appropriate for this client?

☐ Exercise 3. WEB ACTIVITY: Go to the FDA's Web site and find the form to report an ADE (www.fda.gov/medwatch/index.html). Read over the information to be provided. You can find the source for news on drug safety at the same site.

☐ Exercise 4. WEB ACTIVITY: Go to the Web site for the National Center for Complementary and Alternative Medicine (http://nccam.nih.gov), which is a division of the National Institutes of Health. Go to the "Health Information" section, then choose "All Diseases or Conditions." Choose the condition "Bone Health" and look for information on an herb or supplement used for the indication. Answer these questions:

a. How effective is the supplement for this indication?
b. Are there any adverse effects?
c. Are there any drug or food interactions?
d. Are there any warnings about dosing? Who should not use the product? Should the product be used on a chronic basis?
e. What are the Key Points?

☐ Exercise 5. WEB ACTIVITY (Canadian students): Log on to http://www.imshealth.com/vgn/images/portal/cit_40000873/3/31/80063346The_top_200.pdf for drug information data on drugs dispensed in Canada.

2

General Principles of Pharmacology

The science of pharmacology is the study of drugs. The science developed when early individuals observed the effects of herbs and plant extracts on themselves or others. Historically, the clinician was responsible for information about the sources, physical and chemical properties, and compounding and dispensing of drugs. These activities are now delegated to pharmacologists and pharmacists. Today, the practitioner's responsibility relates to the clinical application of this knowledge. Oral health professionals must understand basic prin-

ciples of pharmacology as they apply to drugs used in oral health care as well as other drugs taken by the dental patient. This understanding provides for more efficient communication when explaining drug effects to the patient or when medical consultation is necessary. Important principles include:

- knowing how a drug works, called *the mechanism of action*;
- the potential adverse (or side) effects (ADEs) that are possible;

- oral health education information related to drug effects;
- the risks of taking a drug.

These principles apply to all therapeutic agents (including vitamins, herbs, and nutritional supplements) and pertain to a drug's mechanism of action (pharmacodynamics), the movement of the drug through the body (pharmacokinetics), and potential adverse effects when the drug is taken (pharmacotherapeutic variables).

■ Self-Study Review

1. List four principles of pharmacology that the oral health professional must understand in order to provide information on drug effects.
2. Define *pharmacodynamics* and *pharmacokinetics* as they apply to drugs.

PHARMACODYNAMICS

Pharmacodynamics is the science of molecular interactions between drugs and body constituents. It relates to the biochemical and physiologic actions of drugs. When a drug is delivered to the tissue cells, it goes through several steps. The first step in initiating a drug-induced effect is the formation of a complex, or bond, between the drug molecule and a cell component called the drug **receptor**. The receptor site where a drug acts to initiate a series of biochemical and physiologic effects is that drug's site of action. The molecular event that follows this drug-receptor interaction is called the drug's **mechanism of action**. An example of this process is the action of epinephrine in local anesthetic agents. Following the injection of a local anesthetic solution (delivery), epinephrine binds to its receptor on vascular smooth muscle (complex formation) and causes the muscle cell to constrict (drug-receptor interaction), resulting in vasoconstriction (mechanism of action). Most drugs go through a similar process; however, it should be understood that not all drugs produce their effects by interacting with specific receptors. This concept will become apparent as one considers drug action in future chapters. A number of drugs form chemical bonds with small molecules, chelating agents, or metallic cations. A practical example of this type of drug-receptor interaction is the therapeutic neutralization of gastric acid by antacids. Many other drugs act by mechanisms that are not yet understood.

Receptors

Drug receptors are large, highly specialized molecules, which are components of the plasma membrane or are located intracellularly. A single cell may have hundreds of different receptor sites, and a drug may interact with a variety of different receptor types or subtypes, producing different pharmacologic effects. Drug molecules and their receptors must have similar structures (structural specificity), described as "lock and key" complementary fits. Figure 2-1 illustrates the

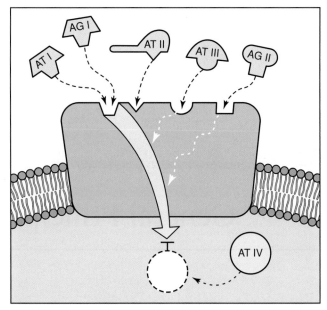

Figure 2-1 Complementary Receptor-Molecule Fit. Major features of classical receptors. Drug molecules (AG, agonist; AT, antagonist) and their receptors must have a similar structure (structural specificity), described as a "lock and key" complementary fit. AT I and AG I compete for the same receptor site, AG I to enhance and AT I to block signal; AG II and AT III enhance or block signal, respectively, by binding to alternative sites that influence signal transmission; AT II binds to an alternative site and blocks AG I activation site. AT IV blocks signal at intracellular signal reception site.

complementary fit and the interaction with different receptors. Only one molecule can bind to a receptor at a time; i.e., two drugs cannot occupy the same receptor at the same time. Receptors have a variety of other features that determine their function, location in the body, relationship to cellular membranes, and binding capacity (Box 2-1), including:

- electrochemical force (either electropositive or electronegative) that functions to attract the drug molecule to the receptor
- the trait of being hydrophilic or hydrophobic to attract or repel a molecule
- are cellular macromolecules

BOX 2-1. Characteristics of Drug Receptors

- Cellular macromolecules
- Location on the cell surface or within the cell
- Hundreds of different receptors on a single cell
- Complementary fit between drug and receptor
- Electrochemical charge
- Hydrophilic or hydrophobic
- Only one drug molecule can occupy a receptor at one time

The drug molecule binds to the complementary receptor and stimulates the receptor to produce a definable pharmacologic response.

Chemical Bonds

Drugs attach to or interact with these receptor sites through various types of chemical bonds. These include ionic, hydrogen, and covalent bonds, and van der Waals forces. Hydrogen bonding and ionic bonding are the most common types between drugs and receptors. The bonds are similar in that both involve an electrochemical attraction. These interactions require little energy and are made and broken easily.

Ionic Bonds

Ionic interactions occur between atoms with opposite charges. An atom with an excess of electrons imparts a negative charge, which causes an attraction to an atom with a deficiency of electrons. A simple example of this type of interaction is reflected in the attraction between sodium and chloride ions (sodium chloride [Na^+/Cl^-]). Applying the concept to the attraction between drug molecules and receptor sites, a positively charged drug molecule is attracted to a negatively charged receptor site. These bonds are weak and are easily reversed.

Hydrogen Bonds

When bound to nitrogen or oxygen, hydrogen atoms become positively polarized and bind to negatively polarized atoms such as oxygen, nitrogen, or sulfur. These bonds are generally weaker than ionic bonds.

Covalent Bonds

Covalent bonds are the strongest type of bond between a drug and its receptor, resulting from the sharing of electrons by two atoms. The energy required to overcome such interactions can be so great that the bond is often irreversible. Fortunately, such drug–receptor interactions are not common. A good example of a covalent bond is the complex formed between tetracycline and dentin to produce a permanent intrinsic discoloration.

van der Waals Forces

These nondescript forces contribute to the mutual attraction between organic molecules through a shifting of electron density in or around a molecule that results in the generation of transient positive or negative charges. This provides for a weak attractive force between some drugs and their receptors.

Attractive Forces Between Drugs and Receptors

Drug molecules move in constant random motion in the cellular area, binding to receptors and breaking away from recep-

tors. The following forces govern the potential for a complex to form.

Affinity

When a drug molecule moves so close to its receptor that the attractive force between them becomes great enough to overcome the random motion of the drug molecule, the drug binds to the receptor. This phenomenon is called **affinity**. The affinity of a drug for a particular receptor and the type of binding that occurs is intimately related to the drug's chemical structure. Because two drug molecules cannot occupy the same receptor site at the same time, the drug with the greater affinity will bind more readily to the receptor. Affinity is expressed by its dissociation constant (K_D), which is the concentration of a drug required in solution to achieve 50% occupancy of its receptors. When two drugs of equal concentrations are competing for the same receptor population, the drug with the greater affinity will bind with more receptors (and stimulate the receptor to cause an action) at any given instant (Fig. 2-2). Thus, a lower concentration of that drug will produce the same level of pharmacologic effect. This means that drugs with good affinity have greater **potency**; i.e., they require a smaller dose to cause a specific effect. Consequently, potency is related to the affinity of a drug.

Figure 2.2 illustrates that when equal concentrations of two drugs are in equilibrium with the same receptor population (square indentations), the drug with the greater affinity (Drug A) will make a greater number of effective bindings at any given instant. The result is that Drug A is more potent, and a lower concentration of Drug A is required to produce the same level of pharmacologic effect as that produced by Drug B.

Agonists

Drugs that have direct stimulatory effects on receptors are called **agonists**. A strong agonist produces a significant physiologic response when only a relatively small number of receptors are occupied. The ability of an agonist to interact with a receptor and initiate a response is the function of its **intrinsic activity**. Using these terms in an example, when a small dose of a drug (agonist) produces a desired effect, the drug has good *affinity* and good *intrinsic activity*. A weak agonist must be bound to many more receptors to produce the same effect, so a much larger dose of a weak agonist will be required to produce the desired effect—i.e., the drug has lower affinity and/or lower intrinsic activity. A partial agonist has affinity for the receptor, but very low intrinsic activity. Therefore, it will never produce the same effect as a strong agonist or a weak agonist, even when all receptors are occupied. This can be illustrated with the log dose–response of three different drugs with affinity to the same receptors, as shown in Figure 2-3, where a low dose of Drug A (strong agonist) produces a full effect, Drug B (weak agonist) must have a higher dose to reach that effect, and Drug C (partial agonist) never reaches the effect produced by Drugs A or B. An example of the above concept would be the use of 5 mg of morphine to relieve strong pain, compared with 50 mg of meperidine (Demerol) to relieve the same degree of pain,

Relationship of Affinity and Potency

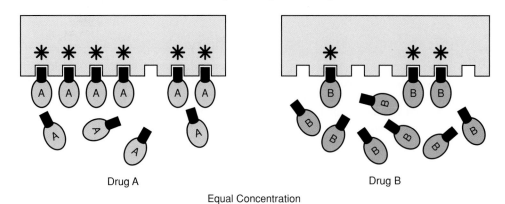

Drug A   Drug B

Equal Concentration

Figure 2-2 Relationship between Drug Affinity to Receptor and Potency. When equal concentrations of two drugs are in equilibrium with the same receptor population (square indentations), the drug with the greater affinity (Drug A) will make a greater number of effective bindings at any given instant. Thus, a lower concentration of Drug A will be required to produce the same level of pharmacologic effect as that produced by Drug B.

and further compared with 65 mg of propoxyphene (Darvon), which will not relieve strong pain, no matter how high the dose given. Thus the affinity and the intrinsic activity of an agonist determine efficacy of a drug.

Efficacy

Efficacy is the maximum response produced by a drug. It is a state of optimal receptor occupancy by the drug molecules; additional doses would produce no further beneficial effect. This concept is often referred to as the **ceiling dose**. As seen with the affinity of a drug for a particular receptor, the efficacy of a drug is also related to its chemical structure. This concept is referred to as the *intrinsic activity relationship*. The quantification of a specific response elicited by a drug given in a range of doses (5 mg, 10 mg, 50 mg, etc.) is called the graded dose–response relationship. This relationship is expressed visually and mathematically with a dose–response curve. The curve is established by placing the logarithmic value for the dose (or log dose) on the x-axis and the quantified response on the y-axis (Fig. 2-4). The upper plateau of the dose–response curve represents the efficacy or the maximal effect of a drug associated with a specific dose. A good example of this concept is acetaminophen, which has a ceiling dose of about 1,000 mg for pain relief. Taking 2,000 mg in a single dose will not produce greater pain relief and may lead to toxicity (overdose). The lowest dose of a drug that will produce a measurable response is called the *threshold dose*. The dose range of acetaminophen for pain relief is 325 mg to 1,000 mg. Therefore, 325 mg would be the threshold dose of acetaminophen.

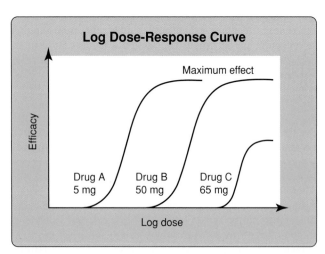

Figure 2-3 Log Dose-Response Curve Illustrating Three Different Drugs (a Strong Agonist, a Weak Agonist, and a Partial Agonist) with Affinity for the Same Receptors. Drugs A and B have the same efficacy, but it takes more of Drug B to produce the effect. Drug C does not have the same efficacy of Drugs A and B, even at a higher dose.

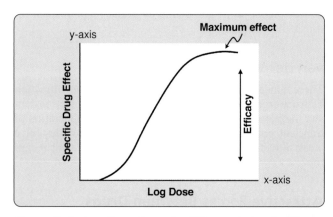

Figure 2-4 Log Dose Curve for Efficacy. A drug's efficacy, or maximum effect, is represented by the upper plateau of the dose–response curve.

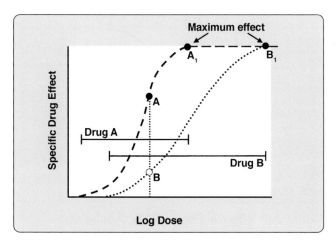

Figure 2-5 Log Dose of Potency and Efficacy. This shows two drugs with same efficacy (A, B), but different potency (A, B). Potency relates to two or more drugs by comparing the doses required to produce a given effect.

Potency

Potency is defined as the relative pharmacologic activity of a dose of a compound compared with a dose of a different agent producing the same effect. The concept provides a mechanism by which to compare the ability of two or more drugs, with affinity for the same receptor, to produce a given effect as a function of dose. Potency *is related to the affinity of a drug to its receptor, whereas* efficacy *is related to the intrinsic activity of that drug once a drug–receptor complex is formed.* It is determined by the relative position of the dose-response curve along the dose axis as illustrated in Figure 2-5. Note that for the maximum effect, the dose of Drug A is smaller than that required for Drug B, illustrating that Drug A is more potent than Drug B, yet they have the same efficacy. An example is the ability of two nonsteroidal agents (ketorolac and ibuprofen) to relieve dental pain. Ketorolac at 20 mg relieves dental pain to the same degree as 400 mg of ibuprofen. Therefore, ketorolac has greater potency and equal efficacy.

Antagonists

An **antagonist** is a drug that interferes with the action of an agonist, but has no effect in the absence of an agonist. Antagonists can be classified as receptor or nonreceptor antagonists.

Receptor Antagonists

Receptor antagonists can bind at the active site (called agonist binding domain) and prevent the binding of the agonist, or they may bind to an adjacent site (overlapping with the agonist binding domain) and prevent the conformational change required for receptor activation by an agonist. Receptor antagonism can be either reversible (competitive) or irreversible (noncompetitive):

- A competitive antagonist binds reversibly to the active site of the agonist and maintains the receptor in its inactive

conformation. In other words, it has affinity for a receptor but no efficacy (i.e., it cannot cause an effect). It competes with the agonist for the receptor, and the outcome depends on the degree of affinity of the competitive antagonist compared with the agonist. A competitive antagonist forms a reversible drug-receptor complex, which can be overcome by increasing the dose of the agonist. Consequently, the inhibition is surmountable. In effect, the presence of a competitive antagonist reduces the potency of the agonist. A practical example of this type of antagonism with relevance to dentistry is the reversal of respiratory depression caused by excessive doses of an opioid analgesic (agonist) with naloxone, an opioid antagonist.

- A noncompetitive antagonist binds either to the active site or to an allosteric (adjacent) site of the receptor. It binds to the active site either covalently or with very high affinity, both of which are effectively irreversible. An allosteric noncompetitive antagonist prevents the receptor from being activated, even when the agonist is bound to the active site. In effect, the presence of a noncompetitive antagonist reduces the efficacy of the agonist. Aspirin is a practical example of a noncompetitive antagonist. It irreversibly affects cyclooxygenase, the enzyme responsible for the process that causes platelets to clump together and produce a clot. This reduces clotting and increases the bleeding time. Normal platelet function can be reestablished only by the generation of new platelets in the bone marrow.

Nonreceptor Antagonists

A nonreceptor antagonist may be either a chemical or physiologic antagonist.

Chemical Antagonist

A chemical antagonist may either bind a molecule at some point in the activation pathway or directly inhibit the agonist. A practical example of this type of antagonism with relevance to dentistry is the one produced by local anesthetic agents. They block sodium channels in the activation pathway of chemicals that promote depolarization of nerve fibers. By blocking depolarization, information about tissue damage (in the form of electrical impulses) is not transmitted to the cortex, and the patient will not experience pain.

Physiologic Antagonist

A physiologic antagonist activates pathways that oppose the action of the agonist. An example of this type of antagonism is reflected in the action of epinephrine on blood vessels (vasoconstriction) following an allergic reaction (anaphylaxis) and histamine release. The effect of epinephrine overcomes the effect of histamine (vasodilation) on the same blood vessel, and the vessel becomes constricted.

Mixed Agonist–Antagonists

Mixed agonist–antagonists are drugs that have both agonistic and antagonistic properties. When used alone, such a drug behaves as an agonist. However, when another drug that competes for the same receptor site is administered concurrently, the agonist–antagonist will also act as an antagonist. A practical example of an agonist–antagonist is pentazocine, an opioid analgesic; when used alone, it interacts with its opioid receptor to produce analgesia, but it antagonizes the action of other opioid agonists.

Receptor Classification

Receptors are classified according to the type of drug they interact with or according to the specific physiologic response produced by the drug–receptor complex. Receptor sites may also be subclassified by evaluating the effects of different agonists in the presence of a given antagonist. The previous example of using epinephrine to counteract the effects of histamine illustrates this concept. Earlier in this chapter, it was noted that drugs can interact with different receptors. Epinephrine can bind to receptors in the bronchioles of the lungs to cause bronchodilation, and it can bind to different receptors on blood vessels to cause vasoconstriction; hence, one drug interacts with two different receptors and causes two different actions.

Similarly, receptors and receptor subtypes exist for many other agents. The number of any given receptor types or subtypes on a cell also may vary. Certain disease states or drugs taken long term and/or in large doses may increase (up-regulate) or decrease (down-regulate) the number of receptors and provide a degree of adaptability in the face of changing physiologic events. Developing tolerance to a drug so the former dose no longer causes an adequate effect and a higher dose is needed to cause the effect illustrates this concept.

Toxicity

Any drug at a high-enough concentration can produce a toxic effect (overdose). In the context of this discussion, **toxicity** refers to undesirable effects associated with the administration of *therapeutic* dosages of drugs. These adverse effects may be:

- An exaggeration of direct effects seen at higher doses. For example, barbiturates may produce sedation, drowsiness, and reduced rate of respiration at therapeutic levels (direct effect), but cause death (exaggerated effect of respiratory depression) at increased dose levels. This is an extension of the intended therapeutic effect of central nervous system (CNS) depression.
- Multiple concurrent adverse, or side, effects occurring at therapeutic dosage levels. For example, the administration of certain antihistamines for hay fever, intended to antagonize histamine action at H_1-histaminic receptors in the respiratory system, can also bind to H_3-histaminic receptors in the CNS and cause drowsiness. In this case, the drowsiness is a concurrent side effect, not an intended response. ADEs are discussed in detail in Chapter 5.

Median Effective Dose or Lethal Dose

The dose of a drug required to produce a desired response in 50% of the individuals within the same population is the median effective dose (ED50), as shown in Figure 2-6. If

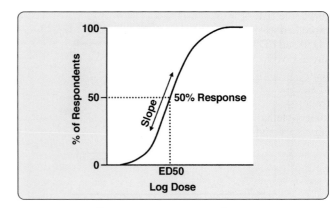

Figure 2-6 Effective Dose in 50% of Subjects.

death is the measured end point, the ED50 is expressed as the median lethal dose (LD50). A steep dose–response curve indicates a narrow dosage range between minimal and maximal effects. Consequently, the risk for toxic or even lethal dosage levels can be greater because of the narrower dosage range. Similarly, the median toxic dose (TD50) is the dose of a drug that produces a specific toxic response in 50% of the individuals within the same population. These concepts are used during drug development to determine the safety of doses. Fortunately, laboratory animals are used to determine the LD50 in drug research centers! The relative safety of a drug for humans is extrapolated from animal data and clinical data during new drug's clinical trials.

Therapeutic Index

When evaluating potential therapeutic agents, dose–response curves provide valuable information relative to their safety. The margin of safety of a drug is expressed by the Therapeutic Index (TI). For example, if the slope of the dose–response curve is steep, it indicates a narrow range between dosages that produce minimal and maximal effects, or between a safe dose and a toxic dose (Fig. 2-7). Using the dose–response

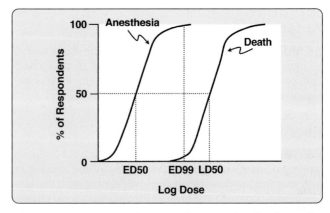

Figure 2-7 ED50 and LD50. The margin of safety of a drug may be expressed by its therapeutic index, the actual ratio of LD50 and ED50, or by comparing the 99% dose–response curve for the therapeutic effect with the curve for the toxic effect.

curve, the risk of a toxic effect may also be calculated and expressed as the drug's TI. The TI is the actual ratio of the LD50 and ED50 (LD50/ED50). The same concept applies to any toxic effect in that the higher the numerical value of this ratio (or the higher the TI), the safer the drug. The margin of safety also may be established by comparing 99% dose–response curve for the therapeutic effect to the curve for a toxic or lethal effect (Fig. 2-7). The farther apart these two curves are, the wider the margin of safety.

■ Self-Study Review

3. Describe the steps a drug follows after being delivered to body cells.
4. List seven features of receptors.
5. Describe the features of the four types of chemical bonds between a drug molecule and the complementary receptor. Which type is most common in drug–receptor complexes?
6. Define the roles of *affinity* and *intrinsic activity* in drug action. Which is related to potency?
7. What is the difference in the effect of a weak agonist when compared to a partial agonist? Identify both in a log dose curve illustration.
8. Describe the relationship of *efficacy* and the *ceiling dose* concept.
9. Compare the *ceiling dose* with the *threshold dose*.
10. Define *ED50* and *LD50*.
11. What is the *therapeutic index* (TI), and how is it used? What is the formula to determine the TI, and what is the significance of a high number?

PHARMACOKINETICS

Pharmacokinetics deals with the movement of drugs through the body. Therefore, pharmacokinetics relates to a drug's absorption; distribution in the body, including to the site of action; metabolism to prepare the drug for removal from the body; and excretion, where the drug is ultimately removed from the body and its effect is terminated. As drugs progress through these various phases within the body to be delivered to their sites of action and, ultimately, to be eliminated from the body, they must pass through biologic barriers (e.g., cell walls, blood vessels) in various tissues.

Passage across Biologic Membranes

To produce an effect, most drugs must pass through cell membranes to gain access to their receptor(s). Passage through biologic membranes affects the amount of the drug that reaches the site of action and influences the time it takes the drug to get to the site of action. The physicochemical properties that influence the movement of drug molecules across biologic membranes are molecular size, lipid solubility, and the degree of ionization (a function of the pH of the environment

and pK_a of the drug). In an acid environment, an acidic drug exists mainly in the nonionized form. Nonionized molecules are lipid soluble and pass through biologic membranes easily. In the same acid environment, a basic drug exists mainly in the ionized form. Ionized drugs are water soluble and must pass through water pores of the biologic membrane or be transported through the membrane by specialized transport mechanisms. These movements are accomplished in a variety of ways.

Filtration

Small, water-soluble substances may pass through aqueous channels or water pores in cell membranes by a process known as *filtration*. Larger water-soluble molecules are in the ionized form and are blocked from moving through small water pore openings. They must rely on specialized transport mechanisms (discussed below) to move through the biologic membrane.

Passive Diffusion

Most drugs are weak acids or weak bases, and drug molecules are too large to pass through most aqueous channels. However, as a function of their lipid solubility, the nonpolar (nonionized) forms of these drugs readily can cross biologic membranes by *passive diffusion* along a concentration gradient (from high concentration to low concentration) until equilibrium is reached across the membrane. Therefore, nonionized lipid-soluble molecules can easily pass through biologic membranes.

Specialized Transport Mechanisms

Large ionized, water-soluble drug molecules require more complex processes to cross biologic membranes. These include facilitated diffusion and active transport mechanisms.

Facilitated Diffusion

The concept of *facilitated diffusion* assumes that the drug forms a complex with a component of the cell membrane on one side. The complex is then carried through the membrane, the drug is released, and the carrier returns to the original surface to repeat the process. Vitamins are known to participate in facilitated diffusion, furnishing the energy to carry large, water-soluble drug molecules across membranes. Facilitated diffusion does not require energy and does not proceed against a concentration gradient. One example is the movement of glucose across cell membranes; it is thought to be *facilitated* by insulin. Another example is that some water-insoluble substances, such as fat-soluble vitamins (vitamins A, D, E, and K), are engulfed by the cell membrane and are released unchanged in the cytoplasm by a process known as *endocytosis*, a form of facilitated diffusion.

Active Transport

Active transport is the movement of drug molecules across biologic membranes against both a concentration and an electrochemical gradient. This activity requires energy. The

---

BOX 2-2. Factors That Influence Absorption

- Degree of ionization
- Formulation (liquid or solid)
- Concentration
- Circulation to area
- Area of absorptive surface
- Route of administration

---

transfer of some drugs through biologic membranes in the kidneys and intestines relies on an active transport mechanism.

Absorption

Regardless of the process by which a drug moves through biologic membranes, it first must be dissolved in the fluids encircling the cells. For this reason, a drug must have some degree of both lipid and water solubility—water solubility to get it to the cell, and lipid solubility to get it through the cell membrane. Factors that influence the rate of absorption of drugs include

- the degree of ionization and pH of tissues;
- the formulation of the drug (liquid or solid);
- the drug's concentration (the greater the concentration of a drug, the faster the rate of absorption);
- circulation to the area (the greater the blood flow to tissue, the faster the rate of absorption);
- the area of absorptive surface (the greater the area to which the drug is exposed, the faster the rate of absorption);
- the route of administration (ROA; Box 2-2).

Degree of Ionization

As mentioned earlier, the ionized form of a drug tends to be more water soluble, and nonionized forms tend to be more lipid soluble. Biologic membranes are composed of

- layers of lipid material and proteins that allow for passage of lipid-soluble molecules;
- small openings or water pores that allow for the passage of water-soluble molecules.

Consequently, the nonpolar, nonionized form of a drug will diffuse across biologic membranes more readily than its polar, ionized form. This phenomenon has clinical implications. For example, if the patient is taking an antacid, which increases the pH of the stomach and upper small intestine, the administration of a weak acid (such as aspirin) may result in increased ionization and poor absorption of the aspirin, giving less-than-optimal pain relief.

pK$_a$ and Ionization

The pH of the area affects drugs' degrees of ionization. Drugs will be ionized or nonionized primarily as a function of their pK$_a$ and the pH of the environment. The *pK$_a$* is defined as that

pH at which a drug is 50% ionized and 50% nonionized. For example, in the highly acidic environment of the stomach, drugs with a low pK$_a$ will exist primarily in their nonionized forms (weak acids in an acidic environment). Ionization occurs when different charges (acids mixed with bases) exist together. Similarly, in the small intestine where the pH is more basic, the same drugs with a low pK$_a$ will be more ionized.

Formulation of Drug

The form in which a drug is administered can affect the rate of absorption. To illustrate this point, let us consider the form in which a drug is administered to a patient. Aqueous formulations of drugs (such as Alka-Seltzer) do not require time to dissolve after oral administration and, therefore, will cover a wider area of the absorptive surface in the gastrointestinal (GI) tract much faster than a tablet, which must go through stages of a dissolving process. In general, the liquid formulation results in an increased rate of absorption of the drug (and more rapid onset of action) than solid formulations of the same drug.

Enteric Coating

Drugs can be modified in various ways that result in delayed absorption. Enteric-coated formulations delay dissolution of tablets until they have moved from the stomach into the upper small intestine, thereby reducing adverse gastric side effects.

Other Modifications

A strategy involved in formulating intraoral topical agents is to combine them with an insoluble agent. This strategy prevents agents applied to the oral mucosa from dissolving in saliva and being removed (e.g., corticosteroid mixed with an insoluble agent [Kenalog in Orabase]). New doseforms and delivery systems are being developed every day. For example, in 2006 the Food and Drug Administration (FDA) approved the very first inhaled insulin, a drug formerly only administered by injection.

Drug Concentration

Highly concentrated drugs are absorbed faster than the same drugs in low concentrations. Absorption of drugs through skin and mucosa by passive diffusion is proportional to the drugs' concentration and lipid solubility. This concept is discussed further when ROAs are presented.

Circulation to Area

The greater the blood flow to tissue, the faster the rate of absorption. Organs with significant blood flow include the heart, the GI tract, and the liver. This concept is illustrated in the discussion related to ROAs.

Area of Absorptive Surface

The upper small intestine has a large surface area and is the site of absorption for most orally administered drugs. Drugs

---

---

must pass through the wall of the small intestine and be absorbed into the bloodstream to be distributed to the body tissues and their receptors.

Routes of Administration

ROAs are classified as **enteral** or **parenteral**. Enteric drugs are placed directly into the GI tract by oral or rectal administration and must pass through the liver before distribution to the site of action. This reduces the bioavailability of some drugs by a process called *first-pass metabolism*. Parenteral drugs bypass the GI tract and include various injection, inhalation, and topical routes, such as direct application to the skin or mucosa and sublingual administration (Box 2-3).

Enteral

The oral route is the safest, most common, most convenient, and most economical method of drug administration. It is also the most unpredictable route because many factors can affect the rate of absorption between the GI tract (Box 2-4).

The rectal route, which is a form of enteric drug administration, may be useful in young children who have trouble swallowing tablet doseforms, and for unconscious or vomiting patients. However, absorption with this route is unpredictable. When a drug is administered enterally, its rate of absorption into the systemic circulation is influenced by

- the inherent characteristics of the drug (lipid soluble, water soluble, molecular weight, pK_a of the drug);
- the pH of the GI tract, which can change the ionization characteristics of a drug molecule;

- the presence of food in the stomach, which slows the rate of absorption because the drug competes for absorption with food components in the GI mucosa;
- gastric motility, which can move the drug through the intestines so fast that it does not have time for complete absorption;
- the degree of splanchnic blood flow (blood flow through intestinal viscera)—i.e., the intestinal viscera have a large surface area and significant vascularity;
- patient compliance in taking the prescribed drug regimen.

First-Pass Effect

The close anatomical relationship between the liver and the GI tract, and the abundant blood supply of these organs, has important effects on the bioavailability of some drugs. Because the liver is situated between enteric sites of absorption and the systemic circulation, it can profoundly influence the amount of drug in circulation when the drug is administered orally—an action that has been described as the *first-pass effect*. A drug given orally is absorbed mainly in the upper small intestine and enters the splanchnic circulation supplying that mucosa. Rectally administered drugs are absorbed via the lower intestinal mucosa. Within the circulation, the drug molecules attach to plasma proteins, called *albumin*. Drugs bind at various ratios to plasma proteins. When the drug binds at a 90:10 ratio, this means that 90% of the molecules are bound to albumin and 10% exist in an unbound form. Albumin serves to carry the molecule in the circulation to be distributed to the site of action. The protein-bound drug is protected from metabolism as the blood moves through the liver. Drugs that are removed efficiently from the liver during "first pass" will have a low bioavailability. Consequently, only that fraction of the drug that reaches the systemic circulation after first-pass metabolism is bioavailable to its receptor site.

Parenteral

Parenteral drugs bypass the GI tract and include various injectable routes, such as intravenous (IV), subcutaneous (SC), intramuscular (IM); inhalation; and topical routes. This ROA often is used for agents susceptible to degradation in the GI tract and those adversely affected by hepatic first-pass metabolism.

Intravenous Administration

The IV route provides for accurate and immediate deposition of drugs into the circulation, bypassing the absorption phase. The effect is rapid, with almost immediate onset of action. This route is considered to be the most predictable ROA. The IV route often is used in emergency situations. The dose of injected drugs can be adjusted to the patient's response; however, once a drug is injected, there is no recall. This makes the IV route less safe than the oral route, where absorption can be manipulated. Sterile formulations of soluble substances and an aseptic technique are required. Local irritation, often referred to as *injection site reactions*, and damage to the inner blood vessel wall can result in thromboembolic complications (Box 2-5).

BOX 2-5. Features of IV Route

- Bypasses absorption, causing immediate effect
- Most predictable route
- Used in emergency situations
- Less safe than oral route
- Injection site reactions are possible

Subcutaneous Injection

Following SC injection, a drug's rate of absorption into the bloodstream is slow and sufficiently constant to provide a sustained effect. The incorporation of a vasoconstrictor into a drug formulation, such as in a local anesthetic agent used in dentistry, can further retard the rate of absorption. Local tissue irritation characterized by sloughing, necrosis, and severe pain are potential complications. Insulin is administered by SC injection.

Intramuscular Injection

The IM injection allows for rapid absorption of aqueous solutions into the bloodstream. Oily or other nonaqueous formulations may provide for slow, constant absorption. This is another example that illustrates the role of drug formulation in the drug's absorption. Substances considered too irritating to administer by IV and SC routes in some instances may be given intramuscularly. The IM injection is usually given in the deltoid or gluteal muscle.

Other Parenteral-Injectable Routes

Intradermal, intrathecal, and intraperitoneal routes are other types of parenteral ROAs given by injection. The tuberculosis skin test uses the intradermal route.

Inhalation

Inhaled drugs are considered to be delivered topically—the drug is inhaled and attaches to pulmonary tissues, where absorption occurs. This direct topical absorption also has an advantage over enteric administration because it circumvents the metabolic first-pass breakdown in the liver. The large pulmonary absorptive surface in the lungs allows for rapid access of gaseous, volatile agents to the circulation. Drugs administered by inhalation may act locally or they may cross the alveoli, enter the circulation, and act at the appropriate receptor site. Concentration is controlled at the alveolar level because most of these drugs are exhaled immediately. Asthma often is treated with inhaled drugs.

Topical Application

This ROA is used to apply drugs directly to tissue. It includes those placed sublingually, supplied via patches, inserted by drops in the eyes or ears, or placed within the gingival sulcus. Absorption of drugs through skin and mucosa by passive diffusion is proportional to their concentration and lipid solubility. Drugs' concentrations may be increased for topical products because the skin is a barrier to absorption. Warnings related to applying topical anesthetic agents include

- limiting the area of application in order to reduce the absorption of these concentrated local anesthetic agents;
- avoiding placement of an occlusive dressing;
- avoiding application over abraded areas or where skin is not intact;
- considering the allergic potential.

Systemic adverse effects can occur if occlusive dressings are placed over the drug or if the drug is applied to abraded or inflamed areas. In these situations, the concentrated drug is absorbed more easily, leading to overdose. For unexplained reasons, the topical ROA is more likely to cause allergic drug reactions.

Sublingual

Topical application of a drug placed under the tongue is absorbed into the lingual venous system through nonkeratinized mucosa. Because venous drainage from the mouth flows into the superior vena cava, and because of the rich vascularity of the oral area, sublingually administered drugs enter the circulation quickly. This direct absorption also has an advantage over enteric administration because it circumvents the metabolic first-pass breakdown in the liver. Absorption of many drugs is immediate, and this ROA is often used when a rapid response is needed, such as when nitroglycerin is used to treat anginal pain.

Transdermal Patch

Transdermal delivery systems are designed to provide for a slow, continued release of medication. The patch is applied to the skin, eliminating the need for multiple doses of the drug. Most patches consist of several layers: An adhesive to stick to the skin, a membrane to control the rate of drug release, a reservoir where the drug is placed, and a backing that keeps the drug from evaporating. Common adverse effects with patches include local erythema and irritation. These are minimized by rotating the location of the patch when it is reapplied. Patches are changed daily, every few days, or weekly, depending on the specific drug.

Other Topical Routes

The recent introduction of locally applied antimicrobial agents into the gingival sulcus utilizes a polymer-based formulation. This keeps the antimicrobial product from leaving the area and increases the duration of the effect. This is discussed in detail in Chapter 9.

■ Self-Study Review

12. Describe the stages a drug goes through from the time of administration to the elimination of the drug.
13. Compare the features of ionized molecules with those of nonionized forms as the molecule moves through tissues to cause an effect.

14. What is the role of specialized transport mechanisms in moving drug molecules across the membrane? Give an example of a specialized transport vehicle.
15. Identify three factors that affect the absorption of a drug.
16. From where in the GI tract are most drugs absorbed?
17. Describe how taking a drug that alters the pH of the stomach can affect the absorption of a drug.
18. Describe two means to alter a drug's absorption through modifying the formulation.
19. Identify features of enteral and parenteral ROAs.
20. How does food in the stomach affect drug absorption?
21. Describe how the first-pass effect influences the onset of drug action.
22. List parenteral routes and identify the route used in most emergency situations.
23. What is the most predictable ROA?
24. What are the precautions to follow when using topical agents?

Distribution of Drugs

Drug absorption is a prerequisite for establishing adequate plasma levels. Next, drugs must reach their target organ(s) in therapeutic concentrations to produce effects. Drug distribution is achieved primarily through the circulatory system. In most cases, the therapeutic effect of a drug in tissues correlates well with the concentration in the circulation.

Tissues and organs vary greatly in their abilities to absorb various drugs and in the proportion of systemic blood flow that they receive. Highly perfused organs, such as the liver, kidney, heart, and CNS, tend to receive the drug within minutes of absorption. Muscles, most viscera, skin, and fat may require a longer amount of time before equilibrium is achieved. When the patient has excess body fat, those drugs that tend to accumulate in fat are slowly released from these fat stores, which can result in high blood levels when multiple doses of the drug are taken. *Redistribution* may affect the duration of a drug effect. For example, if a drug of high lipid solubility accumulates rapidly in the brain and then is redistributed to other tissues, the drug effects in the brain are reduced. The distribution of drugs—their ability to cross biologic membranes and leave the vascular compartment, and ultimately to accumulate in tissues and at their sites of action—relies on the same factors that affect absorption (i.e., molecular weight, concentration in plasma, lipid solubility, pH of the vascular compartment, and pK_a of the drug). In addition, in the circulation, many drugs are bound to plasma proteins and, therefore, are unable to bind to therapeutic receptors.

Plasma Protein Binding

The capacity of tissues (i.e., muscle and fat) to bind and store drugs increases the tendency of drugs to leave the vascular compartment, but this tendency is counteracted to some extent by plasma protein (albumin) binding of drugs. Plasma protein binding is a nonselective process. Many drugs compete with each other and with endogenous substances for albumin-binding sites. Plasma protein binding tends to reduce the availability of drugs for diffusion into target organs because, in general, *only the free or unbound drug is capable of crossing biologic membranes*. Because highly protein-bound drugs cannot leave the circulation, their rate of metabolism and excretion also is reduced. The therapeutic consequence of this phenomenon is taken into consideration when drug dosages are determined. Highly protein-bound drugs, such as aspirin, are also an important mechanism for some drug–drug interactions. When administered concurrently with another drug, highly bound drugs will compete for albumin-binding sites, and the drug with the greatest affinity (e.g., aspirin) will tend to "bump" the other drug off the albumin receptor, effectively increasing its free, unbound form. The increased blood level of the free drug molecules can lead to increased therapeutic and/or toxic effects, even though the drug was administered in therapeutic doses.

Blood–Brain Barrier

The distribution of drugs to the CNS and cerebrospinal fluid is restricted by the blood–brain barrier. However, cerebral blood flow is the only limiting factor associated with highly lipid-soluble, uncharged (nonpolar) drugs.

Placenta as a Barrier

In a pregnant woman, drugs pass across the placenta by simple diffusion (once again, as a function of their concentration in plasma, molecular weight, lipid solubility, pH of the vascular compartment, and their pK_a). The result is that the fetus becomes medicated along with the mother. This is the reason for the restriction of drugs, except prenatal vitamins, during pregnancy.

Metabolism

Rarely does a drug enter the body and leave it without modification. A number of organs (liver, kidneys, GI tract, skin, lungs) are capable of metabolizing drugs using a variety of enzymatic reactions. However, the liver contains the greatest diversity and quantity of metabolic enzymes, and the majority of drug metabolism occurs there. The liver preferentially metabolizes highly lipophilic drugs, rendering the drugs in their metabolite state and inactive, although some drug metabolites maintain a degree of pharmacologic activity. The kidneys easily eliminate the metabolite form, which is ionized (water soluble). These enzymatic reactions, classified as Phase I and Phase II processes, are collectively referred to as *biotransformation* and can alter drugs in four different ways:

1. Convert an active drug to an inactive drug
2. Convert an active drug to an active or toxic metabolite
3. Convert an inactive drug to an active drug
4. Convert an unexcretable (more lipophilic) drug into an excretable (more hydrophilic) metabolite

Phase I Reactions

A drug's chemical structure is modified through oxidation, reduction, or hydrolysis, which require very little energy. The most commonly used pathway is the hepatic microsomal cytochrome P450 (CYP450) enzyme system, which oxidizes lipophilic molecules. Some drugs are biotransformed by CYP450-independent oxidation, hydrolysis, or reduction. These reactions are not limited to the hepatic endoplasmic reticulum. A practical example is the hydrolysis of ester and amide local anesthetic agents and the oxidation of epinephrine, which may be hydrolyzed or oxidized, respectively, at their sites of administration within tissues, thereby limiting their systemic toxicity.

Phase II Reactions

The chemical structure of a drug is modified by conjugation to a large polar endogenous molecule. Some metabolites of Phase I reactions can undergo additional Phase II metabolism. In contrast to a Phase I reaction, Phase II biotransformation almost always results in inactivation of the parent drug. Virtually all Phase II metabolites are pharmacologically inactive.

Cytochrome P450 Induction and Inhibition

The CYP450 enzyme system can be induced to increase drug metabolism or inhibited to reduce the rate of a drug's metabolism, and it is responsible for many adverse drug–drug interactions. For example, chronic ethanol toxicity induces the metabolism of barbiturates, whereas acute ethanol toxicity inhibits the metabolism of barbiturates. Alcohol and barbiturates are additive CNS depressants. These potential drug–drug interactions are the basis for the "DO NOT DRINK ALCOHOL WITH THIS DRUG" warning on a barbiturate prescription. Other drugs (erythromycin, omeprazole, cimetidine, ciprofloxacin) inhibit CYP450 enzymes and decrease the metabolism of many other drugs. This increases the drugs' blood levels and effectively increases their therapeutic and/or toxic effects.

Excretion

Renal excretion is the most common and important mechanism of *drug elimination* from the body. Biotransformation prepares the molecule, and the kidney eliminates it via urination. Consequently, following biotransformation, drugs are intrinsically hydrophilic (ionized) and are excreted more readily than lipophilic (nonionized) compounds. A relatively small number of drugs are excreted primarily in the GI tract via the bile, and only minor quantities are excreted through respiratory (exhalation) and dermal routes (perspiration). Lactation is responsible for minor amounts of drug excretion.

Glomerular Filtration, Tubular Secretion, and Reabsorption from the Tubular Lumen

Renal blood flow represents about 25% of total systemic circulation. Therefore, afferent arterioles in the kidney constantly bring free, unbound, and plasma-protein–bound drugs

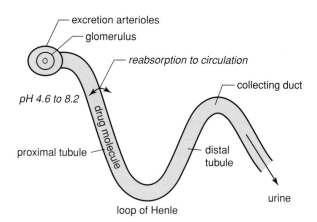

Figure 2-8 Elimination of a Drug in the Kidney

into the glomeruli. The glomerulus is the primary location for drug elimination to occur. Typically, only the free drug is filtered by the glomeruli. A drug may be filtered at the renal glomerulus or secreted into the proximal tubule, and, subsequently, either may be reabsorbed into the tubular lumen and returned to the circulation or may be excreted into the urine where, via urination, it is removed from the body (Fig. 2-8).

The mechanism includes these processes:

- Glomerular filtration depends on renal blood flow, glomerular filtration rate, and plasma protein binding. Reduced renal blood flow, reduced glomerular filtration rate, and increased plasma protein binding all contribute to reduced drug elimination.
- Active tubular secretion facilitates the movement of the drug from the bloodstream into the renal tubular fluid by a nonselective carrier system for organic ions. Some drugs, such as penicillin, aspirin, and probenecid, are actively secreted at the proximal tubule and compete with each other for the same secretory transport mechanisms.
- Passive tubular reabsorption of nonionized drugs results in net passive reabsorption. Although reabsorption can decrease the elimination rate of drugs, many drugs exhibit pH trapping in the distal tubules and are efficiently eliminated in the urine. When drugs need to be retained in the body, the pH of the urine can be manipulated. By alkalinizing the urine (via administration of sodium bicarbonate), the plasma level of weak acids can be decreased; alternatively, by acidifying the urine (via administration of ammonium chloride), the plasma level of weak bases can be decreased.

In summary, drug molecules are removed from the circulation into renal proximal tubules by the glomeruli, or they may be secreted into renal proximal tubules from peritubular capillaries and, if not reabsorbed in the collecting tubules of the kidney, excreted in the urine. Although the kidneys excrete most drugs via glomerular filtration, there are other mechanisms whereby the body eliminates drugs.

Enterohepatic Recirculation

Some metabolites formed in the liver are excreted via the bile into the intestinal tract to be eliminated in the feces. If these metabolites are subsequently hydrolyzed and reabsorbed from the gut (a process called *enterohepatic recirculation*), drug action can be re-established. One could say this is the body's contribution to recycling! Enterohepatic recirculation can result in a significant delay in the elimination of drugs from the body.

Exhalation

Pulmonary excretion is important mainly for the elimination of anesthetic gases and vapors.

Other Mechanisms

Drugs can be excreted in lactation and are potential sources of unwanted pharmacologic effects in nursing infants. Other routes, such as saliva, sweat, and tears, are quantitatively unimportant.

Half-Life of a Drug

The removal of most drugs from the body follows exponential or first-order kinetics. Assuming a relatively uniform distribution of a drug within the body (considered to be a single compartment), first-order kinetics implies that a constant fraction (%) of the drug is eliminated per unit time. The rate of exponential kinetics may be expressed by its constant (k), the fractional change per unit time, or its **half-life** (expressed as $t_{1/2}$), which is the time required for the plasma concentration of a drug to decrease by 50%. This occurs in several ways, such as

- the distribution half-life, which represents the rapid decline in plasma–drug concentration as 50% of the drug is distributed throughout the body;
- the elimination half-life, which reflects the time required to excrete 50% of the drug from the system.

Following the administration of multiple therapeutic dosages of a drug at time intervals equal to or shorter than the drug's half-life, a plateau level of drug accumulates. This is called **steady-state concentration** and involves over four half-lives. For example, if the $t_{1/2}$ of a drug is 1 hour, then it will require the administration of four therapeutic doses at 1-hour intervals to reach steady state (Fig. 2-9). The plateau rep-

resents a rate of drug administration that is equal to the rate of drug elimination. Consequently, fluctuations in the plasma concentration of drugs occur as a function of the dosage interval and the drug's elimination half-life. Assuming first-order kinetics, it takes approximately four half-lives to eliminate a drug from the body. The elimination of some drugs (such as alcohol) may follow zero-order kinetics, implying that a constant amount of the drug is eliminated per unit time. In this case, the enzymes that metabolize the drug become saturated and cannot absorb more drug, resulting in a constant amount of drug being metabolized per unit of time. Small changes in the dose of drugs with this type of kinetics can lead to large serum concentrations and increase the risk for toxicity.

■ Self-Study Review

25. Describe features of distribution that affect a drug molecule reaching the receptor.
26. What is the role of albumin in the blood?
27. Identify the organ responsible for most drug metabolism.
28. Describe the four ways drugs are altered during biotransformation.
29. What are the differences between Phase I reactions and Phase II reactions in biotransformation?
30. Which enzyme system is the primary pathway for drug metabolism?
31. In which organ are most drugs excreted? What is the primary area of the organ where this occurs?
32. Describe the process of drug excretion.
33. Define a drug's half-life.

CONCLUSION

After initial administration of a drug, there is a period of time before any perceptible effect of the drug is observed in the patient. The time of onset is determined mainly by the rate and degree of absorption. The effect increases with time until the drug reaches the peak effect. Movement through biologic membranes and drug redistribution influences the peak effect. The effect diminishes as the drug is metabolized and eliminated from the body. The duration of action is affected primarily by the rate of inactivation and excretion of the drug by the liver and kidneys. The onset of action, the peak effect, and the duration of action are all dependent upon the dose administered—i.e., the larger the dose, the shorter the time to reach the peak effect, and the longer the duration of action. An important clinical use of time-effect relationships involves multiple dosing schedules over a period of time that depends on the drug's half-life. To eliminate adverse events, the dosage schedule must be designed to avoid giving more drug than has been eliminated since the last dose.

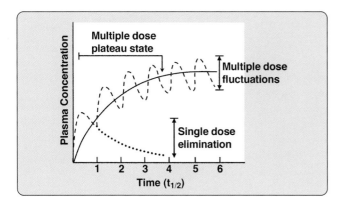

Figure 2-9 Drug Half-Life. This shows the effects of dosing on plasma concentration.

CLINICAL APPLICATION EXERCISES (CAE)

☐ **Exercise 1.** During the review of the health history, it is noted that the patient lists Tums as a current over-the-counter (OTC) medication. The current appointment is for periodontal débridement of one quadrant. The diagnosis of the case is severe chronic periodontal disease, and a recommendation will be made for "saltwater rinse in evening, plus OTC medication for pain relief." How will the current drug history information affect your recommendation for pain relief?

☐ **Exercise 2.** During oral examination, your patient gasps, clutches his chest, and cries out in pain. He reports taking anticholesterol medication due to a recently identified problem with high cholesterol. You tell the receptionist to call 911, and you secure the medical emergency kit. What ROA should be used to get the vasodilating drug to the coronary arteries quickly?

☐ **Exercise 3.** Your patient is an elderly, overweight person who presents to the office in pain. The dentist decides to prescribe a narcotic agent. What considerations are important in determining dosage, and why?

3

Principles of Prescription Writing and Other Pharmacotherapeutic Considerations

The essence of good prescription writing is to ensure that the pharmacist knows exactly which drug formulation and dosage to dispense, and the patient has explicit written instructions for self-administration of the prescribed drug. A prescription is a legal document that carries regulations to ensure safe use and to comply with governmental regulations. Dental hygienists may be asked to participate in the prescription-writing process in a variety of ways.

PRESCRIPTION WRITING AND PRESCRIPTION FOR A CONTROLLED SUBSTANCE

A prescription is a legal document for which the prescriber and pharmacist are both responsible. Prescriptions are regulated by state and federal laws and must be properly written, with specific information included. Online prescribing is currently available, and the same legal requirements must be met for it as for written prescriptions. Other requirements, such as an insurance company's approved list of covered drug products, may be important to consider when prescriptions are

written. This can help the patient avoid having to pay for a drug not included in his or her benefit plan. Many insurance-approved drug plans cover specific branded products, while the same drugs with different brand names may not be covered. Errors in prescribing drugs can occur from a variety of reasons, some of which include

- wrong dose, such as incorrect calculation of a pediatric dose;
- prescription written for a patient whose medical condition creates a contraindication for taking the drug;
- poor handwriting, making the information unclear to the pharmacist;
- incorrect information written from memory, rather than from a reviewed drug reference;
- look-alike drug names that may be confused at the pharmacy.

Rules for Prescription Writing

The following prescription-writing guidelines have been developed to comply with state and federal laws, avoid errors when the prescription is prepared, and prevent misuse of prescription information:

BOX 3-1. Prescriber–Patient Relationship

- The patient record is established
- The diagnosis is established: Medical history, examination, tests, radiographs
- The treatment plan is prepared and the need for medication orders is determined
- The treatment plan is presented, and the patient is counseled
- Follow-up care is provided as needed

- Written prescriptions should be legible, accurate, include complete information, and be written in ink. Chapter 1 includes sources for drug information.
- Prescriptions for Schedule II controlled substances *must* be written in ink, indelible pencil, or typewritten.
- Blank prescription sheets should not have the name of a pharmacy or pharmaceutical company imprinted on the forms, to avoid the appearance of product endorsement.
- Pads should be kept in a drawer or secure location when not in use to avoid theft or loss. If theft is suspected, the loss should be reported to the state drug control agency.
- A duplicate of each written prescription (medicolegal reasons) or a record of drugs prescribed should be kept in the patient's record.
- English instructions should be used, rather than Latin abbreviations, to ensure clarity in filling the prescription and printing patient instructions.

The process starts with establishing a proper prescriber-patient relationship and presenting a treatment plan to the patient (Box 3-1). Most state dental practice acts specify that prescriptions may be written only for patients under active care. Some states stipulate that only those classes of drugs directly involved in dental treatment can be prescribed by a dentist. Prescribing outside the proper prescriber–patient relationship is unprofessional conduct, such as when drugs are prescribed online for patients unknown to the practitioner.

PARTS OF THE PRESCRIPTION

In the past, several Latin terms were used to describe parts of the prescription, including superscription (which included the abbreviation *Rx*, meaning "take thou"), inscription (information about the drug, dose, and doseform), subscription (information to the pharmacist about filling the inscription), and transcription (directions to the patient for taking the drug). However, these terms have been replaced by a more concise, three-part description of the prescription: A heading, a body, and a closing (Fig. 3-1).

Heading

The heading identifies the prescriber (name, phone number, and address), exhibits the date of the prescription, and lists the patient information (name, age and weight [for children],

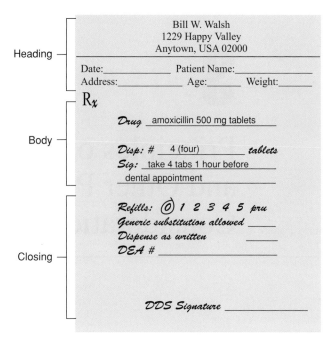

Figure 3-1 Parts of a Prescription

and address). For children, the age and weight should be noted so the pharmacist can monitor the dose prescribed, as a double check to reduce possible errors in prescribing. The prescriber's name and address may be printed on the pad to reduce time when the prescription is written. When a dental practice includes more than one dentist, the names of all dentists in the group may be printed on the pad. In this situation, the name of the appropriate prescriber should be circled when the prescription is written. The telephone number of the prescriber is a convenience to the pharmacist in case clarification of information is needed. The date on which the prescription was written and signed is required when substances controlled by the Drug Enforcement Administration (DEA) are prescribed. The date is used to determine the date on which a prescription will have expired. Prescription pads with printed heading information must be kept secure at the dental office so they will not be stolen and used for fraudulent prescription writing.

Body

The body tells the pharmacist the specific drug, dose or concentration, and amount to be dispensed. It also provides directions to the patient (transcribed by the pharmacist to the packaged drug) that state precisely how the patient is to self-administer the drug. Some drug products are not available in the **doseform** needed and must be mixed by a pharmacist trained to mix or *compound* the product. A good example is a compounded mouth rinse called Miracle Mix that dentists often prescribe for severe oral ulceration. This rinse contains several ingredients to cover ulcerations and reduce pain and inflammation. This product is fully described in Chapter 22.

Closing

The closing provides a space for the signature of the prescriber, the prescriber's U.S. DEA number (if applicable), instructions to the pharmacist about product selection (e.g., if generic can be substituted for the brand-name product), and other items, such as the number of refills allowed. All written prescriptions should be signed by the prescriber, although many prescriptions may be telephoned to pharmacies. However, a signature is required by law for controlled substances (Schedule II drugs), and if a prescription for one of these drugs is telephoned to a pharmacy, it must be followed up by a written and signed order within 72 hours.

Prescription Label Regulations

The label on the prescription container must include the name of the drug (if generic, it will be in lower-case), the number of doses dispensed, and the strength of the doseform. A clearly written label could be important in an emergency situation if the patient were unable to provide information. The pharmacy name, address, phone number, date the prescription was filled, and instructions regarding refills should be on the label. For refill prescriptions, both the date of the original prescription and the date of the next refill should be on the label. This information is useful when a patient is taking medication with a short shelf life. For example, nitroglycerin tablets are to be placed sublingually (under the tongue) to relieve anginal pain. This medication usually has a 3- to 6-month shelf life. The dental hygienist can determine that a prescription is not outdated (and therefore ineffective for the relief of angina) by looking at the refill information that should be on the label. The label also should include directions to the patient on how to take the medication ("Place one tab under the tongue as needed for pain") and any warnings ("Use no more than three tabs").

COMPLIANCE

A **compliant patient** is one who follows the therapeutic regimen recommended by the clinician. In contrast, a patient is considered noncompliant if the regimen is not followed to the extent that therapeutic goals are not achieved. There are several determinants of compliance that take into consideration the disease, the patient, the practitioner, the treatment regimen, economic factors, and the interaction of each of these factors. Patient trust in the clinician and in the treatment plan established during the office visit is important. A patient tends to be more compliant if he or she has a good understanding of the illness and the therapy. Therefore, good communication between the clinician and patient is a major aid to compliance. A positive office visit and attitude, along with individualization of regimens and good follow-up on the clinician's part, improve compliance. The nature of the illness itself also has an important influence on the patient. The patient is more likely to follow the regimen if the illness is serious or disabling. *The patient's perception of the severity of the illness is the major factor influencing compliance.*

The longer the duration of treatment, the more patient compliance diminishes. This is especially true if symptoms are relieved before drug therapy is discontinued. Additionally, noncompliance can result if the regimen itself is discouraging or confusing to the patient because of the number of drugs included, frequency of dosing, side effects, cost, and access to the drug.

Noncompliance in the pediatric patient is complicated by a parent-guardian factor. The major reason for noncompliance in children is a dislike for the taste or smell of the medication. If it is frustrating to the parent-guardian to give the medication, doses are more likely to be skipped or discontinued when symptoms disappear. One must also consider the possibility of a negative parent-guardian attitude transferring to the child. If the child is attending school, the regimen should have a convenient schedule and doses that coordinate with the school schedule. Specific times to take the medication should be communicated to the school authorities, rather than generalizing the schedule.

Noncompliance in the geriatric patient is not uncommon. Geriatric patients may fail to fill prescriptions because of transportation problems, expense, or lack of trust in the doctor or therapy. Poor comprehension of the therapy and concurrent multiple drug therapies are common reasons for omission of doses. Difficulty in opening packages or swallowing pills, poor memory, and visual or hearing impairment may also contribute to confusion in compliance. A good understanding of the patient's needs and fears will help the clinician to individualize drug therapy for better compliance. Verbal repetition of directions, plus written instructions and clear labeling, is helpful.

COUNSELING FOR A PRESCRIPTION

It is estimated that 25% to 60% of patients who receive a prescription for medication do not get the prescription filled or do not take the medication as prescribed. Other noncompliance issues may include

- taking the drug at inappropriate times, such as taking at or before meals when food can prevent absorption of the drug;
- stopping medication too soon and not taking the full course of the drug;
- getting the prescription filled, but never taking the drug.

The reasons behind these noncompliance issues possibly can be avoided with proper counseling and explanations related to

- why the drug is needed;
- what can occur if the drug is not taken;
- clear instructions for when to take the drug (including factors that can cause the drug to be ineffective);
- possible side effects that can occur and how to manage them;
- situations that require notification of the dentist, such as burning mouth, bloody diarrhea, hives or evidence of allergic reactions, and so forth.

ROLE OF THE REGISTERED DENTAL HYGIENIST

Although dental hygienists do not prescribe drugs, knowledge regarding appropriate drugs to prescribe for various indications and properly prepared prescriptions is necessary for several reasons.

Antibiotic Prophylaxis

Occasionally a prescription is provided to the dental patient with instructions to take the medication prior to the appointment. When a prescription has been prepared, the treatment record should include information on the drug prescribed and the specific patient instructions related to the dental appointment. In this situation, the receptionist may have reminded the patient to take the drug when the appointment was verified. However, it is the responsibility of the practitioner to review the treatment record and medical history to verify that the instructions were followed. In other situations, another prescriber may have prepared the prescription. Questioning should include determining compliance in taking the medication according to the most current recommendation for the indication. For example, antibiotic prophylaxis is ordered prior to oral prophylaxis for a patient at high risk for bacterial endocarditis. When the patient arrives for the appointment, the registered dental hygienist (RDH) must ask:

- When was the antibiotic taken? (Was it 1/2 to 1 hour prior to the appointment?)
- Which specific antibiotic was prescribed? (The dose of the antibiotic depends on the specific product prescribed.)
- How much was taken? (Was the correct dose taken?)
- Have any adverse effects developed? (Look for signs of allergy—hives, rash, breathing difficulties—and report signs to the dentist.)

The answers to these questions should be recorded in the treatment record. An example might read as follows: "Four 500-mg tabs amoxicillin taken at 8:00 AM, 1 hour prior to appointment, no complications." Proper documentation in the treatment record of prescriptions written for the dental appointment is essential for medicolegal reasons, as well.

Medication for Emergency Use

Occasionally a medication needs to be available to use if an emergency situation occurs. Two common medications that patients always should bring to each dental appointment are sublingual nitroglycerin tablets when a history of anginal pain is reported, and rescue inhalers when asthma is reported on the medical history. Using sublingual nitroglycerin tablets for an example: The dental hygienist should ask if the patient has brought the nitroglycerin bottle. Generally the patient is told to carry the prescription for sublingually administered nitroglycerin tablets at all times, in case of an acute episode of chest pain. When the bottle is produced, the RDH should examine the label to determine the date the prescription was filled and the date of the next refill. This procedure is necessary to ensure that the nitroglycerin is still active and able to reduce anginal pain. Other responsibilities of the RDH related to prescription writing might include the following:

- A review of the prescription for necessary information prior to the patient's leaving the office
- Discussion with the patient regarding instructions on how to take the medication

These strategies may help prevent delays at the pharmacy if information is missing or unclear.

■ Self-Study Review

1. List rules for prescription writing. Which prescriptions require a written order? Which type(s) of prescription must be written in ink? Which can be called in? In what location should printed prescription pads be kept? How does the dentist know which prescriptions have been written for a patient? Which type of prescription is required by law to be signed by the prescriber?
2. Describe information included in the three parts of a prescription. What does the symbol *Rx* mean?
3. What information should be included on the prescription label? How could this information be used during a dental hygiene appointment? How can one determine if a prescription is past its expiration date?
4. Write out the information to be included in the treatment record when a patient must take amoxicillin prior to the maintenance appointment as a strategy to prevent bacterial endocarditis.
5. What are strategies in the dental office to ensure a properly written prescription has been given to the dental patient?
6. What is the main factor for noncompliance regarding therapeutic medications in an adult? In a child?
7. Describe five principles to include when counseling a patient about a prescription.
8. What questions should be asked when a drug for antibiotic prophylaxis has been prescribed?

METRIC AND HOUSEHOLD MEASURES

The metric system is the language of scientific measurement and should always be used in prescription writing (Table 3-1). Solid drugs are dispensed by weight (mg), and liquid drugs by volume (mL). Although the clinician will direct the pharmacist to dispense a liquid preparation in milliliters (mL), it is generally necessary to convert this dosage to a convenient household measurement in directions to the patient. When greater accuracy is required, the patient may need to use a graduated cylinder or a calibrated dropper to dispense the medication properly.

ABBREVIATIONS

In the past, directions to the patient were written using Latin abbreviations to save time when the prescription was written. Abbreviations are also used in prescription writing to make

Table 3-1	Metric and Household Measures

Weight	
kilogram = kg	1 kg = 1,000 g
gram = g	1 g = 1,000 mg
milligram = mg	1 mg = 1/1,000 g
pound = lb	1 kg = 2.2 lb
grain = gr	1 gr = 65 mg
Volume	
liter = L	1 L = 1,000 mL
milliliter = mL	1 mL = 1/1,000 L
teaspoonful = tsp	1 tsp = 5 mL
tablespoonful = tbs	1 tbs = 15 mL
drop/drops = g+/g++	1 mL = 15 g++
fluid ounce = fl oz	1 fl oz = 30 mL

alteration of a prescription by the patient more difficult (Table 3-2). However, unless a practitioner writes a large number of prescriptions daily, little time is saved by using abbreviations. Use of abbreviations has led to errors in filling the prescription or misunderstandings regarding instructions on how to take the drug. Modern practice is to use the English language when writing prescriptions, although abbreviations commonly are used in progress notes within a patient's treatment record.

DOSE CALCULATIONS FOR THE PEDIATRIC PATIENT

A variety of formulas are used to calculate pediatric dosage in a prescription. The two most common methods of calculating pediatric medications use body weight and body surface area (BSA). The most accurate method for determining the dosage for a child is to use the BSA. The body surface is a function of the height and weight of the child. Tables are available to calculate the surface area and the appropriate dosage (Fig. 3-2). When pediatric dosages are available from the manufacturer, it is best to use the manufacturer's recommendation.

Table 3-2	Commonly Used Abbreviations

English	Abbreviation
before =	a or ā
before meals =	a
dispense =	disp
number =	no
capsule =	cap
tablet =	tab
label =	sig
by mouth =	po
after meals =	pc
at once =	stat
at bedtime =	hs
as needed =	prn
every hour =	qh
every day =	qd
twice a day =	bid
3 times a day =	tid
4 times a day =	qid
discontinue =	d/c

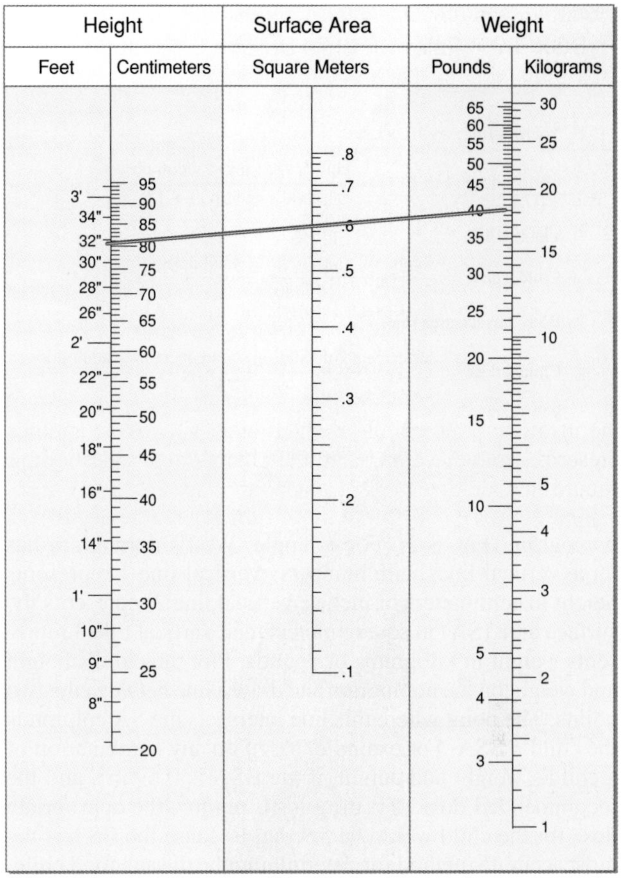

Figure 3-2 West's Nomogram for Body Surface Area. (Reprinted with permission from Molle EA, Kronenberger J, Durham LS, et al. *Lippincott Williams & Wilkins' Comprehensive Medical Assisting.* 2nd ed. Baltimore: Lippincott Williams & Wilkins; 2005:473.)

When reading children's dosage information, the source may refer to milligrams (mg) of drug per kilogram (kg) of body weight. The American Heart Association's recommendation for antibiotic prophylaxis to prevent infective endocarditis in the child is to use 50 mg of amoxicillin per kilogram of body weight. Table 3-1 illustrates that 1 kg equals 2.2 lb. To determine the dose of amoxicillin for antibiotic prophylaxis in a 50-lb child, divide 50 lb by 2.2 to determine the number of kilograms, then multiply that number (~23 kg) by 50 mg to get the milligram dose (1,150 mg) of amoxicillin. Amoxicillin comes in 250-mg and 500-mg tablets. Rounding the dose down to 1 g (1,000 mg) yields instructions that the child should take two 500-mg tablets 30 minutes to 1 hour prior to the appointment. When the child dosage is not specified by the manufacturer, there are several rules for calculating it. These include Young's rule, which uses age for dose calculation, and Clark's rule, which uses the child's weight. Box 3-2 illustrates rules for calculating children's dosage. Weight is the usual basis for determining the dose, but weight can vary in children of the same age. For this reason, the BSA rule is considered the most accurate. Some pediatric medications specify dosages in milligrams or units per square meter (m^2). If the child's BSA is known, the practitioner will multiply the recommended dosage by the BSA. The BSA is determined by plotting a child's height and weight on a graph called a

BOX 3-2. Rules for Child Dosage Calculation

1. Young's rule:

$$\text{Child's dose (1 to 12 y)} = \frac{\text{child's age (in y)} \times \text{adult dose}}{\text{child's age (in y)} + 12}$$

2. Clark's rule:

$$\text{Child's dose} = \frac{\text{weight of child (in lb)} \times \text{adult dose}}{150 \text{ lb}}$$

3. Body surface area rule:

$$\text{Child's dose} = \frac{\text{surface area of child (in square meters)} \times \text{adult dose}}{1.73}$$

y = years

nomogram (Fig. 3-2). For example, West's nomogram has three vertical lines with numbers: Vertical line 1 represents height in centimeters or inches, vertical line 2 represents the surface area (SA) in square meters, and vertical line 3 represents weight in kilograms or pounds. Plot the child's height and weight on the nomogram and draw a line between the two points. The point where this line intersects the SA column is the child's BSA. For example, based on any combination of a child's weight and height, if the BSA is 0.59 m^2, and the recommended dose of a drug is 10 mg/m^2, the appropriate dose for the child would be 5.9 mg. Because the BSA is the most accurate method for determining the dosage for a child, the BSA is most frequently used to calculate anticancer drug dosages.

REGULATIONS FOR PRESCRIBING CONTROLLED SUBSTANCES

Over the years, Congress has enacted more than 50 pieces of legislation related to drug control. The Controlled Substances Act of 1970 (CSA) collects and conforms most of these diverse laws into one piece of legislation. The act is designed to improve the administration and regulation of manufacturing, distributing, and dispensing of controlled drugs, and to provide a "closed" system for the legitimate handlers of controlled substances. Individual states or local governments may enact additional requirements concerning controlled substances. Whenever state and federal laws differ, the more stringent law must be followed.

Every practitioner who administers, prescribes, or dispenses controlled substances must be registered with the DEA's Registration Unit. If a clinician has more than one office from which he or she prescribes drugs listed in the five schedules, then the clinician must register each location. The number on the certificate of registration must be indicated on all prescription orders for controlled substances and must correspond to the specific office location. A certificate of registration also authorizes clinicians to prescribe controlled substances from specific schedules. For example, as mentioned earlier, substances listed in Schedule I are not

for prescription use, but they may be obtained for research and instructional use or for chemical analysis by application to the DEA, supported by a protocol for the proposed use. A clinician with a DEA number is not authorized to prescribe Schedule I drugs. Similarly, if a clinician sees no reason to prescribe Schedule II drugs at a particular office location, a request can be made for a DEA registration number that only authorizes the prescription of drugs in Schedule III, IV, and/or V. The DEA has created a Web site where application forms can be found, as well as laws dealing with controlled substances (www.deadiversion.usdoj.gov). The attorney general has the authority to deny an application for registration if it is determined that the issuance of such registration would be inconsistent with the public interest. In determining the approval or denial of an application for a DEA number, the following factors are considered:

- The recommendation of the appropriate state licensing board or professional disciplinary authority
- The applicant's experience in dispensing or conducting research with respect to controlled substances
- The applicant's conviction record under federal or state laws relating to the manufacturing, distributing, or dispensing of controlled substances

A practitioner who does not follow the laws regulating prescribing controlled substances can lose the authority to write prescriptions for scheduled drugs.

Controlled Substance Schedules

Controlled (C) substances that come under the jurisdiction of the CSA are divided into five schedules according to the abuse potential of the drug. Schedule I (C-I) drugs have the highest risk for abuse and Schedule V (C-V) drugs have the lowest potential for abuse. Schedule I drugs cannot be prescribed and are used for drug research purposes only. Special permission from the DEA is necessary before Schedule I drugs can be obtained for research purposes. Table 3-3 lists the schedules, describes rules for prescribing drugs in the specific schedules, and provides examples of drugs in the schedules.

Rules for Prescribing Scheduled Drugs

All prescription orders for controlled substances

- must be written in ink or typewritten;
- must bear the full name and address of the patient;
- must list the full name, address, and DEA registration number of the practitioner;
- must be dated;
- must be manually signed by the practitioner.

Responsibilities of the Practitioner

When prescribing a controlled substance, the clinician must write out the actual amount, in addition to giving an Arabic number or Roman numeral (e.g., ten [10 or X] tablets), to discourage alterations in written prescription orders. To avoid errors in prescribing, overprescribing, or inappropriate prescribing, clinicians also must be aware of gimmicks and techniques used by drug abusers to obtain controlled substances; for example, clinicians should be cautious of patients

Table 3-3	Drug Schedules	
Schedule	**Description**	**Example(s)**
Schedule I (C-I)	C-I drugs have no legal medical use in the United States and have a high abuse potential. They may be used for research purposes and must be obtained from governmental agencies.	• hallucinogens (LSD) • marijuana • selected opiates (heroin, opium derivatives)
Schedule II (C-II)	C-II drugs have legal medical uses in the United States, but they have a high abuse potential, which may lead to severe psychologic and/or physical dependence. A written prescription order is required for C-II drugs. Refilling C-II prescription orders is prohibited. In the case of a bona fide emergency, a practitioner may telephone a prescription order to a pharmacist. In such a case, the drug prescribed must be limited to the amount needed to treat the patient during the emergency period. Such oral orders must be followed up by written orders within 72 hours.	• amphetamines • selected opiates (morphine and congeners, codeine congeners, methadone) • some barbiturates (secobarbital) • oxycodone
Schedule III (C-III)	C-III drugs have legal medical uses in the United States and a moderate abuse potential, which may lead to moderate psychologic and/or physical dependence. A prescription order for C-III drugs may be issued either orally or in writing to the pharmacist, and it may be refilled up to 5 times within 6 months after the date of issue, if so authorized on the prescription. After 5 refills or after 6 months, a new oral or written prescription is required.	• anabolic steroids • selected opiate combinations (acetaminophen [APAP] with codeine, hydrocodone mixtures [Vicodin])
Schedule IV (C-IV)	C-IV drugs have legal medical uses in the United States and a low abuse potential, which may lead to moderate psychologic and/or physical dependence. A prescription order for C-IV drugs may be issued either orally or in writing to the pharmacist, and it may be refilled up to 5 times within 6 months after the date of issue, if so authorized on the prescription. After 5 refills or after 6 months, a new oral or written prescription is required.	• benzodiazepines (diazepam [Valium]) • selected opiates (propoxyphene [Darvon]) • some barbiturates (phenobarbital)
Schedule V (C-V)	C-V drugs have legal medical uses in the United States and a low abuse potential, which may lead to moderate psychologic and/or physical dependence. A prescription order for C-V drugs may be issued either orally or in writing to the pharmacist and may be refilled if so authorized on the prescription. Some states allow C-V products to be sold over-the-counter (OTC) provided they are dispensed by a pharmacist and the patient is at least 18 years of age. A record of the transaction must be kept by the pharmacist if permitted by law.	• selected opiates (cough and diarrhea preparations)

who self diagnose and self prescribe ("I have an abscessed tooth, and the only drug that helps my pain is oxycodone."), and they should be alert to a series of "new" patients all complaining of similar symptoms. Once a substance abuser is successful in getting a prescription for a controlled substance from a dentist, this person often "sends friends."

Triplicate Prescription Blanks

Some states require triplicate prescription forms when Schedule II drugs are prescribed. The state supplies blanks upon request from the dentist. Blanks are numbered consecutively as a measure to provide additional control of the prescription blanks. After a prescription is written, one copy is placed in the dentist's records and the other two copies are provided to the patient. These two copies then are given to the pharmacist, who keeps one copy and sends the other copy to the state regulatory agency. Triplicate form pads should be kept in a secure place to prevent them from being stolen. When these forms are misplaced or stolen, the appropriate state agency must be notified immediately.

Canadian Drug Schedules

The Controlled Drugs and Substances Act (1996) and subsequent amendments consolidate Canada's drug control pol-

icy. It provides (a) a framework for the control and use of substances that can alter mental processes and that may produce harm to health and to society when distributed or used without supervision; (b) mechanisms to ensure that regulated substances are confined to medical, scientific, and industrial purposes; and (c) enforcement measures available to police and to the courts for the interdiction and suppression of unlawful distribution of controlled substances. Practitioners—defined by the act as "those registered and entitled under the law of a province to practice in that province the profession of medicine, dentistry, or veterinary medicine"—may prescribe controlled substances for medical purposes in accordance with the various provincial mandates. Controlled substances are identified in six schedules, not in five schedules as in the United States. Schedules are I, II, III, IV, V, and VI, and the drugs are placed in schedules according to their perceived abuse potential as determined by Canadian authorities. Table 3-4 illustrates the Canadian controlled substances schedules.

■ **Self-Study Review**

9. Identify the U.S. agency that governs prescriptions for controlled substances.

Table 3-4	Canadian Controlled Substance Schedules

Schedules	Examples

Schedule I	1. Opium poppy, its preparations, derivatives, alkaloids and salts
	   a. Morphine and congeners
	   b. Codeine and congeners
	2. Fentanyl derivatives, their salts, and analogues
	   a. Fentanyl

Schedule II	1. Cannabis, its preparations, derivatives, and similar synthetic preparations a. Marijuana
Schedule III	1. Amphetamines, their salts, derivatives, isomers, and analogues, and salts of derivatives, isomers, and analogs a. Amphetamine

Schedule IV	1. Barbiturates, their salts, and derivatives
	   a. Barbital
	   b. Pentobarbital
	   c. Secobarbital
	2. Benzodiazepines, their salts, and derivatives
	   a. Alprazolam
	   b. Diazepam
	   c. Lorazepam

Schedule V	1. Phenylpropanolamine
Schedule VI	1. Ephedrine 2. Ergotamine 3. Pseudoephedrine

10. Describe how a dentist secures a DEA number. For what reasons would a DEA number be denied?
11. Identify drugs in each of the five DEA schedules. Which schedule has the highest risk for abuse? Which has the lowest? Which schedule is used for research only?
12. List the rules for writing prescriptions for controlled substances. What is done to discourage prescription alterations?
13. What is the purpose of triplicate prescription blanks? Which three individuals or agencies get copies?
14. How does the Canadian scheduled drugs classification system differ from its U.S. counterpart?

CONCLUSION

The dental hygienist uses knowledge of prescription writing to check prescriptions prepared by the dentist and to examine information on the prescription label. The dentist often relies on the dental hygienist for clinical applications of this knowledge. The rules for prescription writing are used to properly prepare a prescription. These regulations must be followed before a pharmacy will accept an order for medication. This is especially true for prescriptions for substances of potential abuse, which must comply with DEA regulations.

CLINICAL APPLICATION EXERCISES

☐ **Exercise 1.** A new patient reports for dental hygiene care. During the medical history review, it is determined that the patient received a total hip replacement 13 months ago and has been told to have antibiotic prophylaxis prior to dental treatment. The patient says a prescription was called in to the pharmacy by the orthopaedist. What questions need to be asked to verify the proper antibiotic prophylaxis regimen? Write out the information to be included in the treatment record following the questioning of the patient.

☐ **Exercise 2.** You have been asked to review a prescription written by the dentist for a controlled substance prescribed for one-time use. Which essential elements on the written prescription will you check?

☐ **Exercise 3.** During the health history review, it is discovered that the patient has a history of chest pain. When the hygienist asks if any medication has been prescribed for the condition, the patient produces a bottle of nitroglycerin tablets. What information on the label will reveal if the drug is still active?

4

Autonomic Pharmacology

KEY TERMS

Adrenergic: A receptor (alpha or beta) or an effect related to the sympathetic nervous system

Afferent: Inflowing; conducting toward an area such as the central nervous system (CNS)

Alpha receptor: A receptor subtype of the sympathetic nervous system

Autonomic nervous system (ANS): The involuntary nervous system that includes the parasympathetic and sympathetic divisions; regulates physiologic function of internal organs

Beta receptor: A receptor subtype of the sympathetic nervous system

Catecholamines: Drugs (agonists) synthesized from tyrosine (dopamine, norepinephrine, epinephrine) that stimulate the sympathetic nervous system

Cholinergic: A receptor (muscarinic or nicotinic) or an effect related to the parasympathetic nervous system

Effector organ: The specific tissue stimulated to act by the postganglionic nerve

Efferent: Outflowing; conducting outward from a given area, such as the CNS

Innervate: To supply with nerves

Muscarinic receptor: A receptor subtype of the parasympathetic nervous system

Neurotransmitter: A small peptide molecule released by presynaptic cells in response to electrical signals that diffuses across the synaptic cleft and subsequently binds to membrane receptors of postsynaptic cells, producing an excitatory or inhibitory effect

Nicotinic receptor: A receptor subtype of the parasympathetic nervous system

Prototype: The first drug in a class of drugs to which all other drugs in the same class are compared

Reflex arc: An automatic motor response to sensory stimuli

Somatic nervous system: A part of the peripheral nervous system that controls voluntary skeletal muscle activity and conducts sensory information

KEY ACRONYMS

Ach: Acetylcholine
ANT: Adrenergic nerve terminal
CNS: Central nervous system
EPI: Epinephrine

Nor: Norepinephrine
PNS: Parasympathetic nervous system
SLUD: Salivation, lacrimation, urination, defecation
SNS: Sympathetic nervous system

The nervous system is composed of two main divisions: The central nervous system (CNS), composed of the brain and spinal cord, and the peripheral nervous system, which includes the **somatic nervous system** and the **autonomic nervous system (ANS)**. The somatic nervous system controls voluntary skeletal muscle activity and conducts sensory information. In the somatic nervous system, fibers pass from the spinal cord directly to the striated muscles. The ANS controls the involuntary automatic activity of smooth muscle, cardiac muscle, visceral organs, and glands. For example, an autonomic response would be blinking the eyes in response to an object quickly brought close to the face. Therefore, the ANS has been called the *involuntary nervous system*, or *automatic nervous system*. The dental hygienist must understand the physiologic effects of the ANS and identify drugs that stimulate or inhibit these effects. Potential adverse reactions related to the ANS can affect management of the dental client.

AUTONOMIC NERVOUS SYSTEM

The ANS regulates physiologic function of internal tissues. For example, it controls the digestion of food and the maintenance of blood pressure. Information is collected about conditions inside and outside the body, and the ANS responds to changes through a **reflex arc**. The reflex arc is the automatic motor response to sensory stimuli. In a reflex arc, nerve impulses transmitted via a nerve fiber (neuron) are the basis of communication of information through the nervous system. Two main functional processes are involved: Sensory *input* (**afferent**) and motor *output* (**efferent**). The first component is the receptor, which detects environmental changes (temperature, blood pressure) and produces a stimulus that transmits a nerve impulse along the afferent neuron to the CNS. The second component occurs within the CNS, which then issues instructions to the tissues innervated by either (a) the somatic system or (b) the ANS via an efferent motor nerve impulse to the peripheral **effector organ** (i.e., blood vessel smooth muscle, sweat gland, etc.). This stimulates the appropriate response of the muscle or gland. Therefore, the reflex arc functions as a feedback mechanism operating from a receptor to an effector organ for the purpose of preventing changes in function that may result in internal disturbances.[1]

There are many drugs that either inhibit or stimulate receptors in the ANS. Several of these drugs are used in oral health care, such as vasoconstrictors (inhibitors) and agents

to stimulate salivation, or sialogogues (stimulators). A basic understanding of the physiologic function of the ANS and changes associated with dysfunction is helpful to understand the effects of drugs on tissues innervated by the ANS.

Subdivisions of the Autonomic Nervous System

The ANS is divided into two subdivisions called the parasympathetic nervous system (PNS) and the sympathetic nervous system (SNS). The PNS influences basic daily life situations, whereas the SNS shocks physiologic processes into action during environmental or internal stress. It is essential to review anatomic features of each subdivision before examining the drugs that influence them. The anatomic arrangement of each system consists of two motor nerves, a preganglionic nerve (or fiber) and a postganglionic nerve. These nerve fibers are connected by a ganglion (group of nerve cell bodies). In the CNS the neuron cell body for each division sends impulses through an axon (nerve fiber) that goes from the spinal cord into the peripheral nervous system and connects with a ganglion, where a synaptic connection is made. These electrical impulses or action potentials traveling along preganglionic nerve fibers stimulate the release of **neurotransmitters**, which are released by the presynaptic cells, diffuse across the synaptic cleft (space), and bind to receptors in the membrane of postsynaptic cells. For this reason, synaptic transmission is often referred to as electrochemical transmission, which is the basis of cellular communication essential for the effective functioning of complex multicellular organisms. Figure 4-1 illustrates the anatomical relationships between the two divisions, from the point of exit from the CNS (brain, spinal cord) to the muscles or glands innervated, called the target tissue or effector organ.

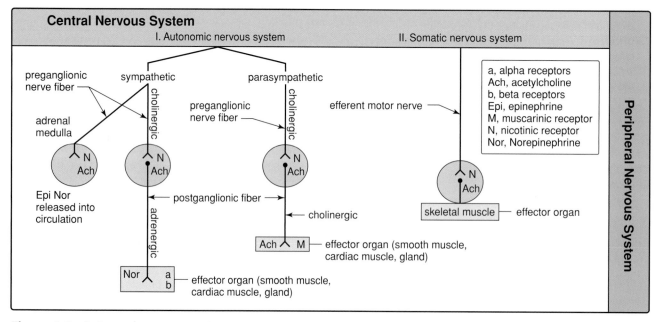

Figure 4-1 Autonomic nervous system

Terminology

There are specific terms used to refer to each division of the ANS. The term associated with parasympathetic activity is **cholinergic**, whereas sympathetic activity is called **adrenergic**. Each division has different receptors, and receptor names are often used to describe the effects of each division. For example, parasympathetic receptors are called **muscarinic** and **nicotinic**. Drugs that interact with muscarinic or nicotinic receptors and stimulate the PNS may be cholinergic, cholinomimetic, or parasympathomimetic, and are called muscarinic or nicotinic agonists. In essence, if one reads a test question about muscarinic receptors, the question relates to the PNS. Sympathetic receptors are classified as either alpha (α) or beta (β) receptors, and these are further subdivided into alpha-1 (α_1), alpha-2 (α_2), beta-1 (β_1), beta-2 (β_2), and beta-3 (β_3) receptors. Drugs that interact with alpha- and beta-receptors and stimulate the SNS are called adrenergic, or sympathomimetic, and may be further defined as alpha-adrenergic and/or beta-adrenergic agonists. Furthermore, some chemicals that interact with SNS receptors are classified as **catecholamines** or sympathomimetics. Antagonists at muscarinic and nicotinic receptors are called parasympatholytics, and antagonists at alpha- and beta-receptors are called sympatholytics.

Receptors

Cholinergic Receptors

Figure 4-2 illustrates the locations of both muscarinic and nicotinic receptors. Note that sweat glands are anatomically within the SNS. Box 4-1 lists the same information. *Muscarinic* receptors are activated by small amounts of acetylcholine (Ach) and are found at the neuroeffector junctions (also called effector organs) of the PNS (the ends of postganglionic fibers). Muscarinic receptors also are located at

---

BOX 4-1. Locations of Cholinergic Receptors

Muscarinic	Nicotinic
Effector organ in PNS	Ganglionic synapse in SNS and PNS
Effector organ in sweat gland	Preganglionic innervation of adrenal medulla
Effector organ in skeletal blood vessel	Skeletal muscle of Somatic Nervous System

---

anatomically sympathetic, but physiologically cholinergic, postganglionic effector organs in sweat glands and skeletal blood vessels. The second type of receptor in the PNS is called a *nicotinic* receptor. Nicotinic receptors require much higher doses of Ach to cause an effect. Nicotinic receptors are found at the ganglionic synapse of both the SNS and PNS, at the sympathetic preganglionic neuroeffector junction to the secretory cells of the adrenal medulla and at the myoneural junctions in the somatic nervous system.

Adrenergic Receptors

Adrenergic receptors are found in many tissues of the body. There are at least two types of alpha-adrenergic receptors (alpha-1 and alpha-2) and three types of beta-adrenergic receptors (beta-1, beta-2, and beta-3). Beta-1 receptors are located in the heart and renal juxtaglomerular cells; beta-2 receptors are located in smooth muscle of the peripheral vasculature and lungs, the liver, and the skeletal muscle; and beta-3 receptors are located in adipose tissue and regulate lipolysis. The following general rule describes nonmetabolic adrenergic effects: Alpha-adrenergic receptor agonists *stimulate*

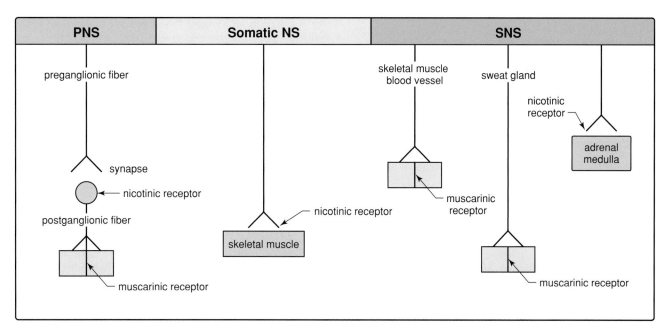

Figure 4-2 Muscarinic and Nicotinic Receptors

(produce contraction of vascular smooth muscles [alpha-1 and alpha-2 receptor activation] and contraction of cardiac muscle [alpha-1 receptor activation]). An exception to the rule is that α_1-adrenergic receptor activation in intestinal smooth muscle results in inhibition, or decreased muscle tone, the effect of which is constipation. β_2-adrenergic receptor agonists *inhibit* (produce relaxation of bronchial smooth muscles). An exception to the rule is that beta-1 receptor agonists in the heart stimulate (both rate and force of cardiac muscle contraction), the effect of which is tachycardia. By learning the general effects, and exceptions, of the SNS, one can predict many pharmacologic effects of adrenergic agents. To anticipate a drug effect, one also must learn which receptors are activated by the specific adrenergic drug. For example, the vasoconstrictor epinephrine (EPI) binds to both alpha- and beta-receptors; another vasoconstrictor, isoproterenol, is selective for only beta-1 and beta-2 receptors; and a third vasoconstrictor, levonordefrin, has only alpha-receptor activity. Applying this concept to drug selection, levonordefrin has less cardiac stimulation and CNS excitation. As various drug classifications are discussed in the text, the specific receptor activation is identified. EPI is used to illustrate the effects of adrenergic drugs.

Neurotransmitters

Cellular communication is essential for the effective functioning of complex multicellular organisms. In excitable tissues such as nerves, rapid intercellular communication relies on the propagation of electrical signals or action potentials. The passage of a nerve impulse (action potential) along a nerve fiber is called *conduction*. While the nerve fiber conducts these electrical impulses along the plasma membrane of cells, it requires a chemical substance to permit the impulse to cross the synapse and stimulate receptors. This event stimulates receptors either on the postganglionic fiber or at the effector organ, causing a response (e.g., blinking an eye) or a physiologic effect (e.g., digestion). These chemical substances, known as **neurotransmitters**, are biosynthesized, stored, and released by special autonomic nerves. The chemical neurotransmitter of the PNS at the effector organ is Ach, and the neurotransmitter of the SNS at the effector organ is norepinephrine (Nor). In general, cholinergic nerves release Ach, and adrenergic nerves release Nor.

Acetylcholine

Ach is the neurotransmitter at the following sites (Fig. 4-1):

* The neuroeffector junction (or effector organ) at the end of the postganglionic fiber in the PNS
* The synaptic junctions between the preganglionic and postganglionic fibers in both the PNS and SNS
* The neuroeffector junction between the preganglionic sympathetic nerve ending and the adrenal medullary secretory cells
* The neuroeffector junction between the postganglionic sympathetic nerve endings and the smooth muscle walls of blood vessels in skeletal muscle
* Postganglionic sympathetic nerve endings in sweat glands innervated by sympathetic, cholinergic postganglionic fibers.

BOX 4-2. Comparison of Features of Parasympathetic and Sympathetic Divisions

Parasympathetic	Sympathetic
preganglionic fibers— long	preganglionic fibers—short
postganglionic fibers— short	postganglionic fibers—long
neurotransmitter at synapse—Ach	neurotransmitter at synapse—Ach
neurotransmitter at effector organ—Ach	neurotransmitter at effector organ—Nor
preganglionic fibers—myelinated	preganglionic fibers—myelinated
postganglionic fibers— nonmyelinated	postganglionic fibers—nonmyelinated
leaves CNS at cranial, sacral level	leaves CNS at thoracic, upper lumbar area
1 to 2 postganglionic fibers (local effect)	1 to 20 postganglionic fibers (generalized effect)
does not fire as a unit	fires as a unit

Ach, acetylcholine; Nor, norepinephrine; CNS, central nervous system

---

Norepinephrine

The only location where Nor acts as a chemical transmitter is at the effector organ of the SNS.

Anatomy

A comparison of features of each subdivision of the ANS is in Box 4-2. The anatomic arrangement of each division includes two efferent motor nerves: A preganglionic nerve or fiber, and a postganglionic nerve, with the two connected by a ganglion, or synapse. As a general rule, in the PNS, preganglionic fibers are long and postganglionic fibers are short; in the SNS, preganglionic fibers are short and postganglionic fibers are long. Preganglionic synapses are found mostly in the paravertebral sympathetic chain near the spinal cord. The neurotransmitter at the synapse between preganglionic fibers and postganglionic fibers in both the PNS and SNS is Ach. Postganglionic fibers in both divisions innervate an **effector organ**—i.e., blood vessel, nerve, gland, or muscle. The neurotransmitter between the postganglionic fibers and effector organs in the PNS is Ach; in the SNS, it is Nor. All preganglionic fibers in the ANS are myelinated, and all postganglionic fibers are nonmyelinated.

Parasympathetic Division

Preganglionic fibers in the PNS leave the CNS at the cranial and sacral levels of the spinal cord. These fibers emerge along with the cranial nerves (III, VII, IX, X [vagus nerve]). The vagus nerve has several branches that supply fibers to the heart, lungs, and most of the abdominal organs. The organs innervated and the major effects produced by the nerves are illustrated in Figure 4-3. The ganglia usually are found

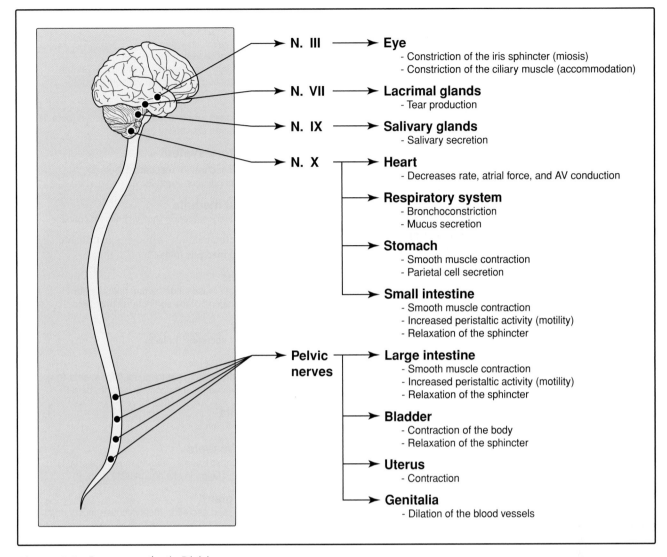

Figure 4-3 Parasympathetic Division

close to or within the effector organ, making the postganglionic fibers very short. There are generally no more than one or two postganglionic fibers branching from a preganglionic fiber, resulting in a localized effect. The PNS does not fire as a unit. Parasympathetic fibers innervate cardiac and smooth muscles, visceral organs, secretory glands, and all neuromuscular junctions.

Sympathetic Division

Preganglionic fibers in the SNS leave the CNS at the thoracic and upper lumbar levels of the spinal cord, as shown in Figure 4-4. They synapse with their specific ganglion and travel to the effector organ. There can be numerous (1 to 20) postganglionic fibers leaving one synaptic ganglion in the SNS. This allows for the innervation of several different effector organs, and can result in either a localized or generalized effect. During acute stress, the SNS fires as a unit, with actions occurring in many areas of the body (increased blood pres-

sure, increased blood sugar, constipation, xerostomia, pupil dilation, increased respiration, etc.).

Exceptions to General Anatomic Rules

One might suspect there would be exceptions to these general anatomic rules. The adrenal medulla is part of the SNS. It has a preganglionic fiber, but it acts as its own postganglionic fiber; anatomically, no postganglionic fiber exists in the adrenal medulla, and the secretory cells are innervated by a preganglionic fiber with Ach as the neurotransmitter. The adrenal medulla secretes EPI and Nor.

Another rule exception is that innervation by the SNS to skeletal muscles, blood vessels, and sweat glands is accomplished via parasympathetic postganglionic fibers, with Ach as the neurotransmitter at the effector organ. When Ach is the neurotransmitter, the fiber is described as *cholinergic*. This means that adrenergic skeletal muscles, blood vessels, and sweat glands are innervated by cholinergic postganglionic fibers.

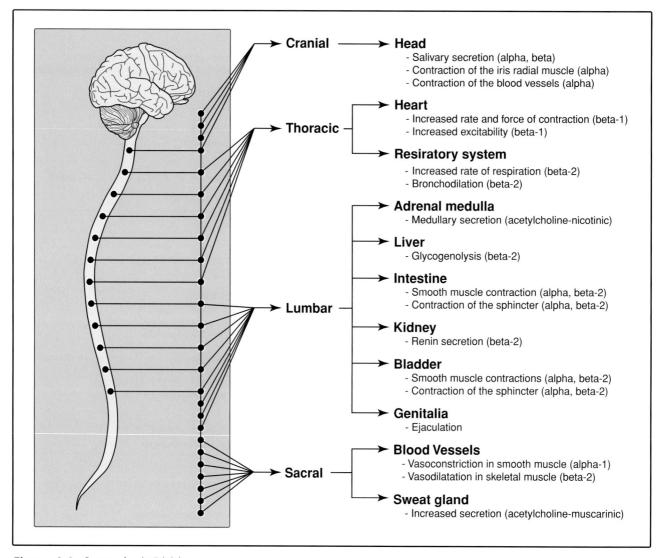

Figure 4-4 Sympathetic Division

Many organs are innervated by both sympathetic and parasympathetic fibers, and the opposing actions of the two systems balance one another. In this case, when one division of the ANS is stimulated, an action (e.g., contraction) results; when the other division is stimulated, the opposite action occurs (e.g., relaxation). The CNS controls the stimulus, and when one division of the ANS is activated, the other division is inhibited. Additionally, when one division of the ANS is inhibited, the other division can take over and stimulate receptors in that division (i.e., inhibition of the SNS results in activation of PNS effects).

■ Self-Study Review

1. Which nervous system is involuntary? Which is voluntary?
2. Identify the divisions of the ANS.
3. Which neurotransmitter stimulates the PNS response? Which neurotransmitter stimulates the SNS response?
4. What terms are associated with the PNS? What terms are associated with the SNS?
5. What are the receptors in the PNS? What are the receptors in the SNS?
6. List tissues involved in "exceptions" to the general rules of the ANS and adrenergic receptors.
7. List areas in the ANS where Ach is the neurotransmitter.

AUTONOMIC NERVOUS SYSTEM RESPONSES IN SPECIFIC TISSUES

The PNS functions to conserve energy and promote rest and digestion. This includes reducing the heart rate, increasing

| Table 4-1 | ANS Responses in Selected Tissues | | | |

Effector Organ		Cholinergic	Receptor	Adrenergic
Eye	Radial muscle iris	Contraction (miosis)	Alpha	Contraction (mydriasis)
	Sphincter muscle iris	Contraction (near vision)	Beta-2	Relaxation (far vision)
	Ciliary muscle			
Heart	SA node/Atria	Decrease in contractility;	Beta-1	Increase in heart rate, increase in
	Vagal nerve	increase in conduction velocity		contractility, and conduction velocity
		Decrease in heart rate		
Blood Vessels	Coronary	Dilation	Alpha, beta-2	Constriction, dilation
	Skin, mucosa	Dilation	Alpha	Constriction
	Salivary glands	Dilation	Alpha	Constriction
Lung	Bronchial muscle	Contraction	Beta-2	Relaxation
Intestine	Motility	Increased (diarrhea)	Alpha, beta-2	Decrease (constipation)
	Sphincters	Relaxation	Alpha	Contraction
Liver			Beta	Glycogenolysis
Urinary Bladder	Detrusor muscle	Contraction	Beta-2	Relaxation
	Trigone and sphincter	Relaxation	Alpha	Contraction
Sweat Glands		Generalized secretion	Alpha	Contraction, gooseflesh
Salivary glands		Profuse, watery secretion	Alpha	Thick, viscous secretion

All cholinergic responses are due to muscarinic receptor activity; adrenergic receptor responses are alpha or beta. (Adapted with permission from Cowan F. *Dental Pharmacology.* 2nd ed. Baltimore: Lippincott Williams & Wilkins; 1992:61–62.)

gastrointestinal (GI) activity for digestion and absorption, and increasing excretion. The SNS mobilizes energy resources in an emergency as part of the stress response, often referred to as the *fight or flight system.* These functions involve increasing blood sugar, heart rate, and blood pressure, and dilating bronchioles to accommodate for increased respiration. Table 4-1 illustrates the anatomic features and responses of the PNS and the SNS. Because all cholinergic responses are activated by the muscarinic receptor, only the adrenergic beta or alpha receptors are illustrated. It should be noted (as explained in the prior section) that adrenergic responses are usually the opposite of cholinergic responses (e.g., adrenergic receptors speed the heart rate and cholinergic receptors slow the heart rate). As well, when both alpha- and beta-receptors in the SNS are activated, alpha responses are generally the opposite of beta responses. For example, in coronary blood vessels where alpha-receptor activation causes vasoconstriction, beta-receptor activation causes vasodilation. The resulting effect relies on the specific pharmacologic receptor that is activated (alpha or beta) and the agonistic potential of the specific drug involved.

In order to predict the specific ANS response, it is necessary to know the class of agents to which the specific autonomic drug belongs. An example is doxazosin, an α_1-blocking cardiovascular drug used to lower blood pressure. Doxazosin blocks alpha-1 receptors in vascular smooth muscles, allowing beta effects to prevail to produce vasodilation, lowering peripheral resistance and leading to lower blood pressure. An example of a PNS blocking agent is atropine, a drug used to decrease salivary secretions. It is classified as a *muscarinic, cholinergic blocking agent,* which means it will block muscarinic receptors. When atropine blocks muscarinic receptors, adrenergic effects predominate. Similarly, when beta-adrenergic receptors are blocked, the effects of alpha-adrenergic responses prevail.

Cholinergic Effects

The acronym SLUD (salivation, lacrimation, urination, defecation) describes the effects of the PNS. The list is not all-inclusive as the PNS also affects other tissues, such as the cardiovascular system and the eye. However, because effects of the SNS are usually *opposite* those of the PNS, memorizing the acronym SLUD helps to remember some effects of the SNS (e.g., xerostomia, dry eyes, and constipation).

Cardiovascular System

The vagal nerve innervates the SA node and the AV node. Stimulation of the vagal nerve causes muscarinic receptors to be activated, and the heart rate slows. The clinical effect of vagal stimulation is bradycardia. Muscarinic receptors also are found in endothelial cells (blood vessels). Cholinergic stimulation of these cells releases nitric oxide, which produces vasodilation.[2]

Eye

The sphincter muscle of the iris and the ciliary muscle in the eye have PNS innervation. When the ocular nerves to these tissues are stimulated and Ach is released, the effect is a contraction of the sphincter muscle, which results in the pupil becoming smaller (miosis). The constriction on the ciliary muscle causes a relaxation of ligaments of the lens of the eye, which results in accommodation for near vision. Constriction of the ciliary muscle opens the canal of Schlemm in the eye and promotes a reduction of internal pressure within the eyeball. This effect of cholinergic drugs is used to treat glaucoma, a disease where pressure builds within the eye. Drugs that mimic the effects of Ach can cause similar results.

Glands

Many glandular cells in the digestive and respiratory systems have postganglionic parasympathetic innervation. When these fibers are stimulated, the cells secrete. In the oral cavity, salivation occurs. Lacrimation, or watery eyes, is caused by cholinergic action on lacrimal glands. As explained previously, most sweat glands have sympathetic *cholinergic* innervation (not adrenergic), and Ach stimulates muscarinic receptors to secrete. This effect can be blocked by atropine.

Urinary Bladder

Parasympathetic innervation of the bladder causes contraction of the detrusor muscle and relaxation of the trigone and sphincter, resulting in urination. These tissues have muscarinic receptors. Muscarinic agonists are used to improve bladder function and reduce urinary retention.

Intestinal Smooth Muscle

Parasympathetic innervation of the smooth muscle in the gastric and upper small intestines results in contraction of the intestinal wall and relaxation of the sphincters. This promotes diarrhea.

Skeletal Muscle

Ach binds with nicotinic receptors at the myoneural junction in skeletal muscles of the somatic nervous system. The somatic nervous system innervates voluntary muscles of the skeleton, which is different from the involuntary visceral muscles of the ANS.

Synthesis and Termination of Acetylcholine

Ach is synthesized in the cytoplasm of the nerve terminals from acetyl coenzyme A (CoA) and choline, and stored in vesicles located within cholinergic neurons at the prejunctional and postjunctional nerve endings (Fig. 4-5). This includes both preganglionic and postganglionic nerves of the PNS, as well as preganglionic nerves in the SNS. When the nerve impulse stimulates the release of Ach at the nerve ending, the neurotransmitter crosses the junction and reversibly binds to Ach receptors on the postganglionic fiber. The effect takes only seconds, and then Ach is released from the binding site and is degraded by an enzyme called *acetylcholinesterase* found in the junctional fluids. Enzymatic action of Ach results in the choline component's being separated from the acetate fraction. Consequently, the choline portion is absorbed by the nerve to be used to form more Ach, whereas the acetate portion enters the metabolic pool. The rapid destruction of Ach results in a short duration of receptor activation.

■ **Self-Study Review**

8. Identify the following tissue responses of the PNS: Cardiovascular system, eye, glands, genitourinary system, and GI system. Define SLUD.

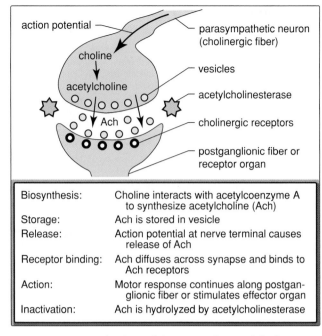

Figure 4-5 Synthesis and Storage of Acetylcholine

9. Identify locations of muscarinic and nicotinic receptors.
10. How is Ach synthesized, where is it stored, and how is it terminated?

Adrenergic Effects

The SNS functions to provide for homeostasis of body function, continually monitoring and readjusting organ systems. For example, changing from a supine to an upright position prompts the SNS to constrict visceral blood vessels and dilate blood vessels in the legs. Dilation of blood vessels in the legs promotes venous return of blood to the heart, and constriction of visceral vessels increases blood pressure, enhancing the blood supply to the brain. The SNS is said to function as a unit, a feature used during the stress response. In this situation the SNS causes glycogen in the liver to be broken down into glucose for energy, respiration is stimulated, bronchioles dilate to promote oxygenation in the lungs, heart rate increases along with the force of contraction to supply blood to body tissues, and vasoconstriction in the viscera shunts blood to skeletal muscles where vessels dilate. As this occurs, GI function is inhibited. This prepares for the ability to "fight or flight." The **prototype** adrenergic stimulant is EPI. EPI, like Ach, also is developed as a drug.

Epinephrine

EPI is used in dental local anesthetics because of its vasoconstrictive properties. Vasoconstriction tends to reduce systemic toxicity (by slowing systemic absorption of the local anesthetic), prolongs the duration of anesthetic action (by slowing absorption from the site of action into systemic circulation), and reduces intraoperative bleeding (by causing vasoconstriction). The evidence suggests that, like Ach (the chemical transmitter for both muscarinic and nicotinic receptors), EPI can activate different receptor sites (both alpha- and beta-receptor sites). This concept is illustrated by the effects of EPI in the treatment of anaphylaxis. EPI binds to a receptor (β_2-adrenergic receptor) in the bronchioles of the lungs to cause bronchodilation (opening the airway), and binds to a different receptor (α_1-adrenergic receptor) on blood vessels to cause vasoconstriction (elevating blood pressure). In this example, the effect of EPI on vascular and bronchial smooth muscle is also a classic example of physiologic antagonism between EPI and inflammatory chemicals associated with the allergic response, histamine and leukotrienes. By interacting with different receptors, EPI produces an effect opposite of that associated with both histamine and leukotrienes. These inflammatory chemicals are the major causes of bronchospasm and vasodilation during anaphylaxis.

Effects in Tissues

Cardiovascular System

EPI has significant cardiovascular effects because beta-1 receptors predominate in the organ. EPI increases the force of the cardiac muscle contraction (referred to as a positive inotropic effect), stimulates the sino-atrial (SA)-node pacemaker cells to increase heart rate (positive chronotropic effect), and increases atrio-ventricular (AV)-node conduction velocity, which affects ventricular muscle contraction. The result is an increased amount of blood pumped out of the heart (referred to as increased cardiac output). The increase in heart rate has a negative effect of decreasing atrial filling because there is less time between beats to accommodate for atrial filling. Other negative effects are that the increase in cardiac workload from the inotropic and chronotropic effects causes an increased need for oxygenated blood by cardiac muscle. The decrease in cardiac efficiency can result in muscle hypoxia. The effects on the ventricular conduction system can result in ventricular arrhythmia and fibrillation when high doses of EPI are administered systemically. In a healthy cardiovascular system, the tissues can adapt to these negative features, but when cardiovascular disease exists, there is a potential for negative effects.

Adrenal Medulla

Ach binds with nicotinic receptors in the adrenal medulla to stimulate the release of EPI and Nor. The adrenal medulla is part of the SNS, but it acts as its own postganglionic fiber.

Peripheral Vascular System

Alpha-1 receptors predominate in the blood vessels in the body, except for blood vessels in skeletal muscle, which have both alpha-1 and beta-2 receptors. The concentration of EPI can affect which receptors are activated and influence sympathetic effects. Generally, one would expect EPI to constrict blood vessels through alpha-mediated effects. However, in vascular beds with beta-2 receptors, adrenergic agents (such as EPI) can cause vasodilation (recalling that beta effects

often are opposite of alpha effects). In the skeletal muscle vascular bed, beta-2 receptors have a greater affinity to EPI than do alpha-receptors, and EPI (in small doses) causes vasodilation and increased blood flow. Large doses of EPI result in activation of alpha-receptors and vasoconstriction, but, as the tissue level of EPI falls, vasodilation again prevails. This is what occurs in the oral mucous membranes when a local anesthetic with EPI is administered (i.e., initial vasoconstriction), but as EPI levels diminish, vasodilation results. Sympathetic drug effects relate to the specific receptors that are stimulated, as illustrated in these examples:

- The adrenergic vasoconstrictor isoproterenol acts on beta-2 receptors to cause vasodilation in blood vessels and bronchodilation in the lungs, but in cardiac muscle it acts on beta-1 receptors to stimulate cardiac muscle.[2,3]
- In salivary glands, stimulation of adrenergic nerves in vascular beds results in vasoconstriction (alpha-receptors), and secretions are inhibited (xerostomia).
- In the peripheral blood vessels where alpha-receptors predominate, EPI causes increased blood pressure due to vasoconstriction.
- In coronary arteries, vasoconstriction usually dominates, but the effect may be obscured by local vasodilation as a result of relative hypoxia that may occur when EPI causes increased myocardial contraction.

All of these events are affected by the SNS, which functions to maintain homeostasis. The net effect of EPI on the cardiovascular system as a whole is the algebraic sum of the beta-mediated vasodilation and the alpha-mediated vasoconstriction, with vasodilation predominating at low doses. However, even small doses of EPI when given intravenously at a rapid rate can cause elevated heart rate, increased blood pressure, and arrhythmia. This can cause adverse effects when the cardiovascular system is compromised by disease. The dental applications of these issues are discussed further in Chapter 6.

Respiratory System

The most significant effects of EPI on the respiratory system are mediated via beta-2 receptors in the smooth muscle of the bronchioles. Beta-adrenergic agonists are powerful bronchodilators and can reverse bronchoconstriction associated with asthma or anaphylaxis. EPI can also interact with alpha-1 receptors in vascular smooth muscle of bronchiolar mucosa and cause vasoconstriction. Bronchodilation and vasoconstriction work together for symptomatic relief of mucosal congestion. The sum result of these actions improves vital capacity and respiration.

Gastrointestinal System

Adrenergic agonists generally inhibit the smooth muscle of the wall of the stomach and intestines, thereby decreasing both the tone and motility, resulting in constipation. This effect is mediated by alpha- and beta-receptors, the alpha-receptor in this case acting as an exception to the general rule (formerly discussed) for alpha-receptor effects. EPI generally causes contraction of the sphincter smooth muscles, and this effect participates in the constipation effect.

Eye

As one might expect, EPI acts in opposition to Ach in the eye. Alpha-1 receptor activation causes contraction of the radial muscle of the iris, resulting in pupil dilation (mydriasis). At the same time beta-2 receptor activation relaxes the ciliary muscle, which increases ligament tension on the lens and results in a decrease of the angle of lens curvature (miosis).

Urinary Bladder

In the bladder, EPI (and other adrenergic agonists) produce retention of urine. This effect is mediated by beta-receptors causing relaxation of the detrusor smooth muscle walls (fundus of the bladder), accompanied by an alpha-mediated constriction of the smooth muscle of the trigone and sphincter.

Salivary Glands

Salivary flow can be increased by EPI and other adrenergic drugs (*not* an opposite effect from Ach), but the characteristics of the secretions are different. The saliva is a thick, mucous type of secretion. These characteristics suggest that alpha-receptors in the mucoid salivary glands (primarily the submaxillary gland) are stimulated rather than the serous gland (parotid). This hypothesis is further supported in that alpha-adrenergic blocking agents antagonize salivation. The significance of increased salivary flow is not well understood and may be an indirect result of vasodilation and increased blood flow to the glands.

Metabolic Effects

EPI affects carbohydrate metabolism both directly and indirectly. The activity of several enzymes involved in glycogen synthesis and storage are affected, with the result that glycogen is metabolized to utilizable glucose in the liver and to lactate in skeletal muscle (direct effect). By actions on other metabolic pathways, new glucose is synthesized. These actions are supported by alpha-receptor–mediated inhibition on insulin secretion (indirect effect). Triglyceride breakdown is influenced by EPI, resulting in the release of free fatty acids and glycerol into the circulation. This increases energy sources.

Synthesis and Termination of Norepinephrine

The chemical mediators of the SNS include both Nor and EPI. The two compounds are identical in chemical structure except that EPI has a methyl group attached to the amino nitrogen. Because of this close structural similarity, both of the agents have many pharmacologic actions in common. Nor is the *official* neurotransmitter of the SNS at the effector organ. These chemicals belong to a class known as **catecholamines**.

Adrenergic Nerve Terminal

The adrenergic nerve terminal (ANT) contains granules, each of which contain several "pools," or compartments (Fig. 4-6).

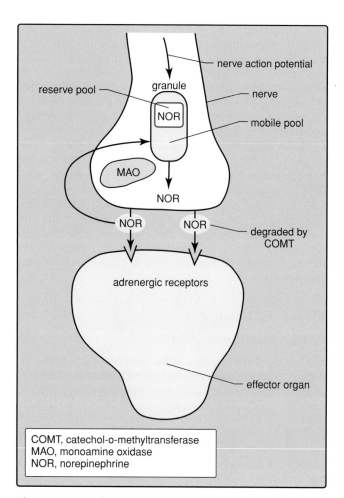

COMT, catechol-o-methyltransferase
MAO, monoamine oxidase
NOR, norepinephrine

Figure 4-6 Adrenergic nerve terminal

Nor is synthesized by cells within the reserve pool and stored in the mobile pool. It is released primarily from the intragranular mobile pool. Following stimulation from the adrenergic nerve impulse, Nor leaves the mobile pool and enters the synapse at the effector organ. As Nor leaves the mobile pool, it is replaced by Nor from the reserve pool. Termination of Nor effects occurs mainly by a unique reuptake process that pumps Nor back into the ANT, although a small portion is degraded by the enzyme catechol-o-methyltransferase (COMT) in the synaptic fluid. This process has the characteristics of a carrier-mediated active transport system. When Nor is returned to the ANT, it enters the cytoplasmic mobile pool. A small portion is degraded by an enzyme, monoamine oxidase (MAO), but most is pumped back into the granules. In summary, Nor release occurs via the nerve action potential at the junction of the postganglionic fiber and the effector organ, binds to a receptor, and, when released from the receptor, is reuptaken into the ANT and stored, ready to be released again for receptor activation. Unlike Ach, the chemical does not have to be resynthesized, allowing the adrenergic effects to have a longer duration. Metabolic inactivation of both EPI and Nor occurs by the action of COMT and MAO. This occurs mainly by the metabolism of catecholamines in the blood.

■ Self-Study Review

11. What is the general rule for effects produced by the receptors in the SNS? Name the prototype adrenergic stimulant.
12. Describe the sympathetic responses in the following tissues: Cardiovascular, peripheral vascular system, respiratory system, GI system, eye, salivary glands, and genitourinary system. How is carbohydrate metabolism affected by EPI?
13. Describe how Nor is synthesized and how it is terminated. Compare this mechanism to that of Ach. What is the effect on duration of Nor effects?

CHOLINERGIC DRUGS

Ach is available as a drug and used in pharmacotherapy. It is applied locally as eyedrops for a miotic effect in some diseases of the eyes. It has the same effects as the endogenous neurotransmitter. Cholinomimetic drugs are used in dentistry (pilocarpine [Salagen] and cevimeline [Evoxac]) to treat xerostomia associated with disease, such as Sjögren syndrome, or from various drug therapies. These cholinergic agonists have parasympathetic effects, but they are not choline esters, so they are not inactivated by acetylcholinesterase. Pilocarpine is also administered as eyedrops for treatment of narrow-angle glaucoma.

Anticholinesterase Drugs

These are drugs that do not act on cholinergic receptors, but instead inhibit the enzyme that degrades Ach. They promote the action of Ach by allowing the chemical to accumulate in the synaptic cleft, thus prolonging its effects. One drug of this type, neostigmine, is useful in the treatment of myasthenia gravis. The nerve gas sarin is a potent irreversible cholinesterase inhibitor.

Cholinergic Blocking Agents

This group of drugs includes agents that affect muscarinic receptor activity and drugs that affect nicotinic receptor activity.

Muscarinic-Receptor Blocking Agents

The prototype antimuscarinic drug is atropine. It blocks muscarinic receptors only and has no effect on nicotinic receptors. Atropine comes from the nightshade plant, *Atropa belladonna*. This is an example of a drug derived from a plant, a concept discussed in Chapter 1; however, products used today are synthetic substitutes for atropine. The action of atropine is competitive antagonism. Atropine has a high affinity for the muscarinic receptor, greater than that of Ach. Atropine has no intrinsic activity. It simply binds to the receptor, thereby preventing Ach from binding. This allows tissue cholinesterase to degrade Ach before it can bind to muscarinic receptors.

Administration of anticholinesterase drugs can override the blocking action of atropine. In dentistry, atropine has been used prior to making a dental impression when a dry field is needed. Recalling the effects of the divisions of the ANS, one can anticipate that when the PNS is blocked, this allows the SNS effects to take over. In this regard, atropine can be used to reverse bradycardia by inhibiting Ach effects on the vagal nerve. In ophthalmology, it is used to dilate the pupil for ocular examination. Toxic doses of atropine have been described in the mnemonic: Dry as a bone (decreased sweating), hot as a hare (increased body temperature when the body is not cooled by sweating), blind as a bat (mydriasis, cycloplegia), and mad as a hatter (CNS stimulation).

Nicotinic-Receptor Blocking Agents

Drugs that block nicotinic receptors include ganglionic blocking agents and skeletal muscle relaxants. They inhibit Ach effects at the synapse between preganglionic and postganglionic fibers in the ANS, at the adrenal medulla, and at the skeletal myoneural junction. Nicotinic-receptor blocking agents are used therapeutically in dentistry as skeletal muscle relaxants. There are two main types of drugs in this category of muscle relaxants: Competitive nondepolarizing agents and noncompetitive depolarizing agents.

Nondepolarizing Agents

Nondepolarizing blockade occurs when an antagonist competes with an agonist for the same receptor site. The blockade may be overcome by administration of higher concentrations of Ach.

Depolarizing Agents

Depolarizing blockade occurs when an agonist binds to the receptor site, causes muscle contraction, and then dissociates slowly from the receptor. During the time that the agonist remains bound to the receptor, other agonists are excluded from binding to the same receptor site. Cholinergic blocking agents are included in Box 4-3.

Other Antimuscarinic Agents

There are several drugs used in dentistry that block muscarinic receptors.

BOX 4-3. Cholinergic Blocking Agents

Muscarinic	Nicotinic
Atropine, scopolamine, methantheline, propantheline	Competitive nondepolarizing agents: Tubocurarine, metocurine, alcuronium, doxacurium, pancuronium, others
	Noncompetitive depolarizing agents: Succinylcholine

Scopolamine

Scopolamine has a more pronounced CNS depressant effect than atropine, and it is used for surgical premedication to gain a dual benefit of CNS depression (amnesia to surgery) and reduced airway secretions. Scopolamine is also used as a motion sickness drug and is administered as a patch, a gel, or an oral doseform. This is a common preventive drug recommended while on a cruise. If a fellow cruise passenger is observed to have a round patch behind the ear, the patch is likely to contain scopolamine. Other agents include the synthetic atropine methantheline (Banthine), used as an antisialagogue in prosthodontics and orthodontics. It has a longer duration of action than atropine which is advantageous. Propantheline (Pro-Banthine) has a strong affinity for muscarinic receptors in the GI tract and is used to reduce GI motility. Other muscarinic blockers are used in the treatment of Parkinson disease to reduce tremors associated with the disease.

Contraindications

Atropine and other antimuscarinic drugs should not be used when narrow-angle glaucoma exists. It blocks the outflow of fluid in the eye, increasing pressure within the eyeball and precipitating an attack. When cardiovascular disease exists, these blocking agents may block the vagus nerve, resulting in SNS effects (tachycardia, hypertension), and should be used only after consultation with the physician managing the condition. Another condition in which these agents are contraindicated is benign prostate hypertrophy due to the urinary retention effect. These drugs are not recommended for the prepuberty age group.

■ Self-Study Review

14. List therapeutic uses of cholinergic drugs and highlight dental uses.
15. Identify cholinergic drugs used for dental applications.
16. How do anticholinesterase drugs extend cholinergic effects?
17. Identify the prototype muscarinic blocking drug and the mechanism of action. What is the plant source for this chemical?
18. Describe the uses of atropine in dentistry. Memorize the mnemonic.
19. What are the indications for using nicotinic blocking agents in dentistry?
20. Describe the uses and action of scopolamine.
21. What are contraindications for using anticholinergic drugs?

ADRENERGIC DRUGS

Sympathomimetic agents are used in dentistry for local vasoconstriction (EPI, levonordefrin) in local anesthetic agents. When applied topically, such as when using EPI-impregnated gingival retraction cord, vasoconstrictors are used to control

---

BOX 4-4.   Uses of Adrenergic Drugs

- Local vasoconstriction to control bleeding
- Local vasoconstriction to prolong duration of local anesthesia
- Relief of nasal congestion via constriction of vessels in the upper respiratory tract (URT)
- Increased blood pressure in treatment of shock
- Bronchodilation in asthma and allergic bronchoconstriction
- Anaphylactic shock (increases blood pressure and dilates airway)

---

minor bleeding from arterioles and capillaries. If the crevicular tissue is denuded or inflamed, EPI easily can be absorbed into the bloodstream and lead to cardiovascular stimulation. Precautions with these agents used in dentistry are discussed in Chapter 6. Topical application of sympathomimetics in the doseforms of drops or sprays is used to relieve nasal congestion. Disadvantages of these doseforms are that they: (a) have a relatively short duration, (b) can irritate the nasal tissues, and (c) can result in rebound congestion of nasal passages.

Other therapeutic uses of sympathomimetics include cardiac pressor effects for treating hypotension and shock in emergency situations, and bronchodilation effects in acute bronchospasm (Box 4-4). Agents used include inhaled short-acting agents (isoproterenol, EPI, albuterol), or EPI given by subcutaneous administration. Long-acting agents are used for treatment of asthma or chronic bronchospasm (salmeterol).

Mechanism of Action

Sympathomimetics act either by direct activation of sympathetic receptors or, indirectly, by actions at the ANT. Some drugs act both directly and indirectly. Indirectly acting sympathomimetics block the reuptake of Nor into the ANT, or they may displace Nor from the mobile pool within the nerve terminal. Both mechanisms result in increased Nor concentration and produce mainly alpha responses. They are not easily degraded by COMT because they have a different chemical structure than directly acting sympathomimetics. When given by parenteral administration, they have a fast onset and longer duration of action than directly acting adrenergic agents.

Cocaine

Cocaine is the prototype of indirectly acting sympathomimetics that block the active uptake of Nor and other catecholamines into the ANT. It has local anesthetic effects as well as CNS stimulant effects. It acts by blocking the active uptake of Nor and other catecholamines into the ANT. This blockade increases the concentration of Nor at the adrenergic receptor and increases the effect. Because alpha receptors are activated by Nor, when cocaine is applied as a local anesthetic, vasoconstriction occurs. Remember that EPI is *added* to a local anesthetic to produce vasoconstriction because most local anesthetics produce vasodilation. In the CNS, the effect of Nor is to elevate the mood. Other drugs, such as tricyclic antidepressants, can block Nor reuptake in the brain.

Amphetamine

Amphetamine is the prototype for indirectly acting drugs that cause a rapid release of Nor from the mobile pool of the ANT. Amphetamine in peripheral tissues causes a sustained pressor effect, increasing both systolic and diastolic blood pressure. Increased heart rate and force of contraction can occur, although compensatory reflexes generally act to slow the heart rate. If the dose of amphetamine is high, arrhythmia can occur. Contraction of the sphincter in the urinary bladder leads to difficult urination and urinary retention. Amphetamines are used therapeutically for narcolepsy, a sleep disorder. However, this drug and similar drugs (methamphetamine) can be abused for their CNS effects. These sympathomimetic agents are among the most powerful CNS stimulants. When used therapeutically, amphetamines

- stimulate the medullary respiratory center in the brain;
- reverse drug-induced CNS depression;
- increase wakefulness and alertness;
- decrease the appetite;
- decrease fatigue;
- elevate the mood, leading to euphoria.

All these effects lead to the high abuse potential. Methamphetamine abusers are known to go for days without eating; if they have small children, the children go without food, as well. The ability of amphetamines to improve physical performance and delay fatigue has led to abuse of the agents. It should be noted that artificial prolongation of performance is followed by fatigue, prolonged sleep, and depression.

Ephedrine

Ephedrine is an example of a sympathomimetic with a mixed action (both direct and indirect effects). Ephedrine products were removed from the market in recent years due to reports of cardiovascular stimulation, in some cases leading to death. The effects of ephedrine are similar to EPI but last up to ten times longer. This is a positive effect for the relaxation of bronchial muscle. CNS effects are similar to amphetamine, but less potent.

Adrenergic Blocking Agents

Drugs that block SNS activity include two groups: (a) inhibitors of catecholamine storage and (b) adrenergic-receptor blocking drugs.

Inhibitors of Catecholamine Storage

The two most important drugs are guanethidine and reserpine, both used in therapy for severe hypertension. They act by depleting the neurotransmitter (Nor) from peripheral adrenergic neuron terminals. Guanethidine displaces Nor from the storage site in the ANT, and reserpine blocks Nor uptake into the storage granule. Reserpine has the ability to reduce catecholamine content in the brain and the adrenal medulla. Both drugs can prevent the response to postganglionic adrenergic nerve stimulation, and both can reduce the effects of indirectly acting sympathomimetics. A major adverse effect of both guanethidine and reserpine is postural hypotension; when either of these drugs is taken and the supine position is used for dental treatment, the practitioner should monitor the blood pressure after placing the patient in an upright position and prior to dismissing the patient from the dental chair.

Adrenergic-Receptor Blocking Agents

Alpha-receptor blocking drugs are used in the treatment of hypertension, and beta-receptor blocking drugs have several effects on cardiovascular tissues (reducing blood pressure, reducing angina, and so forth). They act as competitive pharmacologic antagonists at the receptor. Alpha-blocking drugs can be nonspecific and block alpha-1 and alpha-2 receptors, or they can be specific only to alpha-1 or only to alpha-2 receptors. The same holds true for beta-blocking drugs—they can be nonspecific blocking agents or selective agents. These are discussed in greater detail in Chapter 17.

Contraindications and Precautions

EPI is contraindicated when severe cardiovascular disease and unstable angina is reported. When nonspecific beta-blocking drugs are taken (e.g., propranolol [Inderal]) the use of EPI-containing gingival retraction cord is contraindicated, and other forms of EPI should be used with caution. Most adrenergic drugs and anticholinergic drugs are classified as pregnancy category C and should be used with caution in the pregnant patient. Some patients taking adrenergic-blocking agents experience postural hypotension. This condition is described as dizziness and cerebral ischemia due to low blood pressure when changing from a supine to a sitting or standing position.

■ Self-Study Review

22. Identify examples of adrenergic drugs and their therapeutic uses. What doseform is associated with rebound congestion?
23. Describe the effects of cocaine as a prototype agent.
24. Describe the effects of amphetamine. When is it used therapeutically?
25. Identify two important antiadrenergic drugs. What is a dental consideration when these drugs are taken by a dental patient?

DENTAL HYGIENE IMPLICATIONS

Cholinergic Drugs

Dryness of the mouth, blurred vision, and photophobia (aversion to bright light) can occur with cholinergic agents. Elderly patients may experience confusion. Footstools or furniture that can obstruct walking should be moved out of the walking area. Oral problems related to chronic dry mouth include increased caries, especially cervical decay; burning and lubrication problems; and fungal infection (candidiasis). Previous texts recommended avoidance of alcohol-containing mouth rinses, but recent evidence reveals no adverse effects of alcohol-containing mouth rinses in xerostomic individuals.[4] However, alcohol-based rinses may increase burning of oral mucosa. Saliva is stimulated when gum is chewed, and xylitol-containing gum has an added anticaries effect.[5]

Adrenergic Drugs

Older adults are particularly vulnerable to adverse reactions to adrenergic drugs, especially EPI. Older patients are more likely to have cardiovascular disease and are predisposed to having cardiac arrhythmias. The pulse rate and rhythm of all elderly patients taking an adrenergic drug should be monitored at every appointment, as should their blood pressure. The patient should be monitored for signs of postural hypotension at the end of the dental appointment. Low concentrations of EPI (1:100,000) should be considered for the patient with cardiovascular disease when injectable local anesthesia is planned. Box 4-5 includes dental hygiene management procedures for the patient taking autonomic drugs.

CONCLUSION

The ANS is responsible for the regulation of internal viscera, such as the heart, blood vessels, digestive organs, kidneys, and reproductive organs. A basic understanding of the ANS in health and when dysfunction develops is necessary to understand the pharmacologic agents that affect it. With an understanding of potential adverse drug effects, the practitioner can implement strategies in the treatment plan to reduce potential adverse consequences. Understanding autonomic pharmacology may help to identify potential risks during treatment and assist the practitioner in developing strategies to reduce complications from those risks.

BOX 4-5. Management When ANS Drugs Are Taken

Cholinergic Blocking Agents
- Do not direct overhead dental light into eyes (photophobia)
- Monitor heart rate and qualities before treatment
- Make sure the walkway is unobstructed (blurred vision)
- Examine oral cavity for caries, candidiasis, periodontal inflammation
- Oral health education
  - When chronic dry mouth occurs, recommend home fluoride products on a daily basis
  - Suggest xylitol gum to stimulate saliva and for anticaries effect

Adrenergic Agonists
- Monitor blood pressure and pulse every appointment
- Use vasoconstrictor in low concentrations (1:100,000)

Adrenergic Blocking Agents
- Monitor for postural hypotension
  - Raise chair back slowly
  - Sit upright a few minutes before dismissing from dental chair
  - Monitor for lightheadedness as patient leaves operatory

CLINICAL APPLICATION EXERCISES

☐ Exercise 1. You have a new, 20-year-old patient who has never had dental treatment. He admits to being "a little anxious" about what to expect. How will this anxiety be likely to affect the physiologic status of the patient?

☐ Exercise 2. Your patient presents with a chief complaint of excessive dry mouth and asks, "What can I do about this?" What ANS drugs might the dentist consider to alleviate this oral problem? What is the mechanism of action and classification of the product? What are the clinical implications of this chief complaint?

☐ Exercise 3. Look up the generic drug *propantheline* in a drug reference. List brand names. What is the drug classification? What is the mechanism of action? Why is it used (indication)? What adverse effects can cause modification of the treatment plan and should be followed up? What are the clinical implications for the patient care?

☐ Exercise 4. WEB ACTIVITY: Go to the Web site of the National High Blood Pressure Education Program (www.nhlbi.nih.gov/about/nhbpep/index.htm). Select "Information for Patients & the Public," then select "List of All Publications"; navigate to the document titled "Your Guide to Lowering Blood Pressure." Go to the section on treatment and find the discussion of lifestyle modifications to help lower blood pressure. Write down five ideas you can discuss during oral health education. Check out the information on "Quitting Smoking" for your smoking cessation program.

References

1. Salerno E. *Pharmacology for Health Professionals.* St. Louis: Mosby; 1999:244.
2. Cowan F. *Dental Pharmacology.* 2nd ed. Philadelphia: Lea & Febiger; 1992:55–103.
3. McCann JAS, Pub. *Nursing 2005 Drug Handbook.* Philadelphia: Lippincott Williams & Wilkins; 2005:563–585, 629.
4. Fischman SL, Aguirre A, Charles CH. Use of essential oil-containing mouthrinses by xerostomic individuals: Determination of potential for oral mucosal irritation. *Am J Dent.* 2004;17: 23–26.
5. Milgrom P, Ly KA, Roberts MC, et al. Mutans streptococci dose response to xylitol chewing gum. *J Dent Res* 2006;85(2):177–181.

5

Adverse Drug Effects

Drugs, including herbal remedies and various dietary supplements, seldom exert their beneficial effects without also causing adverse events. This happens because drugs can act on many different tissues at the same time. Those drug effects that are desirable are called *therapeutic effects*, and undesirable drug effects are called **adverse drug effects (ADEs)**, or "side effects." The inevitability of this therapeutic dilemma

lends credence to the statement that there are no absolutely safe biologically active agents. When selecting a drug necessary to obtain a desired therapeutic effect, prescribers must take several factors into consideration:

• The diagnosis of the problem, or "What will the drug be used for?" The Food and Drug Administration (FDA) approves drugs for specific indications, or uses, but occasionally a drug will be prescribed for other conditions. This practice is called "off-label" use. A good example of off-label use is the common use of the antihypertensive drug propranolol to prevent or treat migraines. Sometimes a side effect of a drug is used for a therapeutic effect. For example, an antihistamine (which can cause drowsiness) can be used to treat insomnia. This brings to mind the old TV commercial "Nytol to help you get your ZZZs!"

- Individual variations in **physiologic status**. Adverse drug effects are more likely to occur in the very young and the very old because their organ functions are either not fully developed (very young) or progressively declining (very old).
- Variations in disease states or unusual circumstances, such as pregnancy. An example of a disease state influencing the selection of a therapeutic agent is the contraindication of aspirin use in peptic ulcer disease.
- Drug-related pharmacodynamic and pharmacokinetic variables, which can occur when other biologically active chemicals compete with a drug at the receptor site or during the pharmacokinetic phases of medication action. This can include an exaggerated response, an expected but undesired response (such as losing hair in cancer chemotherapy), and other responses described later in the chapter. Oral health care providers, like other health care professionals, should be aware of examples of drug-induced effects and should be actively involved in monitoring and reporting them. Chapter 1 explains how ADEs are reported to the FDA, and Table 1-2 in Chapter 1 illustrates some recently reported ADEs. Follow-up questioning during the review of the drugs listed on the health history should include monitoring for potential side effects. As well, oral examination for ADEs or for complications that can result due to ADEs should be monitored. For example, chronic xerostomia is a common side effect that can lead to dental decay, especially at the cervical third of the tooth. This finding should lead to the recommendation of a home fluoride regimen in the oral health education plan.

A companion text to this basic pharmacology text is *Lippincott Williams & Wilkins' Dental Drug Reference with Clinical Implications*. This companion text can be used to efficiently complete the clinical application activities in this pharmacology textbook.

ALTERATION OF DRUG EFFECTS

Several factors can influence the effect of a drug. These include

- patient noncompliance in taking the medication as prescribed;
- psychologic factors, such as taking a substance with no pharmacologic activity, called a **placebo**, when the client believes the agent will produce an effect. In this instance, the effect experienced by the client is called "the placebo effect." The placebo effect results from the doctor–patient

relationship, the significance of the therapeutic effect to the patient, and the mental "setting" imparted by the clinician. Although it is usually identified with the administration of an inert substance in the guise of medication, all drugs can produce a placebo effect. This can be both favorable and unfavorable relative to the therapeutic objectives. Exploited to advantage, placebo effects can significantly contribute to the success of therapy[1];

- tolerance to the medication, which can develop when a drug is taken for a long period of time, and greater doses are necessary to cause the same degree of effect. **Tachyphylaxis** is an uncommon condition where tolerance develops rapidly. When tolerance develops, changing to another drug with the same effect often solves the problem;
- time of administration, which can be an issue for drugs that must be taken on an empty stomach. Agents likely to cause a taste disturbance are to be used following meals, such as rinsing with chlorhexidine, an antigingivitis mouth rinse;
- the sex of the client. Women may be more sensitive than men to certain drugs and need a smaller dose to avoid toxicity;
- age and weight, factors that must be considered when determining drug dosage. Pediatric patients and geriatric patients may require reduced doses. The primary reason for the dose reduction in pediatric clients is a smaller body size. Even when the size differential is considered, children may exhibit an unusual (hyperreactivity) response to drugs. Geriatric clients are often hyperreactive to drugs. Decreased kidney and liver function can also be factors. Patients over the age of 65 are twice as likely to experience ADEs than young adults.

The relative distribution of drugs to different body components can influence dosage requirements. For example, a lean but muscular 200-lb man will require a higher dose of a drug than a lean 150-lb man with a smaller muscle mass because the bioavailability of a drug is affected by its accumulation in muscle. Similarly, an obese man will require a higher dose of highly lipid-soluble drugs, such as diazepam, than a man with a lean body mass. A patient with edema will require a dosage modification because larger water-soluble molecules (mannitol) tend to accumulate in the expanded volume of extracellular water. Finally, certain ions, such as fluoride, tend to accumulate in bone, and individuals with large bony frames may require higher dosages of these drugs if the intended site of action is tissue, rather than bone.

ETIOLOGY AND EPIDEMIOLOGY

It is estimated that as many as 75% of office visits to medical practitioners are associated with the initiation or continuation of pharmacotherapy. This magnitude of drug use predisposes patients to adverse drug effects (ADEs). The frequency of clinically important ADEs is difficult to estimate, but it has been reported that between 3% and 11% of hospital admissions could be attributed to ADEs. The incidence of ADEs during hospitalization ranges from 0.3% to 44%, depending on the type of hospital, definition of an ADE, and study methodology. Although the U.S. Food and Drug Administration (FDA) has one of the most rigorous approval requirements in the world to authorize the marketing of new drugs, clinical trials cannot and should not be expected to uncover every potential ADE.

■ Self-Study Review

1. Consider characteristics of drug effects. How does one differentiate between therapeutic effects and adverse effects?
2. Identify an example in which a side effect is used for a therapeutic effect.
3. List four factors to consider before selecting a drug for a therapeutic effect.
4. List factors that can alter drug effects and explain the cause for the alteration.
5. Define *tachyphylaxis*.
6. What two age groups are more likely to experience ADEs?
7. Give two examples of how the registered dental hygienist can monitor for ADEs and how the dental hygiene treatment plan can be affected.

TYPES OF ADVERSE DRUG EFFECTS

ADEs may be classified as Type A or Type B (Table 5-1). They can range from mild to severe reactions and can lead to hospitalization, permanent disability, or death. **Type-A ADEs** generally are associated with the administration of therapeutic dosages of a drug (rather than high doses), usually are predictable and avoidable, and are responsible for most ADEs. Type-A ADEs also can include cytotoxic and toxic reactions that result from a drug overdose, although these are much less common. Some Type-A ADEs occur as a result of interactions with other drugs, interactions due to food components (food–drug interactions), or interactions because of physical changes resulting from disease (drug–disease interaction). **Type-B ADEs** generally are independent of the dose and rarely are predictable or avoidable. These can include immunologically mediated reactions (such as hypersensitivity or allergy-related reactions), situations where tissue is harmed slowly during the chronic administration of a drug, or **idiosyncratic** responses that are associated with genetic

Table 5-1 Classification of ADEs

Type-A Reactions	Type-B Reactions
Predictable	Unpredictable
Cytotoxic reactions	Idiosyncratic reactions
Drug–drug interactions	Immunologic/Allergic reactions
Drug–food interactions	Pseudoallergic reactions
Drug–disease interactions	Teratogenic effects
	Oncogenic effects

variation or age-related variables. While they are uncommon, Type-B reactions are often among the most serious and potentially life threatening of all ADEs. They are a major cause of important drug-induced illness. These reactions seem to affect certain organ systems, most commonly the liver, the hematopoietic system (spleen, bone marrow), or the skin and mucosa. With the exception of immediate hypersensitivity reactions, which can develop in seconds to minutes, Type-B events require longer time periods for the clinical effects to occur, often up to 12 weeks of drug exposure. Some ADEs may be delayed even further and appear a long time after drug therapy has been discontinued. An important example of this type of ADE, with relevance to dentistry, is osteonecrosis of the jaw (ONJ) following bisphosphonate administration for the prevention of bone density changes during cancer chemotherapy or for the prevention and treatment of osteoporosis (Table 1-2). Recent recommendations advise dental hygienists to review the medical history to identify patients taking bisphosphonates and advise them of the possibility of ONJ when the drug is taken.[2,3]

Mechanisms Associated with Type-A Reactions

Type-A reactions involve cell damage and vary from minor side effects to severe organ damage. They include cytotoxic reactions, drug–drug reactions, drug–food reactions, and drug–disease reactions (Table 5-1).

Cytotoxic Reactions

Although cytotoxic reactions can result from a drug overdose, most adverse effects of overdose are extensions of the drug's therapeutic effect. For example, respiratory depression caused by barbiturates can result in oversuppression of respiration, leading to death when too much of the drug is taken. **Cytotoxic reactions** are most commonly caused by the formation of unstable or reactive metabolites following biotransformation and are related to some abnormality that interferes with the normal metabolism and/or excretion of therapeutic dosages of a drug. These events lead to the saturation of hepatic enzyme systems. Two main mechanisms lead to the formation of these intermediate compounds during biotransformation:

- an oxidative pathway, which can produce compounds capable of binding covalently with cellular macromolecules
- a reductive pathway, which gives rise to the formation of such substances as free radicals

These substances react with oxygen and produce reactive metabolites, which overwhelm normal antioxidant defense systems. Both covalent binding to proteins and the oxidation of biologic macromolecules lead to direct cytotoxic effects.

Drug–Drug Interactions

Two or more drugs administered in therapeutic dosages at the same time or in close sequence may (a) act independently, (b) interact to increase or diminish the magnitude or duration of action of one or more drugs, or (c) interact to

Table 5-2	Pharmacodynamic Drug–Drug Interactions	
Type	**Mechanisms**	**Example(s)**
Pharmacologic	Drug A and Drug B compete for the same receptor site and, as a function of their respective concentrations, either produce (an agonist) or prevent (an antagonist) an effect.	• Opioids vs. naloxone • Acetylcholine vs. atropine • Epinephrine vs. adrenergic receptor blocking agents
Physiologic	Drug A and Drug B interact with different receptor sites and either enhance each other's action or produce an opposing effect via different cellular mechanisms.	• Cholinergic agents enhance the action of diazepam. • Epinephrine opposes the action of histamine. • Epinephrine opposes the action of lidocaine.
Chemical	Drug A competes with Drug B and prevents Drug B from interacting with its intended receptor.	• Protamine sulfate inhibits heparin.
Receptor alterations	Drug A, when administered long term, may either increase or decrease the number of its own receptors or alter the adaptability of receptors to physiologic events.	• α_1-adrenergic receptor agonists down-regulate their own receptors. • β_1-adrenergic receptor antagonists up-regulate their own receptors.

cause an unintended reaction. Drug–drug interactions may be complex, and even unexplained, but they all seem to have either a pharmacodynamic or a pharmacokinetic basis; the same pharmacologic mechanisms that account for a drug's efficacy also can account for many of its adverse effects.

Pharmacodynamic Drug–Drug Interactions

In pharmacodynamic interactions, the intended or expected effect produced by a given plasma level of a drug is altered in the presence of a second drug. These types of interactions may be characterized as (a) pharmacologic interactions, (b) physiologic interactions, (c) chemical interactions, or (d) drug-related receptor alterations. Examples of mechanisms and specific drug interactions are illustrated in Table 5-2.

Pharmacokinetic Drug–Drug Interactions

The duration and intensity of a drug's action is based on the amount of drug in the circulation (also called the plasma level of the drug), as explained in Chapter 2. This concentration is directly related to the drug's rate of absorption, distribution, metabolism, and excretion. One or more of these rates may be altered when an additional drug is added, resulting in unexpected differences in the plasma levels of a drug (Table 5-3). As discussed in Chapter 2, the concept of affinity illustrates the effect when two drugs are given together. The drug with the greater affinity for the plasma protein will cause an increase in the free, unbound molecules of the second drug, leading to toxic effects (overdose) of the second drug.

Drug–Food Interactions

An awareness of significant drug–food interactions can help the clinician to identify nutrients that may reduce the efficacy of or increase the duration of certain medications. This information can be used to educate patients on foods to avoid while taking a drug and, as a result, optimize pharmacotherapy. The example of avoiding milk products while taking tetracycline is well known. The following discussion clarifies issues involving drug–food incompatibilities affecting drug absorption, metabolism, and excretion.

Interactions That Affect Absorption

Nutrients can protect the gastric mucosa from irritants, but they also may act as a mechanical barrier that prevents drug access to mucosal surfaces. This can reduce or slow the absorption of some drugs. Conversely, a meal with high fatty acid content actually will increase the absorption of lipid-soluble drugs. Chemical interactions, such as chelating reactions between a drug and food components, can produce inactive complexes that cannot cross the intestinal mucosa during the absorption phase. The interaction of tetracycline with calcium in milk and other dairy products is an example of a chelating reaction. Similarly, ferrous or ferric salts in liver or organ meats can bind with tetracycline and fluoroquinolone antibiotics, preventing their absorption. An interaction between zinc and fluoroquinolones can also result in the formation of inactive complexes, which decreases absorption of the antibiotic.

Interactions That Affect Metabolism

Drinking grapefruit juice or eating the fruit is implicated in several drug interactions. Components in grapefruit juice inhibit the CYP450 3A4 isoenzyme in the liver. This causes plasma levels of drugs metabolized by this isoenzyme to greatly increase (up to threefold) and result in overdose or toxicity. Common examples relevant to dentistry include some antibiotics, calcium channel blocking agents, benzodiazepines, and warfarin (Table 5-4).

Interactions That Affect Excretion

Changes in the pH of kidney fluids can inhibit excretion of some drugs. For example, a large dose of ascorbic acid (vitamin C) can lower the pH in the glomerulus and cause acidic drugs to be reabsorbed in the kidney, thereby delaying the excretion and placing the vitamin back into the circulation. This strategy is sometimes used therapeutically to prolong the duration of drug action. For instance, in the treatment of sexually transmitted diseases, administration of high doses of penicillin G can be maintained by giving probenecid simultaneously. Probenecid inhibits renal tubular excretion of penicillin, thereby increasing the duration of action.

Table 5-3	Pharmacokinetic Drug–Drug Interactions	
Type	**Mechanisms**	**Example(s)**
Interactions that affect absorption	Drug A, by causing vasoconstriction, interferes with the systemic absorption of Drug B.	Epinephrine vs. lidocaine (or other local anesthetic agents)
	Drug A, by forming a complex with Drug B, interferes with the systemic absorption of Drug B.	Calcium vs. tetracycline
	Drug A, by delaying gastric emptying, delays the systemic absorption of Drug B, which is absorbed primarily in the intestine.	Opioids vs. acetaminophen
	Drug A, by elevating gastric pH, prevents the absorption of Drug B (a weak acid).	Antacids vs. acetylsalicylic acid
Interactions that affect distribution	Drug A (a weak acid), by competing for plasma protein binding with Drug B, increases the plasma level of Drug B.	Acetylsalicylic acid vs. sulfonylureas and many other drugs
Interactions that affect metabolism	Drug A, by increasing or decreasing hepatic microsomal enzyme activity responsible for the metabolism of Drug B, increases or decreases the plasma level of Drug B, respectively.	Macrolides, azole antifungals, and ethanol (chronic use) increase the plasma level of many drugs; H_2-receptor antagonists decrease the plasma level of many drugs.
	Drug A, by decreasing hepatic nonmicrosomal enzyme activity responsible for the metabolism of Drug B, increases the plasma level of Drug B.	MAO-inhibitors increase the plasma level of benzodiazepines.
	Drug A, by inhibiting the enzyme acetaldehyde dehydrogenase, interferes with the further metabolism of intermediate metabolites (oxidation product) of Drug B.	Disulfiram and metronidazole inhibit the metabolism of intermediate metabolites of ethanol.
Interactions that affect renal excretion	Drug A, which competes with Drug B for the same excretory transport mechanisms in the proximal tubules, increases the plasma level of Drug B.	Acetylsalicylic acid and probenecid increase the plasma level of penicillin and other weak acids.
	Drug A, by alkalizing the urine, decreases the plasma level of Drug B.	Sodium bicarbonate decreases the plasma level of weak acids.
	Drug A, by acidifying the urine, decreases the plasma level of Drug B.	Ammonium chloride decreases the plasma level of weak bases.
Interactions that affect biliary excretion	Drug A, by increasing bile flow and the synthesis of proteins, which function in biliary conjugation mechanisms, decreases the plasma level of Drug B.	Phenobarbital decreases the plasma level of many drugs.
	Drug A binds to Drug B, which would undergo extensive enterohepatic recirculation, and decreases the plasma level of Drug B.	Activated charcoal and cholestyramine decreases the plasma level of many drugs.

Drug–Disease Interactions

A drug prescribed for the treatment of one disease or condition may have an adverse effect on a different medical condition. Additionally, certain disease states affecting the liver or the kidneys can interfere with the metabolism and/or excretion of drugs in general. These drug–disease interactions can also involve mechanisms related both to pharmacodynamic and pharmacokinetic principles.

Table 5-4	Grapefruit–Drug Interactions Relevant to Dentistry	
Drug Class	**Example**	**Effect**
Antibiotics	Clarithromycin	Arrhythmia
Benzodiazepines	Diazepam Midazolam Triazolam	Decreased psychomotor function, increased sedation
Calcium channel blocking agents	Amlodipine Felodipine Nifedipine	Tachycardia, hypotension
Oral anticoagulants	Warfarin	Increased bleeding

Pharmacodynamic Interactions

There are a variety of drug–disease interactions. Nonselective beta-adrenergic receptor antagonists, such as propranolol (prescribed for the treatment of chronic stable angina, hypertension, or cardiac arrhythmia), can induce an asthma attack in susceptible individuals by blocking β_2-adrenergic receptors that aid in bronchodilation. Blocking these receptors causes the opposite effect and increases airway resistance. β_1-adrenergic receptor antagonists (prescribed for hypertension and other cardiac abnormalities) can also adversely affect glycogen metabolism and inhibit an endogenous epinephrine-mediated hyperglycemic response to excessive insulin levels, thus placing the diabetic patient at risk for hypoglycemia. Cyclooxygenase-1 (COX-1) inhibitors, especially aspirin, can lead to gastrointestinal (GI) bleeding in patients with pre-existing peptic ulcer disease. COX-1 (ibuprofen), COX-2 (celecoxib [Celebrex]), and COX-3 inhibitors (acetaminophen [APAP]), and amoxicillin may induce renal toxicity in patients with pre-existing renal dysfunction. Uncontrolled hypothyroidism increases the sensitivity of patients to sedative/anxiolytic agents and opioids, whereas uncontrolled hyperthyroidism predisposes to epinephrine-induced hypertension and cardiac arrhythmias.

An understanding of these drug–disease interactions will prompt the clinician to modify the relevant treatment plan accordingly.

Pharmacokinetic Interactions

Hepatic dysfunction can affect drug metabolism and biliary (gall bladder) excretion. In addition, kidney dysfunction can be expected to impair renal drug elimination. Cardiac disease can result in reduced metabolic activity in general because of poor tissue oxygenation and organ perfusion. All of these conditions can lead to elevated plasma concentrations of drugs with associated ADEs. Patients with congestive heart failure may experience fluid collection in the lungs while receiving β_1-adrenergic receptor blocking agents because these drugs decrease cardiac output, which leads to reduced glomerular filtration and sodium excretion, increasing the risk of fluid retention and edema. In patients with liver disease, drugs taken on a long-term basis that are metabolized primarily by the liver (such as APAP) may induce further hepatic dysfunction, even at therapeutic levels. For the patient with osteoarthritis who must take APAP chronically, this provides an increased risk for the development of another medical problem completely unrelated to the arthritic condition.

■ Self-Study Review

8. Explain the mechanisms involved in each component of Type-A and Type-B ADEs. Make a list of each, in order to organize the information and avoid confusion. What is the most common type?
9. Which ADEs are related to a genetic determination? Which usually have the most serious manifestations? Which are predictable? Which type usually manifests after long time periods following drug ingestion?
10. List examples of cytotoxic reactions, drug–drug reactions, drug–food reactions, and drug–disease reactions. Describe associated etiologic factors for each.
11. What patient instructions regarding diet should be given when tetracycline is prescribed?
12. Why are some drugs to be taken on an empty stomach?
13. Give an example of a chelating drug–food reaction.
14. Which liver enzymes are responsible for drug–grapefruit interactions?
15. How would an acidic agent affect excretion of other acidic drugs used simultaneously?

Mechanisms Associated with Type-B Reactions

Type-B reactions include idiosyncrasy, allergy, developmental effects, and oncogenic effects related to malignancy.

Idiosyncratic Reactions

An unusual reaction of any intensity observed in a small percentage of individuals is referred to as an **idiosyncrasy**. If a drug produces its usual effect at an unexpectedly high dose, the patient is said to be **hyporeactive**. A patient is said to be **hyperreactive** when a drug produces its effect at an unexpectedly low dosage. These terms are discussed further in Chapter 6. In certain individuals, especially those on the extremes of the age spectrum (children and elderly), some drugs can produce unexpected reactions. These idiosyncratic responses are not fully understood but are most often related to genetic variations affecting the biotransformation activities among CYP450 enzymes in the liver. Among the various CYP450 enzymes, CYP2D6 has been studied the most extensively, and various genetic phenotypes have been identified. Patients who lack CYP2D6 activity will exhibit poor metabolism of certain drugs, patients who have normal enzyme activity will exhibit normal metabolism, those with reduced activity will exhibit intermediate metabolism, and those with markedly enhanced enzyme activity will exhibit ultrarapid drug metabolism. If the consequence is reduced drug metabolism, it leads to excessive therapeutic effects and associated adverse reactions. If the consequence is accelerated metabolism, it results in insufficient therapeutic response.

Allergic/Immunologic Reactions

An inherited predisposition to drug allergy has been reported, and it is suggested that specific human leukocyte antigen (HLA) genes are involved in the reaction to at least some drugs. An *antigen* is a substance recognized as "foreign" to host antibodies. Drugs are immunogenic (antigenic) if the immune system is able to recognize the antigenic determinants as foreign (nonself) and if the molecular weight of the drug is sufficiently large. A *hapten* is a substance (drug) of lower molecular weight than an antigen. It can react with an antibody, but it is unable to induce antibody production unless it is attached to another molecule, usually a protein. Penicillin is an example of a hapten. Penicillin must attach itself to albumin before it can induce antibody synthesis. *The production of antigens occurs in genetically predisposed individuals, is not related to the dose administered, and is unpredictable.* Generally the first time a predisposed individual is exposed to an allergenic chemical, plasma cells form antibodies to destroy the antigen. This process is referred to as *sensitization*. On subsequent exposures to the antigen, the "antigen/antibody" immune reaction occurs. Similar to idiosyncrasy, most allergic reactions to drugs tend to occur in young individuals or older adults. Although it is not clear why, research has shown that drug allergies are observed twice as frequently in women as men. There are four main types of antigen/antibody hypersensitivity reactions: Immediate, cytotoxic, immune-complex, and delayed.

Type I (Immediate) Hypersensitivity Reactions

Exposure to an allergen results in antigen-specific antibody production dominated by the immunoglobulin E (IgE) isotype. IgE antibodies bind to specific sites on mast cells,

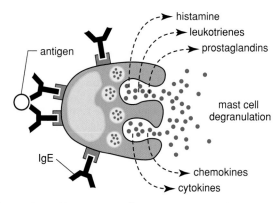

Figure 5-1 Type I Immediate Hypersensitivity

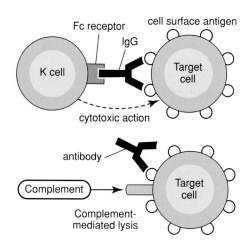

Figure 5-2 Type II Cytotoxic Hypersensitivity

basophils, and eosinophils within mucosal and epithelial tissues. The simultaneous binding of an antigen to adjacent IgE molecules triggers degranulation of mast cells and basophils, resulting in the production and release of inflammatory mediators, including histamine, leukotrienes, prostaglandins, chemokines, enzymes, and cytokines (Fig. 5-1). Histamine causes contraction of bronchial smooth muscle leading to bronchoconstriction. It also causes dilation of arterioles and postcapillary venules leading to redness (erythema). Histamine- and leukotriene-induced contraction of endothelial cells causes separation of these cells from one another, which, along with dilation of arterioles and post-capillary venules, increases capillary permeability and thus allows the escape of plasma proteins and fluid leading to edema. Leukotrienes also cause bronchospasm, increase mucous secretion, and impair mucus clearance from the alveoli. Prostaglandins promote vasodilation, bronchospasm, and increased mucous secretion. Chemokines attract leukocytes, enzymes break down tissue matrix proteins, and the cytokines promote inflammatory activities in target tissues. This is the most dangerous form of hypersensitivity reaction—it includes anaphylactic shock—and reactions develop within minutes of exposure to the allergen.

Type II (Cytotoxic) Hypersensitivity Reactions

IgG antibodies are involved in the basic cytotoxic immune reaction. In this reaction, antibodies bind to antigen-coated host cells, followed by complement activation and cell lysis induced by the active by-products of the complement cascade (Fig. 5-2). Alternatively, specialized lymphocytes called killer-cells (K-cells) cause the lysis of affected cells. A practical example of this type of allergic reaction is drug-induced hemolytic anemia.

Type III (Immune-Complex) Hypersensitivity Reactions

IgG antibodies also mediate immune-complex reactions and result in the formation of large, insoluble antigen–antibody complexes (Fig. 5-3). These immune complexes adhere to target tissues and initiate intense complement activation. As a result, leukocytes and platelets migrate to the affected tissues to form thrombi and occlude arterioles, producing either

localized or systemic complications. Examples of this type of allergic phenomenon include drug-induced mucositis.

Type IV (Delayed) Hypersensitivity Reactions

Delayed reactions are closely related to **cellular immunity** in that specifically sensitized CD4+ T-lymphocytes initiate the reaction (Fig. 5-4). Cellular immunity is associated with T-lymphocyte immune responses rather than B-lymphocyte responses. Initial sensitization occurs slowly, over a 10- to 14-day period. Drugs with small molecular weights (haptens) bind covalently to host cell membrane proteins. Subsequent exposure causes the immunologically committed lymphocytes to react with the allergen (antigens) and release cytokines (lymphokines), which activate macrophages and amplify the inflammatory response. These responses are not life threatening. Examples include dermatitis of the skin, stomatitis affecting oral mucous membranes, and the induration produced in a positive tuberculosis (TB) skin test.

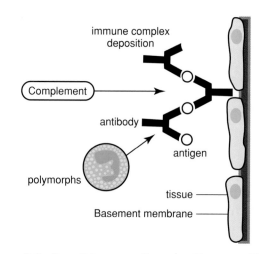

Figure 5-3 Type III Immune-Complex Hypersensitivity

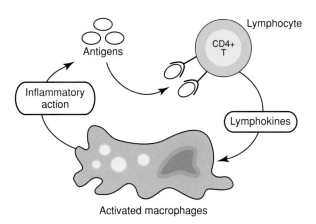

Figure 5-4 Type IV Delayed Hypersensitivity

Pseudoallergic Reactions

Pseudoallergic (also called anaphylactoid) reactions cannot be explained on an immunologic basis. These uncommon ADEs occur in patients with no prior exposure to the drug. Although this ADE is not well understood, possible mechanisms may include direct activation of mast cells through non-IgE receptor pathways, which initiates the release of histamine and other bioactive mediators. Such drugs as penicillin, codeine, morphine, and vancomycin are thought to be involved in this type of reaction. Some drugs, such as penicillin, can produce Type I, Type IV, or anaphylactoid reactions.

Teratogenic Effects

Teratogens are substances capable of causing physical or functional disorders in the fetus in the absence of toxic effects on the mother. Direct teratogenic effects depend on the introduction of drug or metabolite concentrations in the fetus at a critical time period, especially from the 3rd to the 12th week of gestation. Thalidomide, a drug used in Europe to diminish morning sickness associated with pregnancy, caused a variety of teratogenic malformations. These involved a depression of limb formation (no hands, no arms, no legs, etc.), a condition called **phocomelia**. Drugs likely to cause malformations are placed in pregnancy category X (see Chapter 21).

Oncogenic Effects

Oncogenic effects (related to causing malignancy) associated with drug therapy may be primary or secondary. **Primary oncogenic effects** can be produced by certain procarcinogenic drugs, which are converted into carcinogens by polymorphic oxidation reactions. Covalent binding of these oxidized metabolites to DNA leads to mutagenic and carcinogenic effects. **Secondary oncogenic effects** are associated with therapeutic immunosuppression, such as drug-induced immunosuppression to prevent rejection of an organ following organ transplant. This leads to the reactivation of latent infection with oncogenic viruses (e.g., hepatitis B virus [HBV], hepatitis C virus [HCV], Cytomegalovirus [CMV], herpes simplex virus [HSV], human papillomavirus [HPV], and the Epstein-Barr virus [EBV]). The pattern of cancer incidence from secondary effects is distinctly different from cancer in the general population, with a marked excess in the occurrence of (a) carcinoma of the skin and lips, (b) non-Hodgkin lymphoma, (c) Kaposi sarcoma (KS), (d) carcinoma of the uterus, (e) hepatobiliary carcinoma, (f) carcinoma of the vulva and perineum, (g) renal carcinoma, and (h) sarcomas (other than KS associated with HIV infection). The prevalence of *de novo*, or new malignancies, associated with therapeutic immunosuppression ranges from 4% to 18%. The malignancies occur in a relatively young group of patients (average age at the time of transplantation is 42 years), at a fairly predictable time interval, and within a relatively short period of time after transplantation.

■ Self-Study Review

16. Differentiate between *hyporeactive* and *hyperreactive* reactions.
17. Which groups are most likely to have idiosyncratic reactions?
18. Outline the process of the allergic drug reaction from sensitization to production of hives. What is the role of an antigen, a hapten, and a plasma cell?
19. What age groups and sexes are more likely to develop drug allergies?
20. List features of the four types of hypersensitivity reactions. Which is immediate? Which is delayed? Anaphylaxis is an example of which type? Which immunoglobulins are associated with each type? Which reaction involves T-cell activation? Which is most dangerous? Which results from the TB skin test?
21. Differentiate between *hypersensitive* and *pseudoallergic* reactions.
22. What is a *teratogenic reaction*?
23. Differentiate between a *primary* oncogenic effect and a *secondary* oncogenic effect.

CLINICAL MANIFESTATIONS OF ADVERSE DRUG EFFECTS

The clinical manifestations of ADEs may reflect primary (direct) or secondary (indirect) adverse effects. Primary or secondary adverse effects associated with Type-A reactions are those dose-dependent effects that are not desired for the given therapeutic use of a drug. These adverse effects account for most of the ADEs and may be exaggerations of direct effects or multiple concurrent "side" effects. Similarly, the clinical manifestations of ADEs associated with Type-B reactions are either primary or secondary, but they may or may not be dose dependent. Treatments for the various ADEs relate to the specific cause of the clinical manifestation or the symptom. For the following discussion, dental hygiene management considerations are described for symptoms of Type-A reactions. They are the same for Type-B reactions. For example, the management of oral ulceration is the same whether it is a Type-A or Type-B reaction.

Clinical Manifestations of Type-A Reactions

The signs and symptoms of Type-A reactions can develop in some clients with the normal dose of a drug, or they can result from excessive doses.

Cytotoxic Effects

Two main types of cytotoxic effects are presented.

Hepatocellular Toxicity

Drug-induced liver injury is a potential complication of nearly every medication that is prescribed. One such drug, APAP, is one of the most common drugs associated with hepatotoxicity. This usually occurs when high doses of APAP are taken, but it can develop with therapeutic doses in some patient populations (e.g., malnourished or alcoholic patients). Following excessive doses of APAP (>4 g in a 24-hour period), a cytotoxic metabolite accumulates in the liver and binds covalently to cellular macromolecules, thereby disrupting hepatic cell function. This process is accelerated by alcohol. For this reason, the maximum recommended dose of APAP when alcohol is consumed is 2 g, or half the normal maximum dose. Clinical signs and symptoms of liver toxicity include nausea, vomiting, anorexia, and abdominal pain. A few days later, elevated bilirubin causes jaundice (Color Plates 1 and 2).

Methemoglobinemia

Methemoglobinemia is a relatively uncommon toxic reaction to some local anesthetics, including prilocaine, articaine, and benzocaine. In susceptible patients, metabolites of these drugs bind with hemoglobin and interfere with its oxygen-carrying capacity. Cyanosis has been reported in the absence of cardiopulmonary symptoms, nausea, sedation, seizures, and coma. It usually is associated with severe overdose, but it can develop in genetically predisposed individuals.

Cytotoxic Mucositis

Chemotherapeutic agents used to treat malignancies produce extensive injury to certain cancer cells, but they are not selectively tumoricidal and can also arrest the growth and maturation of normal cells. The degree of toxicity usually depends on the specific chemotherapeutic agent, increased dosage levels, the treatment schedule and route of administration, and patient-related predisposing factors. When ulceration of oral mucous membranes occurs during cancer chemotherapy, it is called *mucositis*. Mucositis appears clinically as erythematous or generalized ulcerative lesions. Certain chemotherapeutic agents are more stomatotoxic than others, and chemotherapy-related mucositis provides an entry mechanism leading to systemic infection by the wide variety of oral microorganisms. Other drugs may also produce cytotoxic reactions that affect oral soft tissues (Color Plates 3 to 7).

Management Considerations

The pain associated with cytotoxic ADEs often causes the patient to seek relief. Palliative management strategies include specially prepared mouth rinses containing a topical anesthetic, a liquid antihistamine, and a covering agent (Miracle Mouthwash). Mouth rinses containing alcohol are contraindicated because of the pain and burning sensations that are associated with using them. A nonalcohol chlorhexidine mouth rinse is now available and may be indicated when oral infection is likely.

Gastrointestinal Disturbances

Disturbances in the GI tract are among the most common ADEs listed in drug reference texts. They include nausea, vomiting, and abdominal pain associated with constipation or diarrhea.

Nausea and Vomiting

The physiologic purpose of nausea is to prevent food intake; that of vomiting is to expel food or toxic substances present in the upper part of the GI tract. The chemoreceptor trigger zone found in the medullary area of the brain plays a major role in inducing vomiting. The chemoreceptor trigger zone is outside the blood–brain barrier and, thus, it is accessible to drugs circulating either in the blood or in the cerebrospinal fluid. The vomiting center, which is inside the blood–brain barrier, is activated by impulses that originate in the chemoreceptor trigger zone and induces nausea and vomiting. Protracted vomiting may cause electrolyte imbalance, dehydration, and malnutrition syndrome, and it may result in mucosal laceration and esophageal hemorrhage. A variety of drugs has been implicated in causing nausea and vomiting. Opioid analgesics either can induce (codeine) or block (morphine) emesis, depending on their affinity for opioid-receptor subtypes in the brain. Both the emetic and antiemetic actions can be blocked by an opioid antagonist (naloxone) used to reverse opioid overdose, which suggests that both effects are mediated by opiate receptors.

Constipation

Constipation is defined as the passage of excessively dry stool, infrequent stool, or stool of insufficient size. It involves the subjective sensations of incomplete emptying of the rectum, bloating, passage of flatus, lower abdominal discomfort, anorexia, malaise, headache, weakness, and giddiness. Constipation may be of brief duration (e.g., when one's living habits and diet change abruptly), or it may be a lifelong problem. The administration of many drugs (such as anticholinergic drugs found in many over-the-counter medications, antiparkinsonian drugs with anticholinergic properties, antihistamines, neuroleptics, antidepressants, anticonvulsants, opioid analgesics, and antacids) can lead to constipation.

Diarrhea

Diarrhea, and associated fecal urgency and incontinence, is defined as passage of liquefied stool with increased frequency. Chronic diarrhea can be due to a variety of medical conditions, such as lactose intolerance, inflammatory bowel disease, malabsorption syndromes, endocrine disorders, and irritable bowel syndrome. Drug-associated diarrhea can occur with the abuse of laxatives and antacids. Infection (viral or bacterial), toxins, or drugs (such as antibacterial agents) are the usual causes of acute diarrhea.

Management Considerations

When GI symptoms are reported during the follow-up of drug side effects, a commonly employed strategy is to use a semisupine chair position for treatment. When vomiting occurs, the patient is unlikely to present for a dental hygiene appointment.

Urinary Incontinence

Urinary incontinence is characterized by frequent urination. Urinary incontinence caused by medications can be attributed to a number of mechanisms. Diuretics cause incontinence by increasing urinary flow. Other drugs cause this problem as a result of overflow stemming from urinary retention. Drugs acting in this manner include anticholinergic agents, used to reduce salivary secretions, and adrenergic agonists, such as ephedrine and theophylline.

Management Considerations

When incontinence is reported, suggest a visit to the restroom before initiating treatment, and be aware of the possible need to have a break during treatment.

Mood Alterations

Several agents have been implicated in causing depression in susceptible patients. Depression is a frequent consequence of treatment with antihypertensive agents, beta-adrenergic antagonists, cardiac glycosides, benzodiazepines, barbiturates, levodopa, indomethacin, phenothiazines, and steroids. Delirium (acute confusional states) in some cases may also be attributed to drug therapy. The primary offending agents include anticholinergic agents, antipsychotic agents, cardiac glycosides, opioids, and sedative-hypnotic agents.

Management Considerations

This side effect may be difficult to identify. Depression can lead to poor oral hygiene and associated periodontal inflammation. Encouragement to set specific goals for oral hygiene practices may help the patient to remember to develop effective oral hygiene practices.

Cardiovascular Dysfunction

Several drugs can have adverse effects on cardiovascular function, including postural hypotension, hypertension, and arrhythmia. Postural hypotension occurs when there is a drop in the blood pressure after the patient arises from a prone position, putting him or her at risk for loss of consciousness. Drugs known to produce postural hypotension include antihypertensive agents, antidepressants, drugs for erectile dysfunction and other psychotropic agents, alcohol, and levodopa. Some drugs can cause an increase in blood pressure, such as oral contraceptives and decongestants. Digoxin, a drug used to treat congestive heart failure and atrial arrhythmias, is associated with *causing* cardiac arrhythmias. It is a strange situation: A drug used therapeutically to reduce arrhythmia in some instances causes the ADE. Macrolide antibiotics also are known to cause cardiac arrhythmias (QT interval prolongation). This cardiac effect is amplified when macrolides are used in combination with drugs that cause CYP3A4 isoenzyme inhibition, such as some calcium channel blockers, azole antifungal agents, and protease inhibitors. The serious consequence of this interaction is a type of ventricular arrhythmia that can result in sudden death.

Management Considerations

Monitor the blood pressure and pulse when any drug is reported on the medical history that has cardiovascular effects. Postural hypotension is prevented by raising the chair back slowly following supine positioning and allowing the patient to sit upright for several minutes before dismissal. The blood pressure should be measured at the end of the appointment in patients at an increased risk for postural hypotension (e.g., the elderly).

Equilibrium Problems

Patients at increased risk for falls include those with impaired vision, impaired mobility and cognition, postural hypotension, and peripheral neuropathy. The administration of certain drugs to an individual predisposed to balance difficulties may contribute to falls. Elderly individuals are commonly affected. Drugs frequently implicated in falls include benzodiazepines, antidepressants, neuroleptics, barbiturates, phenytoin, antiarrhythmic agents, and alcohol.

Management Considerations

It may or may not be apparent when the patient experiences balance difficulty. This ADE can occur at the end of the appointment, so the patient should be monitored and assisted if imbalance is observed as the individual leaves the treatment area.

Xerostomia

Qualitative (mucoid, not watery) and quantitative (reduced secretion) changes in saliva lead to a variety of oral problems, some of which can include reduced lubrication; reduced antibacterial, antiviral, and antifungal activity; loss of mucosal integrity; loss of buffering capacity; reduced lavage and cleansing of oral tissues; interference with normal remineralization of teeth; and altered digestion, taste, and speech. The major classes of drugs causing xerostomia include anticholinergic agents, antidepressants, antihypertensive agents, antipsychotics, diuretics, antihistamines, central nervous system stimulants, systemic bronchodilators, and a small number of cancer chemotherapeutic agents (Color Plates 8 and 9). Long-term salivary gland hypofunction leads to an increased risk for periodontal disease and root surface caries. Altered salivary flow and composition is an important predisposing factor in oral candidiasis. Reduced salivary amylase and IgA levels in saliva are also associated with an increased incidence of oral infections from opportunistic bacterial pathogens.

Management Considerations

When signs of chronic xerostomia are observed, the specific oral manifestation must be addressed. If caries is present, a daily home fluoride recommendation should be made. Antibacterial salivary stimulants, such as xylitol gum or mints, may be helpful. A controlled study of older adults revealed that chewing xylitol gum three to four times per day reduced *Streptococcus mutans* levels significantly.[4] Artificial saliva products are available. Periodontal inflammation is managed with effective plaque control and a 3- to 4-month maintenance schedule. Oral fungal infection is managed with antifungal drug therapy.

Bleeding Diatheses

Antithrombolytic agents, such as aspirin and clopidogrel (Plavix), alter the ability of platelets to stick or clump together and form a clot. This can increase the bleeding time and lead to increased intraoperative bleeding in association with invasive procedures (e.g., curettage, extractions). When clopidogrel and aspirin are taken at the same time, the potential for significant bleeding is increased.

The orally administered anticoagulant warfarin (Coumadin) reduces intravascular clot formation by inhibiting the formation of vitamin-K–dependent clotting factors, primarily Factor VII. The parenterally administered anticoagulant heparin interferes with the formation of Factors II and X. *The most common side effect of both warfarin and heparin is hemorrhage.* Hemorrhages may present clinically as gingival bleeding or submucosal bleeding with hematoma formation.

Cancer chemotherapeutic agents can inhibit formation of platelets secondarily and induce profound thrombocytopenia, a condition where platelets are reduced from normal levels of >130,000 mm^3 to <20,000 mm^3. Hemorrhage from thrombocytopenia can occur anywhere in the mouth and can be spontaneous or precipitated by trauma or existing disease (Color Plates 10 to 14).

Management Considerations

When antiplatelet drugs are reported and increased bleeding develops, digital pressure can induce clot formation. Hemostatic agents can be used as needed (e.g., Gelfoam). When drugs that affect clotting factors are reported (warfarin), the prothrombin time or international normalized ration (INR) blood test should be requested. When these drugs are taken, the INR is checked on a routine basis, and the physician's office should be able to provide the most recent lab test results.

An INR of ≤3.5 is acceptable for periodontal procedures likely to involve increased bleeding. When INR levels are >3.5, periodontal treatment should be delayed until values are within an acceptable range.

When cancer chemotherapy affects platelet levels, a physician consult is indicated and a medical release form is obtained from the physician for treatment recommendations. The physician will check platelet levels and determine when oral health care treatment can be provided.

Bacterial Infections

If a patient complains of diarrhea with lower abdominal cramping and is currently taking, or has taken in the recent past, an antibacterial agent, the clinician must consider the possibility of a bacterial **superinfection**. The most dangerous form of such a bacterial superinfection is pseudomembranous colitis, which is associated with an overgrowth of *Clostridium difficile* in the GI tract.[5] While pseudomembranous colitis may be a complication associated with the administration of any antibacterial agent, clindamycin and the broad spectrum penicillins and cephalosporins are implicated most frequently. Bacterial infections often contribute to morbidity and mortality in association with therapeutic immunosuppression. A wide range of bacteria, including odontopathic, periodontopathic, and transient pathogens of the oral flora, may manifest as ulcerative lesions. The normal signs of infection are not always obvious, but the most commonly reported signs include pain, fever, and the presence of an oral lesion (Color Plate 15).

Management Considerations

Patients with ulcerative colitis are unlikely to come for dental treatment because the condition is painful. When the dentist prescribes antibiotics, information about potential ADEs should be provided and the patient advised to contact the dental office if signs and symptoms develop.

Fungal Infections

Antibacterial chemotherapy and therapeutic immunosuppression, including inhaled corticosteroids, often lead to opportunistic infection with *Candida albicans* and other fungal organisms (Color Plates 16 to 17). Oral candidiasis may appear as white, raised, or cottage-cheese-like growths that can be removed with gauze, leaving a red, sometimes hemorrhagic, mucosal area. *C. albicans* can spread to the esophagus or lungs via swallowing or droplet aspiration, or it can cause systemic infection through the hematologic route. This is most likely to develop in immunocompromised individuals. Eventually, all organ systems can be affected.

Management Considerations

When evidence of fungal infection is found, an antifungal drug (nystatin) usually is prescribed. If dentures or removable appliances are worn, instruct the patient to soak them in nystatin solution or a diluted sodium hypochlorite solution (1 tsp to 1 cup water) for 5 minutes. Appliances should be removed at night during sleep.

Viral Infections

Immunosuppression drug therapy can also exacerbate latent viral activity.

Herpes Simplex Virus Infections

Clinical manifestations of secondary HSV infections in patients undergoing therapeutic immunosuppression may be observed on the lips and intraorally on all tissues. This is unlike most recurrent HSV lesions, which affect only mucosa bound to periosteum. The ulcerations are quite painful. The optimal period of observation for the detection of recurrent HSV infections is during the 7- to 14-day period following the administration of immunosuppressive chemotherapy (Color Plate 18). Primary HSV infections, which are the initial infections from HSV, appear to account for fewer than 2% of infections in these patients.

Varicella-Zoster Virus Infection

Recurrent infection with the varicella-zoster virus (VZV), known as herpes zoster or shingles, is a painful, unilateral vesiculation that may follow the distribution of a branch of the trigeminal nerve (Color Plates 19 and 20). The lesions coalesce into large ulcerations and may linger for weeks before remission occurs.

Epstein-Barr Virus Infection

Infection with EBV has been associated with a wide range of syndromes in solid organ transplant recipients. In the oral cavity, EBV has been causally related to hairy leukoplakia, characteristically found on the lateral borders of the tongue in patients with therapeutic immunosuppression (Color Plate 21).

Management Considerations

When oral viral infections are observed in the patient taking immunosuppressants, management usually includes palliative products, such as the oral rinse described earlier (Miracle Mouthrinse). The dentist or physician may prescribe an antiviral drug, such as valacyclovir.

Gingival Hyperplasia

Gingival hyperplasia (GH) in patients taking the anticonvulsant phenytoin (Dilantin) has long been recognized. The gingival condition can also occur in patients treated with cyclosporine (an immunosuppressive agent) and some calcium channel blocking agents (antihypertensive and antianginal agents). The mechanisms responsible for the development of GH are unknown, but they may be related to a factor in calcium metabolism combined with the inflammatory changes resulting from poor oral hygiene. Gingival enlargement is usually noted within 1 to 2 months after the initiation of therapy and appears to affect primarily the labial/facial interdental papillae. Although the enlarged tissue is often firm and painless, it can be associated with erythematous and edematous chronic inflammation. The patient may report pain, gingival bleeding, and difficulty with mastication as a result of the enlarged, hyperplastic tissue (Color Plates 22 to 24).

Management Considerations

Effective removal of bacterial plaque has been shown to decrease the rate of gingival enlargement, although this does not prevent the condition from occurring. A frequent maintenance schedule is suggested to manage inflammation associated with areas difficult for self-cleansing. When possible, the dentist can consult with the prescribing physician and suggest a medication change to a drug that is less likely to cause gingival hyperplasia.

Neurologic Complications

Oral Pain

Oral pain may be secondary to drug-induced mucositis. During therapeutic immunosuppression, acute exacerbations of chronic periodontal or apical infections can also precipitate pain. Finally, pain or paresthesia may be associated with the administration of certain cytotoxic chemotherapeutic agents (e.g., the plant alkaloids vinblastine and vincristine).

Tardive Dyskinesia

Tardive dyskinesia (TD) is an example of an ADE produced by certain psychotropic (antipsychotic) drugs. It is characterized by uncontrolled, repetitive movements of the lips, tongue, and mouth, which can occur after several months on the drug. It is irreversible and can impair the ability of a patient to wear dental prostheses. It complicates the ability to take dental radiographs and to deliver routine dental care.

Taste Alterations

Many drugs, some of which include angiotensin-converting enzyme (ACE) inhibitors, metronidazole, benzodiazepines, chlorhexidine mouth rinse, gold salts, and lithium, have been implicated in **dysgeusia**, or taste disturbances. The mechanism of action in taste alteration is poorly understood but may be associated with drug effects on trace metals.

Management Considerations

Management relies on the specific cause of the neurologic disturbance. Palliative rinses may be helpful to reduce pain. Taste alteration from chlorhexidine rinse is reduced by advising that meals be eaten before the rinse is used. Tardive dyskinesia can complicate performance of dental hygiene procedures. There is no therapy to stop the oral movements, and stopping the drug may not reduce the ADE.

Inadequate Nutrition

Drug therapy may compromise the nutritive and caloric intake of the patient by inducing nausea and anorexia. Excessive nutrients may be lost to vomiting and diarrhea. Enteritis, malabsorption, and impaired liver function further interfere with the nutritional status of the patient. The cytotoxic effects of chemotherapeutic agents on the oral mucosa also predispose the patient to pain, difficulty in mastication, and swallowing. Altered or reduced taste associated with many drugs further contributes to inadequate intake of food.

Management Considerations

Nutritional deficiency can delay the healing response. Questioning about side effects from drug therapy may provide reliable information on the nutritional status. Oral examination for mucosal or tongue changes related to vitamin deficiencies may provide information.

■ Self-Study Review

24. List and describe the various clinical manifestations of Type-A ADEs.
25. List signs of hepatotoxicity.
26. What is a possible ADE associated with benzocaine and prilocaine that can affect blood components?
27. What is *mucositis*, and how can it lead to systemic infection?
28. What area of the brain induces vomiting?
29. Describe the effects of chronic xerostomia and the dental hygiene implications.
30. Anticoagulant drugs increase the risk for what ADE?
31. Describe the mechanisms by which an infection occurs as a result of an ADE.
32. Describe the various clinical manifestations of ADEs.
33. What is *dysgeusia*?
34. Review dental hygiene management considerations for each Type-A ADE.

Clinical Manifestations of Type-B Reactions

Idiosyncratic Reactions

Clinical manifestations of idiosyncratic responses relate to increased or decreased drug effects. Some of this diversity in rates of response can be attributed to differences in the rates of drug metabolism. For example, the CYP2D6 enzyme converts codeine to morphine. The analgesic, respiratory, psychomotor, and miotic effects of codeine are increased markedly by the CYP2D6 enzyme in people with poor metabolism. Conversely, for people with ultrarapid metabolism, the greater amount of morphine being produced results in exaggerated pharmacologic effects and may lead to life-threatening opioid intoxication. Idiosyncratic reactions are difficult to predict unless the patient has experienced them in the past.

Allergic/Immunologic Reactions

The preferential sites for cellular injury in allergic reactions involve the vascular endothelium, conjunctivae, mucosa of the upper respiratory tract, bronchial mucosa, and epithelial cells of the skin. It is important to know signs of allergy when following up a positive response to allergy on the health history. Sometimes the patient notes an allergy to a drug, but when questioned about signs of the allergy, the patient lists "fainting" or "vomiting." The adverse reaction of fainting often is related to fear of drug administration, such as getting a local anesthetic injection. Vomiting may be a side effect of a drug. The oral health professional must determine if signs described by the patient are related to signs of a true allergy.

Type I Hypersensitivity Reactions

Allergic reactions affecting skin cause *erythematous*, raised areas called a "wheal-and-flare" reaction. Ingestion of an allergenic food element or drug can cause cramping, vomiting, and diarrhea as a result of smooth muscle contraction. If the drug is disseminated to the skin, urticaria (manifested as hives and rash) can occur, and often pruritus (itching) follows (Color Plate 25). Involvement of the nasopharynx and upper airway results in allergic rhinitis. Involvement of the oropharyngeal area can lead to angioedema (Color Plates 26 and 27). Activation of mast cells in the submucosa of the lower airways results in allergic asthma.

Anaphylaxis

Hypotension, a result of vasodilation, may be the first sign of anaphylaxis following exposure to an allergenic substance. It leads to shock, which is followed by bronchoconstriction, asphyxiation, and respiratory collapse. Rapid detection of signs and symptoms with immediate epinephrine administration is necessary to prevent serious complications and death.

Type II (Cytotoxic) Hypersensitivity Reactions

The antibody titer may take 7 to 12 days to rise after exposure to the antigen before a significant fever, urticaria, swelling of the face and feet, lymphadenopathy, and arthralgia occur. These effects may be transient and insignificant, and the patient is usually able to tolerate the reaction without necessity for allergy therapy. A clinical example of this type of allergic reaction is drug-induced hemolytic anemia, which, in addition to the above signs and symptoms, also may cause jaundice in its more severe form.

Type III (Immune-Complex) Hypersensitivity Reactions

Immune complexes attach to host tissue, initiate intense complement activation, and produce either localized (Arthus reaction) or systemic complications (serum sickness). Leukocytes and platelets aggregate to form thrombi, occlude the arterioles, and lead to redness, edema, hemorrhage, and ischemic necrosis of tissues. Deposition of immune complexes can be observed in biopsy specimens, which clinically demonstrate an irregular (lumpy-bumpy) layer of antibody- or complement-coated host tissue (Color Plates 28 and 29).

Type IV (Delayed) Hypersensitivity Reactions

In the sensitized individual, contact with an allergen causes the immunologically committed lymphocytes to react with the drug and release lymphokines, initiating an inflammatory response. Within 24 to 28 hours, the patient develops symptoms such as fever, malaise, erythema, rash, tiny vesicular lesions, and edema in target tissues (Color Plates 30 to 33). With repeated exposure to the antigenic challenge, the response becomes more profound.

Pseudoallergic Reactions

The clinical manifestations of pseudoallergic reactions are similar to those associated with allergic reactions. Angioedema, asthma, and hives can develop with pseudoallergic reactions (Color Plates 34 and 35).

Lichenoid Stomatitis

The clinical appearance of lichenoid stomatitis is indistinguishable from oral lichen planus (LP). Like oral LP, these lichenoid reactions most often affect the buccal mucosa, gingivae, and lateral borders of the tongue, and may be reticular, erythematous, or atrophic (Color Plates 36 to 37). Various drugs—including diuretics (thiazides, furosemide, spironolactone), β_1-adrenergic receptor blocking agents (labetalol, propranolol), ACE-inhibitors (captopril), and COX-1 inhibitors (naproxen)—have been implicated as etiologic agents in the development of lichenoid reactions. It is believed that such agents act as haptens and alter the antigenicity of epithelial self-antigens, resembling an autoimmune response. The diagnosis is confirmed when the condition resolves after the offending drug is discontinued.

Erythema Multiforme and Stevens-Johnson Syndrome

Erythema multiforme (EM) is an acute, frequently recurrent mucocutaneous vesiculobullous erosive disorder. Typically the occurrence is a self-limiting process, and the severity varies from mild (EM minor) to moderate (EM major) to potentially fatal (Stevens-Johnson syndrome [SJS] and toxic epidermal necrolysis [TEN]). The etiology of EM has not been clearly established, although it likely represents a genetically predisposed immunologic host response to antigenic challenge. The majority of cases of EM minor and EM major are related to an infectious agent (typically HSV), whereas most cases of SJS and TEN are related to pharmacologic agents (most frequently sulfonamides, anticonvulsive drugs, and COX-1 inhibitors).

Cutaneous lesions of EM usually begin as erythematous papules that progress to form the more characteristic iris or target lesions (Color Plate 38). Although any oral site can be involved, labile (unattached) mucosal tissues predominate, and hemorrhagic crusting of the lips is highly characteristic and virtually **pathognomonic** (Color Plate 39). In the vast majority of cases, mucosal lesions tend to appear abruptly and manifest as painful vesiculobullous ulcerations and erosions (Color Plate 40). In SJS, the lips and oral mucosa are the most frequently involved, but ocular and genital involvement also may be seen (Color Plates 41 to 43). Ocular involvement manifests as conjunctivitis, periorbital edema, and photophobia (sensitivity of the eyes to light). In this case, the overhead dental light must be directed away from the eyes during treatment. Most mucocutaneous lesions tend to heal completely in 2 to 6 weeks. In severe cases, scarring and permanent visual impairment may ensue. Fatal forms are rare (<1%).

Teratogenic Effects

Drug-related developmental toxicity may produce altered growth (terata), growth retardation, developmental impairments, and/or death of the fetus. Behavioral teratogens disrupt normal behavioral development after prenatal exposure. Fetal abnormalities in the United States occur in 3% to 6% of pregnancies; drugs are considered to be responsible for 1% to 5% of these malformations.

Oncogenic Effects

Malignancies of the Skin and Lips

Skin and lip malignancies are the most frequent ADEs to develop following therapeutic immunosuppression. The reported incidence of lip cancer (squamous cell cancer) in organ transplant patients varies from 7% to 8.1% (versus 0.3% in the general population; Color Plate 44). The average age of patients is 42, and the mean latency from transplantation to malignancy is 5.3 years. Most squamous cell carcinomas (SCCs) are low grade, but a significant percentage behaves aggressively, with lymph node metastasis in 5.8% of the cases, leading directly to the death of 4.9% of all transplant patients (versus 1% to 2% in the general population).

Kaposi Sarcoma

The incidence of KS following therapeutic immunosuppression in organ transplant recipients is 5.6% (compared with 0.02% to 0.07% in the general population). Sixty percent of the patients have KS confined to skin, conjunctiva, or oropharyngeal mucosa. In addition, 24% of patients with visceral KS have no skin involvement, but 3% have oral involvement (Color Plate 45).

Lymphoproliferative Disease, Hodgkin and non-Hodgkin Lymphoma, Leiomyoma, Leiomyosarcoma, and Spindle-Cell Sarcoma

Lymphoproliferative disease (Color Plate 46), Hodgkin and non-Hodgkin lymphoma (Color Plate 47), leiomyoma, leiomyosarcoma, and spindle-cell sarcoma (Color Plate 48) have been associated with therapeutic immunosuppression in solid organ transplant recipients. Lymphoproliferative disease is the most severe and can be life threatening.

■ Self-Study Review

35. List the clinical manifestations of Type-B ADEs.
36. Describe the various clinical appearances of hypersensitivity reactions.
37. Describe clinical signs associated with the four types of hypersensitivity reactions. Which leads to shock? Which includes high fever? Which manifests as diarrhea and vomiting?
38. Which type of ADE includes lichenoid stomatitis?
39. Differentiate between the pathology of erythema multiforme and the ADEs that are similar.
40. Describe pathognomonic signs. What is the management for photophobia?

Table 5-5	A Stepwise Process to the Diagnosis of ADEs
Step 1	Identify the drug(s) taken by the patient.
Step 2	Verify that the onset of signs and symptoms was after the initiation of pharmacologic intervention.
Step 3	Determine the time interval between the initiation of drug therapy and the onset of ADEs.
Step 4	Stop drug therapy and monitor the patient's status.
Step 5	If appropriate, restart drug therapy and monitor for recurrence of ADEs.

PREVENTING ADVERSE DRUG EVENTS

Preventing ADEs is a critical part of clinical practice. Oral health care providers must have an awareness of and access to information related to ADEs. To minimize such events, they must develop a cautious approach to the use of pharmacotherapeutic agents in the management of oral/odontogenic problems and become aware of potential ADEs of drugs used in the delivery of oral care.

Accurate Diagnosis

Diagnosis is the bridge between the study of disease and the treatment of illness. Unfortunately, the establishment of an accurate diagnosis before the initiation of therapy is not always possible. Patients often have vague and multiple somatic symptoms that may be misinterpreted and lead to inappropriate therapeutic interventions. Meticulous documentation of the patient's medical history, questions about recent practices or medications, and an appropriate physical examination are fundamental to establishing the correct diagnosis. Table 5-5 illustrates steps to follow when diagnosing ADEs.

Benefits Versus Risks of Drug Therapy

Practitioners must avoid "symptomatic reflex prescribing." The reflex dental prescriber, referred to as "the agent of brief encounters," is typically concerned with the patient's symptoms and caters to the patient's demands, disregarding the therapeutic balance. Benefits should always outweigh the risks when a drug is prescribed. If clinicians were to follow this basic principle routinely, then the number of unnecessary or inappropriate prescriptions would be reduced, thus minimizing the number of ADEs.

Oral Health Education

The clinician should explain the role of drugs in the treatment of dental disease and provide information regarding potential ADEs. This is a recent recommendation for the dental hygienist when bisphosphonate medications are reported on the medical history.[2] The client should be questioned to ensure compliance in taking the medication. This is especially important when verifying antibiotic prophylaxis compliance. Consideration should be made when impaired intellect, poor vision, or diminished hearing are evident. Simple and clear instructions on how and when to take drugs should be given both by the clinician and the pharmacist, reinforced by clear labeling of containers, and written in the treatment record. Special labels are available for blind or visually impaired patients.

■ Self-Study Review

41. Describe strategies to determine if oral or systemic complications may be the result of an ADE.

CONCLUSION

ADEs evolve through the same physiologic and pathologic pathways as normal diseases, which can make them difficult to distinguish. Prerequisites to considering ADEs in the differential diagnosis of a patient's disease or clinical symptoms include an awareness that an ever-increasing number of patients are taking more and more medications (polypharmacy), recognition that many drugs will remain in the body for weeks after therapy is discontinued, clinical experience, and familiarity with relevant literature about ADEs. It is equally important to recognize that some ADEs occur rarely, and detection, based on clinical experience or reports in the medical literature, is impossible at times. However, timely reporting of ADEs can save lives, reduce morbidity, and decrease the cost of health care.

References

1. Epstein JB. Understanding placebos in dentistry. *J Am Dent Assoc.* 1984;109:71–74.
2. Melo MD, Obeid G. Osteonecrosis of the jaws in patients with a history of receiving bisphosphonate therapy. Strategies for prevention and early recognition. *J Am Dent Assoc.* 2005;136:1675–1681.
3. Pickett F. Bisphosphonate-associated osteonecrosis of the jaw: Literature review and clinical implications. *J Dent Hyg.* 2006; 80(3):1–12.
4. Ly KA, Milgrom P, Roberts MC, et al. Linear response of mutans streptococci to increasing frequency of xylitol chewing gum use: A randomized controlled trial. *BMC Oral Health* [serial online]. 2006;6:6. Available at: http://www.biomedcentral.com/1472-6831/6/6. Accessed 4/29/08.
5. Harder B. Flora horror: Hospitals struggle with a serious new gut microbe. *Sci News.* 2006;169:104–106.

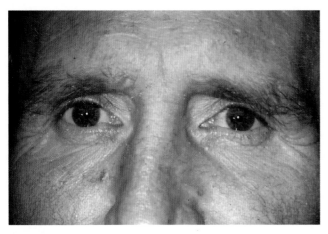

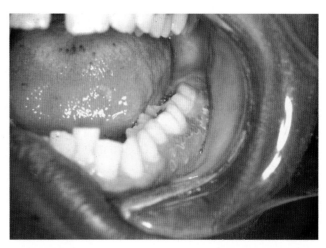

Color Plate 1. Hepatocellular toxicity in a patient with a history of alcohol abuse in association with therapeutic dosages of acetaminophen, manifested as jaundice of the sclera of the eyes.

Color Plate 4. Cytotoxic reaction in response to an overdose of 5% topical lidocaine, manifested as desquamation of the gingival tissues.

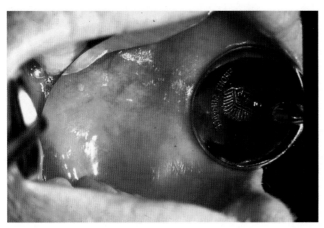

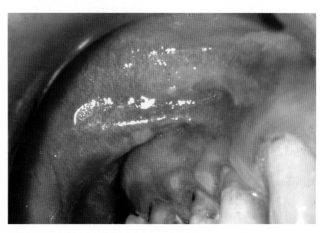

Color Plate 2. Hepatocellular toxicity in a patient with a history of alcohol abuse in association with therapeutic dosages of acetaminophen, manifested as jaundice of the oral soft tissues.

Color Plate 5. Cytotoxic reaction in response to the topical use of acetylsalicylic acid, manifested as erythema and desquamation of the oral soft tissues.

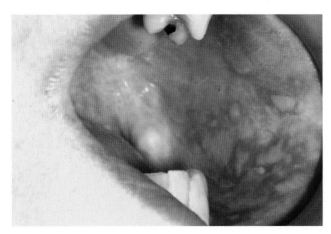

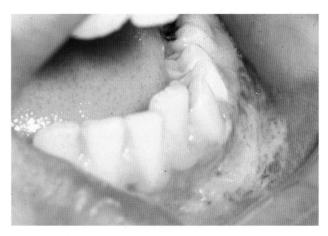

Color Plate 3. Cytotoxic mucositis and xerostomia secondary to a cancer chemotherapeutic regimen that includes methotrexate.

Color Plate 6. Cytotoxic reaction in response to the use of undiluted hydrogen peroxide in the débridement of an oral ulcerative lesion.

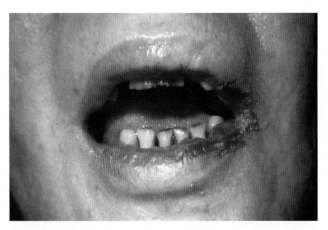

Color Plate 7. Cytotoxic reaction in response to inadvertent overnight contact between the lips and a cotton pellet impregnated with a eugenol-containing over-the-counter topical toothache medication (drops).

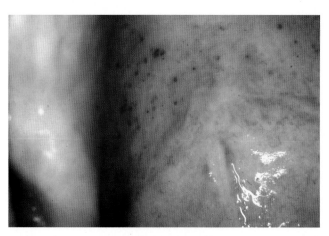

Color Plate 10. Petechial lesions of the oral mucosa in a patient with coronary artery disease being treated with a daily dose (2 mg) of acetylsalicylic acid.

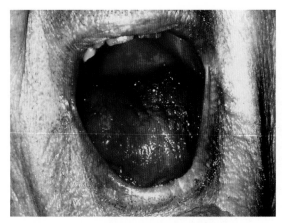

Color Plate 8. Xerostomia and associated candidosis in a patient with congestive heart failure being treated with furosemide.

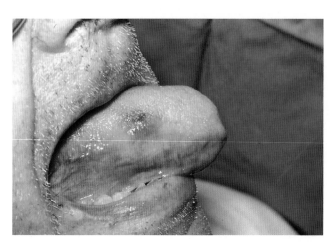

Color Plate 11. Purpuric lesion of the tongue secondary to minor trauma in a patient with an artificial heart valve being treated with warfarin.

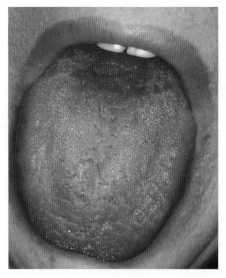

Color Plate 9. Xerostomia in a patient with severe perennial allergies being treated with an antihistamine.

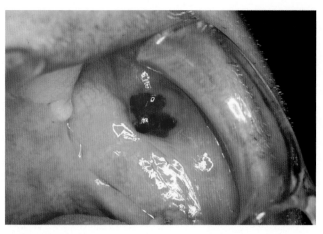

Color Plate 12. Ecchymotic lesion of the buccal mucosa in a patient with acute myocardial infarction being treated with heparin.

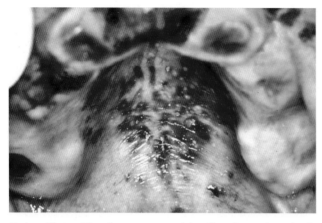

Color Plate 13. Spontaneous bleeding from the gingival tissues of a patient with end-stage renal failure while undergoing hemodialysis with associated heparinization.

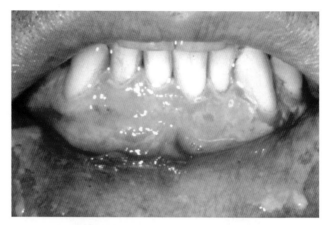

Color Plate 16. Pseudomembranous candidiasis secondary to treatment with a broad-spectrum antibacterial agent.

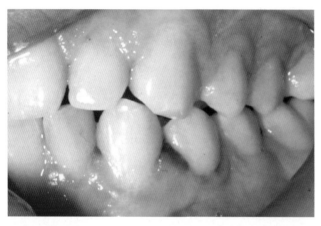

Color Plate 14. Spontaneous gingival bleeding in a patient with profound thrombocytopenia secondary to cancer chemotherapy for leukemia prior to bone marrow transplantation.

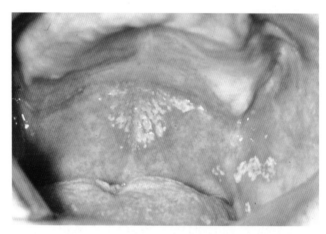

Color Plate 17. Chronic hypertrophic candidiasis in a patient with asthma being treated with inhaled corticosteroids.

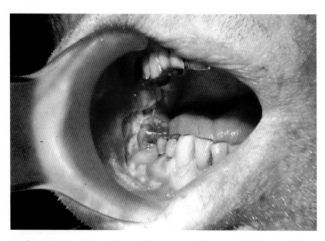

Color Plate 15. Coagulase-negative staphylococcal infection in a patient with leukemia undergoing chemotherapy.

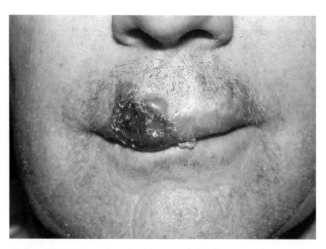

Color Plate 18. Atypical herpes labialis secondary to the reactivation of the latent herpes simplex virus in a patient with leukemia undergoing chemotherapy.

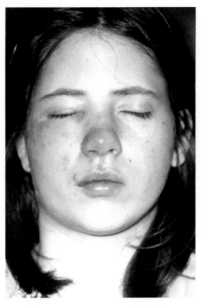

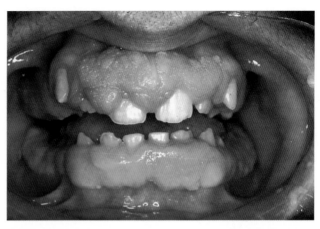

Color Plate 22. Gingival hyperplasia in a patient with a seizure disorder being treated with phenytoin.

Color Plate 19. Herpes zoster infection involving the maxillary and ophthalmic divisions of the trigeminal nerve secondary to the reactivation of the latent varicella zoster virus in a patient with leukemia undergoing chemotherapy.

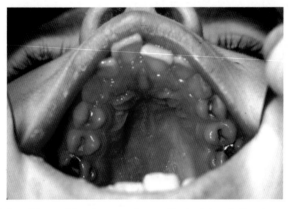

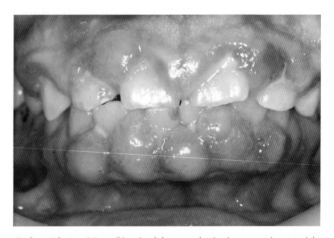

Color Plate 23. Gingival hyperplasia in a patient with hypertension being treated with nifedipine.

Color Plate 20. Intraoral manifestation of the herpes zoster infection.

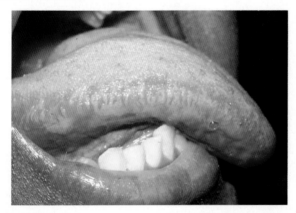

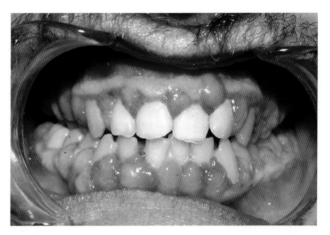

Color Plate 21. Hairy leukoplakia secondary to the reactivation of the latent Epstein-Barr virus in a patient on therapeutic immunosuppression following renal transplantation.

Color Plate 24. Gingival hyperplasia in a patient with a transplanted kidney and renal hypertension being treated with both nifedipine and cyclosporine.

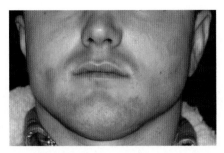

Color Plate 25. Urticaria following the oral administration of cephalexin.

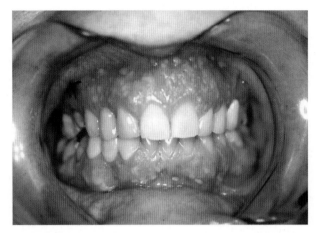

Color Plate 28. Immune-complex hypersensitivity reaction in response to tetracycline therapy for acne.

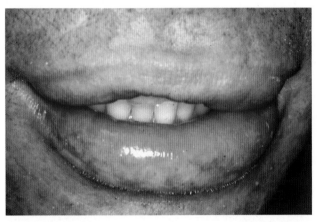

Color Plate 26. Angioedema of the lips following the oral administration of penicillin.

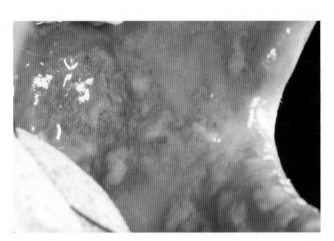

Color Plate 29. Immune-complex hypersensitivity reaction in response to tetracycline therapy for acne.

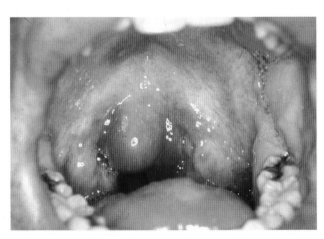

Color Plate 27. Angioedema of the oropharynx following the oral administration of penicillin.

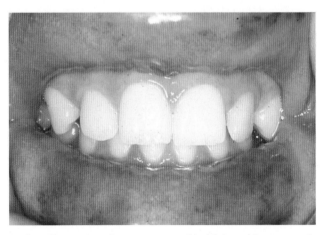

Color Plate 30. Contact mucositis (delayed hypersensitivity reaction) in response to a cinnamon-flavored sugar-free gum.

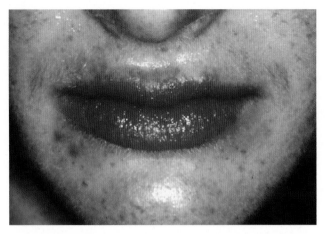

Color Plate 31. Contact mucositis (delayed hypersensitivity reaction) in response to the topical application of bacitracin.

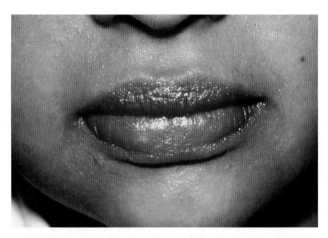

Color Plate 34. Angioedema of the lips in a patient experiencing a pseudoallergic reaction in response to captopril.

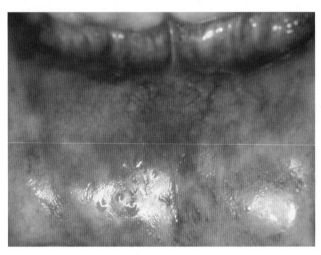

Color Plate 32. Contact mucositis (delayed hypersensitivity reaction) in response to the topical application of bacitracin.

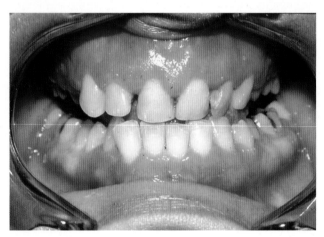

Color Plate 35. Angioedema of the gingiva in a patient experiencing a pseudoallergic reaction in response to captopril.

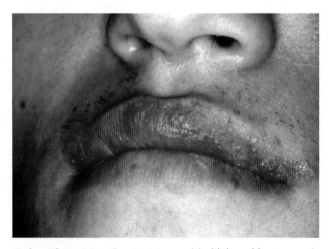

Color Plate 33. Contact mucositis (delayed hypersensitivity reaction) in response to an over-the-counter lip balm containing benzocaine.

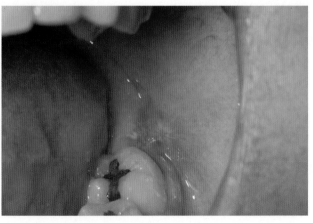

Color Plate 36. Lichenoid stomatitis in a patient with rheumatoid arthritis taking ibuprofen.

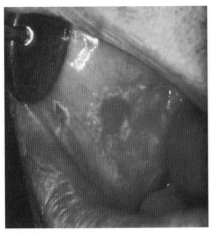

Color Plate 37. Lichenoid stomatitis in a patient with rheumatoid arthritis taking Naprosyn.

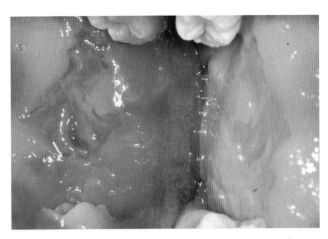

Color Plate 40. Vesiculobullous ulcerations and erosions of the oral mucosa associated with erythema multiforme following the administration of ibuprofen for the treatment of chronic low back pain.

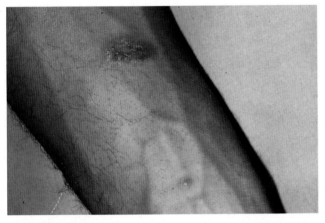

Color Plate 38. Characteristic iris or target lesions of the skin associated with erythema multiforme following the administration of ibuprofen for the treatment of chronic low back pain.

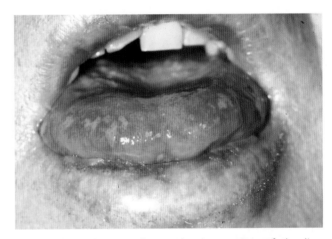

Color Plate 41. Serohemorrhagic crusting of the lips associated with Stevens-Johnson syndrome following the administration of phenytoin for the treatment of a seizure disorder.

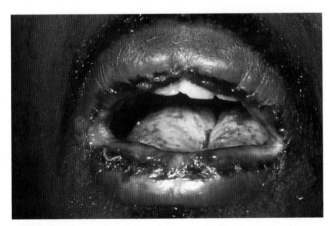

Color Plate 39. Serohemorrhagic crusting of the lips associated with erythema multiforme following the administration of ibuprofen for the treatment of chronic low back pain.

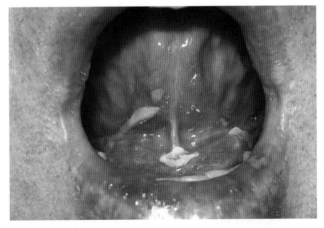

Color Plate 42. Vesiculobullous ulcerations and erosions of the oral mucosa associated with Stevens-Johnson syndrome following the administration of phenytoin for the treatment of a seizure disorder.

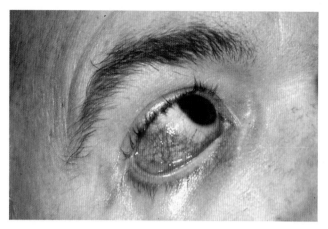

Color Plate 43. Conjunctivitis associated with Stevens-Johnson syndrome following the administration of phenytoin for the treatment of a seizure disorder.

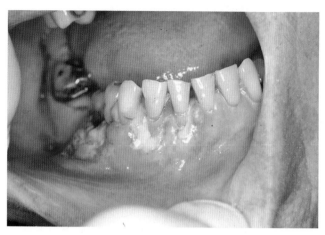

Color Plate 46. Lymphoproliferative disease with gingival infiltration in a patient 3 years after renal transplantation and the initiation of therapeutic immunosuppression.

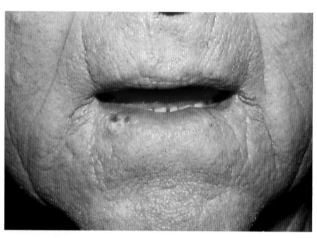

Color Plate 44. Squamous cell carcinoma of the lip, which developed in a patient 2 years after renal transplantation and the initiation of therapeutic immunosuppression.

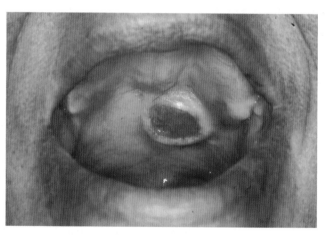

Color Plate 47. Non-Hodgkin lymphoma of the soft palate in a patient 4 years after renal transplantation and the initiation of therapeutic immunosuppression.

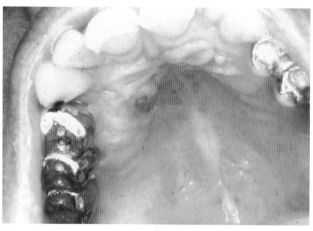

Color Plate 45. Kaposi sarcoma of the palate in a patient 4 years after renal transplantation and the initiation of therapeutic immunosuppression.

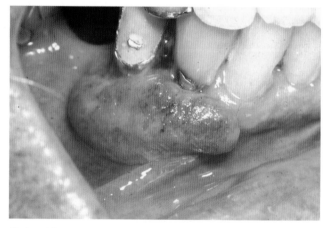

Color Plate 48. Spindle cell sarcoma of the gingiva secondary to the reactivation of Epstein-Barr virus in a patient 4 years after renal transplantation and the initiation of therapeutic immunosuppression.

CLINICAL APPLICATION EXERCISES

☐ **Exercise 1.** Examine the clinical images of various ADEs found in the color insert. Examine the cellular changes described in this chapter for each ADE, and correlate those changes to the clinical changes depicted in the images. This may promote the identification of the ADE when observed clinically.

☐ **Exercise 2.** Read the article on the Web resource material on Bisphosphonate-Associated Osteonecrosis of the Jaw. Review the American Academy of Oral Medicine's

recommendations for the role of the dental hygienist in explaining the possible ADE to the dental client. Prepare an oral health instruction module on this ADE when the client reports taking alendronate (Fosamax) on the health history.

☐ **Exercise 3.** The client reports having an allergy to codeine on the health history. What questions should be asked to verify the presence of a true allergy?

Part 2

Drugs Used in the Provision of Oral Health Care

6

Local Anesthetics: Topical and Injectable

KEY TERMS

Depolarization: A relative reduction in polarity of the nerve membrane, allowing for impulse conduction

Infiltration anesthesia: The injection of a local anesthetic solution directly into or adjacent to the tissue to be treated

Local anesthesia: A reversible loss of sensation in a defined area associated with the transient inhibition of peripheral nerve conduction

Nerve block anesthesia: The injection of a local anesthetic agent into or around peripheral nerve trunks or the nerve plexus

Paresthesia: Numbness or tingling following return of sensation to an area or following injury to a nerve

Prototype: The first drug in a class of drugs to which all other drugs in the same class are compared

KEY ACRONYMS

LA: Local anesthetic

PABA: Para-aminobenzoic acid

Local anesthetics (LAs) are the most commonly used drugs in dentistry. They are not used to treat disease, but are used to manage any pain associated with therapeutic procedures. The management of pain during oral procedures reduces stress and encourages the patient to return for continuing oral health care. In addition, safety is enhanced because pain management reduces the chance that the individual will pull the head away suddenly or close the mouth during intraoral procedures. Although not all states allow dental hygienists to administer LAs, the curriculum is included in all programs of dental hygiene education. Knowledge of the effects and associated risks of the various LA agents is essential in order to use them safely. Understanding the basis for potentially life-threatening systemic reactions when LAs are used, and the specific medical conditions that put individuals at increased risk for adverse reactions, is also important.

HISTORY

For centuries, the natives of the Peruvian and Bolivian Andes have chewed the leaves of the shrub *Erythroxylum coca*. The laborers, who farm land at elevations of 12,000 to 14,000 feet above sea level and carry their harvested crops over the high mountain passes, use the leaves to improve breathing, to make their loads seem lighter, and to relieve aches and pains. Albert Niemann, the German chemist, was intrigued by this increased functional capacity, and in 1860 he successfully isolated cocaine, the alkaloid, from the leaves. He noted that tasting the powder caused a numbness of the tongue and lips and reduced the sense of pain, creating an anesthetic effect. Such was the description given to the world's first LA. As scientists continued to study the effects of cocaine, clinical investigations revealed that when a few drops of 2% cocaine solution were applied to the conjunctival sac, they completely anesthetized the eye area for over an hour. Eye surgeons almost instantly began using the new drug, which is still used in medicine as a topical anesthetic. R. J. Hall, a dental scientist, studied the effects of cocaine as an LA in dentistry. The conservative dental profession, however, did not accept cocaine. There is no doubt that this dental conservatism was beneficial to the patient, because the high dependence liability and toxicity associated with cocaine soon claimed many victims. Clearly, cocaine's mood-altering effects and the development of psychologic and physical dependence in its users negate its use in routine dental practice. In addition, cocaine has inherent sympathomimetic properties—it produces central nervous system (CNS) excitation, profound cardiac stimulation, and vasoconstriction. While other LA agents also produce vasoconstriction (prilocaine, mepivacaine), the intensity of vasoconstriction associated with cocaine is unparalleled.

Procaine

The search for safer alternatives to cocaine resulted in the development of procaine (Novocain). Einhorn reported in 1909 that he had synthesized a diethylaminoethyl ester of para-aminobenzoic acid (PABA), which he named procaine. He described a nondependence-producing product with LA properties. However, procaine's low lipid solubility and inherent vasodilating effects allowed for rapid removal of the drug from the site of administration, resulting in a very short duration of anesthetic effect. In addition, PABA is a known allergen, and the incidence of allergic sensitization with procaine is high. These characteristics reduce procaine's clinical usefulness. Continued research for safer LA agents with longer durations of anesthetic action led to the development of lidocaine, which today is considered to be the **prototype**, or "gold standard," for LA agents.

LOCAL ANESTHETICS

Local anesthesia is defined as a reversible loss of sensation in a defined area of the body associated with the transient inhibition of peripheral nerve conduction. LAs are available in two forms: Topically applied and injectable. Benzocaine is used only as a topical anesthetic. Some agents are used both topically and by injection (lidocaine, tetracaine, prilocaine), while other agents are only available in injectable formulations (mepivacaine, bupivacaine).

General Characteristics of Local Anesthetic Agents

LA agents have many characteristics and general properties in common. To be useful

- the anesthetic effect must occur within a short period of time and last long enough for the procedure to be accomplished;
- the use of an effective LA agent should be followed by complete recovery, without evidence of structural or functional nerve damage;
- LA agents should have moderate lipid solubility, which allows an anesthetic agent to diffuse across lipid membranes of all peripheral nerves (motor, sensory, autonomic), including myelinated nerve fibers.

Consequently, the ideal LA agent should provide profound, reversible local anesthesia with rapid onset; a satisfactory duration of action; and minimal adverse local or systemic effects.

Classification of Agents

Currently available LA agents have three structural domains: An aromatic or thiophene nucleus connected by either an ester or an amide linkage to an aliphatic chain containing a secondary or a tertiary amino group. Because of this, it is agreed that there are two basic types of LA agents: Esters and amides. A few agents do not have this basic chemical structure and are referred to as miscellaneous agents. The length of the aliphatic chain is directly proportional to the potency, duration of action, and toxicity of the LA agent. Those agents connected by an ester (cocaine, procaine, tetracaine, and benzocaine) are referred to as *ester-type* LA agents, and those linked by an amide (lidocaine, mepivacaine, prilocaine, bupivacaine, and articaine [thiophene nucleus]) are called *amide-type* LA agents. The aromatic nucleus of an LA agent provides the lipophilic region, and adding the amino group to the aromatic group alters that lipid solubility by providing the hydrophilic (water-soluble) region on the molecule. This allows the anesthetic agent to remain soluble in interstitial fluid, yet penetrate lipid membranes. Table 6-1 illustrates selected

---

Table 6-1 Classification of Local Anesthetics

	Ester	Amide	Combinations
Water Insoluble	Water Soluble	Water Soluble	Mixed Formulations
benzocaine*	procaine	lidocaine hydrochloride	benzocaine, tetracaine, butamben (Cetacaine)*
	tetracaine†	mepivacaine	prilocaine, lidocaine (Oraqix)*
	butacaine	prilocaine	
	cocaine*	bupivacaine	
	butamben*	articaine	

*only used topically
†used topically in dentistry, injection used for spinal anesthesia

LA products in the ester and amide classifications and identifies examples of currently available topical and injectable LAs.

PHARMACODYNAMIC CONSIDERATIONS

Site of Action

LAs act on peripheral nerves by inhibiting the conduction of action potentials initiated by pain-producing stimuli (mechanical, thermal, and chemical) from being transmitted to the brain. These stimuli may be associated with intraoral procedures. The LA agent is placed very close to the nerve by injection or placed by topical application on mucous membranes of the oral cavity. The drug must travel through tissues to reach the nerve and block the nerve impulse carrying the pain message at the local tissue site. It is interesting to note that LA agents do not readily penetrate heavily myelinated nerve fibers and appear to enter into the axoplasm at the nodes of Ranvier. However, LA agents diffuse readily across small *nonmyelinated* fibers. Once in the axoplasm, the sites of action of LA agents are the sodium channels on the axoplasmic side of the membrane. Resting peripheral nerve fibers (A-delta and C fibers) are electronegative on the inside and electropositive on the outside. Painful impulses, which are propagated along the fibers like electrical waves, produce a transient reversal of this polarity. The reversal of polarity (also referred to as depolarization) results from an increase in the permeability of the fiber membrane to sodium ions (Fig. 6-1). When the potential difference between the interior and exterior surfaces of the cell membrane reaches a critical level, called the threshold potential or firing level, depolarization reverses the potential so that the nerve interior is positively charged by comparison with the exterior aspect of the cell membrane. At its peak, the intracellular potential reaches about +40 mV. Thereafter, the process of repolarization begins and continues until the intracellular resting potential is restored at about –40 to –60 mV. The membrane behind the traveling impulse is repolarized by the efflux of potassium ions.[1] The ionized form of the LA agent binds to the sodium channels from the inside surface of the neural membrane. This decreases or prevents a large transient increase in permeability to sodium ions essential for the transmission of nerve impulses. Figure 6-2 illustrates this concept in a slightly different way by showing the nerve impulse direction. Consequently, the sequential loss of pain and temperature, proprioception, touch and pressure, and ultimately motor function is typical.

Physiologic Nerve Conduction

In most neurons, the balance between voltage-gated Na^+ and K^+ channels regulates the action potential. The voltage-gated Na^+ channels conduct an inward current (influx of Na^+ ions) that depolarizes the nerve cell at the beginning of the action potential. The voltage-gated K^+ channels conduct an outward current (efflux of K^+ ions) that repolarizes the cell at the end of the action potential. At rest, sodium and potassium ions

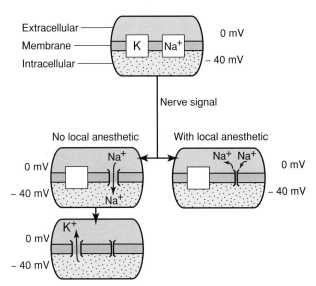

Figure 6-1 Single Nerve Fiber with Impulse Conduction. LAs are believed to block nerve conduction by interfering with the inward movement of Na^+, which is essential for normal transmission. The resting nerve fiber is electronegative on the inside and electropositive on the outside. An action potential generated by a stimulus causes a transient reversal of this polarity by increasing the permeability of the nerve fiber to sodium ions (depolarization). The membrane behind the traveling impulse is repolarized by the influx of potassium ions. LA agents bind to and inactivate the voltage-gated sodium channels, prevent the inward movement of Na^+, and, therefore, prevent depolarization of the nerve fiber.

are distributed on either side of the nerve fiber membrane so that sodium ions are in higher concentrations on the outside and potassium is higher on the inside. This ionic disequilibrium across semipermeable membranes, which is maintained by the Na^+K^+ ATPase (a membrane-bound enzyme), provides the potential energy for impulse conduction. Consequently, resting nerve fibers are electronegative on the inside and electropositive on the outside. The nerve impulse, which is propagated along the fibers like a wave, causes a transient reversal of this polarity. The reversal of polarity, referred to as **depolarization**, results from an increase in the permeability of an area of the nerve fiber membrane (voltage-gated Na^+ channels) to sodium ions (Fig. 6-1). During depolarization, Na^+ ions move into the nerve axoplasm. When the difference in polarity between the interior and exterior surfaces of the cell membrane reaches a critical level, called the threshold potential, depolarization reverses the potential so that the interior of the nerve is electropositive in comparison with the exterior aspect of the cell membrane. At its peak, the intracellular potential reaches about +40 mV. Thereafter, the process of repolarization begins and continues until the intracellular resting potential is restored at about –60 to –80 mV. While the inward Na^+ current dominates the depolarization phase of the action potential, the outward K^+ current dominates the repolarization phase. The membrane behind the traveling impulse is repolarized by the efflux of potassium ions.[1]

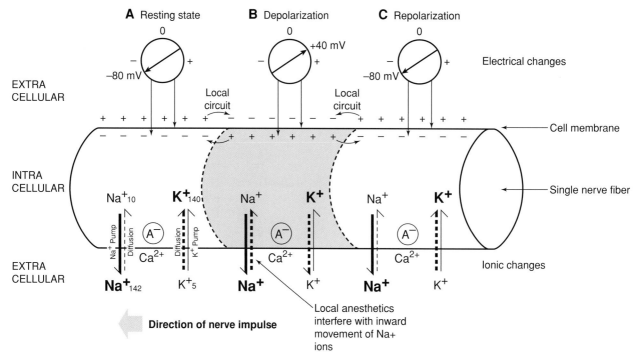

Figure 6-2 Mechanism of Impulse Generation into a Single Nerve Fiber

Mechanism of Action

LA agents prevent impulse transmission (the propagation of action potentials) by blocking individual sodium channels in neuronal membranes (Fig. 6-2). Sodium channels exist in four conformational states: Resting, closed, open, and inactivated. These different conformational states of the target-binding site for LAs (i.e., sodium channels) are a function of the neuronal membrane potential. At resting neuronal membrane potential, the channels are in equilibrium between the resting (most) and the inactivated (some) states. During an action potential, the resting channels move to a closed conformation, and then briefly open to allow Na^+ ions to enter the cell. This sodium influx results in depolarization. Subsequently, the open channels spontaneously close and assume the inactivated conformation. LA agents have high affinities for the closed, open, and inactivated sodium channels, and low affinities for the resting configuration.[1] The binding site for LA agents is near the cytoplasmic opening of the sodium channels. Consequently, an effective LA agent must diffuse through the nerve cell membrane. Once the drug is inside the cell, it rapidly becomes positively charged and binds to the Na^+ channels. This binding of the drug restricts the conformational changes necessary to open the channels. For a drug-bound channel to reopen, the LA must dissociate from the channel and allow the channel to return to its resting state.

Other Mechanisms of Action

In addition to blocking sodium channels, LA agents can have a wide range of other biochemical and physiologic effects. In most cases, these effects are not clinically significant. However, the interaction between an LA and membrane calcium

(Ca^{2+}) ions deserves a short discussion. Historically, it was proposed that the action of an LA is the result of "displacement of calcium ions from the sodium channel receptor sites by competitive antagonism."[2] Current evidence suggests that the interaction between an LA and Ca^{2+} is most likely one of physiologic antagonism. As the concentration of Ca^{2+} ions in the extracellular environment is increased, it appears to relieve (or reduce) the block produced by LA agents.[3] This relief occurs because the increased concentration of Ca^{2+} ions alters neuronal surface potential (the transmembrane electrical field) and, therefore, the threshold at which action potentials are generated. This in turn affects sodium-channel associated depolarization by altering the ratio of sodium receptors between their resting, closed, open, and inactivated configurations. As noted earlier, depolarization is a prerequisite for the conformational change in sodium channels, which favors a drug-receptor interaction and the blockade action potentials by LAs.

■ **Self-Study Review**

1. What was the first injectable LA? First topical agent?
2. List the prototype injectable LA.
3. Describe features of the two forms of LAs and identify examples of drugs in each category.
4. List two main classes of LA agents, identify agents in each class, and state advantages and disadvantages of each.
5. Explain the site of local anesthesia action and the significance of nodes of Ranvier.
6. Explain the mechanism of action of an LA agent.

PHARMACOKINETIC CONSIDERATIONS

The pharmacokinetics of an LA agent is of considerable clinical significance because toxicity depends to a great extent on the balance between the agent's rate of absorption into the systemic circulation and its rate of metabolism and elimination.

Absorption

Topical Agents

Mucous membranes can be anesthetized by the direct (topical) application of aqueous, viscous, gel, cream, or patch formulations (benzocaine, tetracaine, lidocaine, and prilocaine). Because anesthetic agents cross the mucosal membrane by simple diffusion of the nonionized form, lipophilic topical agents are rapidly absorbed locally and, potentially, systemically. When the mucosa is abraded, ulcerated, or desquamated, greater amounts of a topical agent are absorbed more rapidly into the systemic circulation. Consequently, topical application of some LA agents can lead to significant local and systemic toxicity (comparable to that produced by an intravenous (IV) administration of the same drug) as a function of the dose absorbed. Clearly, the greater the concentration of the agent, the greater the surface area to which the agent is applied, and the more rapid the rate of absorption (as may be seen when applied to desquamated mucosal tissues), the more likely that metabolic and excretory pathways will become overwhelmed and toxic accumulation of the drug will occur.

Injectable Agents

Infiltration anesthesia implies the injection of an LA solution directly into or adjacent to the tissue to be treated. In dentistry, there are several modified techniques to conventional infiltration anesthesia (intrapulpal, intraligamental). **Nerve block anesthesia** is associated with the injection of an LA agent into or around peripheral nerve trunks or nerve plexuses. This technique provides anesthesia to a greater anatomical area with a comparatively smaller amount of drug than the other techniques described. The duration of the anesthetic effect is longer with a nerve block than when the same LA is administered by infiltration.

Vasoconstrictors may be added to the LA formulation to constrict blood vessels, thereby reducing local bleeding and delaying diffusion of LA molecules into the circulation. In so doing, vasoconstrictors increase the concentration of the anesthetic around the nerve (an effect that enhances the duration of action of the LA) and decrease the rate of systemic absorption (reducing the risk for systemic toxicity). In summary, vasoconstrictors are added to the LA for the purposes of

- controlling soft tissue bleeding in the local area;
- prolonging duration of the LA;
- delaying systemic absorption of the LA, thereby reducing the risk of toxicity.

Chemical Properties of Agents

The rate of absorption of all LA agents is a function of their inherent chemical characteristics, the vascularity of the absorptive area, and the presence or absence of a vasoconstrictor in the formulation. The vehicle for LA agents is sterile water. Hydrogen chloride is used to adjust the pH. Because LA agents are weak bases, they form water-soluble salts with hydrochloric acid. These solutions are stable at a pH of 4.5 to 6.0. At this pH, LA agents are primarily in their ionized forms. Once an agent is injected, the buffering capacity and pH of the extracellular fluid favors free base formation, allowing for greater tissue penetration of the LA.

Clearly, absorption requires an LA to possess both lipophilic and hydrophilic characteristics. The hydrophilic property serves to keep an LA suspended in water, and the lipophilic property allows an LA to be distributed through tissues (diffuse across biologic barriers) to the nerves and, ultimately, to get through neuronal membranes to interact with sodium channels on the cytoplasmic side of the membrane. Drug molecules with high water solubility do not diffuse through the nerve membrane at all, because their solubility in the lipid bilayer is very low. Such molecules are restricted to the aqueous extracellular environment and never reach the cytoplasmic side of the membrane. Consequently, they are ineffective in blocking peripheral nerves. Molecules with high lipid solubility, on the other hand, easily move into the cell membrane. An ideal LA agent must diffuse across and finally dissociate from the neuronal membrane before it can interact with the LA binding site on the sodium channel.

Factors That Affect Absorption

As mentioned earlier, LA agents are weak bases, formulated in the cartridge as water-soluble salts with hydrochloric acid. This formulation accommodates both water-soluble (charged cation) and lipid-soluble (uncharged base) elements. The proportion of ionic to free base forms varies with the pH of the environment (as in the anesthetic cartridge vs. following injection in tissue) and the pK_a of the drug. The pK_a of the drug is the pH at which a drug is 50% ionized and 50% un-ionized. The pH of LA formulations in the cartridge is between 4.5 and 6.0. The physiologic pH of tissues is 7.4. The pK_a of LA agents varies with the agent and is between 7.6 and 8.9. Consider the example in Figure 6-3 of injecting lidocaine hydrochloride 2% (pK_a 7.9) within oral tissues with a pH of 7.3. Drug molecules disassociate to 106 mg (80%) in the cationic form and 2.7 mg (20%) in the free base form. The water-soluble cationic form of the LA is dispersed in the extracellular environment but cannot penetrate biologic membranes. Only 20% of the agent (nonionized free base) at a tissue pH of 7.3 will be able to penetrate biologic barriers and, ultimately, the nerve sheath to reach the receptor site. As the base leaves the extracellular area, the cationic molecules re-equilibrate, and the newly created lipophilic molecules diffuse through the cell membrane. Once the agent is in the axoplasm (pH 7.0), equilibrium is established between the free base and its cationic form. It is the cationic form that has affinity for the internal receptor sites and blocks the impulse. *So, the cationic form of the LA molecule is actually the more active component of an LA.*

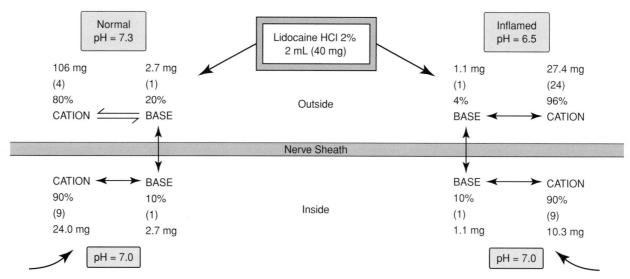

Figure 6-3 Normal Versus Inflamed Tissue pH. The infiltration of LA for normal (left) and for inflamed (right) tissue shows distribution of drug concentrations in both base and cation forms on both sides of the nerve sheath. Note the larger amount of cation form on the inside of the nerve sheath under the normal tissue pH (arrow on left).

Meanwhile, in the area of injection outside the nerve, the LA is absorbed into the circulation and begins to leave the site of administration. As the concentration gradient of the LA in the extracellular tissue is reduced, the intracellular LA molecules diffuse from inside the nerve to the extracellular space and are absorbed into the systemic circulation. The duration of anesthesia depends on the concentration of the cationic form at receptor sites, which in turn depends on the rate of elimination of the LA from the site of action.

Alteration by Apical Infection

In an environment with an acidic pH (e.g., periapical inflammation), the equilibrium shifts to the water-soluble cationic form. Figure 6-3 illustrates a situation of infection or severe inflammation at the apex of the tooth (pH 6.5). The LA effect is reduced by these associated local pH changes because only 4% of the LA is in the base form, resulting in only 10.3 mg in the cationic form versus 24 mg in the normal pH. This can be overcome by using nerve block anesthesia to achieve an anesthetic effect, because the area is sufficiently away from the local pH changes caused by the infection. Another factor to be considered involving infection and inflammation is that inflammation causes dilation of blood vessels, influencing LA molecules to leave the local area more rapidly than the normal situation and reducing the anesthetic effect of the LA. In summary, blockade of nerve conduction is reduced when tissue pH is altered, causing less bioavailability of the base reaching the nerve axoplasm and, consequently, less cation for receptor binding. In addition, dilated blood vessels result in increased removal of LA molecules from the local area.

Distribution, Metabolism, and Excretion

Elimination (redistribution) of an LA agent from its site of action is the consequence of passive diffusion along the concentration gradient and absorption into the systemic circulation. Once in the systemic circulation, LA agents permeate most

tissues (particularly the liver, kidneys, brain, heart, and lungs) and can cross the placenta. The metabolism of ester-type LA agents takes place primarily in the vascular compartment by plasma cholinesterases. The metabolism of amide-type LA agents is more complex. They are metabolized mainly in the liver by CYP450 enzymes and involve oxidation (aromatic hydroxylation, N-dealkylation) and amide hydrolysis. Articaine is metabolized primarily by plasma carboxylesterase and to some extent by hepatic P450 enzymes. The kidney excretes the metabolites of both ester- and amide-type LA agents.

■ Self-Study Review

7. Describe pharmacokinetics of topical LA agents and injectable agents.
8. Identify factors that affect absorption in topical LA application.
9. Describe two techniques for administering injectable LAs and discuss features of each.
10. What are the purposes of adding a vasoconstrictor to an LA?
11. Describe the roles of the base and cation forms of LA agents. Which form promotes access to the site of action? Which form is in the cartridge?
12. Describe factors that affect absorption of an injectable LA.
13. Describe alteration of effects from apical abscess.

PHARMACOTHERAPEUTIC CONSIDERATIONS

For most procedures in dentistry, the use of local anesthesia provides the greatest margin of safety. The major advantage

Table 6-2	Formulations and Other Characteristics of Currently Available Injectable LA Agents				
Drugs and Formulations	pK$_a$	% Free Base at pH 7.4	FDA* Risk Status	mg/mL	Toxic Dose mg/kg (Maximum Recommended Dose)
Procaine (Novocain) 2% plain (medical formulation)	8.9	3	C	20	No longer available for dental use
Lidocaine (Xylocaine, others)					
2% plain	7.9	24	B	20	4.5 (300)
2% with epinephrine 1:50,000	7.9	24	B	20	7.0 (200)
2% with epinephrine 1:100,000	7.9	24	B	20	7.0 (500)
2% with epinephrine 1:200,000	7.9	24	B	20	7.0 (500)
Mepivacaine (Carbocaine, others)					
3% plain	7.6	39	C	30	6.6 (400)
2% with levonordefrin 1:20,000	7.6	39	C	20	6.6 (550)
Articaine (Septocaine)					
4% with epinephrine 1:100,000, 1:200,000	7.8	25	C	40	7.0 (500)
Prilocaine (Citanest)					
4% plain	7.9	24	B	40	8.0 (600)
4% with epinephrine 1:200,000	7.9	24	B	40	8.0 (600)
Bupivacaine (Marcaine)					
0.5% with epinephrine 1:200,000	8.1	17	C	5	2.0 (90)

*Pregnancy risk categories

of LA agents is that they produce loss of sensation in a circumscribed area of the body without loss of consciousness or central control of vital functions. The specific anesthetic agent chosen and the technique used for its administration are important determinants of activity. Injectable LA agents currently available may conveniently be divided into three categories based on their relative duration of anesthetic action: Short, intermediate, and long. Table 6-2 lists available injectable agents. Although it is not currently available for dental injection, procaine is included for comparison. It has a relatively short duration of action. Lidocaine, mepivacaine, articaine, and prilocaine represent agents for dental use that have intermediate duration. Bupivacaine produces anesthesia of long duration. To reduce procedure-related anxiety, local anesthesia may be supplemented with an oral benzodiazepine (antianxiety drug), nitrous oxide sedation by inhalation, or IV sedation.

The Local Anesthetic Cartridge

Each cartridge contains 1.8 mL of an LA formulation. Box 6-1 contains components of the LA cartridge. The vehicle for LA agents is sterile water. Sodium chloride is added to produce

---

BOX 6-1.   Components of an LA Cartridge

- Sterile water
- Sodium chloride
- Hydrogen chloride
- LA agent

---

isotonicity; hydrogen chloride is used to adjust the pH. Because LA agents are weak bases, hydrochloric acid is added to form water-soluble salts. These solutions are stable at a pH of 4.5 to 6.0. Vasoconstrictors (epinephrine, levonordefrin) are included in some formulations to slow the rate of absorption of the LA agent from the site of administration into the systemic circulation, thus increasing the duration of anesthetic action. Metabisulfite, an antioxidizing agent, is included in formulations containing vasoconstrictors to minimize oxidation of the vasoconstrictor. Oxidation causes epinephrine to degrade into a toxic (highly acidic) metabolite, which often causes the clear, aqueous LA solution to turn a brownish color.

All LA cartridges should be examined before use; if the solution is not clear, the cartridge should be discarded. LA agents are supplied in glass cylinders (cartridges) that are sealed at one end with a plunger. The plunger is made of a filler, coloring agent, and paraffin-impregnated rubber compound. The aspirating syringe used to deliver the LA has a barbed projection that engages the plunger so that, when aspirating (or pulling back) on the syringe, the aspiration test draws blood into the cartridge. This alerts the clinician that the needle has been inserted into a blood vessel. A lubricant is added to allow greater ease of plunger movement during aspiration. The opposite end is the diaphragm, a rubber-filler compound sealed with an aluminum cap. Particulate contaminants, or crystal precipitates, in a cartridge should alert the clinician to possible manufacturing problems, extreme temperature changes in transit or storage, oxidation reactions, and loss of sterility. LA agents with epinephrine may also undergo significant reduction in the pH of the solution when exposed to sunlight or to ultraviolet, infrared, or fluorescent light. As the pH of the LA agent decreases, the anesthetic effectiveness of the solution is correspondingly reduced.

Injectable Local Anesthetic Preparations

The following products are used in the primary, secondary, and tertiary lines of treatment (Table 6-2).

Primary Line of Treatment

The following agents are considered agents of first choice for injectable dental analgesia.

Lidocaine Hydrochloride

Lidocaine hydrochloride 2% (Xylocaine, others) with epinephrine 1:100,000 provides for prompt onset and intermediate duration of action. While it has an inherent vasodilating effect, it has a nearly comparable pK_a and a lipid solubility coefficient approximately twice that of mepivacaine, prilocaine, or articaine. This allows for the use of lower concentrations to achieve adequate anesthesia, and makes lidocaine *the LA agent of choice in dentistry*. This is particularly true in the treatment of children and pregnant women, although the lowest dose possible should be considered.

Adverse Effects

Although lidocaine is considered very safe, reversible myotoxicity has been observed following intramuscular (IM) injection. Lidocaine also acts on the heart's electrical conduction system to slow the heart rate, and toxic doses can cause the heart to stop beating. When injected intravascularly, it has a significant antiarrhythmic effect. Lidocaine, like all other LA agents, rapidly crosses the blood–brain barrier. In toxic doses, it initially produces signs of CNS excitation (mild euphoria, tremors, tinnitus, shivers, twitches, and generalized seizures) by selectively blocking inhibitory pathways. As the concentration increases, CNS excitation is followed by depression (inhibition of all neuronal pathways). Death can ultimately result from cardiorespiratory failure.

Mepivacaine Hydrochloride

Mepivacaine hydrochloride (Carbocaine, others) has an onset and duration of action, potency, and toxicity similar to lidocaine. It has a modest inherent vasoconstrictive effect. The advantage this provides is that mepivacaine can be used for short procedures in a 3% concentration without a vasoconstrictor. Levonordefrin, the vasoconstrictor in the 2% formulation, is less likely to cause β_1-adrenergic receptor activation and cardiac stimulation than epinephrine. When injected intravascularly, mepivacaine does not produce a significant antiarrhythmic effect.

Adverse Effects

Mepivacaine is not associated with unique adverse effects.

Prilocaine Hydrochloride

Prilocaine hydrochloride 4% (Citanest) has modest vasoconstrictive activity and will produce a satisfactory duration of anesthesia with or without a vasoconstrictor. It is supplied as a 4% plain or 4% with 1:200,000 solution. Prilocaine plain provides a slightly longer duration (higher concentration of 4% versus 3% mepivacaine) than mepivacaine plain. However, it has been associated with a statistically significant increase in the incidence of **paresthesia** when compared to lidocaine or mepivacaine, and it may produce methemoglobinemia in susceptible patients.

Adverse Effects

Prilocaine is contraindicated in individuals with a history of methemoglobinemia, sickle cell anemia, anemia, or cardiac or respiratory failure associated with hypoxia. High concentrations of prilocaine can increase methemoglobin levels and decrease the oxygen-carrying capacity of red blood cells.[4] Additionally, prilocaine is not a good choice for local anesthesia when concomitant drugs are being taken that can cause increased levels of methemoglobin (acetaminophen). Prilocaine has no apparent advantage over either lidocaine or mepivacaine in routine clinical use.

Articaine Hydrochloride

Articaine hydrochloride 4% (Septocaine) with epinephrine 1:100,000 or 1:200,000 is the newest amide-type LA agent. It is unusual in that it has a thiophene nucleus and it contains an ester group. The presence of the ester group appears to increase the rate of metabolism by plasma choline esterases.

Adverse Effects

Articaine, like prilocaine, is more likely to cause a statistically significant increase in the incidence of paresthesia when compared to lidocaine or mepivacaine, and it may produce methemoglobinemia in susceptible patients. Articaine offers no apparent advantage over either lidocaine or mepivacaine in routine clinical use.

Secondary Line of Treatment

Bupivacaine Hydrochloride

Bupivacaine hydrochloride 0.5% (Marcaine) with epinephrine 1:100,000 is a long-acting LA agent similar in structure to mepivacaine. It has high lipid solubility and, therefore, is the most potent LA currently available. Bupivacaine may be used when more than 90 minutes of anesthesia per appointment are needed, such as in a 2-hour appointment for periodontal débridement. Because it has a longer onset of action, lidocaine is often used prior to the administration of bupivacaine to achieve anesthesia quickly. Bupivacaine will produce prolonged, consistent postoperative analgesia and should be used with caution in the young and the debilitated to minimize the possibility of inadvertent soft-tissue biting and self-mutilation.

Adverse Effects

Bupivacaine blocks cardiac muscle sodium channels and may trigger severe ventricular arrhythmias in susceptible patients. It may also impair psychomotor skills.

Tertiary Line of Treatment

Procaine Hydrochloride

Procaine hydrochloride (Novocain), which is available as a 30-mL medical formulation (1% and 2% without epinephrine), has the shortest duration of action of all available LA agents. It is not available in dental cartridges.

Adverse Effects

While it is associated with a high incidence of allergic reactions, procaine is the LA agent of choice for that rare individual with true hypersensitivity to amide-type but not to ester-type LA agents.

BOX 6-2. Topical LAs for Mucous Membranes

Amides	Peak Effect (min)	Duration (min)
Lidocaine hydrochloride	2 to 5	15 to 45
Esters		
Benzocaine	15 to 30 s	12 to 15
Cocaine	1 to 5	30 to 60
Tetracaine	3 to 8	30 to 60

■ **Self-Study Review**

14. Identify LA agents that have intermediate and long durations of action.
15. Describe the contents of the LA cartridge and the purpose of each component. Which produces the salt form?
16. Discuss what occurs when the metabisulfite is added to an LA formulation.
17. Identify LAs used for primary, secondary, and tertiary lines of treatment. Which is the agent of choice?
18. Identify which vasoconstrictor is used in each formulation.
19. Which LAs are associated with methemoglobinemia?

Topical Anesthetic Agents

The ideal topical anesthetic agent should have a rapid onset of action, duration of action appropriate for the clinical situation, and minimal systemic absorption. Box 6-2 illustrates peak effects and durations of currently available topical agents. Most available topical anesthetic agents produce the intended effect in about 1 to 3 minutes. Benzocaine and lidocaine are the two most widely used topical anesthetic agents. Topical agents are directly applied to oral mucous membranes. The concentration of the LA component in topical formulations is increased to allow for better penetration through the mucosa. When high concentrations of topical lidocaine are applied to nonintact (desquamated) oral mucous membranes, blood levels comparable to those following IV injection are detectable within minutes of application. This is the main reason for limiting the area and amount of drug application. Adding a vasoconstrictor to topical products does not alter the duration of action or affect systemic absorption of a topical LA agent. Table 6-3 lists the concentrations of various topical agents.

Table 6-3 Concentrations of Topical Local Anesthetic Agents

Agents	Formulation	Concentration (%)
Lidocaine		
Xylocaine 10% oral	Spray	10
Xylocaine	Ointment	5
Lidocaine hydrochloride topical, Xylocaine	Solution	4
Lidocaine 2% viscous	Solution	2
Dentipatch	Patch	23/2 cm^2; 46.1/2 cm^2
Benzocaine		
Hurricaine	Gel, liquid, spray, cotton applicator	20
Orabase Gel*	Gel	15
Orajel Mouth Aid*	Liquid, gel	20
Combinations		
Cetacaine	Liquid, spray—benzocaine, tetracaine, butamben	14 / 2 / 2
Oraqix	Gel—prilocaine, lidocaine	2.5 / 2.5
Miscellaneous		
Dyclonine hydrochloride	Solution—dyclonine	0.5

*Over-the-counter product

Benzocaine

Benzocaine (Hurricaine) is a permanently neutral (nonionizable) drug, and it is poorly absorbed through mucosa. Consequently, concentrations in topical formulations are much higher than those in lidocaine (20% vs. 2%, 5%, or 10%). The neutral (nonpolar) drug readily partitions into, diffuses across, and dissociates from the neuronal membrane and is able to block sodium channels and action potentials in submucosal connective tissue; however, the block is weak. Because benzocaine is permanently neutral, it is water insoluble, and its systemic absorption from the site of action is very limited. This feature makes benzocaine *the safest topical anesthetic.* However, in an individual allergic to ester compounds, the risk of a hypersensitive reaction remains (Color Plate 33). The practitioner should be cautious, because tissue sloughing can be related to high concentrations of the topical LA. Benzocaine is the most widely used topical product. Benzocaine 20% is an effective topical anesthetic agent when used before periodontal débridement or the injection of LAs. It has a relatively rapid onset and short duration of action. However, an unusual case of severe methemoglobinemia in a 5-year-old child has been reported in association with the unattended self-use of a benzocaine-containing pain-relief gel for teething.[5] In 2005, the FDA issued a warning for benzocaine products, especially the spray form, because of the high number of methemoglobin reactions reported.

Lidocaine

Lidocaine is available in 2% viscous liquid, 5% ointment and liquid, 10% spray formulations and dental patches. Toxicity related to these agents has largely been attributed to the placement of large doses over a wide area of application resulting in cytotoxic local reactions (Color Plate 4) or excessive systemic absorption. For this reason all topical agents should be placed in small areas of mucosa, but agents with a greater potential for systemic absorption (such as amides) should be used in small amounts and over limited areas. For example, the amount of gels or viscous liquids can be easily controlled, but sprays are difficult to control. The ability of topical anesthetic agents to interfere with the pharyngeal phase of swallowing, causing aspiration, has been documented.

Combination Products

In 2004, the FDA approved a new periodontal anesthetic gel to be used for localized anesthesia prior to periodontal débridement. It contains 2.5% prilocaine and 2.5% lidocaine (Oraqix) and is indicated for adults who require localized anesthesia in the periodontal pocket during scaling. It is marketed as an alternative to injections of local anesthesia. Onset is 20 to 30 seconds, and duration is 14 to 30 minutes. It is supplied within a cartridge with a special applicator device and placed within the sulcus. The manufacturer includes a warning regarding methemoglobinemia with the product, although clinical studies show the product to be safe and effective. A study evaluating efficacy and adverse reactions reported the product did not cause numbness of the tongue, lip, or cheek, and there were no local reactions on oral mucosa.[4]

Another combination product contains three LA agents (benzocaine 14%, tetracaine 2%, and butamben 2%) and is supplied in liquid or spray formulations. Tetracaine is rapidly absorbed when placed on mucous membranes. Because of the risk of toxicity, it should be used in limited areas. The spray form of the combination product containing tetracaine is the most likely to cause toxicity.

■ Self-Study Review

20. List topical agents and their doseforms. Which doseform has the least margin of safety?
21. Which is the safest topical LA? Which is the most widely used?
22. Which topical agents are associated with methemoglobinemia?

ADVERSE DRUG EVENTS

Accurate statistics on the frequency of untoward reactions (morbidity and mortality) to LA agents are not readily available, because few such situations are reported. Estimates range from one death in 1.4 million LA administrations to one death in 45 million. Despite an apparently excellent record of safety with local anesthesia, the clinician must still be aware of potential dangers and must not compromise such precautionary measures as the thorough review of the medical history, the consistent use of an aspiration technique, and the use of minimum effective doses. Most complications associated with the use of LAs are the direct consequences of the pharmacologic properties of the agents, the presence of vasoconstrictors or other additives in the formulations, concomitant interacting drug therapy, client apprehension, and, in rare instances, an allergic phenomenon.

Tachyphylaxis

Tachyphylaxis is a form of rapidly developed tolerance to a drug after the administration of only a few doses of that drug. In dentistry, repeated administration of local anesthesia is the exception rather than the rule; however, if the clinical effectiveness of the local anesthesia dissipates before the completion of a procedure, repeated administration may be unavoidable. In such cases, tachyphylaxis may occur, and it is more likely to develop if nerve function is allowed to return before reinjection. Historically, this was attributed to localized edema, hemorrhage, hypernatremia, and decreased pH of the environment. It was proposed that these factors might restrict the access of the LA to nerve fibers, increase sodium conductance, and reduce free base availability, respectively.[6] However, there appears to be another explanation. Tachyphylaxis is noted primarily when nerve function is allowed to return to normal (i.e., at a time when the nerve assumes the resting state configuration). The concentration of the LA agent in the axoplasm may be in the therapeutic range, but its affinity to the resting state configuration is low. The clinical situation in which the local anesthesia dissipates before the completion of a procedure presents the clinician with two possibilities. It is possible at that late stage of the procedure that: (a) there are fewer action potentials being generated (the time between action potentials is longer than the time required for the LA to dissociate from the sodium channels) and, therefore, only a minority of the receptors are in the closed, open, or inactive configuration; and (b) the concentration of the LA agent in the axoplasm is getting lower. Because drugs interact with receptors as a function of their affinity and concentration, a higher concentration is needed to occupy low affinity receptors.[1]

Toxic Reactions

Toxic reactions are generally a result of the LA agent itself, although additives (preservatives, stabilizers, vasoconstrictors) may also contribute to associated signs and symptoms. Injecting high doses locally, or even therapeutic doses intravascularly, can cause local or systemic toxicity, respectively.

Local Toxicity

Local toxicity in the area of application or injection is primarily due to epithelial, vascular, or neural damage when the recommended dose of an anesthetic agent is exceeded. Table 6-4 includes local toxic reactions of epithelial and nerve tissue. Most of these adverse drug effects are transient, but prolonged anesthesia or paresthesia of the lip or tongue can take 2 to 6 months to resolve. In rare instances, the neurologic deficit may become permanent. Nontoxic local reactions may be due to mechanical nerve injury and hematomas secondary to mechanical vascular damage.

Systemic Toxicity

Systemic toxicity is usually associated with inadvertent intravascular injection, injection into a highly vascular area, altered detoxification of the drug because of drug–drug or drug–disease (e.g., liver disease) interactions, overdose, and injection of an anesthetic without a vasoconstrictor. Systemic toxicity can also result from the application of topical products to large areas of nonkeratinized (especially if desquamated) epithelium. The signs and symptoms of systemic toxicity predominate in the central nervous, respiratory, and cardiovascular systems, and they account for the majority of the adverse reactions (Table 6-5) to LA agents. A practical approach to determine the dosage of LA agents is based on weight. Clinicians should use the minimum dose required to produce profound anesthesia, especially in children, and calculate the maximum recommended dose *before* initiat-

Table 6-4	Clinical Manifestations of Local Toxic Effects
Epithelial Tissue	**Nerve Tissue**
• Tissue edema	• Anesthesia
• Desquamation	• Causalgia
• Necrosis	• Neuritis
• Decreased wound healing	• Paresthesia

Table 6-5	Clinical Manifestations of Systemic Toxic Effects
• Lightheadedness	• Sedation
• Tremors	• Lethargy
• Disorientation	• Coma
• Altered mood	• Dyspnea
• Slurred speech	• Respiratory depression
• Visual and auditory disturbances	• Bradycardia
	• Hypotension
• Clonic seizures	• Cardiac arrest

ing treatment. However, no absolute maximum dose can be unequivocally stated. The general physical condition, emotional state, age, and nutritional status of the patient must also be taken into consideration. As with all drugs, children and elderly individuals are more likely to experience adverse reactions. Another factor involved in variations of individual response is the concept of hyper-responders and hyporesponders, discussed in Chapter 5. Hyper-responders respond even to low doses of LA, but hyporesponders may require higher doses to achieve adequate anesthesia, and the duration of action can be significantly reduced. These accepted practices should be followed:

• be familiar with properties and warnings of the LA agent used
• use an LA agent with a vasoconstrictor
• avoid IV injections by consistently using an aspirating technique
• inject slowly

Methemoglobinemia

Methemoglobinemia is a relatively uncommon toxic reaction to prilocaine, articaine, or benzocaine in susceptible patients. Metabolites of these drugs bind hemoglobin and interfere with its oxygen-carrying capacity. Cyanosis in the absence of cardiopulmonary symptoms, nausea, sedation, seizures, and coma have been reported in severe overdoses. The treatment is a complete transfusion of blood hemoglobin. Both topical and injectable products identified earlier have methemoglobin warnings in product inserts.

Central Nervous System Reactions

All LAs can have serious, dose-related effects on the CNS. LAs rapidly cross the blood–brain barrier. In toxic doses, an LA initially produces signs of CNS excitation (mild euphoria, tremors, tinnitus, shivers, twitches, and generalized seizures) by selectively blocking inhibitory pathways. As the concentration increases, CNS excitation is followed by depression (inhibition of all neuronal pathways). Death can ultimately result from cardiorespiratory failure. CNS toxicity may last longer with lidocaine and, especially, bupivacaine because of their higher lipid solubilities. These LA agents stay attached to their receptors longer than other available LA agents. The management of convulsions from LA overdose includes IM or IV diazepam (Valium).

Cardiovascular Reactions

With its intricate impulse conduction system, the heart is a prime target for an LA. The cardiac effect of an LA is primarily to reduce the conduction velocity of cardiac action potential. General depression of myocardial activity can be expected. For example, lidocaine is used medically as an antiarrhythmic agent because it can prevent ventricular tachycardia and ventricular fibrillation. LA agents can also cause a dose-dependent decrease in cardiac contractility (a negative inotropic effect), which may be related to its ability to alter calcium availability in myocardial cells. Because many adverse effects are extensions of therapeutic effects, myocardial depression can lead to cardiac arrest when high doses of LAs are used.

Sympathetic Nervous System Reactions

LA formulations may contain either of two vasoconstrictors: Epinephrine 1:50,000 (0.02 mg/mL), epinephrine 1:100,000 (0.01 mg/mL), epinephrine 1:200,000 (0.005 mg/mL), or levonordefrin 1:20,000 (0.05 mg/mL), which physiologically is equivalent to epinephrine 1:100,000. Healthy adults can safely receive up to 0.2 mg of epinephrine and 1 mg of levonordefrin per visit. Table 6-6 includes adverse effects of vasoconstrictors. Exacerbation of sympathetic nervous system (SNS) effects can occur due to a variety of situations, including

- the inadvertent intravascular injection of an LA agent containing a vasoconstrictor;
- the use of high concentrations of a vasoconstrictor by injecting too many cartridges;
- the potentiation of the injected vasoconstrictor by endogenous catecholamines;
- concomitant therapy with other sympathomimetic agents (e.g., asthma medications, decongestants).

However, with appropriate monitoring of vital signs before and during LA use, the concomitant use of such drugs presents minimal risk.

Vasoconstrictor Safety

Vasoconstrictors are added to most LAs to reduce blood flow at the area of injection by causing the smooth muscles of blood vessels to contract and slow the rate of removal of the LA. Consequently, vasoconstrictors increase the concentration of anesthetic around the nerve and decrease the concentration that reaches the systemic circulation. These factors enhance the duration of action and depth of anesthesia, reduce

local bleeding, and reduce the potential for systemic toxicity. It is known that the clinical effects of epinephrine 1:100,000 are similar to those produced with epinephrine 1:200,000. Consequently, the routine use of LA agents with epinephrine 1:200,000 may be more appropriate. There is very little justification for using an LA with epinephrine 1:50,000 unless local hemostasis is needed. Occasionally a medical consultation form is returned with an order for "no epinephrine." This may be a reflection of the doses of epinephrine used in medicine (0.5 to 1 mg), which are much higher than those in dental formulations (0.018 mg/cartridge in 1.8 mL of 1:100,000).

There are situations in which vasoconstrictors are contraindicated. For example, vasoconstrictors must be avoided in individuals who have recently used cocaine.[7] Although there is not an absolute contraindication, nonselective beta-blocking drugs (e.g., propranolol, nadolol) can interact with epinephrine. By blocking β_2-vasodilation in blood vessels of skeletal muscles, propranolol causes epinephrine to bind to alpha receptors and cause vasoconstriction, leading to hypertension and reflex bradycardia. In these individuals, vital signs should be monitored before and during treatment. There are also a number of clinical situations in which the use of low concentrations of vasoconstrictors with local anesthesia is imperative; these include patients with blood pressure in excess of 180/110, severe cardiovascular disease (e.g., recent myocardial infarction [more than 7 days but less than 1 month]), unstable angina pectoris, decompensated heart failure, severe valvular disease, symptomatic ventricular arrhythmias in the presence of underlying heart disease, supraventricular arrhythmias with uncontrolled ventricular rate and high-grade atrioventricular (AV) block, and uncontrolled hyperthyroidism.[7,8] In these situations, it is recommended that vasoconstrictors be limited to no more than 0.04 mg (often referred to as the "cardiac dose"), which is in the equivalent of approximately one cartridge of LA with epinephrine 1:50,000, two cartridges of LA with epinephrine 1:100,000 (or levonordefrin 1:20,000), or four cartridges of LA with epinephrine 1:200,000. In the past, some textbook authors have advised against using LAs with vasoconstrictors in certain medical conditions. However, new evidence in two reports provides better direction on the safety of LAs with vasoconstrictors in medical conditions.[9,10]

The first report presents new data to help resolve the issue of safety as it relates to the use of LA agents containing a vasoconstrictor. The investigators started with the premise that exercise capacity is a simple and reliable index to estimate cardiac function in patients with heart disease. They evaluated the cardiovascular effects of infiltration anesthesia (2% lidocaine with epinephrine) compared with those produced by ergometric exercise. The hemodynamic effects of infiltration anesthesia (72 mg of lidocaine and 0.045 mg of epinephrine, which is equivalent to approximately two cartridges of LA with epinephrine 1:100,000) were less than those produced by ergometric stress testing at 25 watts in young patients and at 15 watts in older subjects. In this study, there were no differences in hemodynamic responses (evaluated by echocardiography) between normotensive and hypertensive patients. The workload of ergometric stress testing at these levels is about four metabolic equivalents (METs),[9] which are approximately equivalent to the workload produced

Table 6-6	Clinical Manifestations of Sympathetic Toxic Reactions

Mild Reactions	Severe Reactions
• Restlessness	• Palpitation
• Headache	• Tachycardia
• Tremors	• Chest pain
• Dizziness	• Ventricular fibrillation
• Pallor	• Cardiac arrest

by climbing a flight of stairs, walking 4.8 km/hour, doing light yard work (raking leaves, weeding, or pushing a power mower), painting, or doing light carpentry work. Based on this report, lidocaine 2% with 0.045 mg of epinephrine can be administered safely to patients whose exercise capacity can tolerate the activities noted above with minimal or no adverse symptoms, such as shortness of breath, chest pain, or fatigue. Based on the U.S. formulation of local dental anesthetic agents, 0.045 mg of epinephrine is equivalent to 4.5 mL of a local dental anesthetic agent with epinephrine 1:100,000 (because one cartridge is 1.8 mL, the 4.5 mL above is approximately 2.25 cartridges). This study provides a scientific, rather than an anecdotal, basis to the clinical observation that the patient's ability to tolerate physical and/or emotional stress is a practical determinant for the safe use of LA agents containing a vasoconstrictor.

In another study, investigators recorded the effects of minor oral surgical procedures (tooth extraction, alveoplasty, and soft tissue biopsy) under local anesthesia (lidocaine 2% with epinephrine 1:100,000, or bupivacaine 0.5% with epinephrine 1:200,000) on cardiac rhythm. The epinephrine doses administered ranged from 0.010 to 0.079 mg, or the equivalent of 1 to 7.9 cc (approximately 0.5 to 4.5 cartridges) of an LA agent with epinephrine 1:100,000. The heart rate and rhythm were recorded on 40 patients older than age 60. Twenty of the patients studied were under treatment for such cardiovascular diseases as hypertension, coronary artery disease (angina pectoris and previous myocardial infarction), conduction abnormalities, and heart failure. The remaining 20 patients had no history of cardiovascular disease. Although arrhythmias were detected in 17 patients, they were typically benign in character, and nearly all of the arrhythmias were supraventricular (ventricular arrhythmias are associated with more morbidity and mortality). The incidence of arrhythmia did not increase with age and did not differ between males and females or between patients with or without cardiovascular disease.[10] These findings further support the safety of vasoconstrictors in concentrations found in local dental anesthesia formulations and in dosages used by dental practitioners in some medical conditions.

Allergic Reactions

Allergy to an LA can usually be managed by using a product from a different class. For example, when allergy to an ester-type LA agent exists, an amide can be used. Amides are unique and different from esters in that there is no crossallergenicity within the class. This means if an individual is allergic to lidocaine, one of the other amides could be used. In the past, hypersensitive reactions to LA agents were accurately attributed to procaine; if the individual was allergic to procaine, all other esters were unacceptable for use due to crossallergenicity within the class. The antigenicity of procaine and other ester compounds lies in their structural formula. The breakdown of the ester-type anesthetic agents proceeds via hydrolysis, which is catalyzed by plasma cholinesterase. PABA, one of the breakdown products, is a highly antigenic compound. It is capable of eliciting the formation of antibodies or sensitized lymphocytes. True allergy to amide-type anesthetic agents is rare. In the past, many amide-type LA solutions contained methylparaben,

a germicide with bacteriostatic and fungistatic properties. Methylparaben is structurally similar to PABA, suggesting the mechanism for hypersensitivity. Sulfites, widely used as food preservatives, are used in LA solutions containing vasoconstrictors to reduce their oxidation to toxic metabolites, not as preservatives. Angioedema and urticaria have been reported following the administration of LA agents containing metabisulfite, but there appears to be no crossallergenicity with sulfonamide antibacterial agents. Individuals with asthma have a predisposition to sulfite allergy and may be unable to receive LAs with a vasoconstrictor. In summary

- methylparaben was formerly used as a preservative in LA cartridges, but it was removed due to its high degree of allergenicity;
- LAs with vasoconstrictors all include bisulfite to serve as an antioxidant;
- bisulfite crossallergenicity to other sulfa drugs is uncommon;
- bisulfite allergenicity is uncommon, except in asthmatics.

Psychomotor Reactions

Psychomotor reactions, such as vasopressor syncope and hyperventilation (Table 6-7), are nonpharmacologic, patient-elicited emotional responses likely to occur in the oral health care setting in response to the sudden emotional stress brought on by pain, surgical manipulation, the sight of blood, or needles. Psychomotor reactions are seen most commonly in young adults.

Local Anesthetic Agents, Epinephrine, and Pregnancy

There is no firm evidence that any LA agent is teratogenic in humans; however, drugs in general should be prescribed with caution for pregnant women. To assist practitioners in prescribing drugs for the pregnant patient, the Food and Drug Administration (FDA) has established a pregnancy code for categorizing drugs according to their potential to cause fetal injury (see "FDA Risk Status" in Table 6-2). Issues related to drug use during pregnancy are discussed in Chapter 21.

Lidocaine

Because of its FDA pregnancy category rating of B (animal studies show no risk, but no human studies are available) and

Table 6-7	Clinical Manifestations of Vasopressor (Psychogenic) Reactions
Adrenergic Component	**Cholinergic Component**
• Pallor	• Perspiration
• Tachycardia	• Salivation
• Hyperventilation	• Nausea
• Papillary dilatation	• Bradycardia
• Clonic activity	• Hypotension
	• Syncope

Table 6-8	Clinical Considerations for Vasoconstrictor Safety
Condition	**Management Strategy**
Use of cocaine (known, suspected)	Do not use LA with vasoconstrictor Emergency care only
Use of nonselective beta-blocker or tricyclic antidepressant	Use low doses of vasoconstrictor (concentration 1:200,000) based on the patient's functional capacity Monitor vital signs before and during treatment
Blood pressure >180/110	Use low doses of vasoconstrictor (concentration 1:200,000) based on the patient's functional capacity Monitor vital signs before and during treatment
Severe cardiovascular disease (unstable angina, decompensated heart failure, severe valvular disease, some arrhythmias, AV block) or recent myocardial infarction (<1 mo)	Use low doses of vasoconstrictor (concentration 1:200,000) based on the patient's functional capacity Monitor vital signs before and during treatment
Uncontrolled hyperthyroidism	Do not use LA with vasoconstrictor Emergency care only Monitor vital signs before and during treatment

low concentration, lidocaine 2% with epinephrine 1:100,000 is the drug of choice in the treatment of pregnant women. Whereas epinephrine can adversely affect uterine blood flow in higher doses, studies have not documented adverse fetal effects. The doses of epinephrine in LA agents are unlikely to affect uterine blood flow and, in fact, have a beneficial effect by reducing the systemic absorption of the LA agent while also providing a more profound and longer duration of anesthesia. However, because of the complexity of metabolism and the incomplete development of fetal organs, the anesthetic drug dose should be kept to an absolute minimum to decrease the possibility of fetal toxicity.

■ Self-Study Review

23. Describe the adverse events associated with the use of LAs and how they can be avoided.
24. Which drug reverses seizures from an LA overdose?
25. List the concentrations of vasoconstrictors available, and identify a situation in which each would be selected.
26. List drug/vasoconstrictor interactions.
27. Define the "cardiac dose" of a vasoconstrictor.
28. Identify the medical conditions that pose a risk when using a vasoconstrictor, and describe the management solution.
29. Which LA is indicated for use during pregnancy?
30. Identify how amides and esters are metabolized.

DENTAL HYGIENE APPLICATIONS

The dental hygienist must understand and apply the information in this chapter when providing professional care. When the use of topical LA agents is planned, the area of application

should be limited, and product selection should be based on patient characteristics and health history information. Sprays should be avoided. Consideration of health history information and current drug therapy should guide the selection of injectable LA agents. Doses should be consistent with the maximum safe dose. The practitioner must record any drugs used during dental hygiene care in the written treatment record for medicolegal reasons and so future practitioners will know what medications were given. Clinical considerations related to safe use of vasoconstrictors when LAs are used are listed in Table 6-8. The amount of epinephrine in various doses of LA must be calculated before administration of LA so that the maximum safe dose is not exceeded. The drug, dose administered, method of administration, and amount of vasoconstrictor included in the LA dose must be recorded in the treatment record (Box 6-3). For example, if one cartridge of lidocaine 2% with epinephrine 1:100,000 was administered, the entry would be either "lidocaine 2% with EPI 1:100,000, 1.8 mL, by infiltration (or block)" or "lidocaine 36 mg, EPI 0.018 mg, by infiltration (or block)."

BOX 6-3. Dental Hygiene Applications for Local Anesthesia Use

Topical	Limit the area of application
	Select a safe product, using the health history information
	Avoid using spray formulations
Injectable	Select a safe product, using the health history information
	Use the maximum safe dose of vasoconstrictor
	Record the LA used, vasoconstrictor concentration, number of cartridges used
	Describe the method of administration in the treatment record

CLINICAL APPLICATION EXERCISES

☐ **Exercise 1.** Outline the steps that result in the action of lidocaine when infiltrated apically in normal tissues. Which form actually results in the blockade of nerve conduction? Outline the events that develop when the LA is placed in an abscessed area, and note how this influences the effect of the bioavailable LA concentrations.

☐ **Exercise 2.** Identify the appropriate armamentarium, LA agent, and area of injection for a one quadrant ultrasonic periodontal débridement in the lower right quadrant. The medical history shows no contraindications to

the administration of local anesthesia. Give the rationale for each item selected. Describe the entry in the treatment record when one cartridge of lidocaine 2% with 1:50,000 is administered.

☐ **Exercise 3.** Go to the drug section of a drug store. Find Orajel (look in the baby teething section). What is the active ingredient? What type and class of drug is it? Are there any safety issues? From this information, determine the use for the product.

Calculation of Vasoconstrictor

For the above example, the epinephrine calculation is

$$1:100,000 = \frac{1\,g}{100,000\,mL} \times \frac{1,000\,mg}{1\,g} = \frac{1,000\,mg}{100,000\,mL}$$
$$= \frac{1\,mg}{100\,mL} \times \frac{1,000\,\mu g}{1\,mg} = \frac{1,000\,mg}{100\,mL}$$
$$= \frac{10\,\mu g}{mL} = 0.01\,mg/mL$$

Two cartridges of 1:100,000 vasoconstrictor is within the limits of the cardiac dose, and four cartridges of 1:200,000 vasoconstrictor are within the cardiac dose limit. The information needed to calculate dosages of the LA is found in Table 6-2. Using the table, 0.5% is 5 mg/mL, 2% is 20 mg/mL, 3% is 30 mg/mL, and 4% is 40 mg/mL.

CONCLUSION

LAs are used frequently in the provision of oral health care procedures. The main goal in administration of an LA is to relieve discomfort and provide less stressful treatment. These drugs are relatively safe if general precautions are followed.

References

1. Butterworth JF, Strichatz GR. Molecular mechanisms of local anesthesia: A review. *Anesthesiology.* 1990;72:711–734.
2. Cowan F. *Dental Pharmacology.* 2nd ed. Philadelphia: Lea & Febiger; 1992:110–111.
3. Hille B. Local anesthetics: Hydrophilic and hydrophobic pathways for the drug-receptor reaction. *J Gen Physiol.* 1977;69: 497–515.
4. Friskopp J, Nilsson M, Isaacsson G. The anesthetic onset and duration of a new lidocaine/prilocaine gel intro-pocket anesthetic (Oraqix) for periodontal scaling/root planing. *J Clin Periodontol.* 2001;28:453–458.
5. Balicer RD, Kitai E. Methemoglobinemia caused by topical teething preparation: A case report. *Scientific World Journal* 2004;4:517–520.
6. Malamed S. *Handbook of Local Anesthesia.* 5th ed. St. Louis: Elsevier Science; 2004:24.
7. Yagiela JA. Adverse drug interactions in dental practice: Interactions associated with vasoconstrictors. *J Am Dent Assoc.* 1999;130:701–709.
8. Eagle KA, Berger PB, Calkins H, et al. ACC/AHA guideline update for perioperative cardiovascular evaluation for noncardiac surgery: A report of the American College of Cardiology/ American Heart Association Task Force on Practice Guidelines (Committee to Update the 1996 Guidelines on Perioperative Cardiovascular Evaluation for Noncardiac Surgery). *J Am Coll Cardiol.* 2002;39:542–553.
9. Niwa H, Satoh Y, Matsuura H. Cardiovascular responses to epinephrine-containing local anesthetics for dental use: A comparison of hemodynamic responses to infiltration anesthesia and ergometer-stress testing. *Oral Surg Oral Med Oral Pathol Oral Radiol Endod.* 2000;90:171–181.
10. Campbell JH, Huizinga PJ, Das SK, et al. Incidence and significance of cardiac arrhythmia in geriatric oral surgery patients. *Oral Surg Oral Med Oral Pathol Oral Radiol Endod.* 1996;82:42–46.

7

Topical Agents: Anticaries, Antigingivitis, and Desensitizing Agents

KEY TERMS

Dentinal hyperalgesia (DH): Extreme tooth sensitivity that causes a painful response to stimuli

Hydrodynamic theory: A theory that the movement of fluid within dentin tubules generates impulse transmission in nerves at the odontoblast connection with dentin

Iatrogenic: A result or effect caused inadvertently by a clinician or a clinician's treatment

Substantivity: The ability to produce a prolonged effect, usually through maintaining a bond with receptors

KEY ACRONYMS

APF: Acidulated phosphate fluoride
NaF: Sodium fluoride

SnF: Stannous fluoride

The most common therapeutic products used by dental hygienists are applied directly to oral tissues and include various fluoride products, antiplaque rinses, and agents to reduce dentin hypersensitivity. Some products have multiple uses; for example, stannous fluoride (SnF) is used to prevent caries, to avoid gingivitis, and to reduce dentin hypersensitivity. Some products produce their therapeutic effects by different modalities; for example, some anticaries toothpastes contain both fluoride and xylitol (Tom's of Maine Natural Toothpaste). The dental hygiene student may be faced with a dilemma in deciding which products to use or recommend for various oral conditions (composite restorations, gingivitis, caries, dentin hypersensitivity, and others). Home care recommendations can involve a variety of agents that are available in a variety of different formulations (pastes, gels, foams, etc.), which makes the situation even more confusing. Patients often ask about products for oral problems, including antigingivitis products, various fluoride formulations (pastes, rinses, gels), and agents to reduce dentin hypersensitivity. In recent years, a large number of new products for both professional use and home use have been developed. Those products that have the American Dental Association (ADA) Seal of

Acceptance can be accessed at (http://www.ada.org/ada/seal/adaseal_consumer_shopping.pdf). The dental hygienist must continually keep updated on the efficacy of the active ingredients of these new products, ask dental product representatives for clinical studies that provide a scientific basis for recommending or using the products, and know the risks associated with the use of the products. In addition, concerns regarding the use of nonpharmacologic agents (sealants, dietary modifications) must be considered. For these reasons, this chapter focuses on product information to be used as part of dental hygiene care.

ANTICARIES AGENTS

On a daily basis, the dental hygienist is faced with situations that involve patients at risk for dental caries, and requests for information on products to reduce this risk. Information on the efficacy of various agents in preventing dental caries is widely available. Only pharmacologic information on products used or recommended by the dental hygienist will be included in this chapter because issues of water fluoridation and fluoride supplementation are discussed thoroughly in textbooks for preventive dentistry.

The risk for caries is associated with a variety of issues: Is the child drinking fluoridated water at optimum levels? Is a drug being taken that puts the individual at risk for caries? When a patient undergoing head and neck radiation comes for caries preventive therapy, which products are safe and most efficacious? The prevention of dental caries by adding fluoride to community drinking water supplies is considered to be a highly successful public health strategy. Professionally applied fluoride products have been developed that add additional cariostatic benefits. Formulations include agents to be professionally applied (gels, foams, fluorides with 5,000 ppm [parts per million], fluoride varnishes) and formulations for home use (over-the-counter [OTC] products, products that require prescriptions). *Fluoride varnish* is the newest professionally applied fluoride formulation that has positive anticaries benefits and a high safety profile. The newest consumer product with strong evidence for effective caries prevention is *xylitol*, a naturally occurring sweetener found in several plants with antibacterial and cariostatic properties. However, there are several issues to be considered prior to recommending a xylitol product. Research is currently being completed to determine therapeutic dose levels of xylitol in children and adults, how often xylitol must be introduced in the mouth to have an anticaries effect, and which dose-forms (gums, mints, toothpastes) are the most efficacious. Chlorhexidine has proven to be the most efficacious antigingivitis agent, but early studies also showed an anticaries effect. Clinical investigations using chlorhexidine varnish, usually at a 40% concentration, have shown a cariostatic effect. Chlorhexidine varnish is not available in the U.S. market, so this topic is not included in this discussion of anticaries agents.

Systemic and Topical Fluorides

Prevention of dental caries and treatment to initiate remineralization of enamel is a primary goal of oral health professionals. The process of tooth destruction involves the dissolution of hydroxyapatite crystals of enamel by acids produced by bacterial fermentation, principally *Streptococcus mutans* and the *Lactobacilli* species. Pharmacologic approaches used by dental professionals include prescribing systemic fluorides during tooth development, professionally applying topical fluoride products, and recommending fluoride products to be used at home.

Pharmacotherapeutic Uses of Fluorides

The use of fluoride is the most common strategy to both reduce demineralization and to remineralize areas of decalcification. The use of sodium fluoride (NaF) varnish is regarded as one of the superior professionally applied topical fluoride agents for young children.[1]

Dental Caries

The recommendation for fluoride therapy is based on whether an individual is at low, moderate, or high risk of caries.

Box 7-1 illustrates caries risk criteria. Low-risk individuals should use fluoridated dentifrices, but there is insufficient evidence to suggest that additional benefit is gained from professionally applied fluorides.[2] Those individuals with a moderate to high risk are the target populations for professionally applied fluoride products. Dental professionals have questioned the efficacy of annual professionally applied topical fluoride treatments for adults. According to the newest guidelines, only adults with active caries in the last 3 years and those with conditions that put the individuals at high risk for caries should receive professionally applied fluoride treatments.[2]

BOX 7-1. Caries Risk Criteria

Low Risk: All Age Groups
- No incipient or cavitated primary or secondary carious lesions during the last 3 years, and no factors that may increase caries risk*

Moderate Risk: <6 Years of Age
- No incipient or cavitated primary or secondary carious lesions during the last 3 years, but presence of at least one factor that may increase caries risk
- One or two incipient or cavitated primary or secondary carious lesions during the last 3 years, OR
- No incipient or cavitated primary or secondary carious lesions during the last 3 years, but presence of at least one factor that may increase caries risk*

High Risk: <6 Years of Age
- Any incipient or cavitated primary or secondary carious lesion during the last 3 years, OR presence of multiple factors that may increase caries risk,* OR
- Low socioeconomic status, suboptimal fluoride exposure, xerostomia†

High Risk: >6 Years of Age (Any of the Following)
- Three or more incipient or cavitated primary or secondary carious lesions during the last 3 years
- Presence of multiple factors that may increase risk*
- Suboptimal fluoride exposure, xerostomia†

---

*Factors that increase the risk of developing caries also may include, but are not limited to, high titers of cariogenic bacteria, poor oral hygiene, prolonged nursing (bottle or breast), poor family dental health, developmental or acquired enamel defects, genetic abnormality of teeth, many multisurface restorations, chemotherapy or radiation therapy, eating disorders, drug or alcohol abuse, irregular dental care, cariogenic diet, active orthodontic treatment, presence of exposed root surfaces, restoration overhangs and open margins, and physical or mental disability with inability or unavailability of performing proper oral health care.

†Medication-, radiation-, or disease-induced

(Reprinted with permission from Council on Scientific Affairs, American Dental Association. Professionally applied topical fluoride: Evidence-based clinical recommendations. *J Am Dent Assoc.* 2006;137;1151–1159.)

Pharmacologic approaches to preventing tooth destruction from dental caries are varied. The two most commonly used approaches involve either fluorides, xylitol, or both. Fluorides are used to reduce the dissolution of enamel from mouth acids and to alter the enzymatic action within biofilm so that less acid is produced. Xylitol reduces the numbers of acidogenic bacteria in the mouth by not providing a nutrient source necessary for bacterial multiplication.

Mechanism of Action

Fluoride ions are chemical substances that interact with mineralized tissue, including teeth and bones. Two effects of the fluoride ion result in the prevention of decay. The first is a direct effect on the hydroxyapatite crystal of enamel. It is theorized that systemic fluorides consumed during tooth development interact with hydroxyapatite crystals of enamel, forming the stable compound calcium fluoride. This chemical structure results in mineralized tissues that are less soluble in acids secreted by acidogenic micro-organisms in the mouth. The same action is thought to occur when fluorides are placed topically. The second action of the fluoride ion is on the individual micro-organisms in biofilm. When SnF is topically applied at appropriate concentrations, bacterial enzyme systems are inhibited, thereby altering the pattern of acid production that would result in demineralization of tooth structure. Early theories explained that when teeth were in the pre-eruptive stage, systemically acquired fluoride was a prime factor in caries prevention. Topically applied fluorides change hydroxyapatite to fluorapatite and also promote remineralization of decalcified enamel, which provides effective protection from progressive cavitation. Topical fluoride absorbed by dental biofilm alters the usual pattern of microbial acid production. These events demonstrate that complete plaque removal prior to topical application is not essential for the benefits of fluoride to occur.

Toxicity

Fluoride has both beneficial and detrimental effects, with beneficial effects outweighing the other. As with all drugs, there can be unwanted adverse effects, and the proper doseform and proper use of an agent is often all that differentiates a remedy from a poison. Acute toxicity from a fluoride overdose is a serious medical emergency and must be managed immediately to prevent death. Chronic fluoride toxicity occurs slowly over time, and management is by medical intervention.

Acute Toxicity

Acute toxicity occurs due to a single overdose of fluoride. This has occurred with a child who received a professionally applied fluoride rinsing agent and was supposed to rinse and expectorate, but swallowed the fluoride instead. There have been three reported incidents of fluoride toxicity fatalities, with one occurring in the dental office. One case followed in-office topical therapy, where inappropriate agents (concentrated 4% SnF rinse) and procedures (a 3-year-old child was given the rinse and not monitored for expectoration) were used. Adequate treatment was not provided to

manage the acute toxicity that resulted, and, within 5 minutes, the child developed convulsive seizures followed by cardiac arrest. He died 3 hours later at the hospital. This incident involved a dental hygienist.[3] The other two incidents resulted from children ingesting chewable fluoride tablets because containers did not have childproof caps. In addition, there have been many cases of nausea and vomiting from unintentionally swallowing fluoride after topical applications before patients left the dental facilities. However, when used properly and with attention to safety, preventive therapy using fluorides is a safe procedure. Signs and symptoms of acute fluoride toxicity include nausea, vomiting, diarrhea, intestinal cramping, profuse salivation, black stools, progressive hypotension, and cardiac irregularities (tachycardia, fibrillation). Death is due to respiratory failure and cardiovascular collapse.

Management

Immediate treatment directed toward inducing vomiting and binding fluoride in the GI tract must be initiated to avoid absorption into the system. After calling 911, oral health professionals should do the following:

- Start with inducing emesis and vomiting to get fluoride out of the stomach
- Have the patient drink several glasses of milk to bind fluoride and prevent absorption
- Monitor vital signs and prepare for CPR until emergency medical services arrive

Chronic Toxicity

During the age of tooth mineralization, drinking water with fluoride >2 ppm can lead to fluorosis of tooth enamel.

Dental Fluorosis

Fluorosis of enamel (often called mottled enamel) is the most common sign of chronic fluoride toxicity during tooth development. Hypomineralization of the outer one third of enamel causes a range of color abnormalities from brown to white. Hypoplastic pitting of enamel occurs in some cases. Children drinking water with fluoride at 1 ppm who also ingest additional fluoride supplements can develop dental fluorosis. For this reason, prescribing daily fluoride supplementation must be carefully determined. In 2004, recommendations were changed to reduce the dosage of fluoride supplementation in the United States for patients younger than 3 years old to 0.25 mg/day. Table 7-1 contains current recommendations of the American Academy of Pediatrics, the American Academy of Pediatric Dentistry, and the ADA Council on Access, Prevention and Interprofessional Relations. In Canada, fluoride supplementation is not recommended until the child reaches age 3 years, and only those at high risk for caries or children who do not use fluoridated dentifrices are recommended to receive fluoride supplementation. The Canadian Dental Association does not recommend fluoride supplementation after age 5 years. Dental management of fluorosis is for esthetic reasons and includes bleaching anterior teeth, as well as covering anterior teeth with porcelain restorations.

Table 7-1	Dosage Schedule (mg/day*) for Fluoride Supplements and Water Fluoridation Ion Concentration in Drinking Water (ppm)		
Child Age (y)	**<0.3 ppm***	**0.3 to 0.6 ppm**	**>0.6 ppm**
0.6 to 3	0.25 mg/day	0	0
3 to 6	0.5 mg/day	0.25 mg/day	0
6 to 16	1 mg/day	0.5 mg/day	0

*2.2 mg of NaF provides 1 mg of fluoride ion
**Drinking water concentrations
(Adapted and reprinted with permission from the American Dental Association Council on Scientific Affairs. Intervention: Fluoride supplementation. In: ADA Council on Access, Prevention and Interprofessional Relations. Caries diagnosis and risk assessment. *J Am Dent Assoc.* 1995;126(6 Suppl):19-S. Copyright 1995, American Dental Association.)

■ Self-Study Review

1. Identify substances with scientific evidence for caries reduction. What is the most commonly used substance for an anticaries effect?
2. Describe the mechanism of action for each anticaries agent.
3. Describe changes in hydroxyapatite when fluoride is ingested during tooth development. Compare to changes following topical application of fluoride.
4. Describe the effects of SnF on biofilm.
5. Describe the signs of *acute* fluoride toxicity and the signs of *chronic* fluoride toxicity.
6. Describe management procedures for acute fluoride toxicity.

Fluoride Preparations

Fluoride preparations used by the dental hygienist can be organized into two groups: Professionally applied topical products and patient-applied topical products.

Topical Agents

The anticaries efficacy of topical fluoride agents depends on their fluoride concentrations, the frequency of application, and the duration of application. Table 7-2 lists fluoride concentrations in a variety of topical agents. For agents used in topical fluoride application, the neutral 2% NaF solution contains approximately 9 mg/mL fluoride ion, and the typical acidulated phosphate fluoride (APF) preparation contains approximately 12 mg/mL fluoride ion. It is this concentration that poses a possible danger of poisoning when large amounts of a topical product are swallowed. If excess fluoride is swallowed and not expectorated during administration of currently available topical products, the most likely event is that nausea and vomiting would occur.

Professionally Applied Topical Agents

Currently accepted agents for professional application include NaF products and APF products. The efficacy for caries prevention between the two fluoride products is similar, but the neutral NaF product is recommended when restorations

are present that could be damaged by acids. Topically applied fluoride products must maintain contact with the tooth surface for a certain length of time to allow the chemical changes to develop. This is the basis for the 4-minute application time. The ionic exchange continues for around 30 minutes, so the patient is instructed not to eat or drink for 30 minutes following the treatment. Fluoride interactions in enamel are not permanent because fluoride leaches from enamel over the 5 to 8 weeks following topical application and returns to its preapplication levels. Because fluorides leach over time, daily applications of low concentrations of fluoride in toothpaste and rinses help maintain fluoride levels in tooth structure.

Annual 4-minute in-office applications of any of the topical preparations available (APF or NaF) provide an average of 26% reduction in decay in permanent teeth of children living in nonfluoridated areas.[4] Some agents are marketed to the dental profession on the basis of claims that only a 1-minute application is needed, versus the traditional 4-minute application. These claims have not been supported by properly designed clinical trials that demonstrate a reduction in caries with this shortened application time. The ADA has only given the Seal of Acceptance to products with a 4-minute application period.

Table 7-2	Fluoride Concentrations in Topical Agents
Preparation	**Fluoride Concentration (ppm)**
Mouth rinse	
Daily	0.05% (230 ppm)
Weekly	0.2% (920 ppm)
Quarterly*	2% (5,000 ppm)
Dentifrice	
Child	250 to 500 ppm (pea-size portion)
Adult	1,000 to 1,500 ppm in strip
Gel	
Daily*	5,000 ppm
Solution, foam, gel, varnish*†	
Sodium 2%	9,050 ppm
Sodium varnish 5%	22,600 ppm
APF 1.23%	12,300 ppm

*prescription product
†professionally applied
(Reprinted with permission from Council on Scientific Affairs, American Dental Association. Professionally applied topical fluoride: Evidence-based clinical recommendations. *J Am Dent Assoc.* 2006;137;1151–1159.)

The concentrations of fluoride products vary widely. Table 7-2 illustrates this variability. The majority of fluoride studies show the higher the fluoride concentration in the topical agent, the better the anticaries effect. How can one apply this information to a clinical situation? Clinical studies reveal that agents used at home can supply up to 5,000 ppm, and those agents would be expected to have superior anticaries effects. This is the product to recommend to the patient with rampant decay or who is at increased risk for caries, such as a client who is undergoing head and neck radiation therapy. A compilation of a variety of clinical trials illustrates average efficacy levels of different professionally applied topical fluoride products.[5] The 5% NaF varnish supplies the highest concentration and has the most efficacious caries reduction (38%), followed by 2% NaF (29%), and 1.23% APF (22%).

The need for coronal polishing preceding the application of fluoride has been questioned because trials show that anticaries efficacy is similar regardless of whether pretreatment polishing was completed.[6] The decision to polish the teeth is based on the presence of extrinsic stains and for supragingival biofilm removal.

Sodium Fluoride

Topical NaF is supplied as a viscous gel or foam and is relatively stable in the 2% solution. It has an agreeable taste, is nonirritating to tissues, and does not stain teeth or restorations. All NaF topical agents have a neutral pH of 7.0. The neutral formulation is the agent of choice when porcelain or composite restorations or sealants are present. These dental materials can be etched by the more acidic APF topical agents.

Early studies recommended that NaF be applied once weekly over 4 weeks for a total of four sessions at ages 3, 7, 11, and 13 years. This protocol resulted in a 30% to 40% caries reduction. In current clinical practice, NaF is applied once or twice a year for 4 minutes. A concentrated 2% NaF rinse is available for in-office use. The product is to be swished for 30 seconds and expectorated, and it is applied four times a year. This product is an alternate selection when porcelain restorations or sealants are present and a 3-month maintenance schedule is followed.

Acidulated Phosphate Fluoride 1.23% Topical Agents

It was found that reducing the pH of the NaF solution resulted in a greater uptake of the fluoride ion by enamel. The acid commonly used is orthophosphoric acid (hence, the name of the product) and the active fluoride ion is derived from both NaF and hydrofluoric acid. The pH of the acidulated fluoride product is 3.5. The APF agents are used in manners similar to the NaF products and are applied every 6 to 12 months following an oral prophylaxis. The product is stable, is nonirritating to oral tissues, does not produce discoloration of teeth or restorations, and produces a slightly astringent feeling in the mouth. This product is indicated for the patient who may be taking medications on a chronic basis that contain sugar (for example, some antiepileptic drugs are supplied as syrups for children who cannot tolerate taking tablets); when the patient is taking a drug for more than a few days that contains sugar (for example, nystatin is used for days to weeks to treat candidiasis, and sugar is added to make the drug palatable); or when drugs are taken chronically that cause xerostomia, such as antidepressants and many others. APF is contraindicated when porcelain, composite, or glass ionomer restorations or sealants are present.

Stannous Fluoride Topical Agents

SnF 10% solutions are no longer marketed for topical application due to their disagreeable taste and staining of decalcified areas and margins of restorations. SnF is unstable and must be freshly mixed immediately prior to use. The only SnF product for professional application is a two-part rinse of SnF 1.64% and APF 0.3%. The manufacturer recommends a 60-second rinse with APF as a pretreatment to enhance stannous uptake, followed by a 60-second rinse with SnF. The product is not ADA accepted, and it is not listed in professional publications that discuss topical fluoride products. It is included in this text only because it is one of the few professionally applied stannous formulations available.

Sodium Fluoride Varnish

Fluoride varnishes are widely used all over the world. European research with 5% NaF supplied as a resin varnish has added a significant body of evidence to support the use of fluoride varnishes to prevent caries (approximately 30% reduction). The first commercially available fluoride varnish in the United States was approved by the Food and Drug Administration (FDA) in 1994 (Duraphat).[1] The active ingredient is 5% NaF. It has been widely accepted, and now there are a variety of products available (Cavity Shield, Duraflor, others) that all contain the 5% NaF formulation with the exception of one, which has difluorosaline in a polyurethane varnish (Fluor Protector). The 5% NaF formulation is FDA approved in the United States as a dentin desensitizing agent and as a cavity liner under the medical device category of approval. Although the FDA has not approved fluoride varnish for an anticaries use, many public health agencies are using the product for caries prevention. For example, school nurses in Tennessee have been directed to paint elementary school students' teeth once a year with fluoride varnish to prevent caries. Use of fluoride varnish for caries prevention has been endorsed by the ADA, but a practitioner who uses fluoride varnish as an anticaries agent is using the product "off label" on the basis of professional judgment.[7]

Fluoride varnish is advocated for moderate- and high-risk caries-susceptible children, particularly children younger than 5 years, as well as for children receiving orthodontic treatment. A recent clinical study demonstrated the varnish's efficacy in primary teeth in young children between the ages of 6 and 44 months.[8] The simplicity of application also makes the varnish suitable for special-needs populations, including very young children with autism and those with management problems, such as mental or physical disabilities.[1]

The varnish has several advantages over topically applied fluoride products that require the 4-minute application:

- Oral prophylaxis prior to application is not needed
- The varnish has a longer retention time than topical fluorides
- It is effective when saliva is present, so there is no need to maintain a dry field during application
- It dries quickly after application (within 10 seconds) and is slowly released in saliva, so there is less systemic absorption
- Chairside application time is short, well tolerated, and safe

Application Procedure

Fluoride varnish is applied to the occlusals or smooth surfaces of teeth, and dries leaving a yellow color on the occlusal surface. One product (Vanish) is marketed as a nonstaining formula to avoid this disadvantage. Varnishes are supplied as a one-application formulation that must be stirred to mix its components in the dispensing cup. The varnish is painted onto teeth with a small brush applicator and dries within 10 seconds. The varnish can be applied quickly and sets rapidly, so gagging is not a problem. Food should not be eaten for approximately 2 hours after application. Because toothbrushing can remove fluoride varnish, brushing on the day of application is not recommended. Varnishes are applied two to four times yearly to susceptible tooth surfaces. In high-risk groups, it is generally recommended that 5% NaF varnish be applied at intervals of 3 to 6 months.

Safety Profile

Fluoride varnish is safe. The 0.9% fluorsilane varnish yields a fluoride concentration approximately one half of conventional APF. The fluoride concentration of 5% NaF (Duraphat, Duraflor) varnish is twice that of APF gels, but the amount used per treatment is ten times less. For applications in the primary dentition, 0.1 mL to 0.3 mL is utilized (2.3 mg to 6.8 mg of fluoride ion). The toxic dose of fluoride varnish is reached with ten times the normal dose. The toxic dose of APF gel is reached with about double the normal dose. An additional advantage of fluoride varnish is its slow release over time. An APF gel not removed by evacuation is swallowed as a bolus, but varnishes dry quickly and are slowly swallowed over many hours. Despite the high fluoride concentration in fluoride varnish, no toxic effect on fluoride plasma levels or renal function was found in preschool children and school children treated with fluoride varnish. This is typical considering the varnish's fast setting time, its slow release of the fluoride, and the small amount required for an application. In essence, there are no alternatives for use of a topical fluoride on very young children. Fluoride varnishes offer the safest topical fluoride treatment available for the young child at risk for dental caries. One manufacturer reports edematous swelling and vomiting as rare side effects (Duraphat, package insert). There is one report of dermatitis in a dental assistant's hand, and one report of stomatitis in a patient.[1]

Patient-Applied Fluoride Products

The purpose of applying fluoride to the teeth is to retard, arrest, and reverse the caries process. To be most effective, fluoride should be used daily and in low concentrations. This requires at-home use of products. With the exception of dentifrices, fluoride products (rinses, gels) come with a warning to expectorate after using, as well as a warning against using in children younger than 6 years.

Fluoridated Dentifrice

Today approximately 98% of toothpastes sold have some form of fluoride in the dentifrice. The first fluoride-containing dentifrice to gain ADA approval for its anticaries effect was a 0.4% SnF product. A NaF formulation with 1,100 ppm fluoride that used a silica abrasive was found to be more effective than the earlier SnF preparations. Some dentifrice formulations include sodium monofluorophosphate (NaMFP) 0.76% (Tom's of Maine) because it is stable when combined with silica abrasives and has a long shelf life. SnF 0.454% (Crest Pro-Health) has a higher concentration of fluoride and is used in a dentifrice for its anticaries effect and its antibacterial effect. One product (Colgate Total) has a combination formula of NaF 0.24% and triclosan 0.3%, an antibacterial agent. The addition of triclosan is responsible for the ADA acceptance of this product as an antigingivitis dentifrice. The 0.454% SnF dentifrice also has ADA acceptance as an antigingivitis dentifrice. These dentifrice products would be the most appropriate to recommend when gingivitis is present. There are many fluoride toothpastes with ADA acceptance for the anticaries effect, and most contain NaF at 0.243%, providing 1,100 ppm fluoride.

The frequency of brushing with a fluoride dentifrice is important. Studies show that individuals ages 10 to 15 years who brushed three times daily with a fluoride dentifrice had a 46% reduction in the decayed-missing-filled (DMF) rate, compared to those who brushed once daily and had a 21% reduction. Children should use a pea-size amount of dentifrice to reduce the ingestion of fluoride.

Fluoride Gels

Prescription gels include 1.1% NaF (PreviDent, Oral-B NeutraCare), 0.4% SnF (Omnii Med, Gel-Kam, Oral-B STOP), and a combination of 1.1% NaF in an acidulated phosphate gel (Phos-Flur Gel). These gels are applied for 1 to 2 minutes with a toothbrush, or they can be placed in custom-fitted trays. A 5-minute application of 1.1% NaF gel supplying 5,000 ppm NaF has been tested for high-risk caries individuals (rampant decay). This is about 40% of the concentration used in the dental office. This procedure was used in school children living in a nonfluoridated area, over a 5-day/week application period while attending school. Caries reduction was 75% after 2 years of treatment. In fluoridated communities, children had approximately a 30% caries reduction. This protocol is for individuals with a high risk for caries and *not for young children*, but it can be used for school children and adults. It is often recommended following head and neck radiation therapy. The FDA has accepted a 0.1% SnF rinse, a SnF dentifrice, and a 0.4% SnF gel (1,000 ppm) for at-home use. These have the ADA Seal of Acceptance for caries reduction but, because the fluoride uptake is time dependent, applying a gel with 1,000 ppm for 1 minute does not provide as much fluoride uptake as applying a gel with 5,000 ppm for 5 minutes via a custom-filled tray.

Fluoride Rinses

In the 1960s, Scandinavian researchers found that rinsing at home with a 0.2% NaF rinse for 1 minute every 2 weeks provided more caries reduction than a 10% SnF professionally applied once a year. When compared to four professional treatments of 2% NaF applied every 3 years at ages 3, 7, 11, and 13, it was equally effective. When compared to the daily use of fluoride dentifrices available, it also was equally effective to prevent caries. Later studies showed that using a more diluted solution of 0.05% NaF rinse once per day gave even greater caries protection, approaching 30% less decay. This 0.05% formulation is available OTC (ACT, generic mouthwashes). The recommended dose is 10 mL, which contains 2.3 mg fluoride. It is to be used in individuals over age 6 years, vigorously swished for 1 minute, and expectorated. Parents should supervise children to ensure the product is not swallowed. Rinses of 0.63% SnF and 0.2% NaF are available with a prescription.

Prophylaxis Pastes with Fluoride

Several manufacturers have added fluoride to prophylaxis paste in order to replace the fluoride removed during polishing. These products are not as effective in preventing caries as are more concentrated topically applied products.

■ Self-Study Review

7. What directions should be provided to the patient for topical home-use fluoride preparations?
8. Which product should be used for topical fluoride application when composites or sealants are present?
9. Which professionally applied fluoride is safest for the very young child?
10. What is the rationale for daily, low-concentration fluoride use? For the 4-minute professional application?
11. List concentrations of fluoride agents used for *professional* application and those for *at-home* application.
12. Describe patient instructions following fluoride varnish application.

Xylitol Products

Xylitol is a naturally occurring sugar alcohol found in various plants that looks and tastes like sucrose but is not fermented by cariogenic bacteria. It has been shown to reduce the level of *Streptococcus mutans* in plaque and saliva. Xylitol also inhibits attachment of biofilm to teeth and transmission from mother to child of oral bacteria, both of which may be involved in the cariostatic effect. The *cariostatic effect* is thought to be related to the inability of *S. mutans* to utilize the sugar alcohol and produce acid. Xylitol is a five-carbon sugar alcohol and cannot be digested by bacteria. Xylitol interferes with the metabolism of *S. mutans* when it is transported into the cell, where it may stay bound to the transport protein.[9] The degree of effect is based on the amount of xylitol ingested and the frequency of use. Most studies have included chewing gum as the delivery vehicle. Gum provides a duel benefit in xerostomic individuals: It stimulates saliva and helps reduce dental caries. Studies show that dose levels between 5.8 g and 10.32 g/day will reduce *S. mutans* levels at a statistically significant level from baseline, with the reduction increasing the more xylitol is chewed. A prospective study series has determined that *S. mutans* reduction required therapeutic dose levels of xylitol ranging from 6.88 g to 10.32 g/day, and that xylitol gum at therapeutic levels must be chewed three to four times per day to reduce *S. mutans* levels in plaque and unstimulated saliva.[10,11] Chewing the gum twice daily, even though it contained 10.32 g of xylitol, did not produce statistically significant reductions of *S. mutans*. At 6 months, *S. mutans* levels in plaque were ten times lower than at baseline. Most studies regarding xylitol have used children, but the two studies above included adults ages 18 to 73 years (mean age 34 years), suggesting the beneficial effects apply to all. Xylitol comes in a variety of forms (granulated sweetener, tooth wipe cloths for babies, gum, mints, toothpaste, spray), and it is unclear if any form other than gum will provide cariostatic effects. Most doseforms do not reveal the amount of xylitol they contain, but one can determine approximate levels by looking at the sugar alcohol grams on the label and comparing that to the listed ingredients. When xylitol is listed first in a product's ingredient list, the product has high levels of xylitol. Several gums (Ice Breakers ICE CUBES, Altoids, Beeches, Spry) contain 1.55 g xylitol or more. Using the clinical studies by Milgrom[10] and others, one can conclude that chewing a stick of gum with at least 1.55 g xylitol four to six times per day will reduce *S. mutans* levels and provide a cariostatic effect (or chewing two sticks [providing 3.1 g] three times a day). The goal for the bacterial reduction is to have at least three exposures and to get a minimum of 5.8 g per day. See Table 7-3 for a list of products that contain xylitol.

Chlorhexidine

Chlorhexidine gluconate 0.2% (Peridex) is a bis-biguanide local anti-infective agent used to kill *S. mutans* bacteria and reduce the harmful effects of biofilm. It is not effective against lactobacilli. Early experimental gingivitis studies revealed a cariostatic effect, along with periodontal benefits. In this early study, chlorhexidine prevented the development of decalcified lesions on enamel. As product development continued, chlorhexidine varnishes were created. A 40% chlorhexidine varnish applied to exposed root surfaces following periodontal surgery was as effective in preventing root caries as 5% NaF varnish (Duraphat).[12] The mechanism appears to be related to reduction of *S. mutans* levels. Chlorhexidine mouth rinse can be an effective anticaries agent when used 10 mL/day for a 2-week period every 2 to 3 months.

Miscellaneous Anticaries Products

A recent strategy to assist in the remineralization of enamel involved using amorphous calcium phosphate (ACP) to replenish calcium removed by demineralization from mouth

Table 7-3 Products Containing Xylitol at Known and Clinically Demonstrated Levels of Efficacy to Reduce Caries

USA Availability: General Consumer Outlets

Amount Xylitol = Gum ≥1.55 g per serving	Category	Brand	Product Position	Xylitol first Ingredient	Also Contains	Finished Product Country of Origin	Manufacturer
X	Gum	Ice Breakers ICE CUBES – All Flavors	Consumer	X	Sorbitol	USA	Hersheys
X	Gum	Starbucks–Peppermint	Brand surround	X	Sorbitol	USA	Richardson Brands
X*	Toothpaste	The Natural Dentist Healthy Teeth Toothpaste	Consumer		No SLB	USA	The Natural Dentist

USA Availability: Dental Offices

Amount Xylitol = Gum ≥1.55 g per serving	Category	Brand	Product Position	Xylitol first Ingredient	Also Contains	Country of Origin	Co-packer or Distributor
X	Gum	Epic Gum	Health/Wellness	X		China	Epic Dental
X	Gum	TheraGum	Therapy	X		Finland	Omnii/3M
	Mints	Epic Mints	Therapy	X		USA	Epic Dental
X	Mints	TheraMint	Therapy	X		Finland	Omnii/3M

USA Availability: Online or Health/Organic Markets

Xylitol = ≥1.55 g per serving	Category	Brand	Product Position	Xylitol first Ingredient	Also Contains	Country of Origin	Manufacturer or Co-packer
X	Gum	V6 Dental Gum	Health/Wellness	X		Sweden	Scanlab
X	Gum	Spry Gum	Health/Wellness	X		China	Xlear, Inc
X	Gum	ElimiTaste	Life-Style	X		USA	Inhale Solutions, Inc.
X	Gum	Zapp	Life-Style	X		USA	Inhale Solutions, Inc.
X	Gum	Xylifresh 100 Cinnamon	Health/Wellness	X		Finland	Leaf
X	Gum	Xylichew Gum	Health/Wellness	X		Finland	Naturemart
X*	Toothpaste	The Natural Dentist Toothpaste	Health/Wellness	X		USA	The Natural Dentist
X*	Toothpaste	Xylifresh	Health/Wellness		Sorbitol	Finland	Finnfoods
X*	Toothpaste	XyliWhite	Health/Wellness		Sorbitol	?	Now Foods–various manufacturers
X*	Toothpaste	Squigle AKA Enamelsaver	Therapy		Sorbitol	USA	Squigle, Inc.

USA Availability: Consumer Outlets, Dental Offices or Health/Organic Markets

Contains Xylitol at levels < 1.0g or unknown	Category	Brand	Product Position	Xylitol first SWEETENER	Also Contains	Country of Origin	Manufacturer or Co-packer
X	Gum	Trident "with Xylitol"	Consumer		Sorbitol	USA	Cadbury Schweppes
X	Gum	Eco-DenT Between	Health/Wellness		Stevia	USA	Lotus Products
X = Confections containing efficacious levels of Xylitol confirmed by at least one clinical study							
X* = Dentifrice containing 10% Xylitol (or higher)							

Brand manufacturers change product names and formulations frequently. Consumers are advised that this listing may be incomplete or inaccurate.
Consumers are advised to review product labeling to evaluate xylitol content.

acids. New products claim to have bioavailable calcium at the tooth surface (Prospec MI Paste, Recaldent). Delivery systems include gum, sealants, and prophylaxis paste, with the last two used as in-office treatments. Clinical studies demonstrate efficacy, and further research will help dental professionals determine the use of these materials as anti-caries products.

■ Self-Study Review

13. Describe patient instructions for using xylitol for caries prevention.
14. Describe instructions for using chlorhexidine rinse for caries control.

ANTIGINGIVITIS PRODUCTS

Epidemiologic data from the United States and around the world suggest that mechanical plaque control procedures fail to achieve their potential to control periodontal inflammation in a significant number of people. In the third National Health and Nutrition Examination Survey, gingivitis was present in 63% of the sampled U.S. adult population. In addition, dental hygienists often notice visible stained plaque following patient-demonstrated brushing and flossing. Because of this inability of many individuals to remove supragingival plaque through mechanical procedures alone, the use of antigingivitis agents is frequently recommended by oral health professionals. Ideally, using the specific plaque hypothesis as a guideline, oral chemotherapeutic agents should target pathogens responsible for periodontal inflammation without affecting harmless oral flora. Box 7-2 identifies properties of the ideal antigingivitis agent. Presently, there is no product available that includes all of these features. Effective agents must be used daily and must remain at the site of action for a sufficient time to cause a therapeutic effect. Clinical studies using antigingivitis/antiplaque agents (mouth rinses or dentifrices) as delivery vehicles have sometimes re-

BOX 7-2. Properties of an Ideal Antigingivitis Agent

- Safe (nontoxic, nonirritating, nonallergenic)
- Efficacious with statistically significant and clinically meaningful reductions in gingival inflammation
- Specific for periodontal pathogens
- Substantitive (binds to and slowly releases active ingredient from oral tissues)
- No microbial resistance formation
- Tastes good and is cost affordable

vealed a reduction in plaque scores, but without a parallel reduction in the gingival index (clinical signs of inflammation or bleeding). Reduction of bleeding is evidence of reduced inflammation.

There are a variety of antigingivitis products available for home use. Within the dental office, some antibacterial solutions are used as irrigants within the gingival crevice. Chlorhexidine 0.12% rinse is the most effective antigingivitis rinse and has been shown to have a 62% to 99% efficacy in reducing the development of biofilm and gingivitis. Other efficacious antigingivitis rinse formulations contain cetylpyridinium chloride (CPC) or a combination of phenol-related essential oils (thymol, eucalyptol, menthol with methyl salicylate). There are numerous mouth rinses available OTC that contain essential oils and have received the ADA Seal of Acceptance. Triclosan, an antibacterial agent, has antibacterial effects and is included in one dentifrice (Colgate Total) with fluoride. SnF 0.454% has antigingivitis effects. Chlorhexidine and essential oils rinses and both dentifrices mentioned above have received the ADA Seal of Acceptance for antigingivitis effects. To get ADA acceptance, research must last at least 6 months and have a minimum of 20% reduction of gingivitis when compared to a placebo or control. Dental professionals should only recommend products that demonstrate scientific evidence of efficacy and safety. For this reason, only ADA-accepted antigingivitis products are included in this discussion.

Chlorhexidine

Chlorhexidine is effective against both gram-positive and gram-negative organisms, and it also has antifungal activity. It has been shown to reduce gingivitis and prevent the development of biofilm. This effect is due in part to a property of high **substantivity**, which allows molecules of chlorhexidine to remain attached to pellicle and mucosa for up to 24 hours. It is a safe product that has no development of bacterial resistance. Used as a supragingival rinse, chlorhexidine does not reach the sulcular area. It is supplied with alcohol (Peridex) and without alcohol (0.12% Chlorhexidine Nonalcohol). Both a 0.2% and a 0.12% concentration produced similar reductions in gingivitis when used twice daily at a 15 mL dose. Studies showed beneficial effects at 21 days and up to 6 months. The rinse is not to be used prophylactically, but as an adjunct to therapeutic treatment up to 6 months. When periodontal disease is controlled, chlorhexidine rinse should be discontinued. Patient instructions should include rinsing with 15 mL for 30 seconds, twice a day. The same 0.12% formulation is used for professional irrigation. Chlorhexidine is also included in a locally applied periodontal chip and, when used following periodontal débridement, has been shown to produce a statistically significant reduction in probing depths when compared to periodontal débridement alone. The difference in probe depth reduction between the two groups was approximately 0.5 mm.

Mechanism of Action

The molecule of chlorhexidine has a high positive charge and is attracted to electronegative surfaces, such as microbial cell surfaces and enamel pellicle. Chlorhexidine binds to the microbial cell membrane and increases its permeability, which results in leakage of essential cellular components and cell death.

Undesirable Effects

The most common adverse effects are tooth and mucosal staining, bitter taste, taste alteration, increased calculus formation, and mucosal ulceration. Because of the taste disturbance, patients are instructed to use the rinse *after* eating breakfast and at night prior to going to bed.

Interactions

Sodium laurel sulfate (SLS) acts as a binding agent and is used in the majority of dentifrice formulations. It binds to chlorhexidine molecules and reduces the antimicrobial effect. To improve the efficacy of chlorhexidine, allow 30 minutes to 1 hour between brushing with a dentifrice containing SLS and rinsing with chlorhexidine.[13]

Essential Oils

The second ADA-accepted antigingivitis mouth rinse formulation contains essential oils (thymol, menthol, eucalyptol), plus other nonactive ingredients. This formulation has been shown to reduce both gingivitis and plaque.[14] In a recent study, an essential oil mouth rinse (Listerine) plus brushing was as effective as brushing and flossing in reducing interproximal bleeding.[15] The rinse is to be used twice a day for 30 seconds following brushing and flossing. The essential oil preparation when compared against chlorhexidine produced an equivalent reduction in bleeding after 6 months' use, although chlorhexidine improvements at 3 months were better.[16]

Undesirable Effects

There are fewer negative features of the essential oil product, which include an astringent or burning sensation to mucosa and an unpleasant taste. Newer formulations have flavors added to them and may be more acceptable. The alcohol component serves to extend the product's shelf life, but it is not necessary for the antigingivitis effect. In the past, it was thought that mouth rinses containing alcohol provided a negative drying effect to the mucosa, but a recent study determined that the essential oil mouth rinse with 21.9% alcohol increased salivation after use and had an extremely low potential for irritation in individuals with xerostomia.[17] However, another issue must also be considered when recommending mouthwashes as part of preventive care. Alcohol, particularly in association with tobacco, has been recognized as an important risk factor for oral cancer for almost a half century. Mouthwashes may contain alcohol concentrations up to 26%. However, a review of the epidemiology of oropharyngeal cancer in six studies that made reference to mouthwash use found that there is no support for the hypothesis that use of alcohol-containing mouthwash increases the risk of oral cancer.[18] The authors concluded that it is unlikely that the use of mouthwashes that contain alcohol increases the risk of developing oral cancer.

Triclosan

Triclosan is a natural substance that has an antibacterial effect, has substantivity, and effectively reduces plaque and gingivitis.[19] It has been used in antimicrobial soaps and has been investigated in mouth rinses and dentifrices as an antiplaque agent with anti-inflammatory effects. Triclosan is bacteriostatic and fungistatic, and it has a broad spectrum range of antimicrobial activity. Research has shown the triclosan formulation to be more effective than other fluoridated dentifrices in the reduction of gingivitis. These factors earned triclosan the ADA Seal of Acceptance as an antigingivitis agent. A polyvinyl methyl ether copolymer delivery system is combined with triclosan to produce substantivity lasting several hours. The only product available in the United States is a dentifrice containing 0.3% triclosan, copolymer, and 0.243% NaF (Colgate Total). It has no side effects and is safe to use.

Mechanism of Action

In vitro (test-tube) data indicate that triclosan exerts its bacteriostatic antiplaque effects by inhibiting growth of various gram-negative oral bacteria and gram-positive *S. mutans*, although other oral streptococci are unaffected.[20]

Stannous Fluoride

The newest antigingivitis dentifrice is a 0.454% SnF dentifrice formulation stabilized with sodium hexametaphosphate. SnF is a broad-spectrum antimicrobial agent. This stabilized SnF dentifrice was given both the anticaries and antigingivitis ADA Seal of Acceptance. Poor aesthetics, undesirable tooth staining, and bitter taste had historically limited the use of SnF products. The stabilized formulation maximizes the anticaries and antigingivitis benefits, and greatly reduces staining and taste issues. In addition, hexametaphosphate is added to provide an anticalculus effect.

Mechanism of Action

The mechanism of SnF includes inhibition and reduction of bacterial plaque biomass, virulence, and metabolism. Numerous clinical studies of 6 months or longer suggest that SnF is clinically effective in the prevention and reduction of gingivitis. The dentifrice is stabilized in a low water formulation to prevent hydrolysis and oxidation of the SnF ion. Sodium hexametaphosphate has been incorporated into the formulation to aid in the control of calculus and extrinsic tooth staining via inhibition of pellicle formation and mineralization.

■ Self-Study Review

15. Identify efficacious antigingivitis products and classify them according to efficacy.
16. Describe patient instructions when 0.12% chlorhexidine rinse is prescribed. How does use of most toothpaste influence its use?

17. List the side effects of the chlorhexidine rinse.
18. Discuss the evidence for the risk factors associated with carcinogenicity when rinses contain alcohol.
19. What dentifrice products are indicated when periodontal inflammation is present?

DENTINAL DESENSITIZATION

Agents in this class are unique because they are used only in dentistry; both in-office and at-home products are available. They may act through different mechanisms, but their common purpose is to reduce painful sensations in dentin called **dentinal hyperalgesia** (DH), or extreme sensitivity or reactivity of the tooth to painful stimuli. There are a variety of causes leading to tooth hypersensitivity, some of which include severe attrition and gingival recession resulting from such factors as abrasion, erosion, abfraction, and abnormal tooth development. The age range of those affected is 20 to 40 years, and the sensitive areas are primarily on buccal/labial surfaces, commonly affecting premolars. Sometimes sensitivity develops following therapeutic procedures. The prevalence of DH is between 60% and 98% in individuals who received treatment for periodontitis.[21] The use of bleaching agents to whiten teeth, a very popular treatment, can also lead to tooth sensitivity; when root surfaces are exposed, bleaching poses an increased risk for sensitivity.[22] This section examines various preparations that can be used to manage dentin hypersensitivity. Product discussion is mainly limited to those that have received the ADA Seal of Acceptance for desensitization, with the inclusion of a few unique products developed recently. A recent literature review discusses issues related to dentin hypersensitivity and the efficacy of preparations used to manage dentin hypersensitivity.[23]

Dentinal Hyperalgesia

Gingival recession results in root tissue being exposed to the oral environment. Cementum normally covers dentin on the tooth root. Occasionally, areas of exposed dentin with open tubules are found where cementocytes did not deposit cemental matrix. In approximately 10% of teeth, cementum and enamel do not meet, thus exposing dentin. Cementum is thin at the cementoenamel junction and can be easily removed by abrasive dentifrices or by professional instrumentation, leaving exposed dentin. Root caries, abrasion, erosion, and abfraction lesions can leave areas of dentin exposed. All of these conditions leave the area at risk for DH, but dentin tubules (exposed root surfaces) due to gingival recession are the most significant contributing factor.[22]

Pathophysiology

Microscopic examination reveals that dentin tubules in sensitive teeth are wider and more numerous than in nonsensitive dentin.[22,23] It is widely accepted that dentin hypersensitivity is a result of outward fluid movement within the dentino-

pulpal interface. Two phases lead to sensitivity: (a) gingival recession exposes root surface and (b) stimulation of fluid within predisposed dentin tubules provokes pain.[22,23] This occurs when the smear layer of dentin tubular plugs is removed, opening the outer orifice of the tubule. In fact, it has been shown that few exposed dentin tubules were present in teeth that were *not* responsive to physical stimuli. Acid erosion associated with gastrointestinal reflux disease may be a factor in exposing dentin tubules. Acid erosion associated with plaque is less of a factor in most cases, because most individuals with dentin hypersensitivity practice effective plaque control.[24] The impact of exposed dentin is that nerves at the dentinopulpal interface within the dentin tubule can be stimulated by hydraulic conduction within the tubule to cause pain (Fig. 7-1). Currently, the most accepted theory for the mechanism of pain is the **hydrodynamic theory**, which proposes that outward movement of fluid within the dentin tubule stimulates nerve endings surrounding the odontoblast at the dentinopulpal interface and generates an impulse transmission interpreted in the brain as pain.[24]

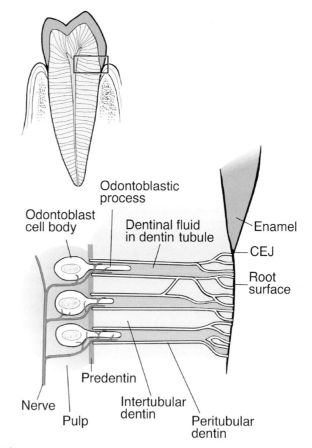

Figure 7-1 Anatomy of Dentin Tubule and Nerve Innervation. (Reprinted with permission from Wilkins EM. *Clinical Practice of the Dental Hygienist*. 9th ed. Baltimore: Lippincott Williams & Wilkins; 2005:713.)

Natural Desensitization

Reports of dentin hypersensitivity decline as people age. Gradual exposure of dentin results in sclerosis within the dentin tubule, as well as the formation of secondary and tertiary dentin. This may block the tubule, interrupt the pain-provoking stimulus, and provide a natural desensitization to protect against pain. Calculus formation over an area of exposed dentin can also naturally desensitize a tooth, the evidence of which is the common occurrence of pain following calculus removal. A smear layer is sometimes formed over dentin that occludes the orifice of dentin tubules and prevents conditions leading to pain. Toothpaste contents and the burnishing action of root instrumentation help create a smear layer. It has been suggested that burnishing dentin with a wood point can induce this smear layer.[23] The smear layer is not permanent, however, and is broken down very easily by dietary acids.

Exciting Factors

Mechanical stimuli (professional instrumentation, toothbrushing), thermal stimuli (hot and cold), evaporative stimuli (blast of air from air/water syringe), osmotic stimuli (sugar, salt), and chemical stimuli (sweets, sours, acids) can incite painful responses. Less frequently, acids produced by biofilm are thought to cause dentin hypersensitivity. When gastroesophageal reflux (GERD) is responsible for acids in the mouth, clinicians should recommend the use of an alkaline baking soda/salt/lukewarm water mixture (1 tsp baking soda, 1 tsp salt, and 1 cup water) to reduce the pH of oral fluids.

Preparations and Mechanisms of Action

The selection of a therapeutic agent should be based on the following factors: effectiveness, caries risk, amount of tooth structure present, patient tolerance or acceptance, cost, and aesthetics. The treatments provided to relieve acute dental hyperalgesia involve placing a barrier between the vital exposed nerve at the area where the pulp interfaces with the dentin tubule and the orifice of exposed dentin tubules that open to the oral cavity. Therefore, a desensitizing agent can be defined as a substance that seals the dentin tubule and prevents irritants from stimulating the nerve when it is topically applied to exposed dentin. Presently, the agents used (a) occlude the orifice of the tubule, (b) act directly on the nerve fiber within the tubule, or (c) provide a physical barrier over the tubule. The preparations discussed here are organized according to at-home use or in-office use for simplicity.

Preparations for At-Home Treatment

The most common agent recommended for home use is a dentifrice. The vast majority of desensitizing toothpastes contain 5% potassium nitrate. Potassium ions are thought to diffuse along dentin tubules and decrease the excitability of intradental nerves by altering their membrane potential and decreasing repolarization.[23] Low concentrations of fluorides (1,100 ppm, or products that contain approximately 0.2% fluoride) are often found in desensitizing dentifrices, but, according

to the product manufacturers, they are added for caries protection and not for DH. There are three products with the ADA Seal of Acceptance for desensitization. One dentifrice contains 0.454% SnF (Crest Pro-Health) for the desensitizing effect, and two products include 5% potassium nitrate (Orajel Sensitive Pain Relieving Toothpaste for Adults, Crest Sensitivity Protection) for desensitization, plus low concentrations of fluoride for the anticaries effect. The 0.454% stannous dentifrice acts by sealing dentin tubules. Another desensitizing dentifrice contains strontium chloride (Thermodent), which seals the dentin tubule orifice. A 0.4% SnF gel to be used at home (Gel-Kam) acts by sealing the tubules. Research continues to find more efficacious preparations. Recently a formulation was introduced (PreviDent 5000 Sensitive) that contains 5,000 ppm NaF to help remineralize root surfaces and prevent root caries, plus 5% potassium nitrate to soothe sensitive teeth. Another combination product that contains 5% potassium nitrate with 0.454% SnF was significantly more effective in reducing dentin hypersensitivity than 5% potassium nitrate combined with 0.24% NaF, or 5% potassium nitrate and 0.2% sodium monofluorophosphate.[22] These products are not yet available in the United States, but they would be the appropriate recommendation when exposed root surfaces are present. Triclosan and zinc citrate, antiplaque agents, do not reduce the efficacy of potassium nitrate.[23]

Preparations for In-Office Treatment

Preparations made for professional application include fluoride (sodium, stannous), adhesives and resins, potassium oxalate (Protect), glutaraldehydes, or calcium phosphates. Because many topical desensitizing agents do not adhere to the dentin surface, their effects are temporary. Stronger, more adhesive materials, such as resins, improve and extend the duration of desensitization. Lasers have been used with varying levels of success. Their desensitizing effect is attributed to the deposition of insoluble salts into the exposed dentin tubules. However, because lasers are not a pharmacologic therapy, no discussion of laser treatments for dentin desensitization is included in this textbook.

Sodium Fluoride

The mechanism of action of fluoride is thought to be the formation of insoluble calcium fluoride within dentin tubules. The ADA list of accepted products for desensitization includes 33.3% NaF applied as a paste or solution and burnished onto the sensitive dentinal area. NaF combined with SnF and hydrogen fluoride (DentinBloc) is an option for rapid but temporary relief of sensitivity. NaF products act by forming crystals to block the orifice; however, the varnish also produces a physical barrier to provide an added layer of protection.[25] These therapies are not permanent and must be repeated as needed for an extended effect. All NaF varnish products have FDA approval for dentin desensitization.

Oxalates

Oxalate products reduce dentin permeability and occlude tubules. This effect occurs more consistently in laboratory studies than in clinical trials involving human teeth. Although several studies show clinical effectiveness, other studies report that the results from using oxalates did not differ significantly from the placebo.[23] A dual-action oxalate combined with potassium nitrate (Centrix) has demonstrated effective desensitization properties. This product both occludes the open dentin tubules and prevents repolarization of the nerve.

Adhesives and Resins

When a loss of tooth structure and contour from abrasion, erosion, and/or abfraction has left notches in the roots, consideration should be given to restoring the area with an adhesive composite resin or glass ionomer restoration. Many topical desensitizing agents do not adhere to dentin, so their effects are temporary. Adhesive products offer longer-lasting desensitization. These include cavity varnishes, bonding agents, and the restorative resin materials described above. Cavity varnishes provide a barrier between dentin tubules and the oral environment, but the acids in saliva ultimately dissolve them, causing the need for reapplication. Restorations seal the tubule or cover it, thereby providing an opportunity for permanent protection from pain.

Miscellaneous Agents

An aqueous solution of 5% glutaraldehyde and 35% HEMA (hydroxyethylmethacrylate) is available in several products created for professional application. It has been shown to be effective for up to 9 months.[26]

■ **Self-Study Review**

20. List and describe contributing factors that lead to dentin hypersensitivity.
21. Describe the pathophysiology of DH.
22. Describe the hydrodynamic theory of dentin hypersensitivity.
23. List the factors related to natural desensitization.
24. Describe recommendations to reduce DH in the patient with GERD.
25. Identify desensitization agents for in-office use and for home use.

DENTAL HYGIENE APPLICATIONS

Caries Prevention

An adequate flow of saliva is recognized as a protective mechanism from caries. When chronic xerostomia occurs, a recommendation to use daily anticaries products (fluoridated toothpaste, low concentrations of 0.05% NaF rinse, xylitol gum) should be included in the oral health education treatment plan. Instructions for the 0.05% NaF rinse should include rinsing for 1 minute daily and expectorating after use.

Xylitol gum, at therapeutic doses (6 to 10 g/day) and used at least three times daily, will stimulate salivation and reduce the levels of pathogenic bacteria in the mouth.

When caries is found in the dental examination, professional application of a topical fluoride agent should be offered to the patient, along with instructions to brush two to three times daily with a fluoridated dentifrice or gel and rinse daily with a 0.05% NaF rinse. For rampant caries, a NaF varnish can be applied, and a fluoridated dentifrice with 5,000 ppm can be prescribed. Fluoride varnishes for caries control should be considered for very young children and for special-needs patients. Safety precautions about not ingesting the product should be provided, and the procedure should be monitored. Conditions associated with caries development (GERD, use of specific medications, others) are cause to recommend the home-use fluoride products described above.

Clinical Procedures for Safe Use

Because professionally applied topical products have high levels of fluoride concentration, care must be taken so that the patient does not swallow large amounts of the product during and after the application procedure. This is done by having the patient in an upright position in the dental chair, using a saliva ejector during the procedure, wiping the fluoride from the teeth at the completion of the procedure, and giving instructions to expectorate for 1 minute following the application. If trays are used, dispense only a small amount sufficient to cover the occlusals of teeth. Box 7-3 illustrates a safe procedural protocol.

BOX 7-3. Safe Procedure for Topical Fluoride Application with Tray

1. Place the patient in a seated, upright position
2. Place a properly functioning saliva ejector in the floor of the mouth
3. Use a properly sized tray; try it in the mouth for size before use
4. Provide a napkin or tissue to catch oral fluids during fluoride application
5. Use a ribbon of gel or foam to cover no more than half the tray's depth
6. Warn the patient NOT to swallow and to lean his or her head forward so fluids flow to the front of the mouth
7. After the manufacturer's recommended time period of application:
   Remove the tray and suction oral fluids and excess fluoride
   Wipe the teeth, tongue, and mucosa thoroughly with gauze
   Have the patient expectorate thoroughly for 1 minute

Parental Instructions for Children

To avoid unintentional ingestion of fluoride by children from fluoride-containing dentifrices, the following steps are recommended for parents:

- Supervise the child's toothbrushing, or do parental brushing
- Store dentifrice out of the reach of children
- Use a child-size toothbrush with a pea-size amount of dentifrice
- Instruct the child to spit out dentifrice after brushing and to avoid swallowing

When natural water supplies contain >2 ppm fluoride levels, recommend drinking water from another source (such as bottled water) to avoid fluorosis. When community water is at the optimum level, fluoride supplements should not be prescribed. If the medical provider has prescribed systemic fluoride, the dentist should consult with the physician and provide American Academy of Pediatric Dentistry recommendations regarding fluoride supplementation.

For young children without the ability to "swish and spit," in-office NaF varnish application may be safer than topical solutions in commercial trays because less fluoride ingestion is likely. They can be used two to four times annually at maintenance appointments. Table 7-4 contains dental hygiene clinical practice recommendations for fluoride use.

Antigingivitis Products

Antigingivitis products, such as chlorhexidine, are prescribed by the dentist or used OTC. When chlorhexidine is prescribed, instructions must include proper rinsing directions (30-second rinse, twice daily; rinse after meals) and the warning to separate the use of toothpaste containing sodium laurel sulfate and the chlorhexidine rinse by 30 minutes to 1 hour. The potential side effects should be explained so the patient is not alarmed if they occur. Although research shows that mouth rinses with alcohol can be recommended for antigingivitis effects when xerostomia is present, some individuals may experience a burning sensation. A nonalcohol antigingivitis mouth rinse is indicated for clients who cannot tolerate mouth rinses with alcohol, for those recovering from alcohol-related substance abuse, or for those taking drugs that interact with alcohol (metronidazole, Antabuse). They are indicated when severe mucositis develops following cancer chemotherapy, as well as for clients with *severe* xerostomia. Antigingivitis toothpastes should be recommended when periodontal inflammation is present, rather than traditional dentifrices. See Box 7-4 for dental hygiene applications.

Desensitization

The development of a sound treatment plan must consider causative factors that influence tooth sensitivity. Often, sensitivity will stop on its own when the etiologic factor is removed. Questioning the patient about current dietary or toothbrushing practices, considering the clinical procedure that caused the painful response (e.g., exploration at the cervical area), and considering recent dental therapy may help the practitioner recognize specific etiologic factors that can affect appropriate management strategies. Dietary sources (citrus juices and wines) contain acids that can remove smear layers and open dentin tubules through erosion. When palatal tooth surfaces are sensitive, the clinician should question the patient about his or her history of gastric reflux or vomiting. In these cases, the patient should avoid toothbrushing for 2 to 3 hours after consuming acidic foods or beverages in order to avoid the effects of acids and abrasion.[22] In addition, the patient should be instructed to rinse with baking soda/salt/water solution after vomiting to help neutralize the acidic environment.

When asking about oral hygiene methods, consider that the recession precedes sensitivity in most cases, and improper

Table 7-4 Dental Hygiene Recommendations for Fluoride Use

Condition	Home-use Product	In-office Product
Children <6 y (low risk for caries)	Fluoridated dentifrice (pea-size amount on brush)	Additional anticaries benefit not established
Children >6 y, adults >18 y (low risk for caries)	Fluoridated dentifrice	Additional anticaries benefit not established
Young children (mod. risk), children with special needs	Fluoridated dentifrice 3 times daily (pea-size amount on brush)	5% NaF varnish, 6-mo intervals
Children >6 y, adults >18 y (mod. risk)	Fluoridated dentifrice 3 times daily, daily 0.05% NaF rinse	5% NaF varnish, 6-mo intervals OR fluoride gel application,[†] 6-mo intervals
Children <6 y (high risk)	Fluoridated dentifrice 3 times daily (pea-size amount on brush)	5% NaF varnish, 3- to 6-mo intervals
Children >6 y, adults >18 y (high risk)	Fluoridated dentifrice 3 times daily (pea-size amount on brush)	5% NaF varnish, 3- to 6-mo intervals OR fluoride gel application,[†] 3- to 6-mo intervals
Head and neck radiation, chronic xerostomia	1.1% NaF (5,000 ppm) gel or paste	5% NaF varnish[‡]
Medications containing sugar, taken chronically	Fluoridated dentifrice, daily 0.05% NaF rinse	APF or NaF gel[‡]
Exposed roots, periodontal patient, GERD*, porcelain restorations, sealants	Fluoridated dentifrice, daily 0.05% NaF rinse	2% NaF gel, foam, rinse

*GERD, gastroesophageal reflux disease
[†]4-min application
[‡]Recommend xylitol gum to stimulate salivation
NaF, sodium fluoride; APF, acidulated phosphate fluoride

BOX 7-4. Antigingivitis Agents and Clinical Applications

Agent	Clinical Application
Chlorhexidine (CHX)	Separate toothpaste use and CHX rinse by 30 minutes to 1 hour Side effects: Staining, calculus, taste disturbance Rinse for 30 seconds, twice daily, after meals Nonalcohol formulation recommended for severe xerostomia, mucositis, or individuals with history of alcohol abuse
Essential oils	Alcohol formulation: Not recommended for severe xerostomia, mucositis, or alcoholic individuals
Triclosan or SNF	Recommend when periodontal inflammation exists

BOX 7-5. Causes of Dentin Hypersensitivity and Clinical Applications

Cause	Management Strategy
Dietary acid, gastric reflux	Historical questions to identify risk, source Avoid acidic foods No toothbrushing for 2 to 3 hours after reflux Rinse with baking soda/salt/water mixture immediately after vomiting
Toothbrushing, abrasive dentifrice	Assess toothbrushing technique Inform about relationship of vigorous brushing, recession, sensitivity Recommend desensitizing dentifrice for sensitive teeth, used routinely
Clinical procedure	Avoid overinstrumentation Recommend desensitizing dentifrice to avoid sensitive teeth, 2 weeks, twice daily use If ineffective, professional application of desensitizing agent Restoration with aesthetic dental material (final recommended procedure)

toothbrushing techniques and abrasive dentifrices can open dentin tubules. Because DH develops more frequently following treatment for periodontal disease, this may occur as an **iatrogenic** result of root instrumentation. Avoid overinstrumentation when possible. Inform the patient that sensitivity may occur after treatment, and either apply an in-office desensitizing agent or recommend use of a desensitizing dentifrice at home. Box 7-5 organizes clinical applications for management of hypersensitivity. Before initiating tooth examination, inquire if any teeth are sensitive as a strategy to identify "at risk" teeth before inciting a painful response. When DH is an acute event, unrelated to recent dental therapy, start the questioning strategy by asking, "What have you done or eaten recently that is not part of your normal routine?" The following considerations are offered:

1. Avoid the stimulus. One may remember the humorous joke, "Doc, it hurts when I do this!" and the medical reply, "Well, don't do that!" This strategy applies to dentin hypersensitivity caused by eating or drinking dietary products that lead to sensitivity. Sometimes foods can be moved to the opposite side of the mouth to avoid eliciting the painful response. When instrumenting, the instrument tip should not contact the hypersensitive area, which is usually at the CEJ. An air/water syringe should not be used to dry a sensitive area; instead, a 2×2 gauze or cotton roll would be less likely to cause pain.
2. Recommend home therapy. Because there is a high risk for the development of DH following periodontal treatment, a plan to address the risk should be implemented. The same is true when tooth whitening procedures are provided in the dental office. Dentifrices to reduce sensitivity, used at home, are the first strategy to prevent DH. The dentifrice should be used for 1 minute twice daily. Desensitization

usually will occur within 2 weeks. The client should be informed that he or she should continue to use the dentifrice once desensitization is reached, because once it is discontinued, sensitivity may return. In the past, some sources recommended applying a desensitizing dentifrice with the finger, rather than with a toothbrush, but there is no scientific base for this recommendation.[23] If no relief occurs after 2 to 4 weeks, advise a return visit for in-office desensitization treatments. If those are ineffective, the final option is to place a restoration over the hypersensitive area.

3. When applying topical NaF paste, burnish the agent onto the dentin to plug the tubule opening and form a smear layer. This layer is broken down easily by dietary acids, however, and the procedure may need to be repeated in the future. Longer-lasting desensitization may result from using oxalates or resin therapies. New product development may provide agents for long-lasting pain relief.
4. Decrease intradental nerve excitability. Potassium nitrate dentifrices are available for this modality. Lasers have also been used for this purpose, but this treatment must be performed in the dental office.

A proper diagnosis of the etiologic agent(s) associated with hypersensitive teeth must be established in order to select the correct therapeutic product. When clinical procedures associated with causing dentin hypersensitivity are planned, a desensitizing dentifrice should be recommended the day of the treatment, with appropriate instructions given on how to

CLINICAL APPLICATION EXERCISES

☐ **Exercise 1.** Your patient reports using a new, non-alcohol mouth rinse by Proctor & Gamble (Crest Pro-Health Nonalcohol Rinse) to "kill bacteria in my mouth that causes gingivitis." She asks if it has the ADA Seal of Acceptance for that use. She also purchased the same brand of toothpaste (Crest Pro-Health Toothpaste) and wonders if it has the ADA Seal of Acceptance for an antigingivitis effect. Where and how will you find this information? How will you respond?

☐ **Exercise 2.** Describe patient instructions for your periodontal patient who is being given a prescription for a chlorhexidine rinse that contains alcohol.

☐ **Exercise 3.** When dentin hypersensitivity is reported, the dental hygienist is often asked, "What can I do?" List a variety of products sold at the drugstore for sensitive teeth. Look at the labels and write down the active ingredient(s) in the dentifrice. Get a dental product catalog and find agents sold to the dental office for dentin hypersensitivity treatment. Write down their active ingredient(s). This will give the clinician useful information for product recommendations and products for professional use.

---

use it. It may take a few weeks for the effect to manifest, but in-office treatment therapies can be provided if needed.

■ Self-Study Review

26. Outline dental hygiene management strategies for using fluorides in clinical practice, including patient instructions following topical applications of fluoride.
27. Outline dental hygiene management strategies for recommending anticaries agents given the age of the patient and individual needs.
28. Outline dental hygiene management strategies for using or recommending antigingivitis agents.
29. Outline dental hygiene management strategies for identifying hypersensitive teeth and for preventing DH following associated clinical procedures, including patient instructions for using agents at home.

CONCLUSION

Topical products are used by the dental hygienist on a routine basis. The rationale for using these agents, plus knowledge of safe practices when using them, is essential. Many therapeutic topical agents are sold OTC, and patients often inquire about various ingredients in products. Knowledge of available products for professional application and their proposed mechanisms of action is essential. Oral health practitioners must continue to review published clinical studies to identify those products that are most likely to be efficacious and have benefit to the dental client.

Web Resources: Featherstone J, et al. Caries risk assessment in practice for age 6 through adult. *J Cal Dent Assoc* 2007;35(10):703–713. http://www.cda.foundation.org/

library/docs/jour1007/featherstone.pdf Accessed May 10, 2008.

References

1. Chu CH, Lo ECM. A review of sodium fluoride varnish. *Gen Dent.* 2006;54(4):247–253.
2. Council on Scientific Affairs, American Dental Association (ADA). Professionally applied topical fluoride: Evidence-based clinical recommendations. *J Am Dent Assoc.* 2006;137:1151–1159.
3. Church LE. Fluorides—use with caution. *J Md State Dent Assoc.* 1976;19:106.
4. Ripa L. An evaluation of the use of professionally (operator-applied) topical fluorides. *J Dent Res.* 1990;69:786–796.
5. Newbrun E. Anticaries agents. In: *Pharmacology and Therapeutics for Dentistry.* 5th ed. St. Louis: Elsevier Science; 2004: 736.
6. Ripa LW. Need for prior tooth cleaning when performing a professional topical fluoride application: Review and recommendations for change. *J Am Dent Assoc.* 1984;109:281–285.
7. Wakeen L. Legal implications of using drugs and devices in the dental office. *J Public Health Dent.* 1992;52:403–408.
8. Weintraub J, Ramos-Gomez F, Jue B, et al. Fluoride varnish efficacy in preventing early childhood caries. *J Dent Res.* 2006;85 (2):172–176.
9. Rothen M. The wonder of xylitol. *Dimensions of Den Hyg.* 2005;3:18–20.
10. Milgrom P, Ly K, Roberts M, et al. Mutans streptococci dose response to xylitol chewing gum. *J Dent Res.* 2006;85(2):177–181.
11. Ly K, Milgrom P, Roberts M, et al. Linear response of mutans streptococci to increasing frequency of xylitol chewing gum use: A randomized controlled trial. *BMC Oral Health* [serial online]. 2006;6:6.
12. Schaeken M, Keltjens H, Van der Hoeven J. Effects of fluoride and chlorhexidine on the microflora of dental root-surface caries. *J Dent Res.* 1991;70:150–153.
13. Barkvoll P, Rolla G, Svendsen AK. Chlorhexidine interactions with sodium lauryl sulfate in vivo. *J Dent Res.* 1989;68(special issue):1722–1723.

14. DePaola LG, Overholser CD, Meiller TF, et al. Chemotherapeutic inhibition of supragingival dental plaque and gingivitis development. *J Clin Periodontol.* 1989;16:311–315.

15. Bauroth K, Charles C, Mankodi S, et al. The efficacy of an essential oil antiseptic mouthrinse vs. dental floss in controlling interproximal gingivitis: A comparative study. *J Am Dent Assoc.* 2003;134:359–365.

16. Overholser CD, Meiller TF, DePaola LG, et al. Comparative effects of 2 chemotherapeutic mouth rinses on the development of supragingival dental plaque and gingivitis. *J Clin Periodontol.* 1990;17:575–579.

17. Fischman SL, Aguirre A, Charles CH. Use of essential oil-containing mouth rinses by xerostomic individuals: Determination of potential for oral mucosal irritation. *Am J Dent.* 2004;17:23–26.

18. Cole P, Rodu B, Mathisen A. Alcohol-containing mouthwash and oropharyngeal cancer. *J Am Dent Assoc.* 2003;134(8):1079–1087.

19. Terdphong T, Rustogi KN, Volpe AR, et al. Clinical effect of a new liquid dentifrice containing triclosan/copolymer on existing plaque and gingivitis. *J Am Dent Assoc.* 2002;133:219–225.

20. Bradshaw DJ, Marsh PD, Cummins D. The effects of triclosan and zinc citrate, alone and in combination, on a community of oral bacteria grown in vitro. *J Dent Res.* 1993;72:25–30.

21. von Troll B, Needleman E, Sanz M. A systematic review of the prevalence of root sensitivity following periodontal therapy. *J Clin Periodontol.* 2002;20(3 suppl):173–177.

22. Canadian Advisory Board on Dentin Hypersensitivity. Consensus-based recommendations for the diagnosis and management of dentin hypersensitivity. *J Can Dent Assoc.* 2003;69:221–226.

23. Orchardson R, Gillam DG. Managing dentin hypersensitivity. *J Am Dent Assoc.* 2006;137(7):990–998.

24. Yoshiyama M, Noiri Y, Ozaki K, et al. Transmission electron microscopic characterization of hypersensitive human radicular dentin. *J Dent Res.* 1990;69:1293–1297.

25. Ritter AV, Dias W, Miguez P, et al. Treating cervical dentin hypersensitivity with fluoride varnish: A randomized clinical study. *J Am Dent Assoc.* 2006;137:1013–1020.

26. Duran I, Sengun A. The long-term effectiveness of five current desensitizing products on cervical dentine sensitivity. *J Oral Rehabil.* 2004;31:351–356.

8

Nonopioid and Opioid Agents

KEY TERMS

Adjuvant: An additional therapy given to enhance or extend the effect of the primary therapy

Algogenic substances: Substances liberated by the body during phases of inflammation that can produce pain

Analgesia: Insensibility to pain without loss of consciousness

Analgesics: Agents that relieve pain by inhibiting specific pain pathways

Antipyretic: Capable of reducing fever

Endogenous: Originating or produced within the organism or one of its parts

Equianalgesic: Equal in the ability for giving pain relief

International normalized ratio (INR): A test to determine risk of bleeding

Ischemia: Reduction of circulation to an area

Loading dose: An initial high dose to quickly achieve a therapeutic blood level

Nociception: Sensory detection and neuronal transmission of pain stimuli

Noxious: Injurious or harmful

Opioid: Derived from opium; a strong dependence-producing analgesic

Pathognomonic: Characteristic or indicative (diagnostic) of a particular disease or condition

Somatic pain: Pain caused by the activation of pain receptors in mucocutaneous and musculoskeletal tissues

Visceral pain: Pain caused by the activation of pain receptors in internal organs

KEY ACRONYMS

AA: Arachidonic acid
APAP: Acetaminophen
ASA: Aspirin
COX: Cyclooxygenase

COX-I: Cyclooxygenic inhibitors
LP: Lipoxygenase
NSAIDs: Nonsteroidal anti-inflammatory drugs

The most common complaint causing a person to seek the services of an oral health care provider is pain. Conversely, the fear of pain may also keep an individual from seeking dental care. Gentleness to prevent pain during oral health care is a common goal, not only to be considerate to the individual, but also to reduce the risks associated with precipitating a medical emergency. Removal of disease is another way to reduce pain from an inflammatory origin. Effective control of pain has several advantages. It facilitates delivery of care, lowers anxiety about treatment, and can promote the patient's return for preventive and maintenance care. In contrast, some chronic oral disease conditions are not associated with pain,

and, therefore, necessary dental care may not be sought. This may lead to habits of sporadic dental visits, dental neglect, and episodic care only for acute pain. Consequently, the primary obligation and ultimate responsibility of every clinician is not only to restore function, but also to relieve or prevent pain. Proper management of pain requires an understanding of its complexity, an appreciation for the causative factors that bring the individual for clinical services, and the implementation of sound clinical and pharmacological strategies. For this reason this chapter begins with a basic explanation of the physiology of and influences on pain perception by the patient. This is followed by an explanation of pharmacological therapy directed toward relief of dental pain and associated side effects that could develop.

PHYSIOLOGY AND EPIDEMIOLOGY OF PAIN

Analgesia is defined as relieving pain by inhibiting specific pain pathways. Pharmacologic agents for this purpose are called **analgesics**. These drugs are taken for a variety of medical conditions, including arthritis, dysmenorrheal, and inflammatory conditions. Frequently they are consumed on a daily basis and for extended time periods for pain relief. *Pain* is an unpleasant sensory and emotional experience associated with actual or potential tissue damage.

Activation of Acute (Nociceptive) Pain Pathways

Nociception is the sensory detection, transduction, and neural transmission of **noxious**, or painful, events. Nociceptors (pain receptors) are found in most tissues and are especially dense in oral mucosa and in the dental pulp. Any stimulation of the pulp is painful whether the stimulation comes from heat, cold, vibration, or pressure. Stimuli that provoke pain receptors can be mechanical, thermal, or chemical—the same stimuli discussed in the desensitization section in the previous chapter. Most pain of dental origin is associated with a recent onset of pain, called acute pain. Chemical agents that occur naturally in the environment of pain receptors following acute tissue damage are called **algogenic substances**. Algogenic substances include substances liberated by the body during phases of inflammation such as adenosine, adenosine triphosphate, serotonin, histamine, bradykinin, cytokines, prostaglandins, and other neuroactive substances (Box 8-1). These chemicals initiate the release of substance P, calcitonin-gene-related peptide (CGRP), and glutamate from nerve terminals. Whereas substance P and CGRP are considered to be neuromodulators involved in evoking neurogenic inflammation, *glutamate* is now thought to be the primary pain neurotransmitter. It activates nociceptive receptors, which generate impulses that are transmitted along peripheral fibers to the central nervous system (CNS). The detection

---

BOX 8-1. Algogenic Substances

- Adenosine
- Adenosine triphosphate
- Serotonin
- Histamine
- Bradykinin
- Cytokines
- Prostaglandins
- Neuroactive substances

---

of pain stimuli in the orofacial region is conveyed by cranial nerves, primarily by nerves in the trigeminal system.

Intrinsic Expression of Inflammatory Pain

Initial Stimulus of Pain

Following tissue injury, macrophages and other cells of the immune system invade the damaged area in an attempt to remove cellular debris and to prevent or combat infection. The inflammatory process triggers the formation of prostaglandins, which enhance the negative effects of other algogenic substances on pain receptors. Traumatic injury may also provoke vasoconstriction, an efferent sympathetic reflex that decreases microcirculation in the injured tissue, producing **ischemia** and further amplifying pain impulses. At the same time, physiologic CNS effects are initiated. Central control systems, by means of efferent fibers leaving the CNS at the trigeminal nerve, modulate signal transmission and inhibit nociceptive impulses. Within the brain, **endogenous** peptides (enkephalins, endorphins, dynorphins) are released to cause analgesia. This pathway is responsible for feelings of analgesia and euphoria in athletic individuals following intense workouts.

The Role of the Higher Central Nervous System in Pain

When applied to pain, the term *perception* (attention and cognition) refers to the awareness of a noxious sensation, appreciation of negative emotions, and interpretation (with attribution of meaning) of the experience. While patients are surprisingly uniform in their perceptions of pain, they differ greatly in their reactions to it. Attention and cognition, along with cultural, emotional, and motivational differences, will alter or modulate the intensity of a patient's response to noxious stimuli. The result is that a level of pain that may not require drug treatment in one individual may necessitate extreme analgesic therapy in another.

Attention

The process of *attention* is largely under conscious (or mind) control. The patient experiencing pain has a choice: Attend to the noxious sensations to the exclusion of other incoming signals from the brain, or attend to signals that can exclude pain perception from conscious awareness. Manipulation of attention for pain control has been used with varying degrees of success. The following are examples of attentional control:

- Most hypnotic procedures involve the clear control and redirection of attention away from pain
- Music used during dental procedures distracts the patient
- Patients who hold a leg up while dental radiographs are being taken use attentional control effectively to suppress the gag reflex

Cognition

A nociceptive afferent outflow from the CNS may elicit different perceptions in different patients and, even within the same patient at different times, if the thought processes associated with the experience are different. These processes include memory of past experience, discrimination between oral procedures, and judgmental function; the matching of present circumstances or experiences against expectations; and the attribution of meaning to the experience. Cognitive factors described above explain many of the individual responses to painful stimulation seen in clinical practice.

Acute Odontogenic Pain

Complaints of anguish, postural displays, groaning, wincing, and grimacing are all equated with pain, along with limitation of normal activity (function), excessive rest, social withdrawal, and medication demand or intake. Patients in pain tend to behave in ways appropriate to their cultural heritage. For example Americans tend to want quick relief (pills, other remedies), while other cultures may accept pain as a natural process. Therefore, it is important for practitioners to recognize that what works with one individual may not relieve the pain of another. Expressed another way, one patient may not need an analgesic following a procedure, whereas another may require a strong analgesic. When cost is an issue, a prescription for analgesic drugs may not be filled by the individual. Ultimately, the choice of a therapeutic intervention for acute odontogenic pain is determined largely by (a) the nature of the patient's problem, (b) the resources available (elimination of infection, analgesics), (c) the individual's acceptance and attitude toward pain, and (d) the cost to the patient. Most patients can attain satisfactory relief of acute odontogenic pain through an approach that incorporates primary dental care (removing the dental cause of the pain, usually infection) in conjunction with local anesthesia and analgesics.

■ Self-Study Review

1. Define the term *analgesia* and list influences associated with pain.
2. Differentiate between the influences of *acute* pain and *chronic* pain on dental care.
3. List algogenic substances.
4. List the primary neurogenic substances involved in transmitting pain responses.
5. Which cranial nerve transmits orofacial painful stimuli to the CNS?
6. Describe what occurs from the *stimulus* of pain to the *perception* of pain.
7. List endogenous peptides that relieve pain.
8. Identify features of attention and cognition in the pain response.
9. List signs of acute odontogenic pain.
10. Describe three methods to relieve most odontogenic pain.

ANALGESICS

Three types of analgesics are available for the management of acute odontogenic pain: Nonopioid analgesics (which include a variety of cyclooxygenase- [COX-] inhibitors; Table 8-1), **opioid** analgesics derived from opium (Table 8-2), and **adjuvant** drugs. An older term used to describe nonopioid analgesics (except acetaminophen [APAP]) is *nonsteroidal anti-inflammatory drugs* (NSAIDs). There are several differences between the nonopioid analgesics (which are not derived from opium) and the opioid agents (which are derived from opium). All nonopioids can reduce fever (antipyresis), but opioids do not have this effect. Another difference between the two types of analgesics is that they have completely different mechanisms of action. The nonopioids inhibit prostaglandin synthesis (peripherally and centrally), and the opioids act as agonists at opioid receptors (peripherally and centrally). It was formerly thought that only opioids acted in the CNS, but recent evidence reveals that all COX inhibitors (COX-I), to variable degrees, also act within the CNS to inhibit pain and reduce fever. For our purposes the nonopioid agents are grouped into one classification called COX-I, because they all inhibit COX in various areas of the body as part of their action. Table 8-1 includes those COX-I used to manage dental pain, and identifies the analgesic dose (some include an initial **loading dose**), maximum dose, and pregnancy risk category associated with each. Table 8-2 includes

Table 8-1 Selected COX-Inhibitors for Analgesia			
Drugs	**Usual Oral Dose**	**Maximum Daily Dose**	**Pregnancy Risk Category***
acetylsalicylic acid (ASA [OTC], Anacin [OTC], others)	500 to 1,000 mg	4,000 mg	D
APAP (Tylenol [OTC], others)	500 to 1,000 mg	4,000 mg	B
ibuprofen (Advil [OTC], Motrin, others)	200 to 800 mg	2,400 mg	B D (third trimester)
naproxen (Naprosyn)	500 mg loading dose, then 250 mg	1,250 mg	B C (third trimester)
naproxen sodium (Aleve [OTC], Anaprox, others)	550 mg loading dose, then 275 mg	1,375 mg	B C (third trimester)

*Refer to Chapter 21
OTC, over the counter

Table 8-2	Selected Opioid-Receptor Agonists		
Drugs	**Formulations**	**Pregnancy Risk Category**[a]	**Restrictions**[b]
Codeine	With ASA, 30/325 mg (Empirin with codeine) With APAP, 30/325 mg (Tylenol with codeine)	C D (if used for a prolonged period or in high doses at term)	C-III
Hydrocodone	With ASA, 5/500 mg (Lortab ASA) With ibuprofen, 7.5/200 mg (Vicoprofen) With APAP, 5/500 mg (Vicodin)	C	C-II
Tramadol	50 mg (Ultram) With APAP 37.5/325 mg (Ultracet)	C	Rx
Oxycodone	With ASA, 5/325 mg (Percodan) With APAP, 5/500 mg (Percocet) With ibuprofen, 5/400 mg (Combunox)	C	C-II

[a]Refer to Chapter 21
[b]Refer to Chapter 3, Controlled Substances Schedule
APAP, acetaminophen; ASA, acetylsalicylic acid (aspirin)

selected opioid-receptor agonists used to manage moderate to severe dental pain. Other opioids, less effective for oral pain and not included in the table, include meperidine, morphine, hydromorphone, and propoxyphene.

An adjuvant agent may either enhance the efficacy of an analgesic or it may have an analgesic activity of its own. Caffeine, in doses of 65 to 200 mg, enhances the analgesic effect of acetylsalicylic acid (aspirin [ASA]), APAP, and ibuprofen in dental and other acute pain syndromes. It is sometimes added to an analgesic agent (Anacin). The antihistamine hydroxyzine (Apo-Hydroxyzine), in doses of 25 to 50 mg, enhances the analgesic effect of opioids in postoperative pain and significantly reduces the incidence of opioid-induced nausea and vomiting. Corticosteroids, through their anti-inflammatory and phospholipase-inhibitory effects, can produce analgesia when pain is of an inflammatory origin.

Pharmacodynamic Considerations

Cyclooxygenase Formation

One of the key elements of cell damage is the formation of *arachidonic acid* (AA) from cell membrane phospholipids. AA is metabolized further by two different pathways. One pathway uses COX, and the other uses lipoxygenase (LP). Almost all cells in the body contain the COX enzymes, whereas LP is found only in inflammatory cells (neutrophils, mast cell, macrophage). COX breaks AA down to various prostaglandins, also known as prostanoids (prostacyclin I_2, thromboxane A_2, prostaglandin E_2, prostaglandin F_2, and prostaglandin D_2). Prostaglandins are endogenous substances known to lower the pain threshold to painful stimuli (making one more likely to feel pain), promote inflammation and fever, and affect vascular tone and permeability (edema). At least two COX isoforms (COX-1, COX-2) and a variant of COX-1 (referred to as COX-3 in this text for simplification,

but more specifically termed COX-1b or COX-1v in other sources) are known to play a role in the rate-limiting step in prostaglandin synthesis. Nonselective COX-inhibiting analgesics inhibit both COX-1 and COX-2 pathways, whereas COX-2 inhibitors only inhibit the COX-2 pathway, leaving the COX-1 pathway free. While all COX-inhibiting drugs increase the pain threshold to noxious stimuli (making one less likely to feel pain), they all reach a ceiling dose for their maximum analgesic effect (Table 8-1). Figure 8-1 illustrates physiologic roles of COX isoforms, which are explained in the next section.

Cyclooxygenase Inhibitors

COX-1 is the major isoform expressed (synthesized and, therefore, available to act at all times, in virtually all normal tissues, including platelets). It is involved in several homeostatic, or "housekeeping," activities throughout the body. For example, physiologic COX-1-induced prostaglandins (PGE_2) protect the gastric mucosa by enhancing gastric blood flow, increasing mucous and bicarbonate secretion, and inhibiting acid output. Physiologic COX-1-induced thromboxane A_2 biosynthesis promotes platelet aggregation and clot formation. Nonselective COX-1 inhibitors (ASA and other NSAIDs, such as ibuprofen) increase the pain threshold to noxious stimuli by reducing prostaglandin synthesis, but they also interfere with thromboxane A_2-induced platelet aggregation and increase bleeding. This may lead to gastric irritation and affect renal function. COX-2 is expressed (synthesized and, therefore, available to act at all times) primarily in the brain, kidneys, female reproduction system, and bones. Synthesis can be induced by inflammatory cytokines in other tissues, including endothelial cells. COX-2 is not found in abundance in platelets, but COX-2 in endothelial cells induces prostacyclin, which prevents platelet aggregation and promotes vasodilation. The COX-2 inhibitor celecoxib (Celebrex), which selectively blocks only the COX-2 arm of COX,

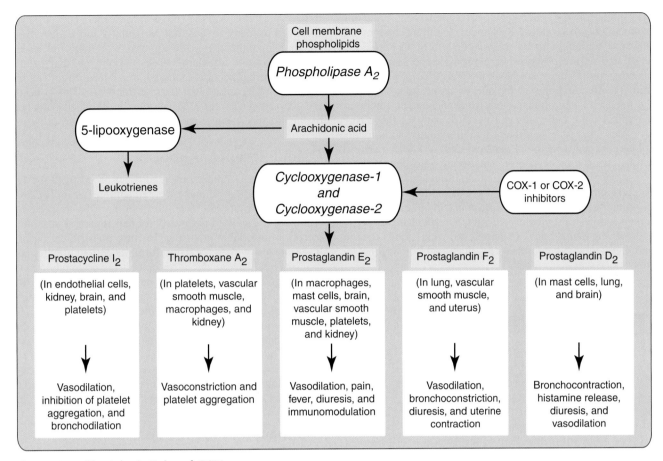

Figure 8-1 Physiologic Roles of COX.

also increases the pain threshold to painful stimuli by reducing prostaglandin synthesis. While COX-2 inhibitors do not inhibit thromboxane A_2-induced platelet aggregation, they do block endothelial prostacyclin synthesis, which leads to platelet aggregation and vasoconstriction (a dangerous combination in patients with cardiovascular disease, as was discovered in those taking rofecoxib [Vioxx]).

COX-3 isoforms are expressed (synthesized and, therefore, available to act at all times) primarily in the CNS. APAP, a COX-3 inhibitor, is a relatively weak inhibitor of peripheral prostaglandin biosynthesis. While it increases the pain threshold to noxious stimuli, it has no clinically relevant anti-inflammatory properties. However, APAP is highly effective in inhibiting COX-3 in the CNS, and its analgesic efficacy and antipyretic effect is related to the ability to inhibit prostaglandin synthesis in the CNS. APAP has no clinically relevant effect on platelet function.

Opioid-Receptor Agonists

Opioid-receptor agonists produce analgesia by interacting with opioid receptors in the CNS (Table 8-3) that are also the natural binding sites for a number of **endogenous** peptides (which include endorphins, endomorphins, enkephalins, and dynorphins). These endogenous chemicals are responsible for the "high" and the "lack of pain" long-distance runners feel when they compete. Opioid-agonist drugs produce

analgesia by virtue of their interaction with opioid receptors in the brain, brain stem, spinal cord, trigeminal nucleus, and peripheral terminals of primary afferent neurons. Consequently, opioid receptors are found in both the central and peripheral nervous systems, although the primary site of action is the CNS. When opioid receptors interact with their natural ligands (endorphins, endomorphins, enkephalins, and

Table 8-3 Opioid Receptors

Receptors	Primary Endogenous Ligands	Effects
Mu	Endorphins and endomorphins	• Analgesia • Euphoria • Decreased respiration
Delta	Enkephalins	• Analgesia • Decreased respiration
Kappa	Dynorphins	• Analgesia • Dysphoria • No respiratory effect
Opioid-receptor-like	Orphanin FQ or nociceptin	• Analgesia • No respiratory effect

dynorphins) or with exogenous opioid agonists (e.g., codeine, hydrocodone, oxycodone), they appear to inhibit calcium influx into neurons, impede presynaptic neurotransmitter release, and reduce postsynaptic neuronal responses. Consequently, opioid analgesics block the activation of peripheral primary afferent fibers at the site of tissue injury; inhibit the release of neurotransmitters from presynaptic fibers in the spinal cord and trigeminal nucleus; increase the activity of cells that provide efferent inhibitory innervation to the spinal cord and trigeminal nucleus; and, in higher cortical levels, alter the mood and the reaction to pain. The affinity of a particular opioid-receptor agonist to a specific opioid-receptor subtype explains the therapeutic and adverse effects of opioid-receptor agonists. Most pain can be relieved with opioid analgesics if the drugs are given in adequate dosages. Most severe dental pain can be relieved with various opioid and COX-inhibitor combinations, such as hydrocodone or oxycodone with ibuprofen.

Self-Study Review

11. Describe the features of the three types of COX-I analgesics for odontogenic pain.
12. List differences between *nonopioid* analgesics and *opioid* analgesics.
13. Note the therapeutic doses of each product in Table 8-1 and the maximum dose.
14. List adjuvant products used for analgesic effects.
15. Describe the role of AA in cellular damage leading to COX formation.
16. How do prostaglandins cause pain?
17. Describe the features of COX-1, COX-2, and COX-3 chemicals in pain; give examples of drugs in each category.
18. List opioid receptors.
19. Describe the mechanism of action of opioid agonists to reduce pain, compared to that of COX-I.

Pharmacokinetic Considerations

Cyclooxygenase Inhibitors

COX-I are rapidly absorbed from the stomach and the upper small intestine. They reach appreciable plasma concentrations in 30 to 60 minutes and peak values at about 2 to 3 hours. As with most orally administered drugs, the rate of absorption is determined by the formulation (liquids are absorbed faster than tablets) and pK_a of the drug, the pH at the mucosal surface of the intestine, the vascularity of the absorptive surface, and gastric emptying time when food is present. Because absorption occurs primarily by passive diffusion of lipid-soluble molecules across the gastrointestinal (GI) mucosal membranes, the rate of absorption of an acidic COX-I is decreased in an alkaline GI environment. The presence of food also delays absorption, so the analgesic should be taken 30 minutes before or several hours after eating. After absorption, COX-I are distributed throughout most body

tissues and fluids, and they cross the placenta. They are metabolized in many tissues, but particularly in the liver. The metabolism of therapeutic doses normally follows first-order kinetics; however, after larger doses, the enzymes that metabolize these drugs become saturated, which leads to zero-order kinetics and increased half-lives of the drugs. This concept is discussed in Chapter 2. Metabolites are excreted primarily by the kidneys as water-soluble conjugates.

Opioid-Receptor Agonists

Opioid-receptor agonists are readily absorbed from the GI tract, but not all are suitable for oral administration because of significant first-pass metabolism in the liver. Meperidine (Demerol), once used frequently for dental pain, is an example of an unsuitable oral drug; because meperidine plasma levels are low with the oral doseform. Its current primary administration is by injection. All opioids are protein bound to some degree in plasma. The free molecules readily leave the blood and accumulate in vascular organs, such as the kidney, liver, lung, and spleen. Although the primary site of action of opioids is in the CNS, only small quantities pass through the blood–brain barrier. During pregnancy, placental transfer occurs. As biotransformation occurs and opioid plasma levels fall, a decline in opioid analgesia occurs. The major route of elimination of opioids and their metabolites is by glomerular filtration.

Pharmacotherapeutic Considerations

The optimal dose of an analgesic that will provide adequate pain relief must be established by titration or individualized according to patient variability, and the drug should be administered on schedule. "By-the-clock" administration of analgesics is much more effective than waiting for pain to return before giving the next dose. "By-the-clock" administration may actually *reduce* the total dosage required for the management of a painful episode. Put simply, once pain is perceived, it is harder to relieve. In addition, some patients may respond better to one COX-I or COX-I/opioid combination than to another. Also, currently available formulations may not be optimal in the management of all pain of odontogenic origin, emphasizing the importance of an individualized approach to pain control. At times, clinicians may have to prescribe more than one analgesic to be administered concurrently to achieve maximal results. Prescribing two drugs (at therapeutic doses) with similar mechanisms of action has no rational pharmacological basis, but prescribing two drugs (at therapeutic doses) with *different mechanisms of action* is "good medicine." It has been shown that combining an opioid with a nonopioid analgesic is more effective in relieving pain than administering a larger amount of opioid alone. Hydrocodone with APAP, the opioid/nonopioid combination analgesic, is an example of the latter and is among the most widely prescribed drugs, appearing in the top ten most widely prescribed drugs for several years.

Primary Line of Treatment

ASA is the standard for the comparison and evaluation of orally effective analgesics. APAP is as effective as ASA,

Table 8-4	ASA Interactions and Clinical Considerations	
ACE-inhibitors	Decreased antihypertensive effect (decreased prostaglandin synthesis)	Monitor blood pressure
Anticoagulants, oral	Increased bleeding (platelet inhibition)	Avoid concurrent use
Cimetidine and nizatidine	Possible salicylate toxicity (decreased metabolism)	Avoid concurrent use
Clopidogrel	Increased GI bleeding (additive effect on platelet function)	Avoid concurrent use
Heparin	Increased bleeding (platelet inhibition)	Avoid concurrent use
Ibuprofen	Inhibition of antiplatelet effect of ASA (blocks access to active site on platelets)	Administer ibuprofen 8 hours before or 30 minutes after immediate release ASA, or avoid concurrent use
Lithium	Lithium toxicity (decreased renal clearance)	Avoid concurrent use
Methotrexate	Possible methotrexate toxicity (decreased renal clearance)	Avoid concurrent use
Naproxen	Inhibition of antiplatelet effect of ASA (blocks access to active site on platelets)	Administer naproxen 2 hours before or 2 hours after immediate release ASA, or avoid concurrent use
Quinidine	Increased bleeding (additive antiplatelet effect)	Avoid concurrent use
Spironolactone	Decreased antihypertensive effect (decreased prostaglandin synthesis)	Monitor blood pressure
Valproate	Possible valproate toxicity (displacement from binding site)	Avoid concurrent use
Zafirlukast	Possible zafirlukast toxicity (decreased metabolism)	Avoid concurrent use

with similar potency and time-effect curve. Six hundred fifty milligrams of ASA or APAP are **equianalgesic** to 200 mg of ibuprofen; 200 mg of ibuprofen is equianalgesic to 275 mg of naproxen sodium. Consequently, over-the-counter (OTC) formulations of ASA, APAP, ibuprofen, or naproxen sodium are the drugs of choice for the management of *mild odontogenic pain*.

Aspirin

In doses of 650 or 1,000 mg, ASA is effective against dull, throbbing pain of odontogenic origin, which is invariably associated with inflammation. Despite its proven efficacy, ASA has gained a bad reputation with many clinicians and patients. This reputation seems to be based more on an exaggerated notion of the drug's potential adverse effects than on its pharmacological properties. The traditional adult single dose of ASA is 650 mg every 4 hours (two 325-mg tablets). It is supplied in both 325-mg tablets and 500-mg tablets. Either dose is effective for mild pain relief. Single doses larger than 1,300 mg (four 325-mg tablets) are above the ceiling dose (discussed in Chapter 2), do not appreciably increase pain relief, and may prove toxic in some clients. Differences in the amount of a single dose and the interval between doses have only a minor effect on the steady state of ASA, which is produced by the total daily dose of the drug the patient takes. What this means is that if one takes ASA around the clock for several days (650 mg q4h), the clinical effect is not determined by the size of a single dose, but by the total dose (not to exceed 4,000 mg) in a 24-hour period. For children, the appropriate dosage is 10 to 20 mg/kg of body weight, given in four to six doses. For adults, the maximum daily dose of ASA for pain management should not exceed 4,000 mg; for children, the maximum dose is 1,200 mg.

Interactions

ASA interacts with many drugs due to its high affinity for protein-binding in the plasma. Recalling information in Chapter 2, ASA binds to plasma protein and may prevent a second drug from binding. This can cause high plasma levels of the second drug, resulting in increased effects. Table 8-4 identifies the most common drug interactions with ASA and the effects of the interactions. It includes the recommended clinical considerations for the treatment plan.

Most drugs used in dentistry or prescribed by the dentist are not adversely affected when the patient is taking ASA. However, when a client is taking a drug prescribed for a medical condition that interacts with ASA, the clinician must not recommend ASA for odontogenic pain relief.

Acetaminophen

One thousand milligrams of APAP is equianalgesic with 1,000 mg of ASA for the relief of mild-to-moderate odontogenic pain, but it has no clinically appreciable anti-inflammatory effect. The main analgesic mechanism appears to be inhibition of prostaglandins in the CNS, and this fact may account for its ability to reduce fever and to induce analgesia with minimal effects on inflammation. The frequency of adverse reactions with therapeutic doses is somewhat less than that associated with ASA. Its main danger is primarily in overdose, which causes a toxic, highly reactive metabolite to accumulate in the liver and results in serious, irreversible, and occasionally fatal liver damage. The traditional adult single dose of APAP is 650 mg every 4 hours. A ceiling dose of 1,000 mg is usually more effective than 650 mg. For children, the single dose is 60 to 120 mg, depending on the patient's age and weight. The daily dose should not exceed 4,000 mg for adults and 1,200 mg for children.

APAP is recommended by the American Arthritis College of Rheumatology as the drug of choice for long-term control of pain associated with osteoarthritis (bone-to-bone damage rather than joint inflammation), not to exceed the daily maximum dose. This recommendation is based on APAP's established analgesic effect and the lack of GI side effects associated with ASA or other COX-1 inhibitors. APAP has no appreciable anti-inflammatory effect and is not the recommended drug for the treatment of inflammatory conditions, such as rheumatoid arthritis. Some sources state that in patients with chronic alcoholism, the 4,000 mg daily dose should be halved to no more than 2,000 mg to avoid possible toxicity.[1] However a randomized, double-blind, placebo-controlled trial showed that alcoholic patients and patients who drink alcohol could safely consume up to 4,000 mg/day of APAP.[2] Alcoholics frequently have problems with GI bleeding, which is aggravated by ASA and other COX-1 inhibitors. New research shows that APAP can be used safely in patients with liver disease and is the preferred analgesic because of the absence of platelet impairment, GI toxicity (ulcerations, bleeding), and nephrotoxicity associated with other COX-I.[3] Therapeutic APAP doses (4,000 mg/day) are safe for treating dental pain in the patient with alcohol-related liver disease.[4]

Interactions

There are no significant drug interactions between APAP and drugs used by the dentist. However, patient self-medication can result in toxic effects when several different APAP products are taken for pain relief. Take, for example, the individual who is given a prescription of Lorcet 10/650 (10 mg hydrocodone, 650 mg APAP) for dental pain, to be taken twice daily, and whose pain is not relieved. The patient then self-medicates with four doses of 1,000 mg of APAP for a few days, along with Lorcet. The result is a daily dose of 5,300 mg of APAP, a toxic dose. This scenario appears to be a common one in case reports of APAP toxicity. Some interactions between APAP and other commonly taken drugs are discussed in the next section. Table 8-5 identifies common drug interactions with APAP and the effects of the interactions. It includes the recommended clinical considerations for the treatment plan.

WARFARIN (COUMADIN)   There is one report of increased anticoagulation leading to excessive bleeding when warfarin (Coumadin) is taken with therapeutic doses of APAP for 6 days. The risk for hemorrhage with warfarin is measured with a blood test referred to as the International Normalized Ratio (INR). Safe levels of the INR are between 2 to 3 for surgical procedures, and 3.5 for periodontal débridement. The patient's INR levels increased after a daily intake equivalent to only four regular-strength (325-mg) tablets of APAP was ingested during 1 week.[5] When warfarin is reported on the health history and an analgesic is needed for oral pain, APAP is appropriate, with the warning that the INR levels be checked when analgesic therapy exceeds 4 to 5 days.

Secondary Line of Treatment (Moderate-to-Severe Odontogenic Pain)

Ibuprofen and naproxen sodium are both COX-1 inhibitors and can be used for either the first line of analgesic treatment or second line of treatment, depending on the dosage. The cardiovascular safety profile is not statistically significantly different between the two drugs, but it is clearly better than that of COX-2 inhibitors.[6] OTC formulations of ibuprofen (Advil, Motrin IB, Rufen) contain 200 mg per dose, while naproxen sodium (Aleve) contains 220 mg per dose. Prescription formulations of ibuprofen may contain 400, 600, or 800 mg per dose. Prescription formulations of naproxen sodium may contain 275 mg (Anaprox); 550 mg (Anaprox DS); 375 or 500 mg (EC Naprosyn); or 250, 375, or 500 mg (Naprosyn). Prescription formulations with increased doses are indicated for increased anti-inflammatory effects and are used for conditions involving inflammation, such as rheumatoid arthritis. The analgesic efficacy of these formulations increases as the dose increases, not to exceed the ceiling dose within a 24-hour period. Both the analgesic and anti-inflammatory efficacy of ibuprofen and naproxen increases with each incremental dose, up to a maximum daily dose of 2,400 mg (ibuprofen) and 1,375 mg (naproxen sodium). The anti-inflammatory efficacy may increase with doses above these ceiling doses, but so will the adverse effects.

COX-1 Inhibitors

COX-1 inhibitors alone, in combination with APAP, or in combination with codeine or hydrocodone are the *drugs of choice for the management of moderate-to-severe odontogenic pain*. In the management of acute moderate-to-severe odontogenic pain, ceiling doses of COX-1 inhibitors (ibuprofen, 2,400 mg; naproxen sodium, 1,375 mg) are as effective

Table 8-5	APAP Interactions and Clinical Considerations	
Cholestyramine	Decreased APAP effect (unknown mechanism)	Administer APAP 1 hour before cholestyramine
Contraceptive, oral	Possible decreased analgesic effect (increased metabolism)	Monitor analgesia
Isoniazid	APAP toxicity (increase in toxic metabolites)	Avoid concurrent use
Phenytoin	Possible increased APAP toxicity (increase in toxic metabolites)	Avoid concurrent use
Probenecid	Possible APAP toxicity (decreased metabolism and renal excretion)	Avoid concurrent use
Sulfinpyrazone	Possible decreased APAP effect (increased metabolism)	Monitor analgesia

---

BOX 8-2. List of Nonselective COX-1 Inhibitors

Propionic Acid Derivatives
- Ibuprofen
- Flurbiprofen
- Fenoprofen
- Naproxen
- Naproxen sodium
- Ketoprofen

Acetic Acid Derivatives
- Indomethacin
- Sulindac
- Tolmetin
- Diclofenac
- Etodolac
- Ketoprofen
- Ketorolac

Others
- Nabumetone
- Mefenamic acid
- Diflunisal
- Piroxicam

---

as, or more effective than, full doses of ASA (4,000 mg) or APAP (4,000 mg). Some have also been shown to be as effective as, or more effective than, oral opioids, such as codeine, hydrocodone, propoxyphene, and pentazocine, in combination with ASA or APAP. Propoxyphene and pentazocine, even in combination with ASA or APAP, offer no clinically relevant advantage for dental pain over codeine or hydrocodone combinations.

Other COX-1 inhibitors are listed in Box 8-2. Agents in the class, such as diclofenac, diflunisal, etodolac, fenoprofen, flurbiprofen, ketoprofen, and meclofenamate, offer no apparent advantage over ibuprofen or naproxen for dental pain. The oral administration of ketorolac, which is also available in a parenteral formulation, is restricted to those patients who might benefit further from the drug following its parenteral administration. COX-1 inhibitors are the drugs of choice for dental pain when substance abuse (other than alcohol) is suspected or when an individual has a history of substance abuse and is in recovery. Prescribing an opioid analgesic can cause substance abuse recovery to fail. A COX-2 inhibitor may reduce some of the adverse effects associated with COX-1 inhibitors; however, recent evidence of potential cardiovascular events associated with COX-2 inhibitors mandates caution in their use in the oral health care setting. The only COX-2 inhibitor currently on the market is celecoxib (Celebrex).

Interactions
Before recommending a COX-inhibitor analgesic, potential drug interactions should be checked in a drug reference.

Ibuprofen

Four hundred milligrams of ibuprofen has been shown to be more effective for dental pain than ceiling doses of ASA or APAP. It has been shown to be more effective than 60 mg of codeine, 650 mg of ASA with 60 mg of codeine, or 600 mg of APAP with 60 mg of codeine. Ibuprofen, in doses between 400 to 800 mg, has a longer duration of action and appears to have a dose-dependent increase in its analgesic and anti-inflammatory efficacy. It has also been shown that 650 mg of APAP in combination with 200 mg of ibuprofen is more effective than either 650 mg of APAP or 200 mg of ibuprofen alone, inferring a synergistic effect.

Interactions
Table 8-6 identifies common drug interactions with ibuprofen and the effects of the interactions. It includes the recommended clinical considerations for the treatment plan.

Naproxen

The following represents the efficacy and duration of naproxen formulations. Naproxen 250 mg is equianalgesic with 650 mg of ASA, but it has a longer duration of action. Naproxen 500 mg is superior in analgesic effect to 650 mg of ASA. Naproxen sodium (Anaprox) 220 mg is equianalgesic to 650 mg of ASA, with a longer duration of action. Naproxen sodium 550 mg is superior to 650 mg of ASA. Naproxen sodium, 220 mg and 440 mg, is equianalgesic with 200 and 400 mg of ibuprofen, respectively, but has a longer duration of action.

Interactions
Table 8-7 identifies common drug interactions with naproxen and the effects of the interactions. It includes the recommended clinical considerations for the treatment plan.

COX-Inhibitor/Opioid Combinations

In some clinical situations, when the patient response to ceiling doses of a COX-I is inadequate, the administration of a COX-1 (ASA or ibuprofen) or COX-3 (APAP) inhibitor, in combination with codeine or hydrocodone, may be appropriate. Codeine and hydrocodone are converted by the CYP2D6 hepatic microsomal isoenzyme into their active morphine analogs. Because of genetic polymorphism, this may lead to severe toxicity or lack of analgesic response in some patients. The analgesic, respiratory, psychomotor, and miotic effects of codeine and hydrocodone are markedly diminished by the CYP2D6 enzyme in people with poor metabolism. Conversely, for people with ultrarapid metabolism, the greater amount of morphine being produced will result in exaggerated pharmacological effects and may lead to life-threatening opioid intoxication. In prescribing codeine or hydrocodone formulations, clinicians should also be conscious of the fact that 60 mg of codeine and 10 mg of hydrocodone are no more effective than 650 mg of ASA, 650 mg of APAP, or 200 mg of ibuprofen, and they are much more expensive.

Interactions
Table 8-8 identifies a common drug interaction with COX-inhibitor/opioid combination products and the effect of the

Table 8-6	Ibuprofen Interactions and Clinical Considerations	
ACE inhibitors	Decreased antihypertensive effect (decreased prostaglandin synthesis)	Monitor blood pressure
Anticoagulants, oral	Increased bleeding (platelet inhibition)	Avoid concurrent use
ASA	Inhibition of antiplatelet effect of ASA (blocks access of ASA to active site)	Administer ibuprofen 30 minutes after ASA, or administer ASA 8 hours after ibuprofen
Beta-adrenergic blockers	Decreased antihypertensive effect (decreased prostaglandin synthesis)	Monitor blood pressure
Corticosteroids	Increased risk of peptic ulcer disease (additive)	Avoid concurrent use
Furosemide	Decreased antihypertensive effect (decreased prostaglandin synthesis)	Monitor blood pressure
Lithium	Lithium toxicity (decreased renal excretion)	Avoid concurrent use
Methotrexate	Possible methotrexate toxicity (decreased renal excretion)	Avoid concurrent use
Naltrexone	Possible increased hepatotoxicity (mechanism unknown)	Avoid concurrent use
Thiazide diuretics	Decreased antihypertensive effect (decreased prostaglandin synthesis)	Monitor blood pressure
Valproate	Possible increased valproate toxicity (displacement from binding site)	Monitor clinical status

interaction. It includes the recommended clinical consideration for the treatment plan. Opioid-receptor agonists are additive with other CNS depressants. ASA, ibuprofen, and APAP interactions must be considered when the combination product is used.

Tramadol

Tramadol (Ultram) is a nonopioid agent that binds to opioid-receptors to produce an analgesic effect. It also blocks the reuptake of norepinephrine and serotonin, which can result in mood elevation. The therapeutic benefit is that it appears to have fewer associated adverse effects than opioid analgesics. In the management of acute odontogenic pain, 50 mg of tramadol was equianalgesic to 60 mg of codeine. In patients with dental pain, two 37.5/325-mg tablets of tramadol/APAP were more effective than one tablet, and they were as effective as hydrocodone/APAP (10/650 mg). Tramadol in combination with APAP may be an appropriate alternative for the management of acute odontogenic pain in those situations where COX-1 inhibitors or opioid analgesics are contraindicated, such as peptic ulcer disease or substance abuse recovery.

Table 8-7	Naproxen Interactions and Clinical Considerations	
Alendronate	Increased risk of gastric ulcers (additive)	Avoid concurrent use
ACE-inhibitors	Decreased antihypertensive effect (decreased prostaglandin synthesis)	Monitor blood pressure
ASA	Inhibition of antiplatelet effect of ASA (blocks access to active site on platelets)	Administer naproxen 2 hours before or 2 hours after immediate release ASA, or avoid concurrent use
Famotidine and ranitidine	Possible decreased naproxen effect (unknown mechanism)	Monitor analgesia
Diazepam	Possible decreased onset of action of naproxen (delayed absorption)	Monitor analgesia
Cholestyramine	Possible decreased naproxen effect (delayed absorption)	Monitor analgesia
Clopidogrel	Increased GI bleeding (additive antiplatelet effect)	Avoid concurrent use
Corticosteroids	Increased risk of peptic ulcer disease (additive)	Avoid concurrent use
Furosemide	Decreased antihypertensive effect (decreased prostaglandin synthesis)	Monitor blood pressure
Misoprostol	Ataxia (unknown mechanism)	Avoid concurrent use
Naltrexone	Possible increased risk of hepatotoxicity (unknown mechanism)	Avoid concurrent use
Probenecid	Possible naproxen toxicity (decreased renal excretion)	Avoid concurrent use
Thiazide diuretics	Decreased antihypertensive effect (decreased prostaglandin synthesis)	Monitor blood pressure

Table 8-8	Codeine/Hydrocodone Interaction and Clinical Consideration	
Bupivacaine	Possible respiratory depression with codeine (unknown mechanism)	Use bupivacaine with caution

Table 8-10	Oxycodone Interaction and Clinical Consideration	
Sertraline	Possible increased serotonin syndrome (unknown mechanism)	Monitor clinical status

Interactions

Table 8-9 identifies common drug interactions with tramadol and the effects of the interactions. It includes the recommended clinical considerations for the treatment plan. Opioid-receptor agonists are additive with other CNS depressants. APAP interactions must also be considered.

Tertiary Line of Treatment (Severe Pain)

The opioid meperidine (Demerol) is not recommended for oral administration and is not used for the management of acute postoperative dental or medical pain in ambulatory patients. Oral doseforms of the opioids morphine, hydromorphone, methadone, levorphanol, and oxycodone are all effective in the management of severe pain. These drugs can relieve practically all forms of pain, both **somatic pain** (caused by the activation of pain receptors in mucocutaneous or musculoskeletal tissues) and **visceral pain** (caused by the activation of pain receptors in internal organs). Of these, oxycodone in combination with a COX-1 (ASA or ibuprofen) or a COX-3 (APAP) inhibitor is the *drug of choice for the management of severe odontogenic pain*. In oral doses, 10 mg of oxycodone is equianalgesic with 90 mg of codeine. A single dose of 5 mg of oxycodone with 400 mg of ibuprofen has been shown to be more effective than 5 mg of oxycodone alone, 400 mg of ibuprofen alone, or a placebo in the management of acute odontogenic pain following extractions.

Interactions

Table 8-10 identifies a common drug interaction with COX-I/opioid combination products and the effect of the interaction. It includes the recommended clinical procedure to include in the treatment plan. Opioid-receptor agonists are additive with other CNS depressants. ASA, ibuprofen, and APAP interactions must also be considered.

■ Self-Study Review

20. List factors that can delay absorption of COX-I.
21. Why are some opioids given by injection?
22. Describe the purpose of "by-the-clock" administration of analgesics.
23. Identify analgesics for mild odontogenic pain and their appropriate doses.
24. What is the main potential problem with ASA when other drugs are taken?
25. Can APAP be recommended to individuals who drink alcohol? If so, what are the dosing instructions?
26. What is the ceiling dose of APAP? What is the maximum dose (child, adult)?
27. What is the drug of choice for moderate-severe dental pain for an individual with a history of substance abuse?
28. List available COX-2 inhibitor(s).
29. Identify the agent(s) most effective for relieving dental pain. What dosage is most efficacious?
30. Which COX-I is most efficacious when a long duration of analgesia is desired?
31. Describe the indication, classification, benefits, and dose of tramadol for dental pain.
32. Discuss agents for the tertiary treatment of odontogenic pain.

Table 8-9	Tramadol Interactions and Clinical Considerations	
Warfarin	Bleeding into skin (unknown mechanism)	Avoid concurrent use
Antidepressants, tricyclic	Increased risk of seizure (additive proconvulsants)	Avoid concurrent use
Carbamazepine	Decreased tramadol effect (increased metabolism)	Avoid concurrent use
Citalopram	Increased risk of seizure (additive proconvulsants)	Avoid concurrent use
Fluoxetine	Increased risk of seizure (additive proconvulsants)	Avoid concurrent use
Fluvoxamine	Increased risk of seizure (additive proconvulsants)	Avoid concurrent use
Monoamine oxidase inhibitors	Increased risk of serotonin syndrome (reduced uptake of monoamines)	Avoid concurrent use
Olanzapine	Increased risk of serotonin syndrome (unknown mechanism)	Avoid concurrent use
Ondansetron	Possible decreased tramadol effect (antagonism at serotonin receptors)	Monitor analgesia
Paroxetine	Increased risk of seizure (additive proconvulsants)	Avoid concurrent use
Sertraline	Increased risk of seizure (additive proconvulsants), serotonin syndrome (additive serotonergic effect)	Avoid concurrent use

Adverse Drug Events

Cyclooxygenase Inhibitors

Intolerance

Intolerance to COX-I (except APAP) is most likely to occur in individuals with a history of asthma, nasal polyps, and chronic urticaria. A single dose of these agents can precipitate asthma in susceptible patients, probably related to increased levels of leukotrienes that result when COX inhibition occurs. A history of rhinorrhea, urticaria, angioedema, or bronchospasm occurring within 3 hours after exposure to a COX-I is an acceptable method of determining intolerance. There is a cross-sensitivity between ASA and other COX-1 inhibitors, so when an allergy to ASA is reported, COX-1 inhibitors should not be recommended. APAP is usually well tolerated. However, an erythematous or urticarial skin rash has occurred with APAP, accompanied at times by fever and mucosal lesions. The mechanism of intolerance to APAP is unknown. Uncommonly, COX-inhibitors can cause IgE-dependent hypersensitivity reactions leading to vasomotor collapse (hypotension, cardiac arrest). Lichenoid reactions (Color Plates 36 and 37) and erythema multiforme (Color Plates 38 to 40) have occurred with COX-I.

Gastrointestinal Effects

Therapeutic doses of ASA and other COX-1 inhibitors may cause epigastric discomfort, nausea, and vomiting. They can exacerbate the symptoms of peptic ulcer disease and with chronic use, bleeding, ulceration, and perforation can occur. Gastric bleeding induced by ASA and other COX-1 inhibitors is painless and may lead to iron-deficiency anemia. In this patient population, APAP appears to be a suitable alternative to COX-1 inhibitors in the management of acute odontogenic pain. The COX-2 inhibitor celecoxib (Celebrex) has been associated with abdominal pain, diarrhea, and dyspepsia, although this class of drugs was originally thought to have a protective effect on gastric mucosa.

Antithrombotic Effects

COX-1 inhibitors impair platelet adhesion to tissue components and platelet aggregation, primarily through the inhibition of thromboxane A_2 synthesis, a component of the COX cascade. ASA is available OTC as a tablet, buffered tablet, effervescent tablet, or caplet in immediate-release formulations, and as a tablet in enteric-coated formulations in strengths ranging from 81 to 500 mg. Any of these ASA formulations, even a single dose, will result in a prolongation of the bleeding time (BT) because ASA prevents platelets from adhering to the site of injury and the subsequent aggregation of platelets from forming a clot. This may be identified as petechia on oral mucosal surfaces (Color Plate 10). This effect, which is dose independent, lasts for the life span of the affected platelets (~8 days) and increases the bleeding time for 4 to 7 days after the last dose of ASA. In contrast to ASA, with therapeutic doses of other COX-1 inhibitors (ibuprofen, naproxen) platelet inhibition is reversible and short lived because platelet function returns to normal when most of these drugs have been eliminated from the body. It has been demon-strated that 100 mg of ASA did not increase the bleeding time over the level of safe use (<20 minutes), making low-dose ASA safe for oral procedures involving bleeding.[7]

In general, it can be anticipated that antiplatelet drugs used in the secondary prevention of thromboembolic disease can cause intraoperative and postoperative hemorrhagic complications. However, discontinuation of these drugs before an invasive procedure exposes the patient to thromboembolic episodes with the potential for significant morbidity. It is well documented that therapeutic doses of ASA do not significantly increase intraoperative and postoperative bleeding in association with dental surgical procedures.[7–9] When intraoperative or postoperative bleeding does occur, local hemostatic measures are usually effective in resolving the problem. Clearly, oral surgical procedures can be carried out safely without stopping long-term low-dose ASA therapy.[7] However, high hemorrhagic risk has been documented in patients taking ASA with concomitant severe hepatic disease, vitamin-K deficiency, hereditary coagulopathies, and in those treated with anticoagulants (warfarin, heparin). Such patients should have a medical consultation to determine their overall risk for excessive bleeding preoperatively. Currently available tests to evaluate hemostasis include the prothrombin time (PT), converted to the INR, and the partial thromboplastin time (PTT), which are discussed in greater detail in Chapter 17 (Box 8-3). In the past, the primary screening test for platelet dysfunction was the bleeding time (Ivy technique normal range: 2 to 10 minutes). However, many medical laboratories are no longer offering the test, and several national organizations have issued position statements against its routine use as a presurgical screen. The bleeding time is not sensitive or specific, and it does not necessarily reflect the risk or severity of surgical bleeding. It is poorly reproducible, can be affected by the skill of the individual performing the test, and frequently leaves small thin scars. The Platelet Function Analyzer-100 (PFA-100) is the test that many medical laboratories are now using as a platelet function screen in place of the BT. The PFA-100 (normal range: 85 to 176 seconds) is a rapid, simple, reproducible screening tool that reflects the bleeding tendency for ASA and other antiplatelet therapy agents.

Risks in Pregnancy

Although there is no evidence that therapeutic doses of ASA cause any fetal abnormalities other than reduced birth weight, the drug should be avoided throughout pregnancy (putting it in pregnancy category C). In addition, excessive intrapartum and postpartum maternal bleeding, with a potential for life-threatening hemorrhage, has been noted when ingestion has occurred within 5 days of delivery. As with ASA, an increased incidence of postpartum bleeding has been observed in patients taking other COX-1 inhibitors. In addition, the administration of COX-1 inhibitors (ibuprofen) during pregnancy may lead to fetal cardiac failure (premature closure of the ductus arteriosus between the pulmonary artery and the aorta).[10] As gestation progresses, the sensitivity of the ductus to the dilating effect of prostaglandins decreases, yet at the same time its sensitivity to constricting agents (COX-I) increases. This effect is least likely to occur in response to ASA; however, all COX-1 inhibitors should be avoided

BOX 8-3. Strategies for the Management of a Patient Taking ASA or Other COX-1 Inhibitors

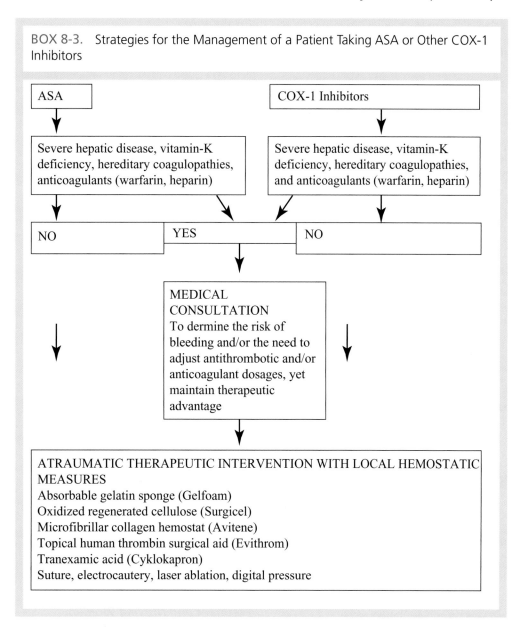

during pregnancy.[9] For pregnant patients, APAP is a suitable substitute for ASA and other COX-1 inhibitors in the management of mild-to-moderate pain.

Local and Systemic Salicylate Toxicity

Local toxicity of ASA is often seen in patients who place a tablet of ASA on the mucosa adjacent to a painful tooth, causing a chemical burn (Color Plate 5). In its free acid form, ASA destroys epithelial cells by producing cellular edema and desquamation and may damage peripheral nerve fibers. In an overdose, ASA causes salicylate toxicity, called *salicylism*, which represents an acute medical emergency. Clinical symptoms and signs include tinnitus, headache, mental confusion, sweating, thirst, and hyperventilation. Hyperthermia, dehydration, and renal dysfunction are associated with ASA

overdose and can lead to delirium, convulsions, and coma, which may result in death. In the young, ASA intoxication is easily diagnosed and is associated with low mortality (2%). Patients with delayed diagnosis of ASA intoxication are usually older, more often become accidentally intoxicated while ingesting ASA for a medical illness, and have a higher mortality risk (25%).

Hepatic Toxicity

Adverse hepatic reactions have been reported in association with ASA and most other COX-1 inhibitors. They appear to be idiosyncratic and often dose-related. Predisposing factors for toxic reactions include advanced age, decreased renal function, and collagen vascular diseases. Lower doses of the drugs should be used when factors predisposing to liver toxicity are present and monitoring liver function tests with chronic use is reasonable. An association has also been reported between Reye syndrome (acute hepatic necrosis) and the administration of ASA to children and teenagers with acute viral illnesses (influenza, chickenpox). For this reason ASA is contraindicated in children when viral infection is suspected.

APAP is metabolized primarily by hepatic conjugation. In high doses, APAP is converted by the CYP2E1 isoenzyme into a hepatotoxic metabolite. Alcohol in the presence of malnutrition may enhance this toxicity in some individuals (Color Plates 1 and 2). When this occurs, nausea, vomiting, anorexia, diarrhea, and abdominal pain occur during the first 24 hours. Clinical evidence of hepatic damage may be noted in 2 to 6 days (jaundice). When the drug's half-life exceeds 12 hours, hepatic coma and death are likely.

Renal Toxicity

COX-I decrease the synthesis of renal prostaglandins, decrease renal blood flow, cause fluid retention, and may precipitate renal failure in susceptible patients. Risk factors include old age, chronic renal insufficiency, congestive heart failure, hepatic cirrhosis, and concurrent diuretic use. Renal toxicity is uncommon even with high therapeutic doses and prolonged use of ASA. However, nephrotic syndrome, acute interstitial nephritis, and an increased incidence of end-stage renal disease have been reported in patients treated chronically with other COX-1, COX-2, and COX-3 inhibitors.

■ Self-Study Review

33. Identify potential adverse drug events associated with COX-I.
34. Describe the mechanism for antithrombotic effects of COX-I and dose levels resulting in an increased bleeding time. When will normal bleeding time resume?
35. Identify conditions that contraindicate use of ASA.
36. Identify safe levels for coagulation tests.
37. Describe the risks of taking COX-I during pregnancy. Which analgesic is indicated during pregnancy?
38. List potential toxic effects of salicylates.
39. Describe the potential for renal toxicity when COX-I are taken.

Opioid-Receptor Agonists
Gastropathy

Nausea, vomiting, and constipation are the most common adverse effects of opioid analgesics. Nausea and vomiting directly results from stimulation of the chemoreceptor trigger zone in the medulla. Depression of the vomiting center occurs late in intoxication. Opioid-induced constipation is a result of decreased GI motility. Some opioid preparations, such as loperamide (Imodium), are effective and fast-acting antidiarrheal agents, although they do not produce analgesia.

Intolerance

Allergic reactions to opioid analgesics are rare. However, some opioids are able to induce histamine release from mast cells and cause peripheral vasodilatation and orthostatic hypotension (pseudoallergic reaction). The cutaneous blood vessels tend to dilate around the "blush areas," such as the face, neck, and upper thorax.

Cardiovascular Effects

Opioids promote the release of histamine, which leads to vasodilation. In the supine patient, this may lead to orthostatic hypotension. In patients with coronary artery disease, opioids will decrease oxygen consumption in cardiovascular muscle, making them the preferred analgesics in patients with ischemic heart disease.

Respiratory Effects

Opioids depress respiratory sensitivity to carbon dioxide. Concurrent administration of oxygen may cause apnea. Carbon dioxide retention produces intracranial vasodilatation and may aggravate increased intracranial pressure. Opioids should be used with great caution in patients with head injuries, the elderly, the debilitated, and those with pulmonary disease, particularly severe asthma. Precautions are because of cough reflex suppression, impairment of ciliary activity, and aggravation of bronchospasm. Respiratory depression is the most common cause of death in an opioid overdose.

Central Nervous System Effects

Opioids modulate mood and behavior, causing drowsiness and euphoria in some, and anxiety and dysphoria in others. They produce miosis as a result of an excitatory action on the autonomic segment of the nucleus of the oculomotor nerve. The miosis is marked and pinpoint pupils are **pathognomonic** of opioid use/abuse, such as with heroin overdose.

Pregnant and Nursing Women

The use of opioids in the pregnant or nursing patient is discouraged because of their general CNS-depressant effects on the fetus and infant. However, short-term use of therapeutic doses of codeine in combination with APAP is appropriate for the management of moderate-to-severe odontogenic pain.

Geriatric Patients

A paradoxical sensitivity to CNS-depressant drugs in the elderly is not uncommon. Because of this, dosages must frequently be reduced by as much as one half to one fourth of the usual therapeutic dosage to avoid both toxic and paradoxical effects (dizziness, hallucination).

Tolerance

Tolerance is a feature of some drugs whereby one needs increased doses of the agent to achieve the former effect of the drug. It is influenced by dose, frequency (chronic use), and the specific opioid administered. *Cross-tolerance* is the resistance to one or several effects of a compound as a result of tolerance developed to a pharmacologically similar compound. Cross-tolerance among opioids has been observed. Tolerance develops to most of the adverse effects of opioids, including respiratory and CNS depression, at least as rapidly as tolerance to the analgesic effect. The result is that usual therapeutic doses will be less likely to cause some of the adverse effects. However, no tolerance develops to their GI (constipation) and papillary (miosis) actions.

Dependence

Patients who take opioids for acute pain rarely experience euphoria and even more rarely develop psychological dependence or addiction to their mood-altering effects. Clinically significant dependence develops only after several weeks of chronic treatment with relatively large doses. Because the duration of therapy for dental pain is short (<6 days), addiction is unlikely to develop from dental use of opioids. Opioids should not be prescribed, however, when a history of drug abuse is suspected or reported. Withdrawal symptoms from opioid abuse include dilated pupils, rapid pulse, gooseflesh, muscle jerks, a flulike syndrome, vomiting, diarrhea, tremors, yawning, and sleep. Opioid prescriptions for dental pain should be given for a short duration with no refills allowed.

Overdose

Opioid overdose is characterized by a variety of features, including constricted pupils (miosis), depressed-to-absent respiration with cyanosis (due to a depressed respiratory chemoreceptor sensitivity to carbon dioxide), hypotension (sometimes leading to shock), hypothermia, sedation, stupor, coma, and convulsions. The respiratory depressant effects of various opioid analgesics are comparable with equivalent doses (e.g., 10 mg of morphine, 20 mg of oxycodone, 130 mg of codeine), meaning equivalent doses will cause an equal degree of respiratory depression. The narcotic antagonist naloxone, administered by mouth, will reverse apnea and other effects of opioid toxicity. Seizures are managed with intramuscular or intravenous benzodiazepines, such as diazepam.

■ Self-Study Review

40. List common adverse effects of opioid analgesics.
41. Identify conditions that contraindicate use of opioids for odontogenic analgesia.
42. Identify the most likely cause of death from opioid toxicity.
43. Describe the effect of opioids on the CNS.
44. Are opioids appropriate for the pregnant or lactating woman?
45. Describe rules for opioid use in the elderly patient.
46. Describe effects of tolerance and dependence during opioid use.
47. Describe prescribing recommendations for opioids when used for dental pain.
48. What are symptoms of withdrawal from opioid intoxication?
49. Describe signs of opioid overdose.
50. Identify the opioid antagonist used for opioid toxicity.

DENTAL HYGIENE APPLICATIONS

The dental hygienist does not prescribe drugs. However, following therapeutic services that might result in pain, it is not uncommon to recommend OTC analgesics. When determining which product to recommend, the health history information and the analgesics contraindicated for various medical conditions should be considered. The drugs being taken should be investigated for drug interaction information before recommending an analgesic. Information should include a warning to not exceed the maximum dose of any drug recommended. A warning to check labels for ingredients included within products should be given to avoid overdosing by the patient. Warnings of significant side effects (such as GI bleeding or signs of allergy) associated with any drug should be provided to the client with notification to call the dental

CLINICAL APPLICATION EXERCISES

☐ **Exercise 1.** WEB ACTIVITY. Complete a Google (or any other search engine) search for the Top 200 Drugs for 2007. Print out the information for future reference.

☐ **Exercise 2.** Secure a dental drug reference. Find the drug monograph for APAP/hydrocodone bitartrate (combination products). List the clinical implications (or dental considerations) when the drug is prescribed by a dentist. Describe patient instructions when a hydrocodone/APAP analgesic combination is prescribed for pain following periodontal débridement (deep scaling).

☐ **Exercise 3.** Secure a drug reference and identify brand names for drugs containing ASA and brand names for APAP.

☐ **Exercise 4.** The medical history of a client includes asthma. A two-quadrant periodontal débridement with local anesthesia has just been completed, and postoperative discomfort is probable. What follow-up question should be asked before recommending a COX-I analgesic for orodental pain?

office should the adverse reaction occur. When APAP is already being taken and the dentist prescribes an APAP/opioid combination, warnings should be given about the need to refrain from taking additional APAP from OTC products due to the risk for exceeding the maximum dosage. When a GI side effect, such as pain in the stomach area, is reported, a semisupine chair position should be used during treatment for client comfort. GI bleeding is a potential adverse side effect with some analgesics and should be reported to the physician. Before recommending any drug, questioning to determine if the drug has been taken in the past should be completed.

CONCLUSION

In practice, the efficacy of any particular analgesic in a specific patient will be determined by the degree of analgesia produced following the use of minimum to maximum doses and limited by the development of adverse effects and medical conditions contraindicating the use of the analgesic. After determining the appropriate analgesic, clinicians should prescribe an adequate dose, and give it soon enough, often enough, and long enough for the specific pain. They should prescribe as they would receive. Potential side effects should be communicated to the patient, as well as clear dosing instructions.

References

1. Drug Facts & Comparisons. Wolters Kluwer Health. 2008:820a.
2. Kuffner EK, Dart RC, Bogdan GM, et al. Effect of maximal daily doses of acetaminophen on the liver of alcoholic patients: A randomized, double-blind, placebo-controlled trial. *Arch Intern Med.* 2001;161:2247–2252.
3. Benson GD, Koff RS, Tolman KG. The therapeutic use of acetaminophen in patients with liver disease. *Am J Ther.* 2005; 12(2):133–141.
4. Glick M. Medical considerations for dental care of patients with alcohol-related liver disease. *J Am Dent Assoc.* 1997;128:61–69.
5. Hylek EM, Heiman H, Skates SJ, et al. Acetaminophen and other risk factors for excessive warfarin anticoagulation. *JAMA.* 1998;279:657–662.
6. McGettigan P, Henry D. Cardiovascular risk and inhibition of cyclooxygenase: A systematic review of the observational studies of selective and nonselective inhibitors of cyclooxygenase 2. *JAMA.* 2006;296(13):E1–E12.
7. Ardekian L, Gaspar R, Peled M, et al. Does low-dose aspirin therapy complicate oral surgical procedures? *J Am Dent Assoc.* 2000;131:331–335.
8. Sonksen JR, Kong KL, Holder R. Magnitude and time course of impaired haemostasis after stopping chronic low and medium dose aspirin in healthy volunteers. *Br J Anaesth.* 1999;82:360–365.
9. Rogerson KC. Hemostasis for dental surgery. *Dent Clin North Am.* 1999;39:649–662.
10. Schessl B, Schneider KT, Zimmerman A, et al. Prenatal constriction of the fetal ductus arteriosus related to maternal pain medication. *Z Geburtshilfe Neonatol.* 2005;209(2):65–68.

9

Antibacterial Drugs

KEY TERMS

Aerobic: An organism that can live only in the presence of oxygen

Anaerobic: An organism that can live in the absence of oxygen

Antibacterial: A drug used to kill or suppress the growth of bacteria

Antibiotic: A chemical substance produced by one microorganism (or semisynthetic substances prepared in the laboratory) that is capable of killing or suppressing the growth of other microorganisms (bacteria, virus, and fungus)

Antibiotic drug resistance: A trait acquired by microorganisms, either through genetic mutation or by the acquisition of genetic material from other organisms, that allows microorganisms to resist the action of specific antibiotics

Autogenous infection: An infection caused by normal flora bacteria

Bactericidal: An antibacterial agent capable of killing bacteria

Bacteriostatic: An antibacterial agent capable of suppressing the growth/multiplication of bacteria

Facultative: An organism able to live in either the presence or the absence of oxygen

Loading dose: An initial dose of a drug (larger than subsequent maintenance doses) that is administered to achieve therapeutic levels with only one or two doses of the drug

Suprainfection: Opportunistic infection caused by the overgrowth of microorganisms that are not susceptible to antibacterial therapy

KEY ACRONYMS

IE: Infective endocarditis

TJR: Total joint replacement

Dental hygienists need to understand general information about infection, conditions that determine when antibacterial agents are indicated, signs of adverse reactions that should be reported to the dentist, and patient instructions on how to take antibacterial agents. In addition, the dental hygienist must monitor the use of antibacterial agents for antibiotic prophylaxis and record a description of "what, when, and how much?" in the treatment record. Antibacterial agents taken for medical reasons should be investigated with attention paid to the reason for which the antibacterial agent was administered (Is there risk for cross-contamination to the clinician?) and to identify potential adverse drug effects that may influence the treatment plan, such as stained mucosa (minocycline), candidiasis, or nausea (erythromycin, tetracycline). Although dental hygienists do not prescribe antibacterial agents, many states allow the dental hygienist to place antibacterial agents by topical application. Understanding the indications for and limitations of antibacterial agents will assist the practitioner in fulfilling these duties.

INDICATIONS FOR ANTIBACTERIAL AGENTS

An **antibacterial** agent is destructive to or prevents the growth of bacteria. The term is often used synonymously with **antibiotic**, although the term antibiotic applies to antiviral and antifungal agents as well. Antibacterial agents are used in dentistry for two basic purposes: For the treatment of infection not resolved after removing the causative factors with primary dental care (débridement, endodontics, tooth extraction) and for antibiotic prophylaxis. Many classes of antibacterial agents are available; however, only a few classes are used in dentistry. This chapter focuses on those agents used for dentoalveolar infection, as well as on the roles of the dental hygienist in antibacterial therapy, including patient-questioning issues regarding antibiotic prophylaxis prior to dental treatment. The dental hygienist does not prescribe drugs; therefore, most pharmacokinetic information is not relevant to clinical dental hygiene practice. Pharmacology texts in the past have focused on drug information necessary for prescribing antibiotics, but this text focuses on clinical applications of pharmacologic information, which is considered to be most relevant to the dental hygienist.

Normal Flora and Infection

The human fetus is free of microorganisms. After initial exposure at birth, most organisms are soon eliminated, but others become permanently established, and the dynamic process of colonization begins. The adult body harbors a dense, diverse, indigenous flora that includes bacteria, viruses, fungi, and protozoa. Interaction between these various microbial ecosystems determines the normal flora, which represents the population of microorganisms inhabiting both the internal and external surfaces of healthy individuals. Microorganisms of the normal flora establish symbiotic relationships (mutualist, commensal, or parasitic) with their human host and with each other.

Factors that modify or shift the balanced environment of the normal flora (age, altered anatomy, diet, local and systemic conditions, or pharmacotherapy) may predispose an individual to infection. *Infection* may be defined as the invasion and multiplication of microorganisms in body tissues, resulting in local cellular injury due to competitive metabolism, toxin production, or immune-mediated reactions. An infection may be an **autogenous infection**, caused by the body's normal flora. In this situation, normal flora has become pathogenic. A common example is candidiasis, which can develop following the use of antibacterial agents (which reduce the numbers of flora organisms that usually prevent the overgrowth of *Candida albicans*). Or it may be a cross-infection, commonly related to the proliferation of transient microorganisms obtained from other humans, animals, or the environment.

PHARMACOTHERAPEUTIC BASIS OF ANTIBACTERIAL CHEMOTHERAPY

In treating bacterial infections, the common thread in pharmacologic strategies is to target differences between prokaryotic (bacterial) and eukaryotic (host or body) cells. Selective toxicity to bacterial cells that preserves host cells can be achieved by (a) attacking targets unique to bacteria that are not present in host cells, (b) attacking targets in bacteria similar but not identical to those in host cells, and (c) attacking targets in bac-

teria that are shared by the host cells, but vary in importance between bacteria and host cells.

- Unique target: Because human cells do not have cell walls, the bacterial cell wall, which is essential for the survival of growing bacteria, is a unique target for antibacterial drugs.
- Similar targets: While many bacteria have metabolic pathways similar to those of host cells, they possess different enzyme or receptor isoforms.
- Shared targets: Both bacteria and host cells synthesize proteins, but they utilize different-sized ribosomes, different ribosomal RNAs, and different amino acids.

Drugs exhibit the least toxicity to host cells when they target unique differences in the two cell types and increasingly more toxicity when they target shared pathways. The ratio of the toxic dose to the therapeutic dose (therapeutic index), therefore, is an indication of the degree of selectivity of a drug in producing the desired effect.

Rules for Antibacterial Drug Selection

Before focusing attention upon the selected groups of chemotherapeutic agents, it is important to review basic rules for prescribing antibacterial agents (Box 9-1). First, it is important to realize that even the most effective antibacterial agent will not generally "cure" an infection simply by virtue of its action on the microorganism. Débridement to remove infectious debris and the actions of an appropriate host immune response (chemotaxis, phagocytosis, and antibody formation) are also essential for resolution of the infection. **Bactericidal** agents, which can kill bacteria, depend less on the host immune response than **bacteriostatic** agents, which do not kill but slow the growth of microorganisms. Second, it is important to select an antibacterial agent based on its efficacy against specific bacteria (i.e., to select an antibacterial agent to which the infecting organism is susceptible). Third, when selecting an antibacterial agent from several equally effective alternatives, the one with the narrowest spectrum of activity should be selected. When broader spectrum antibacterial agents are used and harmless bacteria in the normal flora are killed or inhibited, the risk increases for overgrowth of unaffected microorganisms in the normal flora. This can result in **suprainfection**, a term used to describe opportunistic infection caused by the overgrowth of microorganisms that are not susceptible to antibacterial chemotherapy. It has been stated that 90% of oral infections are associated with gram-positive microorganisms. However, the preponderance of clinical studies in the recent past reveal that oral infections are polymicrobial, caused by gram-positive

facultative cocci and gram-negative bacilli that are strict anaerobes. In fact, by the time an antibacterial agent is indicated (fever, spreading infection, lymphadenopathy), **anaerobic** gram-negative bacilli predominate. Therapy may start with a **loading dose**, which is a higher than normal dose, to achieve adequate blood levels of the antibiotic quickly. This is followed by a maintenance dose regimen consistent with the drug's half-life.

Factors That Influence Antibacterial Effectiveness

Several factors influence the effectiveness of antibacterial agents.

Spectrum of Micro-Organisms

The *spectrum* refers to the relative range of the drug's antibacterial action. *There are three general spectrums: Narrow, extended, and broad. Narrow spectrum* antibacterial agents are effective on limited bacterial species (i.e., on some gram-positive organisms; on some gram-negative organisms; on some **aerobic**, facultative, or anaerobic organisms; or on various narrow combinations of the above). *Extended spectrum* agents are effective on a greater number of micro-organisms, such as most gram-positive organisms and many gram-negative organisms, including some aerobic, facultative, or anaerobic organisms. *Broad spectrum* agents can kill or suppress the growth of a wide variety of both gram-positive and gram-negative aerobic, facultative, or anaerobic organisms. While the oral environment of an average adult harbors more than 300 bacterial species, and most odontogenic infections are polymicrobial (mixed), the number of isolated strains in any given odontogenic infection ranges from one to ten with an average number of approximately four isolates per infection. Based on statistical evidence, the most common organisms responsible for odontogenic infections include viridans streptococci (*Streptococcus oralis, Streptococcus sanguis,* and *Streptococcus mitis*) and *Peptostreptococcus* (both are all gram-positive); and *Fusobacterium,* pigmented and nonpigmented *Prevotella* (*Bacteroides intermedius/P. intermedia*), *Gemella,* and *Porphyromonas* (all gram-negative).↓ In mixed infections, the predominant flora creates an ecosystem of synergism that promotes the growth and proliferation of its members. This is achieved by providing a more favorable acidic environment (which may reduce the efficacy of a local anesthetic agent) by consuming oxygen to support the growth of anaerobes and by producing metabolites that facilitate selective bacterial survival. Ultimately, facultative gram-positive cocci (particularly viridans group streptococci), anaerobic gram-positive cocci, and gram-negative bacilli predominate in all types of odontogenic infections. Based on this information, rather than delaying antibiotic therapy while performing culture and sensitivity testing on infections, dentists prescribe antibacterial agents empirically (i.e., antibacterial agents that are effective against facultative cocci, anaerobic gram-positive cocci, and anaerobic gram-negative bacilli).

Effective Plasma Concentration

The onset and duration of action of an antibacterial agent is strongly influenced by how quickly and efficiently the agent can enter the circulation and remain at the site of action. The absorption, distribution, and elimination of the agent (discussed in Chapter 2) influence these factors.

Age of Infection

As mentioned earlier, in mixed odontogenic infections, the predominant flora creates an ecosystem of synergism that promotes the growth and proliferation of its members. This is achieved by consuming oxygen (which provides a more favorable acidic environment to support the growth of anaerobes) and by producing metabolites that facilitate selective bacterial survival. Consequently, the number of bacterial species actually *declines* as an infection matures and becomes clinically manifest as either an acute or a chronic condition. Acute odontogenic infections tend to be poorly localized (thus becoming spreading infections) because the body's immune response is unable to contain it. When this occurs, antibacterial therapy is often indicated. Chronic infections tend to be more localized, yet they may change into an acute exacerbation if the immune response is overwhelmed. When the immune response is aggressive, an infection can become localized and form an abscess that can be incised and drained (or, within the sulcus, debrided). Débridement reduces the bioburden (microorganisms, infectious debris), enhancing the ability of the immune system to contain the infection and improving the odds that the antibacterial agent will reach its intended site of action. Low-grade chronic infections may become "walled-off" by fibrous connective tissue, as is the case with periapical granulomas or periapical cysts. This makes it difficult for the antibacterial agents to penetrate the site of infection unless infected fibrous tissue is removed through débridement. Significantly, optimal débridement of an odontogenic infection, in the presence of a competent immune system, often eliminates the need for the administration of an antibacterial agent. This concept is verified by a systematic review of the treatment of apical odontogenic infection that found that an antibacterial agent is not necessary in most instances (http://www.cda-adc.ca/en/dental_profession/practising/clinical_practice_guidelines/index.asp).

Host Response

Individual antibacterial agents cannot destroy all bacteria, nor are they expected to. Successful treatment of an infection is based on débridement to remove infectious debris and the presence of a functioning immune system to remove necrotic cells. Antibacterial agents enhance the immune response. When leukocyte function (chemotaxis, phagocytosis, T-cell differentiation, and antibody formation) is suppressed, this can adversely affect the therapeutic outcome. The host defense mechanism can be adversely affected by a variety of diseases and by some medications, such as corticosteroid therapy. Corticosteroids can suppress the immune response to the point that clinical signs of infection (redness, heat, swelling) can be masked and lymphocyte function significantly be reduced. In this situation, selection of a bactericidal drug rather than a bacteriostatic drug is recommended (see the following section).

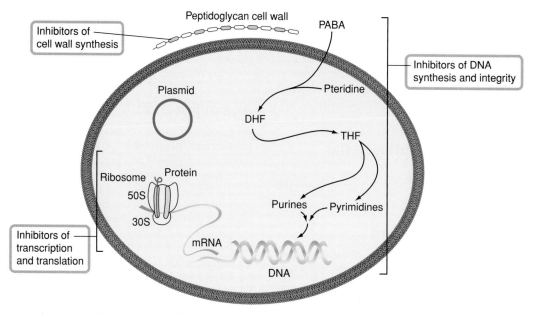

Figure 9-1 Mechanisms of Action of Antibacterial Agents. (Courtesy of the UT Health Science Center at San Antonio, Multimedia & Web Services. Created by Chris McKee.)

Mechanisms of Action

Currently available antibacterial drugs act in three basic ways: They may interrupt (a) bacterial cell wall synthesis, (b) bacterial DNA replication or repair, or (c) protein synthesis (inhibiting transcription or translation; Fig. 9-1).

Table 9-1 illustrates commonly used antibacterial agents for dental infection and their mechanisms of action.

Depending on the role of the drug's target in bacterial physiology, an antibacterial drug can be described as either bactericidal or bacteriostatic.

Bactericidal Drugs

Bactericidal drugs target metabolic pathways essential for bacterial survival. For bacteria to multiply and divide into daughter cells, the bacterial cell wall must be broken and then repaired. The penicillins and cephalosporins interrupt the synthesis of the cell wall during cell division. Consequently, antibacterial agents that act by inhibiting synthesis of the cell wall cause the cytoplasmic contents to spill out through the defects in the cell wall. This effect is bactericidal in susceptible organisms. Metronidazole is bactericidal

against most anaerobes. It causes DNA inhibition in the microbe that leads to cell death not associated with cell division. This is the action of metronidazole, a drug.

Bacteriostatic Drugs

Bacteriostatic drugs target metabolic pathways that are necessary for bacterial growth but not for survival. This leads to inhibition of multiplication and cell division, which is reversible once treatment is terminated. Most antibacterial agents that interrupt protein synthesis (inhibitors of transcription or translation) produce a bacteriostatic effect. Erythromycin, clindamycin, and the tetracycline agents (minocycline, doxycycline, tetracycline) are examples commonly used for oral infections. Bacterial infections in immunocompetent hosts (i.e., the host response to infection is normal) can often be treated with bacteriostatic drugs, whereas the treatment of bacterial infections in immunocompromised hosts often requires a bactericidal agent. This illustrates the important role of the immune response: White blood cells act as scavengers to clear away cellular debris and phagocytize microorganisms to act in support of antibacterial therapy. Bacteriostatic protein synthesis inhibitors retard cell growth

Table 9-1	Sites and Mechanisms of Action of Selected Antibacterial Agents	
Inhibitors of Cell Wall Synthesis	**Inhibitors of Protein Synthesis (Translation)**	**Inhibitors of DNA Synthesis and Integrity**
Penicillins	Macrolides	Metronidazole
Cephalosporins	Clindamycin	Fluoroquinolones
Bacitracin Vancomycin	Tetracycline (doxycycline, minocycline) Neomycin	

Table 9-2	Bacterial Cell Wall Inhibitors and Their Spectra

- Penicillins
  - Narrow-spectrum penicillins (penicillin G, procaine penicillin G, benzathine penicillin G, penicillin VK)
    - Gram-positive cocci and most gram-negative oral anaerobes
      - Beta-lactamase susceptible
  - Penicillinase-resistant penicillins (methicillin, oxacillin, cloxacillin, dicloxacillin, nafcillin)
    - Gram-positive cocci
      - Beta-lactamase resistant
  - Broader-spectrum penicillins (ampicillin, amoxicillin, amoxicillin with clavulanic acid)
    - Gram-positive cocci and most gram-negative oral anaerobes
    - Beta-lactamase susceptible
    - With clavulanic acid, mostly beta-lactamase resistant
  - Antipseudomonal penicillins (carbenicillin, ticarcillin, ticarcillin with clavulanic acid, piperacillin, mezlocillin)
    - Gram-negative organisms
      - With clavulanic acid, mostly beta-lactamase resistant
- Cephalosporins
  - First-generation cephalosporins (cephalexin, cephradine, cefadroxil)
    - Gram-positive cocci and some gram-negative oral anaerobes
      - Beta-lactamase susceptible
  - Second-generation cephalosporins (cefaclor)
    - Gram-positive cocci and extended spectrum to gram-negative oral anaerobes
      - Some beta-lactamase resistance
  - Third-generation cephalosporins (cefixime)
    - Gram-negative bacilli
      - Greater beta-lactamase resistance
- Vancomycin
  - Many gram-positive cocci and gram-negative bacilli
    - Beta-lactamase resistant

and division. The combination of a bacteriostatic drug with a bactericidal drug can result in antagonistic effects. For example, penicillin is most efficient when cell division is rapid, and bacteriostatic drugs slow cell division, thereby producing an antagonistic effect.

Pharmacodynamic Considerations

Bacterial Cell Wall Inhibitors

The cell wall is a common feature of nearly all clinically important pathogens. The cell wall, which provides tensile strength, is critically important in allowing bacterial cells to maintain their intracellular osmotic pressure. A number of drugs have been identified that inhibit various steps in the biosynthesis of the bacterial cell wall. Because human cells lack cell walls, they are generally unaffected by these drugs. Of these, vancomycin and beta-lactam antibiotics (penicillin, cephalosporin) are the most important clinically.[2,3] Beta lactams are true antibiotics because they were originally synthesized from micro-organisms (penicillin from mold, cephalosporins from bacteria). Furthermore, for bacteria to grow and divide into daughter cells, the bacterial cell wall must be broken and then repaired. To accomplish this, bacteria use autolysins to punch holes in the cell wall that allow for expansion or remodeling. The beta-lactam antibiotics interfere with cell wall synthesis and/or loss of autolysin-inhibitor activity, which affects the integrity of the cell walls and allows for the cytoplasmic contents to spill out through the defects. Bacterial cell wall inhibitors are bactericidal in susceptible organisms. Penicillins and several cephalosporins are used as drugs of choice for antibacterial prophylaxis. When a beta-lactam allergy exists, clindamycin or some

macrolide antibacterials (azithromycin, clarithromycin) are recommended. Table 9-2 illustrates examples of various drugs in the penicillin and cephalosporin classes.

Penicillins

The first agent in the penicillin class was penicillin G, generally administered by injection. It is the prototype for the class. The first oral doseform was penicillin V. Potassium was added to enhance absorption; the most common agent used today is penicillin VK. Amoxicillin and ampicillin are penicillins used in specific circumstances. When the client cannot swallow a drug, ampicillin can be administered parenterally. Ampicillin has been associated with causing a nonallergenic rash, most commonly in the patient with mononucleosis.

Penicillinase-Resistant Agents

When an infection is suspected of containing micro-organisms that liberate penicillinase, an enzyme that degrades the penicillin molecule and thereby eliminates the therapeutic effect, penicillinase-resistant agents are used. Dicloxacillin is the prototype penicillinase-resistant agent. Clavulanic acid is added to some penicillins (amoxicillin and others) to make the penicillin combination penicillinase resistant.

Cephalosporins

Cephalosporins are structurally related to penicillins and, therefore, can cause an allergenic response in about 10% of individuals with penicillin allergies. There are first, second, and third generations of cephalosporins. Many agents in the class are administered parenterally. The oral doseforms are relatively acid stable in the GI tract and are resistant to penicillinase, but they are destroyed by cephalosporinase, an enzyme liberated by some micro-organisms. Cephalexin is a first-line agent (with amoxicillin) for antibiotic prophylaxis in selected individuals with a total joint replacement (TJR).

Inhibitors of DNA Synthesis and Repair

Cell wall inhibitors cannot kill all bacteria because some bacteria do not have cell walls (*Mycoplasma pneumoniae, Chlamydia trachomatis*). Other bacteria have unique structures that resist the action of cell wall inhibitors. However, bacteria, like human cells, must synthesize intracellular proteins for self-maintenance and replication. The central dogma of molecular biology states that DNA contains all the information necessary to encode these cellular macromolecules. A single DNA strand can be up to several hundred million nucleotides in length. Two DNA strands form a double helix and serve as an "instruction manual." In its sequence, it provides all the genetic information needed for self-maintenance and replication. Fluoroquinolones (Cipro, Levaquin) inhibit DNA gyrase function, which results in a break in DNA strands, leading to cell death. A common drug used for periodontal infection is metronidazole. Activated intermediates of metronidazole (Flagyl) bind bacterial DNA and inhibit its synthesis. Inhibitors of nucleic acid synthesis have a bactericidal effect. Metronidazole is quite effective against obligate anaerobes. It can be combined with amoxicillin or penicillin VK for an effective therapeutic effect in mixed infections.

Inhibitors of Transcription or Translation

As suggested earlier, like mammalian cells, bacteria must synthesize proteins for self-maintenance and replication. While the DNA serves as the "instruction manual" and provides all the information necessary for protein synthesis, the actual work of translating the information into a medium that can be used directly by cells is a function of ribonucleic acid (RNA). Consequently, the first step in protein synthesis is *transcription*, which involves the synthesis of a single-stranded RNA from a DNA template. The newly synthesized RNA has three major functions: (a) it may serve as a messenger (mRNA) that tells cells (ribosomes) which proteins to synthesize, (b) it may serve as part of ribosomes (rRNA) that synthesize proteins, and (c) it may carry or transfer (tRNA) specific amino acids from the cytoplasm to ribosomes for protein synthesis. Translation continues until the newly synthesized protein is released from the ribosome. Antibacterial agents that inhibit transcription or translation interfere with this physiologic process to cause a bacteriostatic effect.

The macrolides (erythromycin, clarithromycin, azithromycin), lincosamides, chloramphenicol, tetracyclines, and aminoglycosides target bacterial ribosomes that synthesize protein from the mRNA code. The macrolides, lincosamides, and chloramphenicol bind to 50S ribosomal subunits. The tetracyclines bind to 30S ribosomal subunits and reversibly block the attachment of aminoacyl-tRNA. The aminoglycosides (gentamicin, neomycin, streptomycin, and others) also bind to 30S ribosomal subunits, block the formation of the 70S initiation complex, and affect the production of abnormal polypeptides (Table 9-3).

Table 9-3	Protein-Synthesis Inhibitors and Their Spectra

- 50S ribosomal inhibitors
  - Macrolides
    - Erythromycin base, stearate, estolate, ethyl succinate, and dirithromycin
      - Gram-positive and some gram-negative aerobes
    - Clarithromycin and azithromycin
      - Gram-positive and some gram-negative aerobes and anaerobes
  - Lincosamides
    - Clindamycin
      - Gram-positive cocci and most gram-negative oral anaerobes
- 30S ribosomal inhibitors
  - Tetracyclines (minocycline, doxycycline, tetracycline)
    - Gram-positive and gram-negative organisms
  - Aminoglycosides (gentamicin, tobramycin, amikacin, and others)
    - Aerobic and facultative gram-negative bacilli

Bacterial Resistance to Antibiotic Drug Therapy

Mechanisms of Bacterial Drug Resistance

Antibiotic drug resistance may be associated with genetic or nongenetic causes. Genetic mechanisms of resistance may be natural or intrinsic, or they may arise from chromosomal mutations. These mechanisms confer drug-resistance by vertical transmission (daughter cells) of genes that affect altered drug targets, drug transport, or drug metabolic systems. Bacteria may also acquire drug resistance by horizontal transmission (gaining genetic material from other bacteria). A factor thought to significantly influence the development of antibiotic resistance is the indiscriminate use of antibacterial agents, such as taking antibiotics for viral infections (colds, flu) where they are not effective.

Genetic Drug Resistance

Natural or intrinsic resistance is inherent in the molecular or species characteristics of bacteria. Oral organisms with natural or intrinsic resistance to metronidazole (an antibacterial drug specific to gram-negative microorganisms) include certain *Streptococcus* species, *Actinomyces* species, and *Actinobacillus actinomycetemcomitans*. They lack the enzyme *nitroreductase*, which is necessary to convert metronidazole to its active metabolites. Alternatively, certain isolates of *Prevotella* (*Bacteroides*) do not take up metronidazole as readily as do susceptible isolates. Many oral gram-negative anaerobes appear to be resistant to erythromycin because the structure of the outer bacterial cell membrane restricts entry of the drug.

Chromosomal resistance may also result from spontaneous mutation. The synthesis of enzymes that lyse beta-lactam antibacterial agents (beta-lactamase) has been related to chromosomal mutations. Certain species of oral microorganisms are involved in this form of antibiotic resistance. The addition of clavulanic acid to certain antibacterials, such as amoxicillin with clavulanic acid (Augmentin), will inactivate beta-lactamase and protect beta-lactam agents, such as penicillins and cephalosporins.

Acquired Drug Resistance

Most organisms acquire resistance by gaining genetic material from other bacteria. This involves three main mechanisms: transformation, transduction, or conjugation. Susceptible bacteria may acquire segments of free DNA (carrying resistance) from the surrounding environment (released by dead bacteria) by the process known as transformation. Transduction is defined as the transfer of bacterial DNA, from one organism to another, carrying the resistance gene by a bacteriophage. In conjugation, extrachromosomal plasmid DNA is transferred directly between bacteria (i.e., one organism "infects" the other). There is much less species specificity required between donor and recipient for the transfer of genetic information by conjugation than by either transformation or transduction. Because of this reduced specificity, conjugal transfer appears to be the most important mechanism whereby resistance genes are spread among bacteria within and between various ecosystems. For example, resistance information could be transferred from tetracycline to penicillin, two different classes of antibacterial agents and agents that act by two different mechanisms. In addition, transposons may carry genes for resistance from plasmids to chromosomes. Due to selectivity, during antibacterial chemotherapy, resistant micro-organisms face reduced competition and multiply rapidly, giving rise to progeny that carry genes capable of resisting antibacterial challenges.

Biofilm-Related Drug Resistance

Bacteria isolated with standard microbiologic techniques tend to be the free-swimming or planktonic form (the opposite of biofilm), and most of what we know about bacteria is limited to their individual characteristics. If bacteria are resistant to an antibiotic, it is because they carry a gene that confers resistance. But in nature, bacteria live in biofilms, a state that allows them to work together.[4] As bacteria move onto a surface, the dynamic process of biofilm formation begins. The bacteria stack up and encase themselves in a hydrated matrix of polysaccharide and protein. As the cells grow, multiply, and produce more matrixes, they form towerlike structures called "mushrooms." These mushrooms, which are about 85% matrix material, typically contain several thousand bacteria and are pierced with channels that allow nutrients to reach the interior and waste products to be carried away.

Once they are in a biofilm, the bacteria are protected from antibodies and leukocyte phagocytosis and appear to be exponentially more resistant to antibacterial agents than when they are in their free-swimming planktonic form. The mechanisms of resistance to antibacterial agents in biofilms appear to have three plausible explanations. The first hypothesis suggests slow and incomplete penetration of antibacterial agents into the biofilm. The second hypothesis is predicated on an altered chemical microenvironment within the biofilm from bacterial metabolic waste products and oxygen anomalies that result in anaerobic predominance in the deeper layers of the biofilm. The third possibility is that a subpopulation of bacteria in biofilm differentiates into a unique phenotype, which assumes a very low metabolic state that is almost spore-like. Because most antibacterial agents target rapidly dividing cells, cells in this quiescent state may survive exposure and become reactivated when the antibacterial drug is withdrawn.

Pharmacokinetic Considerations

Pharmacokinetics refers to issues related to absorption, distribution, bioavailability, metabolism, and elimination of drugs. The access of antibiotics to the site of infection depends on such factors as (a) their route of administration, (b) the degree of plasma protein-binding in the circulation, (c) the concentration of the free drug in plasma and extracellular fluid, and (d) passive diffusion into foci of infection. The oral route of administration is the most common route used in dentistry. Some antibacterial agents (tetracycline) cannot be taken with some foods (such as those containing calcium) or with minerals (iron, magnesium). In this instance, the tetracycline molecule binds to the mineral and is not absorbed from the GI tract. Erythromycin base is inactivated by gastric acid and is covered with an enteric coating to protect it as it moves through the stomach. The absorption of most agents is slowed when food is in the stomach, although many agents can be taken with food (amoxicillin). A practical approach to this problem is to instruct patients to take the antibacterial agent 30 minutes before or 2 hours after a meal. Renal excretion is the main route of drug elimination from the body.

■ Self-Study Review

1. Identify two reasons for using antibacterial agents in dentistry.
2. Describe primary dental care and when it is used.
3. Describe how the normal flora is established.
4. Differentiate between *autogenous* infection and *environmental* infection or crossinfection.
5. Differentiate between *prokaryotic* and *eukaryotic* cells.
6. Identify an example of an agent that attacks a property of a microbe that is not present in the host.
7. List the rules for prescribing an antibiotic.
8. Differentiate between *bactericidal* and *bacteriostatic* antibacterial agents.
9. Define *suprainfection* and causative factors.
10. List four features that indicate an antibacterial agent is indicated.
11. What is the purpose of the loading dose in antibacterial therapy?
12. Differentiate between microorganisms in each spectrum of activity.
13. Most odontogenic infections can be resolved with an agent in which spectrum?
14. Describe changes that occur as an infection ages into the acute stage. Into the chronic stage.
15. Describe the role of the immune response in managing odontogenic infection.
16. Describe the mechanisms of action for agents in Table 9-1.

17. Compare features of bactericidal agents with bacteriostatic agents.
18. Identify the beta-lactam antibiotics, prototypes, and doseforms.
19. Identify agents that inhibit DNA mechanisms and their dental uses.
20. Identify agents that act on cellular RNA to produce a bacteriostatic effect.
21. Specify the area of the ribosome affected by macrolides and tetracyclines.
22. Identify examples of *aminoglycosides*.
23. Identify three mechanisms of bacterial resistance and give examples of bacterial resistance that affects therapeutic uses of antibiotics.
24. What are dosing instructions when an antibacterial agent cannot be taken with food?

ODONTOGENIC INFECTION

Microorganisms can be described as cocci, rods, spirochetes, or bacilli; culturing provides information about their metabolic characteristics (i.e., whether they are aerobic, anaerobic, or facultative). As was stated earlier, most odontogenic infections are polymicrobial and facultative gram-positive cocci, particularly viridans streptococci; anaerobic gram-positive cocci and gram-negative bacilli predominate in all types of odontogenic infections. Consequently, antibacterial agents used in dentistry that target those organisms would be selected. Like most odontogenic infections, periodontal infections are also polymicrobial, with gram-negative, anaerobic organisms predominating. This evidence is a major consideration in the selection of an antibacterial agent, when indicated, as an adjunct to conventional periodontal therapy.

Indications for Antibacterials in Oral Infection

Odontogenic infections are usually *autogenous*, caused by the body's normal flora that has become pathogenic. Oral bacterial infections primarily affect the teeth (caries) and pulpal, periodontal, or pericoronal tissues. Patients commonly present with localized pain, erythema, and edema, and they can report difficulty chewing. When the infection involves the pulp of the tooth, periapical area, or area within a periodontal pocket, the formation of purulent exudate can block antibacterial therapy from reaching the infection. In this instance the infection should be removed by débridement, endodontic therapy, tooth removal, or with incision and drainage (primary dental care). When primary dental care is provided, antibacterials are often not needed to resolve the infection. However, when patients present with malaise, chills (fever), trismus, rapid respiration, lymphadenopathy, swelling, and/or hypotension, or when transient bacteremia may adversely affect the general health of the patient, appropriate adjuvant antibacterial chemotherapy is indicated.

Therapeutic Strategies in the Treatment of Odontogenic Infections

Most odontogenic infections can be resolved satisfactorily with timely débridement in conjunction with local anesthesia.[5,6] The routine use of antibacterial agents for the management of odontogenic infections is not effective. Table 9-4 outlines principal considerations associated with the administration of antibacterial agents in the oral health care setting.

Odontogenic infections that have not been treated in a timely manner or that have failed to respond to removal of the infection by primary dental care may spread into anatomical spaces contiguous with fascial planes and lead to serious, even life-threatening situations (e.g., cavernous sinus thrombosis, Ludwig angina, mediastinitis, osteomyelitis). This is especially true in immunocompromised patients. Patients presenting with a serious infection typically exhibit swelling, trismus, lymphadenopathy, chills, and fever. Rapid respiration and hypotension are more ominous signs of a life-threatening condition with cardiorespiratory compromise.

Primary Line of Antibacterial Chemotherapy

Most often, primary dental care is successful in resolving odontogenic infection. However, occasionally antibacterial agents are indicated. Unless the patient has an allergy to penicillin, the appropriate empirical drug of choice for the treatment of an uncomplicated odontogenic infection is penicillin VK. It is effective against most causative microorganisms and is a narrow-spectrum antibacterial. Most odontogenic infections will require only 5 days of antibacterial chemotherapy if débridement has removed much of the infectious debris and exudate (rather than 10 days for internal infections). A loading dose is used, followed by maintenance doses identified in Table 9-5. All agents in Table 9-5 can be taken with meals. Resolution of symptoms should be apparent within 2 to 3 days, and the patient should be instructed to notify the clinician if symptoms do not resolve in that time period. In such circumstances, it is prudent to re-evaluate the patient because this may indicate noncompliance in taking the agent or nonresponse due to bacterial antibiotic resistance. If antibiotic resistance develops, a culture and susceptibility test would be completed to identify the infecting organism, and the therapeutic regimen would be modified.

Bacterial Resistance

Some gram-positive (*S. oralis*, *S. sanguis*, and *S. mitis*) and gram-negative organisms exhibit resistance related to structural changes in penicillin-binding proteins. In addition, staphylococci and many gram-negative bacteria can synthesize beta-lactamase enzymes, which inactivate beta-lactam antibiotics. A therapeutic strategy to counter such resistance might be to administer a wider-spectrum penicillin (such as amoxicillin) in combination with clavulanic acid, a chemical that inhibits the formation of beta-lactamase enzymes. Unfortunately, amoxicillin is beta-lactamase susceptible, and certain beta-lactamase enzymes produced by gram-negative bacteria are resistant to clavulanic acid as well. Consequently,

Table 9-4	Principal Considerations in Antibacterial Chemotherapy

- Establish a clear indication for antibacterial chemotherapy
  - The patient presents with malaise, fever, chills, trismus, rapid respiration, swelling, lymphadenopathy, or hypotension
    - Signs and symptoms of infection escalate rapidly (within 24 to 48 h)
    - Oral soft tissue swelling appears to be spreading into adjacent anatomical spaces and affects breathing and swallowing
- Determine the patient's health status
  - Systemic considerations (heart disease, neutropenia, splenectomy, diabetes mellitus, end-stage renal disease, organ transplant, HIV infection, total joint replacement and other implanted devices, hepatic dysfunction, pregnancy)
  - History of adverse drug reactions
  - Potential drug–drug interactions
- Select an appropriate antibacterial agent with a narrow spectrum and low toxicity.
  - Immune status of the patient
    - Bactericidal versus bacteriostatic antibacterial agent
      - Empirical therapy (correlate to most likely organisms associated with odontogenic infections)
      - Focused therapy (correlate to culture and susceptibility tests)
- Establish dosage regimen, duration of therapy, and route of administration
  - Consider the seriousness of the illness
  - Consider potential compliance issues
- Follow-up in 48 to 72 h (note that patients initially presenting with signs of impending airway compromise, marked trismus [<25 mm], or dehydration [e.g., marked malaise, disorientation, tachycardia] should be admitted to the hospital for urgent or emergent care)
  - Determine efficacy
    - Inadequate bacteriologic information
    - Administration of suboptimal doses of the antibacterial agent
    - Inadequate débridement
      - Ability of the drug to reach the site of infection
  - Monitor patient for adverse drug effects

the administration of a wider-spectrum penicillin may offer little therapeutic advantage over penicillin VK in the management of odontogenic infections.

Secondary Line of Antibacterial Chemotherapy

If significant improvement is not noted with penicillin VK in 48 to 72 hours, the empirical addition (for 7 days) of metron-

idazole (to kill the anaerobic component of infection) to penicillin VK is reasonable because it is beta-lactamase resistant (Table 9-5). Consequently, penicillin is still effective against the nonpenicillinase producers. So, metronidazole is added to the regimen, and the penicillin is continued.

Metronidazole

The spectrum of metronidazole, an amebicide, includes bactericidal action against most obligate anaerobes, such as the *Bacterioides* species, making it useful in periodontal infections. While certain oral microorganisms such as *Streptococcus* species, *Actinomyces* species, and *Actinobacillus actinomycetemcomitans* exhibit natural or intrinsic resistance to metronidazole—they lack the enzyme nitroreductase necessary to convert metronidazole to its active metabolites—metronidazole, in combination with penicillin VK, provides excellent coverage for mixed odontogenic infections dominated by obligate anaerobes.

Erythromycin

Erythromycin, a member of the macrolide class of antibiotics, has been suggested as the empirical drug of choice for the treatment of uncomplicated odontogenic infections in patients who are allergic to beta-lactam antibiotics. However, many oral gram-negative anaerobes have natural or intrinsic resistance to erythromycin because the structure of the outer bacterial cell membrane restricts entry of the drug. Resistance to erythromycin has also been related to the ability of certain microorganisms to block ribosomal erythromycin-receptor sites. Unfortunately, this mechanism contributes not only

Table 9-5	Antibacterial Agents of Choice for the Treatment of Odontogenic Infections

Primary Line of Treatment

R$_X$
  Penicillin VK, 500-mg tabs
  Disp. 21 tabs
  Sig. Take two tabs stat, then one tab qid until all are taken.

Secondary Line of Treatment

R$_X$
  Metronidazole, 250-mg tabs
  Disp. 29 tabs
  Sig. Take two tabs stat, then one tab qid until all are taken.

R$_X$
  Azithromycin, 250-mg tabs
  Disp. 21 tabs
  Sig. Take two tabs stat, then one tab qid until all are taken.

Tertiary Line of Treatment

R$_X$
  Clindamycin, 300-mg tabs
  Disp. 29 tabs
  Sig. Take two tabs stat, then one tab qid until all are taken.

to erythromycin resistance, but also these micro-organisms will be resistant to clindamycin. Finally, certain bacteria have developed resistance to erythromycin by activating efflux pumps, which act to remove intracellular erythromycin. These efflux pumps can also affect the intracellular concentration of beta-lactam antibiotics and beta-lactamase inhibitors. Other disadvantages of erythromycin involve the large number of drugs that interact with erythromycin, making it less safe than other antibacterials, as well as common adverse effects involving the gastrointestinal tract (nausea, abdominal pain, diarrhea). Erythromycin is commonly taken four times/day (to maintain therapeutic blood levels) due to the pharmacokinetics of the drug, and this frequency promotes noncompliance in taking the drug.

While there is a paucity of data demonstrating the efficacy of other macrolides (clarithromycin and azithromycin) in the treatment of odontogenic infections, these newer macrolide antibacterial agents may be better alternatives to erythromycin because of their extended spectrum against facultative and some obligate anaerobes, more favorable tissue distribution, not being affected by gastric acids, fewer side effects, and a once daily (azithromycin) or twice daily (clarithromycin) dosage schedule (Table 9-5). However, their substantially higher cost and the association of drug-interaction-related sudden death from cardiac causes following the oral administration of macrolides (with the exception of azithromycin) are compelling reasons to recommend clindamycin as a more appropriate alternative for patients allergic to beta-lactam antibacterial agents.

Tertiary Line of Antibacterial Chemotherapy

When a patient presents with an unresolved odontogenic infection following treatment with a beta-lactam antibacterial agent, the administration of a beta-lactamase-stable antibacterial drug, such as clindamycin, should be considered (Table 9-5). Similarly, the initial empirical drug of choice for the treatment of a complicated or long-standing odontogenic infection is also clindamycin. It is not only beta-lactamase resistant, but it also has excellent activity against gram-positive cocci and most oral gram-negative anaerobes. Some authorities also point to clindamycin as an increasingly attractive choice in the treatment of all odontogenic infections, but concerns about associated gastric side effects (e.g., pseudomembranous colitis, also called antibiotic-associated colitis), higher cost, and, importantly, reports of drug-resistance to clindamycin should prompt caution in using it as a primary line of treatment.

Pseudomembranous Colitis

Pseudomembranous colitis is caused by the bacterium *Clostridium difficile* liberating toxins that desquamate the epithelial lining of the intestines, resulting in bloody diarrhea and systemic infection. This condition has been associated with lincomycin and clindamycin and has resulted in fatalities. Antibiotic-associated colitis can occur with other antibiotics (tetracycline, ampicillin, cephalosporins) and is treated with intravenous (IV) antibiotics (vancomycin). There are reports that many formerly effective agents are now ineffective because *C. difficile* has developed resistance to those agents.

Treatment Failure

Other available antibacterial agents are not indicated as initial empirical choices in the treatment of odontogenic infections. The prescription of other drugs should be predicated on the results of susceptibility testing. When culture and susceptibility results are available, the empirical agent should be changed to an effective narrow-spectrum antibacterial drug. Lack of adequate bacteriologic information, the administration of suboptimal doses of antibacterial agents, and the reliance on chemotherapy with omission of surgical drainage all contribute to failure of therapy. In selecting an antibacterial agent (bactericidal vs. bacteriostatic), one must also consider the state of the immune system and the ability of the drug to reach the site of infection. Furthermore, in considering potential causes of treatment failure, clinicians must be aware of the fact that the high cost of an antibacterial agent may affect compliance in getting the prescription filled.

Locally Applied Antibiotics

There are two locally applied tetracycline formulations (doxycycline and minocycline) that are placed within the periodontal sulcus to achieve a bacteriostatic effect. There is very little systemic absorption of the topical tetracycline, which reduces side effects. These products are highly concentrated and are combined with bioabsorbable polymers that allow the tetracycline product to be maintained within the sulcus (bioadhesive and self-retentive) and slowly released to achieve an antibacterial effect for 7 (doxycycline) to 14 (minocycline) days. An anti-inflammatory side effect of tetracycline (inhibition of matrix metalloproteinase) is thought to inhibit breakdown of collagen in connective tissue. These agents have resulted in approximately 0.5 to 1 mm probe-depth reduction over periodontal débridement alone. They appear to be most efficacious in deeper pockets (≥ 7 mm). Patient instructions include delaying brushing/flossing in the area of insertion for up to 7 days following insertion of the product (doxycycline gel) to avoid dislodging it.

Other Agents

There is a low-dose doxycycline hyclate oral doseform (Periostat) available in a 20-mg tablet taken twice daily (bid) that uses the matrix metalloproteinase inhibitory effect as the primary mechanism to slow the progression of periodontal inflammation. The 20-mg dose is said to be subantimicrobial, in that the dose is too low to affect microorganisms. It is prescribed for 3 months, the response is evaluated, and then the medication can be continued for up to 1 year.

■ **Self-Study Review**

25. Identify indications for antibacterial agents in oral infection.

26. What is the antibacterial agent of choice for most uncomplicated odontogenic infections?
27. Describe advantages and disadvantages of *secondary* and *tertiary* lines of therapy.
28. Describe locally applied agents used in periodontal therapy.
29. Describe the low-dose doxycycline product features and dosing information.

ANTIBIOTIC PROPHYLAXIS

A significant percentage of antibacterial agents prescribed by dental practitioners are for the prevention rather than the treatment of an established infection. In general, chemoprophylaxis is frequently successful when a single effective drug is used to prevent infection by a specific microorganism or to eradicate it immediately or soon after it has become established. Consequently, chemoprophylaxis may be appropriate to prevent secondary bacterial infection in patients who are ill with other diseases.

Antibiotic prophylaxis prior to dental treatment is an *unproven* use of antibiotics to prevent infective endocarditis (IE) in susceptible individuals. It has been recommended because it was thought antibiotics might reduce the risk for distant infection from oral bacteria. However, no studies have proven the efficacy for antibiotics used in this manner. There are a variety of adverse effects that can develop when an antibiotic is taken (Color Plates 16, 25 to 29, 31, and 32). It has been reported that more people have died from penicillin allergies than from developing IE. The practice may also be contributing to the development of antibiotic resistance. So, before prescribing antibacterial agents to prevent illness, the clinician should weigh the benefits and risks not only to the patient, but also to the community.

The Patient with Total Joint Replacement

The American Dental Association (ADA), in cooperation with the American Academy of Orthopedic Surgeons, published guidelines, updated in 2003, for the dental management of patients following TJR.[7] Under these guidelines, only patients during the first 2 years following joint replacement are recommended to have antibiotic prophylaxis before dental treatment. Other high-risk patients who should be considered for antimicrobial prophylaxis prior to invasive dental procedures involving significant bleeding include those who are immunocompromised and those with comorbidities, such as previous prosthetic joint infections, malnourishment, hemophilia, HIV infection, type I diabetes, and malignancy. The drugs to recommend first are cephalexin, cephradine, or amoxicillin (2 g orally 1 hour prior to the dental procedure). It should be noted that these guidelines, similar to those set forth by the American Heart Association (AHA), represent a consensus and, as such, are not absolute. There is one difference between the two regimens related to the specific drug therapy: Macrolides (azithromycin, clarithromycin) are not included in recommendations for TJR prophylaxis. Table 9-6 identifies the potential at-risk patient, the dental procedures associated with causing bacteremia, and the current recommendations for antibiotic prophylaxis in the individual with a TJR.

Other implanted devices include intraocular lenses and breast and penile implants. While there have been anecdotal reports of infection related to an oral source and subsequent recommendations to provide antimicrobial prophylaxis, no validated studies exist that demonstrate a need or justification of providing antimicrobial prophylaxis prior to dental procedures in these situations.[8] Given the lack of data and diversity of opinion on the subject, it is recommended that the patient's physician be consulted regarding the need for antibiotic prophylaxis prior to the initiation of invasive dental procedures.

Prophylaxis for the Prevention of Infective Endocarditis

In 2007, the AHA published new guidelines for the prevention of IE.[9] The AHA recommends that patients be advised of the importance of maintaining meticulous oral hygiene and to receive regular dental care to avoid formation of transient bacteremias. The new recommendations state that oral health is more important than antibiotics to prevent IE. However, antibiotic prophylaxis is recommended for those at the highest risk for endocarditis. The recommendations stratify cardiac conditions according to the risk of developing endocarditis and the severity of the ensuing morbidity (Table 9-7). Antibacterial prophylaxis in the individuals described in Table 9-7 is recommended prior to all dental procedures that involve manipulation of gingival tissue or the periapical region of teeth or perforation of the oral mucosa. It has been demonstrated that significant bacteremia can develop following these procedures. In the former 1997 regimen, only oral procedures that involved significant bleeding were recommended for prophylaxis, but later research showed that most oral procedures, especially toothbrushing, flossing, and chewing, resulted in bacteremia. Oral procedures or events that do not need prophylaxis (in a client with indicated conditions identified in Table 9-7) include routine anesthetic injections through noninfected tissue, taking dental radiographs, placement of removable prosthetic or orthodontic appliances, adjustment of orthodontic appliances, placement of orthodontic brackets, shedding of deciduous teeth, and bleeding from trauma to the lips or oral mucosa. Table 9-8 identifies drug regimens for antibiotic prophylaxis prior to dental procedures in indicated cardiac conditions, which may result in significant transient bacteremia.

Dosing Instructions

The selected antibacterial agent is to be taken 30 minutes to 1 hour prior to the dental procedure. When the client *inadvertently* fails to take the antibiotic, the 2007 recommendations advise that animal studies suggest protection may be gained if it is taken within 2 hours of the procedure. This should only be considered if the patient failed to take the antibiotic prior to coming for the appointment.

Table 9-6	Antibiotic Prophylaxis for Total Joint Replacement

Joint advisory statement of the American Dental Association and the American Academy of
 Orthopaedic Surgeons

Patients at Potential Increased Risk of Hematogenous Total Joint Infection
- All patients during first 2 years following joint replacement
- Immunocompromised/immunosuppressed patients
  - Rheumatoid arthritis
  - Systemic lupus erythematosus
  - Drug or radiation-induced immunosuppression
- Patients with comorbidities
  - Previous prosthetic joint infections
  - Malnourishment
  - Hemophilia
  - HIV infection
  - Insulin-dependent (type I) diabetes
  - Malignancy

Conditions shown for patients in this category are examples only; there may be
 additional conditions that place such patients at risk of experiencing hematogenous
 total joint infection.

Incidence Stratification of Bacteremic Dental Procedures

HIGH incidence*	Tooth extraction
	Periodontal procedures (surgery, subgingival placement of fibers/strips, scaling, probing, recall maintenance)
	Implant placement and replantation of avulsed teeth
	Endodontic instrumentation; surgery beyond apex of root
	Initial placement of orthodontic bands (not brackets)
	Intraligamentary and intraosseous local anesthetic injection
	Oral prophylaxis (teeth and implants) where bleeding is anticipated
LOW incidence†‡	Restorative dentistry with or without retraction cord
	Local anesthetic injections
	Intracanal endodontic treatment; post placement, buildup
	Rubber dam placement
	Post operative suture removal
	Placement of removable prosthodontic/orthodontic appliances
	Taking of impressions
	Fluoride treatment
	Taking radiographs
	Adjustment of orthodontic appliances

Suggested Antibiotic Prophylaxis Regimens

PATIENT TYPE	SUGGESTED DRUG	REGIMEN
For patients not allergic to penicillin	cephalexin, cephradine, or amoxicillin	2 g orally 1 h prior to dental procedure
Patients unable to take oral medication and not penicillin allergic	cefazolin or ampicillin	cefazolin 1 g or ampicillin 2 g IM or IV 1 h prior to dental procedure
Patients allergic to penicillin	clindamycin	600 mg orally 1 h prior to dental procedure
Patients allergic to penicillin and unable to take oral medication	clindamycin	600 mg IV 1 h prior to dental procedure

*Antibiotic prophylaxis indicated
†Antibiotic prophylaxis not indicated
‡Clinical judgment may indicate antibiotic prophylaxis in selected circumstances involving significant bleeding
[Adapted from American Dental Association, American Academy of Orthopaedic Surgeons. Antibiotic
prophylaxis for dental patient with total joint replacements. *JADA.* 2003;134(7):895–898. Copyright 2003,
American Dental Association. Reprinted with permission.]

Patients Currently Taking an Antibiotic

For at-risk patients identified in Table 9-7 who are already taking one of the indicated antibacterial agents, it is recommended that a drug from a different class be used for chemoprophylaxis to counter the possibility of antibiotic resistant microorganism formation. To illustrate this recommendation, if a dental client with a cardiac valve replacement needs an oral prophylaxis and is taking amoxicillin for a respiratory infection (resistant organisms to penicillins may have developed), the drug of choice for antibiotic prophylaxis would be clindamycin or one of the macrolides in the regimen. Cephalosporin would not be used because it has a chemical structure closely related to amoxicillin. If it has been 10 days since the antibiotic was last taken, the same antibiotic can be prescribed because resistant microorganisms would be unlikely to be present.

Table 9-7	Cardiac Conditions Associated with the Highest Risk of Adverse Outcome from Endocarditis for Which Chemoprophylaxis with Dental Procedures Can be Considered

Prosthetic cardiac valves
Previous infective endocarditis
Congenital heart disease (CHD)*
    Unrepaired cyanotic CHD, including palliative shunts and conduits
    Completely repaired CHD with prosthetic material or device, whether placed by surgery or
        by catheter intervention, during the first 6 months after the procedure[†]
    Repaired CHD with residual defects at the site or adjacent to the site of a prosthetic patch or
        prosthetic device (which inhibits endothelialization)
Cardiac transplant recipients who develop cardiac valvulopathy

*Except for the conditions listed above, antibiotic prophylaxis is no longer recommended for any other form of CHD.
[†]Prophylaxis is recommended because endothelialization of prosthetic material occurs within 6 months after the procedure. (Reprinted with permission from Wilson W, Taubert KA, Gewitz M. Prevention of infective endocarditis. *Guidelines from the American Heart Association Circulation.* 2007:115:Table 3-Cardiac conditions.)

Patients Taking Anticoagulants

The 2007 AHA guidelines advise against intramuscular (IM) injections for IE prophylaxis in patients who are receiving anticoagulant therapy. In these circumstances, orally administered regimens should be given whenever possible. For individuals unable to tolerate or absorb oral medications, IV-administered antibiotics should be used.

Coronary Artery Bypass Grafts or Stents

There is no evidence that the individual who has had surgery to replace a coronary artery or arteries is at an increased risk for IE. Therefore, chemoprophylaxis is not recommended prior to dental procedures in this group, nor is chemoprophylaxis prior to dental procedures recommended for those who have coronary artery stents.

Special Considerations

There are areas of concern that are not directly addressed or sufficiently amplified in the AHA guidelines. Prior expo-

sure to the diet drugs fenfluramine or dexfenfluramine has been linked to the development of cardiac valvulopathy and increased risk of IE. The Centers for Disease Control and Prevention (CDC) advised that patients with a history of exposure to these drugs for several months should have an echocardiogram to rule out residual valvular damage. Patients with systemic lupus erythematosus (SLE) often manifest immune-mediated cardiac valvular damage and may have an increased risk for developing IE. As a consequence, several authorities recommend their inclusion in the moderate- to high-risk category for IE. Given that these conditions were not included in the highest risk category in the 2007 guidelines, it is logical to assume that antibiotic prophylaxis prior to dental procedures is not warranted.

Removal of the Spleen

The spleen plays a significant role in the function of the host immune system. Removal of the organ can result in sepsis. Organisms not typically found in the oral cavity cause the

Table 9-8	AHA Antibiotic Regimen to Prevent IE

Situation	Agent	Regimen: Single Dose 30 to 60 min Before Procedure	
		Adults	Children
Oral	Amoxicillin	2 g	50 mg/kg
Unable to take oral medication	Ampicillin OR	2 g IM or IV	50 mg/kg IM or IV
	Cefazolin or Ceftriaxone	1 g IM or IV	50 mg/kg IM or IV
Allergic to penicillins or ampicillin—oral	Cephalexin* OR	2 g	50 mg/kg
	Clindamycin OR	600 mg	20 mg/kg
	Azithromycin or Clarithromycin	500 mg	15 mg/kg
Allergic to penicillins or ampicillin and unable to take oral medications	Cefazolin* or Ceftriaxone* OR	1 g IM or IV	50 mg/kg IM or IV
	Clindamycin	600 mg IM or IV	20 mg/kg IM or IV

*Cephalosporins should not be used in an individual with a history of anaphylaxis, angioedema, or urticaria with penicillins or ampicillin. (Reprinted with permission from Wilson W, Taubert KA, Gewitz M. Prevention of infective endocarditis. *Guidelines from the American Heart Association Circulation.* 2007:115:Table 5-Regimens.)

vast majority of cases of postsplenectomy sepsis syndrome. Antibacterial prophylaxis prior to dental treatment is not routinely recommended for these clients. However, due to the patient's impaired immune status, when an oral infection occurs, the patient's physician should be consulted to determine the patient's overall medical status. Consultation is particularly important if the patient had a splenectomy within the past 2 years and/or is a child. Asplenic patients should be advised of the importance of maintaining meticulous oral hygiene and be placed on a frequent maintenance schedule to monitor compliance for oral health.

Uncontrolled Diabetes Mellitus

Uncontrolled diabetes is associated with poor wound healing and increased risk for cardiovascular events. The increased risk of infection associated with poor glycemic control and the potential for poor wound healing observed in uncontrolled diabetes has led some to advocate the administration of antibacterial prophylaxis prior to dental therapy.[10] A recent qualitative systematic review to determine the level of evidence for antibiotic prophylaxis in type I diabetes mellitus (DM) concluded no scientific evidence supports this practice.[8] It is clear that any infection, including periodontal disease, in the diabetic patient must be managed promptly and aggressively. In addition, the patient must practice meticulous oral hygiene and have frequent maintenance visits to monitor oral health and compliance. As a general rule, patients with DM who are under good glycemic control can be treated the same as normal patients, while diabetic patients with poor glycemic control and those suspected of having undiagnosed DM should be referred for medical evaluation prior to elective oral health care. Medical consultation is further recommended when the planned dental therapy is expected to adversely impact glycemic control, such as when dental therapy interferes with the patient's ability to have an adequate intake of food.

End-Stage Renal Disease

The increased risk of dialysis catheter infection and the increased risk of IE in patients undergoing hemodialysis have led to the recommendation for antibacterial prophylaxis prior to invasive dental procedures. The most frequently recommended regimens follow those established by the AHA. For dialysis patients *with an underlying AHA-defined cardiac risk condition*, such recommendations are logical and prudent. However, there have been no studies directly addressing the impact of orally related bacteremia on dialysis patients. A recent qualitative systematic review to determine the level of evidence for antibiotic prophylaxis concluded no scientific evidence supports this practice.[8] More importantly, the dramatic increase in bacterial drug resistance observed in this patient population warrants caution. Therefore, the decision to use antibacterial prophylaxis and the specific regimen chosen should be determined in consultation with the client's physician.

Organ Transplant

There exist no studies addressing either the need for or benefit of providing antimicrobial prophylaxis to cover dental procedure-induced bacteremia in the organ transplant recipient.[8] The 2007 AHA recommendations include antibiotic prophylaxis only for the transplanted heart that develops valvulopathy *after* the transplant. It could be argued that the patient's drug-induced immunosuppression and increased infection risk support a need to provide prophylaxis to cover invasive dental procedures. However, the complexity of the decision-making process is further complicated by the fact that the transplant patient may already be on a prophylactic antibiotic regimen. It is therefore recommended that the oral health care professional consult closely with the patient's physician to determine the need for and specifics of the antimicrobial prophylactic regimen.

HIV Infection

There exist no studies addressing either the need for or the benefit of providing antibiotic prophylaxis to cover bacteremia-producing dental procedures in patients with HIV infection. Due to the complex and ultimately progressive nature of HIV-related diseases, antibacterial prophylaxis prior to invasive dental procedures should be undertaken only after consultation with the patient's physician. Antibiotic prophylaxis should be considered when <500 PMN/mm^3 is reported, and elective dental treatment should be delayed until blood values improve above this level.[11] Patients with little or no evidence of immunosuppression or other HIV-associated complications can usually be treated in a routine manner. They must practice meticulous oral hygiene and should be recalled frequently to monitor their oral health status, which may reflect progressing immune impairment.

■ Self-Study Review

30. Identify indications for and describe the prophylactic antibiotic regimen for selected TJR patients.
31. List dental procedures requiring antibiotic prophylaxis in these TJR patients.
32. Identify indicators for and describe the chemoprophylaxis regimen to prevent IE prior to dental procedures.
33. How important is oral health in preventing IE?
34. List dental procedures requiring chemoprophylaxis to prevent IE in the patient at risk.
35. Describe dosing instructions for the prevention of IE.
36. When the client is currently taking an antibacterial agent in the class indicated for chemoprophylaxis, what change should be made in the agent selected?
37. Identify other indications or conditions for chemoprophylaxis prior to dental procedures.

ANTIBIOTIC-ASSOCIATED ADVERSE DRUG EVENTS

Drugs seldom exert their beneficial effects without also causing adverse side effects. The inevitability of this therapeutic dilemma lends credence to the statement that there are no "absolutely" safe biologically active agents. In the recent controversy on the efficacy for antibiotic prophylaxis to prevent distant site infections, it was reported that more individuals died from taking an antibiotic than died from developing IE.[8,9]

Drug–Drug Interactions

Two or more drugs administered in therapeutic dosages at the same time or in close sequence may act independently, may interact to increase or diminish the effect of one or more drugs, or may interact to cause an unintended reaction. Drug–drug interactions may be complex and even unexplained, but they all seem to have either a pharmacodynamic or a pharmacokinetic basis because the same pharmacologic mechanisms that account for a drug's efficacy account for many of its adverse effects. Potentially serious drug–drug interactions can occur between antibacterial agents and other medications. By reviewing the patient's medical history, the clinician can identify drugs taken by the patient and seek necessary information in a drug reference to avoid prescribing antibacterial agents that may produce potential drug–drug interactions. Metronidazole is known to interact with alcohol to cause a disulfiram (Antabuse) effect of nausea, abdominal cramps, and vomiting. Patients should be informed that both alcohol ingestion and use of mouth rinses containing alcohol (such as some chlorhexidine preparations and most essential oil mouth rinses) should be avoided when metronidazole is taken.

Antibacterial Agents and Oral Contraceptives

There are no pharmacokinetic data at this time to support the contention that antibacterial agents reduce the efficacy of oral contraceptives, except for rifampin, an antituberculin drug. In a recent decision, the United States District Court for the Northern District of California also concluded, "scientific evidence regarding the alleged interaction between antibacterial agents and oral contraceptives did not satisfy the '*Daubert* standard' of causality."[12] However, according to the American Medical Association (AMA), such interactions cannot be completely discounted. The AMA recommends that women taking oral contraceptives be informed of the possibility of such interactions.[13] Similarly, the ADA Council on Scientific Affairs recommends that women be advised of the potential risk of an interaction between the antibacterial agent and the oral contraceptive. In this case, an alternative nonhormonal contraception method should be used during periods of antibacterial chemotherapy, and affected women should be advised of the importance of compliance with their oral contraceptive regimen while taking the antibiotic.[14]

Gastrointestinal Disturbances

Oral antibacterial agents, especially the macrolides, often cause gastrointestinal disturbances characterized by acute onset of nausea, retching, and vomiting. Antibacterial agents are also a common cause of diarrhea. If the patient has been taking the antibacterial agent for 1 to 2 days, diarrhea is probably due to the mild irritating action of the antibacterial agent. If the patient complains of bloody diarrhea with lower abdominal cramping and is currently taking (or has taken in the recent past) clindamycin or a broader spectrum penicillin or cephalosporin, the clinician must consider the possibility of superinfection with *C. difficile*. The most dangerous and potentially fatal presentation of this infection is pseudomembranous colitis.

Oral Side Effects

Metronidazole is associated with having an unpleasant taste disturbance. It can cause a reddish color in urine (which, although not an oral side effect, could cause anxiety to the patient). Several of the antibacterial agents can cause a brown to black staining of mucosa and teeth (mechanism unknown). Tetracyclines should be avoided during tooth development (age <9) and during pregnancy to avoid intrinsic staining of teeth. Minocycline can cause black pigmentation in mucosa and bone, leading to a bluish color of mucosa bound to periosteum. Intrinsic staining of permanent teeth following minocycline therapy (long term for acne) has been reported. Superinfection is possible with most antibacterial agents taken for more than a few days.

Oral Candidiasis

Superinfections with *C. albicans* organisms commonly occur in association with antibacterial chemotherapy (Color Plate 16). The oral mucosal lesions appear as white, raised, or cottage-cheese-like growths that can be scraped off, leaving a red, sometimes hemorrhagic base. Candidiasis may also appear as an erythematous lesion, commonly associated with chronic dry mouth or found under a dental prosthesis. Once an infection develops, *C. albicans* can spread to the esophagus or lungs via swallowing or droplet aspiration. In immunosuppressed patients, it may spread systemically via the bloodstream. Oral candidiasis is treated with antifungal therapy.

Antibacterial Drugs and Pregnancy

There is no firm evidence that any antibacterial agent is teratogenic in humans; however, drugs in general should be prescribed with caution for pregnant women (Chapter 21). Table 9-9 summarizes the known prenatal risks of antibacterial agents recommended for the empirical treatment of odontogenic infections.[15]

Allergic Reactions

In general, the topical administration of an antibacterial agent is more likely to sensitize a patient than is parenteral drug administration, and parenteral drug administration is more likely to sensitize than an orally administered drug. Most allergic reactions tend to occur for the first time in young or middle-aged adults. The dose, duration, and frequency of drug administration are further confounding factors, and single doses tend to produce less sensitization than prolonged treatment (Chapter 5). Penicillin is the most allergenic drug and can lead to simple rash, urticaria, itching, or anaphylactic

Table 9-9 Safety of Antibacterial Drugs in Pregnancy

Drug	FDA Pregnancy Category	Fetal Toxicity	Recommendation
Penicillins	B[1]	None known	Probably safe
Metronidazole	B[1]	None known; carcinogenic in rats and mice	Caution; use only for strong clinical indication in the absence of a suitable alternative
Azithromycin	B[1]	None known	Probably safe
Clindamycin	B[1]	None known	Caution; use only for strong clinical indication in the absence of a suitable alternative

[1]Category B: Either animal studies do not indicate a risk to the fetus and there are no controlled studies in women, or animal studies have shown an adverse effect, but controlled studies in women failed to demonstrate risk.

shock, which can be fatal. The drug treatment for anaphylaxis is 1:1,000 epinephrine, injected IM.

■ Self-Study Review

38. Identify potential adverse effects of antibacterial therapy.
39. Describe the ADA policy on antibiotics and oral contraceptives.
40. What is the most allergenic drug?

DENTAL HYGIENE APPLICATIONS

Agents Prescribed in the Dental Office

The role of the dental hygienist in antibacterial therapy may include providing or verifying instructions on how to take a specific product prescribed in the dental office. The client should be given warnings regarding taking the product with or without meals, warnings about potential side effects, products to avoid when taking the medication, and side effects that should concern the patient, such as bloody diarrhea or signs of candidal infection. When these signs occur, the patient should be instructed to notify the dentist. For women taking an oral contraceptive, a warning should be given about the rare possibility of a drug–drug interaction with the antibacterial agent and that additional nonhormonal forms of birth control should be used while taking an antibiotic with an oral contraceptive.

Agents Prescribed in a Medical Facility

When antibacterial agents are reported on the health history, the oral cavity should be examined for oral side effects. The client should be assessed for infectiousness to the clinician. The dental hygienist should verify compliance when antibacterial agents have been taken for antibiotic prophylaxis.

Antibiotic Prophylaxis

The recommendations for prevention of IE are different from the recommendations for prevention of a joint infection. The clinician should be familiar with the drugs and doses recommended in each regimen. Information to place in the treatment record includes which antibiotic was taken, what dose was taken (2 g for amoxicillin or cephalosporin, but only 600 mg for clindamycin and 500 mg for clarithromycin or azithromycin), when the dose was taken, and whether the patient has developed any adverse effects from taking the medication. Amoxicillin and cephalosporins come in a 500-mg doseform, so four 500-mg tablets would be taken to make 2 g. Clindamycin comes in a 300-mg doseform, so two tablets would be taken to make 600 mg. Azithromycin and clarithromycin come in 500-mg tablets, so one tablet would be taken for antibiotic prophylaxis. Following verification of dosing information, this should be recorded in the treatment record. See Chapter 3 for legal recording guidelines. Box 9-2 summarizes the dental hygiene applications for antibacterial therapy.

CONCLUSION

Most infections of the orofacial region are odontogenic in origin and can be resolved satisfactorily through an approach that incorporates appropriate, timely débridement (primary dental care) in conjunction with local anesthesia. The routine use of antibacterial agents for the management of odontogenic infections has not been shown to be effective. Before instituting antibacterial chemotherapy, clinicians should consider (a) the diagnosis, (b) the need for antibacterial chemotherapy, (c) the benefits versus the risks of drug therapy, (d) individualization of the drug regimen, (e) education of the patient, and (f) the importance of follow-up. This takes on added importance if one considers the fact that drugs seldom exert their beneficial effects without also causing adverse side effects, including drug resistance. The widespread and ever-increasing use of antibacterial agents has contributed to the development of antibacterial drug resistance. Current evidence suggests that unless health care providers change

BOX 9-2. Dental Hygiene Applications for Antibacterial Therapy

For Agents Prescribed in a Dental Office
- Provide or verify instructions on how to take the antibacterial agent
- Provide warnings as appropriate to the agent
- Describe potential adverse effects and advise the patient to notify the dentist if adverse effects, such as bloody diarrhea or candidal infection, develop
- Identify products to avoid while taking the antibacterial agent
- Advise women taking an oral contraceptive to use an additional nonhormonal form of birth control while taking the agent
- Place information on the drug prescribed and dosing instructions in the treatment record

For Agents Prescribed in a Medical Facility
- Monitor for side effects relevant to oral health care
- Determine if a risk for crossinfection to the operator exists

Antibiotic Prophylaxis
- Monitor compliance for antibiotic prophylaxis and place verification information in the treatment record regarding the drug taken, how much, when it was taken, and any adverse effects
- Record information in the treatment record

their practices, many of the currently available antibacterial agents may become ineffective. Fortunately, after antibacterial chemotherapy is terminated, the normal bacterial flora tends to regain its survival advantage because the resistant strains must compete with susceptible strains for essential nutrients and at the same time reallocate valuable energy from reproduction to maintenance of their resistant traits.

References

1. Kuriyama T, Karasawa T, Nakagawa K, et al. Bacteriologic features and antimicrobial susceptibility in isolates from orofacial odontogenic infections. *Oral Surg Oral Med Oral Pathol.* 2000;90(5):600–608.
2. Wright AJ. The penicillins. *Mayo Clinic Proc.* 1999;73:290–307.
3. Wilhelm MP, Estes LP. Vancomycin. *Mayo Clinic Proc.* 1999; 74:928–935.
4. Socransky SS, Haffaajee AD. Dental biofilm: Difficult therapeutic targets. *Periodontol 2000.* 2002;28:12–55.
5. Sandor GKB, Low DE, Judd PL, et al. Antimicrobial treatment options in the management of odontogenic infections. *J Can Dent Assoc.* 1998;64:508–514.
6. American Dental Association (ADA) Council on Scientific Affairs. Antibiotic use in dentistry. *J Am Dent Assoc.* 1997;128: 648.
7. The ADA/American Academy of Orthopaedic Surgeons Expert Panel. Advisory statement: Antibiotic prophylaxis for dental patients with total joint replacement. *J Am Dent Assoc.* 2003; 134(7):895–899.
8. Lockhart PB, Loven B, Brennan MT, et al. The evidence base for the efficacy of antibiotic prophylaxis in dental practice. *J Am Dent Assoc.* 2007;138(4):458–474.
9. Wilson W, Taubert KA, Gewitz M, et al. Prevention of infective endocarditis: Guidelines from the American Heart Association. *J Am Dent Assoc.* 2007;138(6):739–760.
10. American Academy of Periodontology Research, Science and

CLINICAL APPLICATION EXERCISES

☐ **Exercise 1.** Your patient for tomorrow has a notation on the treatment record that antibiotic prophylaxis is needed prior to dental treatment. Upon reading the medical history and physician consultation form, it is noted that the patient has had a cardiac valve replacement. The patient is allergic to penicillin. Drug history includes warfarin to reduce complications with the valve replacement. Which antibacterial drug is the most likely agent to be prescribed by the physician? You will need to use a drug reference.

☐ **Exercise 2.** Describe pretreatment instructions you would give for the patient who received a prescription for amoxicillin to be used for antibiotic prophylaxis. What questions will you ask when the patient arrives for treatment?

☐ **Exercise 3.** WEB ACTIVITY: Log on to http://www.cda-adc.ca/en/dental_profession/practising/clinical_practice_guidelines/index.asp. Read the two systematic reviews (SR) on clinical practice guidelines for managing apical periodontitis and apical abscess. These guidelines were established based on reliable science and are still current, although the Canadian Dental Association has no plan for updating the guidelines.

☐ **Exercise 4.** WEB ACTIVITY: Go to http://www.ada.org and enter "antibiotic prophylaxis" in the search box. Print the guidelines for your use.

☐ **Exercise 5.** WEB ACTIVITY: Go to http://www.americanheart.org/presenter.jhtml?identifier=11086 and print patient information to give to patients with cardiovascular conditions who formerly were told to use antibiotics prior to dental procedures.

Therapy Committee. Position paper: Diabetes and periodontal diseases. *J Periodontol*. 2000;71:664–678.

11. DePaola LG. Managing the care of patients infected with bloodborne diseases. *J Am Dent Assoc*. 2003;134:350–358.

12. LaCasa C. California court denies wrongful birth claim. *J Law Med Ethics*. 1996;24:273–274.

13. American Medical Association. Policy H-75.986: Drug interactions between oral contraceptives and antibiotics. Available at: http://www.ama-assn.org/apps/pf_new/pf_online?f_n=browse &doc=policyfiles/HnE/H-75.986.HTM. Accessed June 8, 2007.

14. American Dental Association Council on Scientific Affairs. Antibiotic interference with oral contraceptives. *J Am Dent Assoc*. 2002;133:880.

15. Abramowicz M, ed. Safety of antimicrobial drugs in pregnancy. In: *Handbook of Antimicrobial Therapy*. 6th ed. New Rochelle, NY: The Medical Letter on Drugs and Therapeutics; 2002:182–188.

10

Antifungal and Antiviral Drugs

Antibacterial agents are used to treat infections caused by bacteria. Antifungal agents are used to treat fungal infections. Antiviral agents are used to treat viral infections. This chapter describes situations in which the dentist would use antifungal and antiviral drugs and identifies potential drug interactions and adverse drug effects. Instructions on how to take the medication are included. The dental hygienist may be involved in identifying clinical manifestations of both fungal and viral infections, as these are common in the oral cavity. Specific clinical management guidelines for these infections and the role of the dental hygienist in the management of oral fungal and viral infections are described. The chapter ends with a discussion of various viral infections, including common hepatitis infections and the human immunodeficiency viral disease (HIVD), and their potential oral complications.

ANTIFUNGAL AGENTS

Fungi are free-living mycotic organisms that exist as yeasts or molds. There are over 100,000 fungal species, but only a few are pathogenic in humans. Most of the organisms as-

sociated with human disease are **saprophytic** members of the soil microbial flora. Others exist as **commensals** (meaning they obtain benefit without causing harm), typically on oral, vaginal, or gastrointestinal (GI) mucosa or as harmless residents of the skin and, at times, the respiratory epithelium. When events occur that allow for overgrowth of numbers of commensal organisms and disease develops, this is called **parasitism**, or *superinfection*. The latter are the organisms of interest to dental professionals. **Mycotic infection** is usually associated with opportunistic infection due to an impaired immune system and generally affects individuals with a compromised immune response. In recent years, the incidence of mycotic infections has increased. This is mainly due to situations related to suppression of the immune system, such as the following:

- the HIV epidemic
- the increased use of therapeutic immunosuppression drugs for organ transplantation
- the treatment of malignant diseases

Because of the slow rate of fungal growth, mycoses tend to be **subacute** (meaning they are infections without clinical signs and symptoms) to chronic in nature, with a tendency

Table 10-1	Antifungal Agents and Indications	
Drug Class	**Specific Agents**	**Clinical Use**
Polyenes	Amphotericin B	Systemic fungal infections Fungal meningitis Fungal urinary tract infections
	Nystatin	Oral and intestinal candidiasis, thrush
Imidazoles	Ketoconazole	Paracoccidiomycosis Chronic mucocutaneous candidiasis Dermatophyte skin infections
	Fluconazole	Systemic histoplasmosis, blastomycosis, coccidiomycosis, sporotrichosis, and opportunistic cryptococcosis and candidiasis Oral, esophageal, and vaginal candidiasis
	Itraconazole	Aspergillosis, histoplasmosis, blastomycosis, coccidiomycosis, sporotrichosis, and paracoccidiomycosis Oral, esophageal, and vaginal candidiasis
	Clotrimazole	Oral, esophageal, and vaginal candidiasis Dermatophyte skin infections
	Miconazole	Vaginal candidiasis
Other	Flucytosine	Severe, refractory oral and esophageal candidiasis Cryptococcosis
	Griseofulvin	Dermatophytes of hair, skin, and nails
	Terbinafine	Toenail infections due to *Trichophyton* species *Tinea pedis* infections

for relapse. They may present as superficial, cutaneous (skin or mucous membrane), subcutaneous, or systemic disease. Infection by *Candida* species, especially *Candida albicans*, represents the most common fungal infection (candidiasis, thrush) affecting the dental profession's anatomical area of responsibility.

Pharmacologic Basis for Antifungal Therapy

Fungal and human cells have similar metabolic pathways for protein synthesis and cell division. Consequently, unlike with antibacterial therapy, only a small number of unique targets for antifungal therapy have been identified, and antifungal pharmacologic therapy can be more complex. Table 10-1 contains available antifungal agents, some of which include griseofulvin, flucytosine, amphotericin B, nystatin, imidazole agents (ketoconazole), triazole agents (clotrimazole, voriconazole, fluconazole, itraconazole), echinocandins (micafungin sodium), and allylamine antifungals (terbinafine hydrochloride).

Formulations include tablets, creams, liquids, pastilles, troches (pronounced tro'kee; lozenges), and intravenously (IV) administered agents. Only those antifungal products used by dentists are reviewed in this chapter.

Currently available antifungal agents can be divided into drugs with a variety of mechanisms of action, including those that: (a) inhibit ergosterol synthesis, (b) disrupt fungal plasma membrane by binding to ergosterol, (c) inhibit DNA synthesis, and (d) inhibit microtubule function (Fig. 10-1). Antifungal agents used in dentistry act by the first two mechanisms.

Inhibitors of Ergosterol Synthesis

Ergosterol is synthesized within fungal cells from acetyl coenzyme A *and is necessary for cellular activity*. Ergosterol-synthesis inhibitors block a fungus-specific cytochrome P450 (CYP450) enzyme that is responsible for ergosterol forma-

tion. Table 10-2 lists the azole antifungal agents, which are the most common agents of this class used in dentistry to treat fungal infection. Unfortunately, the azoles are not entirely selective for fungal enzymes. They also inhibit hepatic CYP450 enzymes, and this inhibition is responsible for many drug–drug interactions. The extent of hepatic CYP450 enzyme inhibition is variable. It is most pronounced with ketoconazole and decreases in order of magnitude with itraconazole, voriconazole, and, finally, fluconazole. Hepatotoxicity is the major adverse effect of all systemic azole antifungal agents.

Ergosterol-Binding Drugs

Nystatin

Nystatin, an antifungal agent that binds to ergosterol in the fungal plasma membrane, increases membrane permeability and results in leakage of essential cellular components, leading to cell death. The use of nystatin is *strictly limited* to the treatment of superficial candidal infections of the skin, as well as oral and vaginal mucosa with topical formulations. It is used as a cream on skin or on vaginal mucosa, and as a rinse or lozenge in the oral cavity. Sugar is added for palatability when it is supplied as a liquid. The liquid or lozenge formulations must contact the fungal organisms to be effective, which requires that the product be held within the mouth for 5 to 7 minutes. For children or individuals who may find this difficult, the liquid can be frozen into "popsicles" and held in the mouth over a prolonged time as it melts. To reduce the risk for dental caries from frequent exposures to sugar, one can recommend a daily fluoride product to be used during nystatin therapy.

■ Self-Study Review

1. Describe the difference between *commensalism* and *parasitism* of C. albicans.

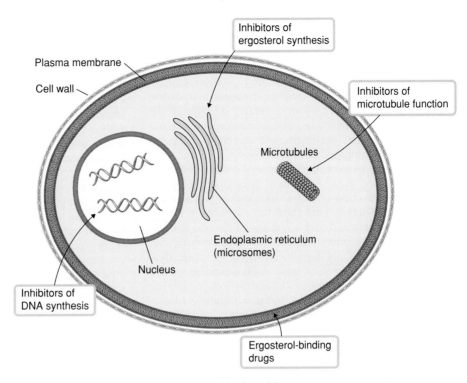

Figure 10-1 Mechanisms of Antifungal Action. (Courtesy of the UT Health Science Center at San Antonio, Multimedia & Web Services. Created by Chris McKee.)

Cellular Targets of Antifungal Drugs

2. List three conditions that are primarily responsible for mycotic infection.
3. Identify the most common example of mycotic infection in the oral cavity.
4. What is the relationship to the host response?
5. Examine agents Table 10-1. Which agents are relevant to oral infection?
6. Explain the mechanisms of action for antifungal agents used in dentistry.
7. List antifungal agents and classifications used to treat oral candida infection.
8. What is the major adverse effect of systemic azole antifungals?
9. Describe the doseforms of agents for topical application and the dosing instruction to the patient (infant, child, adult).
10. What antifungal is given for thrush in infants? What happens if the liquid is swallowed?
11. How is the increased caries risk managed when nystatin is used?

Pharmacotherapeutic Considerations

When managing fungal infections, various pharmacotherapeutic considerations are important. Because infection by the *Candida* species represents the most common fungal infection affecting the dental profession's anatomical area of responsibility, oral health care providers have a primary responsibility to diagnose and treat candidal infections.

Clinical Manifestations of Oral Candidal Infections

C. albicans is a normal inhabitant of the oral cavity. The presence of blastophores (budding yeasts) without hyphae (which may be viewed on a microscopic slide) in the absence of clinical signs or symptoms denotes a commensal status. It can also exist as a commensal organism of the skin, GI, and genitourinary tracts. Candidiasis is an infection, although it is not an infectious disease (i.e., it cannot be transmitted from patient to patient), that is caused primarily by the overgrowth of *C. albicans*. *C. albicans* is an opportunistic organism, and

Table 10-2	Inhibitors of Ergosterol Synthesis

Drugs	Comments
Ketoconazole	Available as an oral agent only Absorption depends on its conversion to a salt, which is predicated on an acidic environment in the stomach Not well transported into CSF and urine
Itraconazole	Available as oral and IV formulations As with ketoconazole, oral bioavailability is unreliable, which favors IV administration Not well transported into CSF, urine, and saliva
Voriconazole	Available as oral and IV formulations
Fluconazole	Available as oral and IV formulations Absorption following oral administration is not influenced by gastric pH; oral bioavailability is nearly 100% Diffuses freely into CSF, urine, and saliva
Clotrimazole	Available as topical formulations only (troche [lozenge], cream, vaginal insert)

alterations in host homeostasis precede the metamorphosis from commensalism to parasitism (Color Plate 16).

Predisposing systemic factors leading to alterations in host homeostasis include acquired and therapeutic immunosuppression (HIVD, cytotoxic drugs, corticosteroids), endocrinopathies (diabetes mellitus, hypoparathyroidism, hypoadrenalism, pregnancy with secondary infection of the infant), nutritional deficiencies, a high carbohydrate diet, use of antibacterial agents, qualitative and quantitative changes in salivary flow (drug-induced, radiotherapy, Sjögren syndrome), poor oral hygiene, the presence of dental prostheses, advanced age, and smoking. In most instances, candidiasis is a localized infection of oral tissues with a potential for systemic dissemination. Oral candidiasis appears in a variety of clinical forms and may affect any of the oral soft tissues (tongue, cheek, pharynx). It is often asymptomatic, but patients may periodically describe a burning sensation, dysphasia, or an altered sense of taste. A classification system based on clinical criteria provides a clear distinction between primary oral candidiasis and the oral manifestations of secondary systemic mucocutaneous candidiasis.[1]

Pseudomembranous Candidiasis

Pseudomembranous candidiasis is characterized by the presence of a white pseudomembrane, which can be wiped away with gauze, leaving a painful, red, and sometimes bleeding mucosal surface. This form can affect all oral soft tissues and may be either acute or chronic in nature. It is frequently observed in **neonates** (as thrush), immunosuppressed patients, and those patients with HIV infection.

Erythematous Candidiasis

Acute and chronic erythematous candidiasis (also called atrophic) appears as a red patch, usually on the palate or dorsum of the tongue, with concurrent loss of the filiform papillae. It can present as a generalized erythema covering mucous membranes. A burning sensation may be reported. This form is seen in HIVD and may follow exposure to broad-spectrum antibiotics.

Hyperplastic Candidiasis

Hyperplastic candidiasis is characterized by persistent (chronic) white plaques, which may be seen on most oral tissues. This form infiltrates the epithelium but when wiped away does not cause severe pain or bleeding. It is also known as candidal leukoplakia and is the least common variant. However, it is differentiated from leukoplakia in that once antifungal therapy is initiated, the lesion disappears. This form is often seen in association with inhaled corticosteroids used in the management of respiratory diseases.

Candida-Associated Denture Stomatitis

Denture stomatitis appears as an erythematous area beneath a denture-bearing surface. These lesions are asymptomatic and are frequently associated with poor oral hygiene and chronic wearing of dental prostheses (i.e., not taking them out during sleep). Similar lesions may be seen under the ridge-lap area

under the pontic in association with fixed prostheses. This illustrates the importance of cleaning the mucosa under the pontic.

Other Candidal Infections

Median rhomboid glossitis appears as an erythematous patch with loss of filiform papillae confined to the dorsal aspect of the tongue located anterior to the circumvallate papillae. Angular cheilitis appears as erythematous fissures at the commissures of the lips. It represents a mixed infection of *C. albicans* and coagulase-positive *Staphylococcus aureus*. Predisposing conditions may include poor oral hygiene, a decrease in the intermaxillary space, or nutritional deficiencies. At times these lesions may be more extensive, especially in children. They tend to lick their lips, resulting in a "chapped lips" appearance that then predisposes them to mixed candidal–bacterial infections, most often associated with the lower vermilion–skin interface.

Diagnosing Oral Candidal Infections

In most cases, the diagnosis of oral candidiasis is based on clinical signs and symptoms.[2] When the clinical diagnosis is unclear, such additional tests as exfoliative cytology, culture, or tissue biopsy may be useful to confirm a diagnosis.

Exfoliative Cytology

Exfoliative cytology involves scraping the suspected lesion with a sterile instrument or a tongue blade and smearing the sample on a glass slide. A wet prep consists of the application of potassium hydroxide (KOH) to the fresh cytologic smear. This allows for immediate examination of the sample for *Candida* hyphae and blastospores under a microscope. If the cytologic smear is allowed to dry, it may be fixed with ethanol and stained with periodic acid Schiff or Gram stain for microscopic evaluation.[1,2]

Culture

To obtain cells for culture, a sterile cotton swab is scraped over the suspected area, placed in a tube containing sterile saline, and mixed vigorously. Following inoculation of an agar plate with the solution and incubation for 48 to 72 hours, the agar plate is evaluated for the presence of fungal colonies.

Biopsy

If tissue invasion has occurred, microscopic examination of the infected tissue may reveal hyphae or pseudohyphae.

Therapeutic Strategies in the Treatment of Orolabial Candidal Infections

Normally a benign inhabitant of oral mucous membranes, *C. albicans* in most instances produces a localized oral infection. However, it may reflect a serious, even life-threatening infection in special patient populations. The goals of treatment are to identify and eliminate possible contributing factors, prevent systemic dissemination, and eliminate any associated discomfort. Appropriate medical treatment to eliminate predisposing systemic factors along with local measures, such as meticulous oral hygiene, management of xerostomia, and the maintenance of optimally functioning and clean dental prostheses, may prevent or minimize oral candidiasis.

Local Treatment

These measures should include proper cleaning of all oral tissues and all surfaces of prostheses, removing prostheses at regular intervals to allow for circulation in the supporting tissues, and periodically evaluating the prostheses for proper tissue adaption. A chlorhexidine rinse may be used in conjunction with antifungal agents to disinfect prosthetic devices.

Pharmacologic Treatment

Pharmacologic treatment should be individualized based on the patient's health status and the clinical presentation and severity of infection.

Topical antifungal therapy (nystatin, clotrimazole) is available via pastilles and troches, creams, ointments, or oral suspensions and remains the cornerstone of treatment in mild, localized cases of oral candidiasis in the healthy patient. After initiation of the empirical antifungal therapy described above for 7 days, a follow-up appointment is recommended to assess response. Some authors have recommended that antifungal medications be continued for at least twice the time required to produce resolution of clinical signs and symptoms. This is done not only to eliminate visual and clinical signs of infection, but also to reduce the mycologic levels of *Candida* to normal oral levels. If initial topical therapy has not produced significant resolution or improvement in clinical signs and symptoms at the follow-up appointment, the use of systemic (tablet doseform) antifungal medications is warranted. In a seemingly healthy patient, failure to respond to conventional therapy might be the initial sign of an underlying, undiagnosed immunologic problem or other systemic disease.

Primary Line of Antifungal Chemotherapy

Nystatin (Mycostatin) is the traditional drug of first choice for the treatment of oral candidiasis. Box 10-1 includes available formulations, including oral suspension, pastilles, creams, and oral and vaginal tablets. Nystatin pastilles, used as a lozenge five times daily, are the formulation of choice. To reduce the risk of relapse, treatment generally should be continued for at least 48 hours after the elimination of all signs and symptoms associated with the infection. The aqueous suspension (100,000 units per mL) may be used as a rinse and expectorated (rinse with 5 ml [500,000 units] five times a day) and is ideal as a holding solution for prostheses when they are removed from the oral cavity.[2] It also can be frozen and used as a "popsicle" (250,000 units per pop). Swallowing the solution would not harm the individual (because nystatin is not absorbed in the GI tract), but it would not resolve pharyngeal candidal infection either. Infant formulations of nystatin suspension are administered by dropper. The pediatric dose is 200,000 units (100,000 units in each side of the

---

BOX 10-1. Methods of Using Nystatin

Doseform	Method of Use
Pastille	Dissolve in mouth five times daily
Suspension liquid	Rinse and hold 5 mL in mouth for 5 minutes, five times daily; expectorate
	Freeze 2.5 mL into popsicles and allow to dissolve in mouth, five times daily
	Infants: Administer 15 drops (total) by dropper five times daily; 3 drops in each side of mouth
Cream	Apply to area of infection and to tissue-based area of denture; insert denture
Vaginal tablet	When used as an oral lozenge, allow to dissolve in mouth; use four times daily

---

mouth) four times a day (for a total daily dose of 800,000 units). This means that 1 mL (15 drops) is administered by a dropper in each side of the mouth four times a day.

Denture stomatitis can be treated by the application of a thin layer of nystatin cream to the tissue side of a denture base. Nystatin vaginal tablets (over-the-counter [OTC] formulation) can be used as oral lozenges five times a day. Unlike other topical formulations, nystatin vaginal tablets do not contain sucrose, which may be preferred in caries-prone patients. Nystatin has minimal side effects.

Clotrimazole

Ten milligrams of clotrimazole (troche) five times a day improves resolution of candidiasis refractory to nystatin. It is recommended that the troches be allowed to dissolve slowly over a period of 15 to 30 minutes. Clotrimazole is an effective way of treating oral and chronic mucocutaneous candidiasis with few adverse effects. Denture stomatitis can be treated by the application of a thin layer of clotrimazole cream to the tissue side of a denture base. Nausea and vomiting may occur rarely, and abnormal liver function tests have been reported in 15% of the patients in clinical trials. Clotrimazole is not recommended for the treatment of candidiasis in pregnant women or children under the age of 3 years.

Secondary Line of Antifungal Chemotherapy

Systemic antifungal agents, such as fluconazole, are generally reserved to treat severe localized, disseminated oral candidiasis or infections in immunosuppressed individuals. Additionally, candidal infections that respond poorly to topical therapy may be treated with systemic antifungal medications. A biopsy, culture, or cytologic smear may help confirm the clinical diagnosis in such cases. Patients with dry mouth or sensitive tissues may report difficulty in dissolving tablets or lozenges and may be candidates for systemic therapy. Other systemic agents include ketoconazole and itraconazole.

Fluconazole

The clinical activity of fluconazole is well established for the treatment of mucocutaneous candidiasis. The initial recommended therapeutic regimen is a 200-mg loading dose, followed by 100 mg/day for 14 days. The treatment should be continued for at least 48 hours after all signs and symptoms associated with the infection are resolved. Fluconazole has been evaluated in several studies for the treatment of denture stomatitis. These studies were initially successful in reducing clinical signs and symptoms; however, relapse usually occurred shortly after cessation of therapy. Resistance to fluconazole may occur with long-term usage and could potentially be problematic in some patients.

Tertiary Line of Antifungal Chemotherapy

Reports indicate that 88% of isolates of *Candida* species are susceptible to flucytosine. Flucytosine resistance in fungi may arise from mutations that affect the synthesis of enzymes essential for the drug's metabolism and ultimately its ability to interfere with DNA synthesis. When flucytosine is used in combination with amphotericin B, the altered fungal cell membrane permeability allows enhanced uptake of flucytosine by strains that are usually resistant.

Drug Interactions and Adverse Effects

The polyene nystatin, by virtue of the fact that it is not absorbed systemically, does not interact significantly with other drugs. Other antifungal agents have many potential drug–drug interactions that mandate ready access by dental prescribers to reliable drug reference books.

Warfarin

One potential drug–drug interaction with immediate relevance to the practice of dental hygiene is the interaction of fluconazole, ketoconazole, or itraconazole with the anticoagulant warfarin sodium, which may increase blood levels of warfarin and increase the risk of bleeding. The International Normalized Ratio (INR) is the standard blood test to measure the risk for hemorrhage when warfarin is taken. The INR should be monitored in those patients. Safe levels for periodontal débridement and oral prophylaxis are 3.5 INR or less.

Drug–Disease Interactions

Prolonged use of systemic antifungal drugs may potentially result in renal or hepatic dysfunction in some patients. As such, fluconazole, ketoconazole, and itraconazole should be administered with caution in individuals with underlying hepatic disease taking other hepatotoxic medications (acetaminophen). If prolonged systemic antifungal therapy is anticipated, liver function tests should be ordered prior to the initiation of therapy and evaluated frequently during treatment.

12. Describe the role of *C. albicans* in the normal flora and changes that promote the development of candidiasis.
13. List conditions that predispose an individual to develop opportunistic infections.
14. Describe features, signs, and symptoms of the various forms of candidiasis.
15. Which three groups are most likely to develop pseudomembranous candidiasis?
16. Consider therapeutic strategies to manage oral candida infection. Differentiate between primary and secondary therapies; describe local treatment strategies that involve the dental hygienist.
17. Identify possible drug interactions with systemic antifungal agents and the dosing regimen suggested when an interaction is possible.
18. When nystatin is ineffective, what is the second line local agent used for candidiasis?
19. Are topical antifungal agents likely to cause drug–drug interactions?

ANTIVIRAL AGENTS

Compared to the high number of antibacterial drugs (Chapter 9) that became available during the past 5 decades, so few antiviral drugs have been developed for oral viral disease that there is no specific treatment for most viral infections affecting the oral cavity. The one exception involves treatment for HIVD. The chief reason for this paucity of drugs is that viruses require a host cell in order to replicate, and most agents capable of interfering with the reproductive processes of viruses are likely to be toxic to host cells as well. Infection by the herpes simplex 1 virus (HSV-1) represents the most common viral infection affecting the dental profession's anatomical area of responsibility. This section will discuss the management of HSV-1 infection, referred to as primary herpetic gingivostomatitis, herpes labialis, or intraoral herpes simplex when it affects mucosa within the oral cavity. Antiviral agents taken by individuals with HIVD and various forms of hepatitis are identified at the end of the chapter, and adverse drug effects that could affect the dental hygiene treatment plan are discussed.

The Clinical Manifestations of Orolabial Herpetic Infections

The transmission of herpes simplex viral organisms (HSV types 1 and 2) occurs via direct contact with contaminated secretions from an infected individual. HSV-1 is transmitted by contact with oral secretions or vesicular fluid, and HSV-2 is usually transmitted sexually, although HSV-2 can be translocated to the oral cavity. There are approximately a half million new cases of mucocutaneous herpetic infections (primary infection) per year in the United States, and most occur in children between the ages of 2 and 3 years old.[3] Both HSV-1 and HSV-2 may be associated with primary HSV infections, with HSV-1 accounting for 75% to 90% of the cases. Over 90% of primary exposures result in either asymptomatic or mildly symptomatic illness. The late effects of herpetic infections are characterized by general disintegration of host cells and the release of infectious viral units into the extracellular environment. These viruses, in turn, can infect nearby cells or can be transported to regional sensory ganglia (trigeminal), where they establish latency in neuronal cell bodies.

Recurrent infection in immunocompetent individuals with HSV-1 involves the skin, the lips (herpes labialis), and intraoral mucosa bound to the periosteum. Lesions are fluid-filled blisters or vesicles for the skin and lips and small pin-point ulcerations of attached gingivae. During the prodromal phase, the only sign of infection may be tingling in the affected area. It has been suggested that oral health care services should not be completed when clinical vesicular lesions are present, because manipulation of lips can promote the spread of the viral particles and also because of the risk of transmitting viral particles to the operator (eyes, nasal mucosa, fingers). However, there may be instances where urgent care is necessary when a lesion in present. Standard precautions, including glasses with side shields, masks covering the nose and mouth, and gloves, are recommended to avoid transmission. Immunocompromised patients (e.g., AIDS patients, organ transplant recipients, chemotherapy patients, and so forth) often have a more severe form of viral infection, and intraoral lesions can affect labile mucosa, as well as mucosa bound to periosteum. For example, lesions can be found in the floor of the mouth.

Pharmacologic Therapy

Primary Line of HSV-1 Antiviral Chemotherapy

Most cases of HSV-1 infection are self-limiting and can be resolved with OTC or prescription agents. For herpes labialis, a topical antiviral agent, such as penciclovir (Denavir), is available by prescription. However, in cases of complicated primary herpetic gingivostomatitis and in the management of immunocompromised patients, systemic antiviral chemotherapy should be added to the primary line of treatment. Systemic acyclovir, in oral or parenteral form, accelerates the resolution of viral shedding and healing time and reduces pain. A generally accepted oral regimen is 400 mg taken three to five times/day for 10 days. Acyclovir is generally well tolerated. Adverse effects include nausea, vomiting, light-headedness, diaphoresis, and rash.

Valacyclovir (Valtrex), a prodrug of acyclovir, has been shown to reduce pain and to speed lesion healing by about 1 day when patients take 2 g of valacyclovir at the onset of prodromal symptoms and 2 g 12 hours later. In doses of 500 mg taken three times/day for 5 days, famciclovir (Famvir), a prodrug of penciclovir, has been reported to have a 2-day reduction in healing time compared to controls. Immunocompromised patients who are either intolerant to acyclovir or are infected with an acyclovir-resistant strain of HSV may respond to foscarnet (Foscavir).

Topical Antiviral Agents

Topical agents are most effective if applied during the early prodromal stage of a herpes outbreak. Penciclovir (Denavir), 1% cream, appears to be helpful in the treatment of recurrent herpes labialis in healthy adults. Penciclovir reduces both the duration of the herpetic lesions and the pain associated with lesions.[4] It is used for both primary and recurrent HSV infection. Penciclovir is preferred over topical acyclovir because it has better entry into infected cells and remains within the cell longer than acyclovir. The recommended treatment regimen, starting with the first prodromal symptoms, is to cover the lip lesion every 2 hours during the day for a period of 4 days. Although the systemic absorption of penciclovir after topical use is negligible, application to intraoral mucous membranes is not recommended.

Docosanol (Abreva), an OTC product, is FDA approved to shorten the healing time and reduce symptoms and pain associated with herpes labialis, but it is not indicated for intraoral herpetic lesions. Other OTC topical agents available for the management of recurrent herpes labialis contain a variety of ingredients, such as menthol, camphor, emollients, and anesthetics. As the claims on the labels indicate, these agents may aid in relieving the symptoms of herpes labialis, but they do not have any antiviral activity and do not alter the course of the infection.

Strategies to Prevent Cross-Infection in the Oral Health Care Setting

Although it is the vesicular fluid that contains the most infectious inoculum, and infectivity diminishes as the vesicles rupture, spontaneous shedding can occur from a resolving or subclinical (prodromal phase) herpetic lesion. HSV is contagious and can be transmitted to others. Patients presenting for dental care with an active herpetic infection should be rescheduled; in emergency situations, isolation of the lesions during dental care may be appropriate. This can be achieved by using a rubber dam. Since the institution of standard body fluid precautions, the occupational risk of herpetic whitlow (herpetic infection of the finger area) and keratoconjunctivitis (herpetic infection in the eye) in the oral health care setting has been dramatically reduced.

ANTIVIRAL TREATMENT FOR HIV INFECTION AND HEPATITIS

With minor variations, all viruses have the same general life cycle (Fig. 10-2). Infection begins when a virion attaches to a host cell. The attachment is mediated by viral proteins that bind specific receptors on the host cell membrane. Once the virus has gained entry into the host cell, it becomes available for genome replication. In most instances, the viral DNA or RNA itself is replicated. The process continues until the newly formed virion becomes infectious and is released from the host cell membrane. The most common forms of infectious hepatitis are caused by the hepatitis B virus (HBV) and

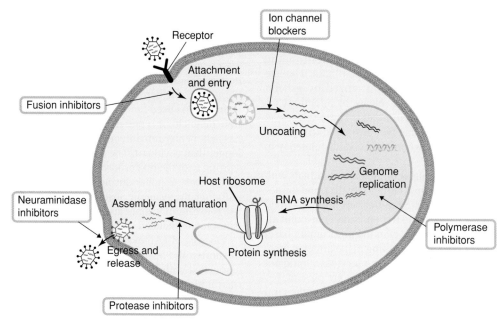

Figure 10-2 Stages of the Viral Life Cycle Targeted by Antiviral Drug Classes. (Courtesy of the UT Health Science Center at San Antonio, Multimedia & Web Services. Created by Chris McKee.)

hepatitis C virus (HCV) organisms. The liver infection results in reduced function of the organ. The main clinical implication for dental hygiene care relates to increased bleeding due to the reduction of vitamin-K clotting factors and the potential for disease transmission in the oral health care setting (exposure to blood and other potentially infectious material). Hairy leukoplakia has been associated with HIV infection (Color Plate 21).

Inhibitors of Viral Attachment and Entry

All viruses must infect cells to replicate. Therefore, inhibiting the initial step of viral attachment and entry could limit the spread of the virus within the body. Active and passive immunization can inhibit viral infection by providing antibodies against viral envelope proteins. These antibodies can then block viral attachment and penetration into cells and increase viral clearance. Alternatively, immunization can be directly virucidal, causing the virus to be destroyed or inactivated before the virus can interact with its receptor on target cells.

Enfuvirtide is the first antiviral agent that inhibits viral entry into host cells. It is an anti-HIV peptide structurally similar to a segment of the HIV protein (gp41) that mediates membrane fusion. It is approved for the treatment of HIV infection in combination with other drugs.

Anti-HIV and Anti-HBV Nucleoside Analogs

HIV is a retrovirus. All retroviruses contain a ribonucleic acid (RNA) genome, and their capsids contain an enzyme

(reverse transcriptase) essential for HIV replication. Reverse transcriptase is a DNA polymerase, which copies the RNA retrovirus genome into double-stranded DNA. Once the viral DNA is integrated, cellular RNA polymerase copies it into the various viral proteins. Nucleoside analogs mimic reverse transcriptase. This information is provided as an introduction to the various drug classifications developed to manage HIV infection. These analogs illustrated in Table 10-3 inhibit reverse transcriptase and terminate elongation as they become incorporated into the growing DNA chain. Some also inhibit HBV-encoded DNA polymerase. Table 10-3 also includes the clinical implications for HIV drugs. Each drug has different potential adverse effects and should be investigated in a drug reference. In general, antiviral HIV agents suppress the hematopoietic blood-forming cells, such as platelets and white blood cells. A recent trend has been to combine anti-HIV drugs into a single doseform. Box 10-2 contains the current HIV combination products. The drug effects can be investigated by looking up each product in the combination in a drug reference. Some dental drug references have a single monograph for the combination product.[5]

Other Antiviral Drugs

Oligonucleotides are capable of base pairing to virus-specific segments of RNA and may disrupt transcription or translation or promote RNA degradation. If the viral RNA is an mRNA, oligonucleotides prevent the synthesis of proteins encoded by the mRNA. Fomivirsen is designed to bind to mRNA that encodes a specific gene regulatory protein and is active against the cytomegalovirus (CMV). Ribavirin (Rebetol) appears to inhibit viral RNA polymerase. The drug is available in aerosol

Table 10-3	Anti-HIV, Anti-HCV, and Anti-HBV Drugs

Classification	Clinical Use	Clinical Considerations
Nucleoside analogs: Abacavir (Ziagen) Emtricitabine (Emtriva) Didanosine (Videx) Lamivudine (Epivir) Stavudine (Zerit) Tenofovir (Viread) Zalcitabine (Hivid) Zidovudine (Retrovir) Nonnucleoside agents: Efavirenz (Sustiva) Delavirdine (Rescriptor) Nevirapine (Viramune) Protease inhibitors: Amprenavir (Agenerase) Atazanavir (Reyataz) Fosamprenavir (Lexiva) Indinavir (Crixivan) Nelfinavir (Viracept) Ritonavir (Norvir) Saquinavir (Invirase) Tipranavir (Aptivus)	HIV	Monitor for ADEs in drug reference Caution to prevent instrument or needle sticks Antibiotic prophylaxis is when PMN/mm are <500; delay elective treatment until values improve Anticipate oral candidiasis Oral health education implications Frequent maintenance prophylaxis Encourage strict plaque control to prevent periodontal inflammation Used in combination anti-HIV therapy
Fusion inhibitor: Enfuvirtide (Fuzeon)	HIV	Used in combination anti-HIV therapy
Antivirals: Adefovir (Hepsera) Entecavir (Baraclude)	HBV	HBV is highly contagious; follow universal precautions on a strict basis Acetaminophen may be contraindicated
Ribavirin (Rebetol)	HCV	Used in combination with interferon for the treatment of chronic HCV infections

form for the treatment of severe respiratory syncytial virus (RSV) infections and, in combination with interferon, for the treatment of chronic HCV infections.

Drugs for HIVD/HAART Therapy

Currently available anti-HIV drugs exploit structural and functional differences between viral and human proteins. These include (a) a fusion inhibitor; (b) inhibitors of viral genome replication (nucleoside reverse transcriptase in-hibitors [NRTIs], a nucleotide reverse transcriptase inhibitor [NtRTI], and nonnucleoside reverse transcriptase inhibitors [NNRTIs]); and (c) protease inhibitors (PIs). The treatment of HIV infection requires combination therapy known as highly active antiretroviral therapy (HAART). HAART regimens currently recommended for the treatment of naïve patients (those who have not been previously exposed to anti-HIV drugs) may be NNRTI-based (one NNRTI and two NRTIs); PI-based (one or two PIs and two NRTIs); or triple NRTI-based (three NRTIs). The treatment of patients with acute HIV infection, HIV-infected adolescents, injection drug users, HIV-infected women of reproductive age and pregnant women, and patients with coinfections (HBV, HCV, and tuberculosis) require special antiretroviral regimens.

BOX 10-2. Anti-HIV Combination Products

Nucleoside reverse transcriptase inhibitor combination products:
- abacavir/lamivudine (Epzicom)
- abacavir/lamivudine/zidovudine (Trizivir)
- emtricitabine/tenovir (Truvada)
- lamivudine/zidovudine (Combivir)

Protease inhibitor combination:
- lopinavir/ritonavir (Kaletra)

■ Self-Study Review

20. Identify the most common viral infection in the oral cavity.
21. Compare HSV-1 oral lesions in healthy and in immunocompromised individuals.
22. Identify systemic agents used for primary therapy in complicated primary herpetic gingivostomatitis.
23. List the "1-day" antiviral treatment.

24. Describe patient instructions for the various antiviral agents.
25. Describe treatment plan modifications for herpes labialis.

DENTAL HYGIENE APPLICATIONS

Although the dentist would prescribe antifungal and antiviral therapy, the dental hygienist must ensure that instructions on how to use the agents are fully understood by the patient so that the chance for successful treatment is increased. Some individuals come to a dental appointment even though they have a herpetic lesion on the lips. Delay in treatment for dental hygiene services is recommended to reduce the risk of spreading the lesion within client tissues. Proper use of protective barriers should protect the clinician.

Fungal infections are usually treated initially with topical doseforms that must contact the organism to act against it, which requires holding the doseform in the mouth for several

---

BOX 10-3. Clinical Implications for HIVD

1. Comprehensive intraoral assessment for opportunistic disease
   a. Antifungal therapy may be needed
   b. Examine for HIV-associated malignancies
2. Question about current drug therapy
   a. Investigate side effects in drug reference
   b. Consider dental clinical implications of HIVD
3. Question about disease control, healing problems, and increased bleeding; blood values
   a. Antibiotic prophylaxis, if severely neutropenic (below 1,000 cells/mm^3)
      i. Use regimen recommended by American Heart Association
   b. CD4 count is not an indicator for antibiotic prophylaxis
   c. Elective procedures contraindicated when PMN <500 cells/mm^3
   d. Use analgesics as recommended by MD, as needed
4. HAART drug therapy can predispose the patient to cardiovascular and diabetes symptoms
   a. Monitor blood pressure and pulse pressure, rate, and rhythm each appointment
   b. Question about blood sugar levels
5. Follow established infection control and standard precautions

(Reprinted with permission from DePaola, LG. Managing the care of patients infected with bloodborne diseases. *JADA.* 2003;134:350–358.)

BOX 10-4. Clinical Implications for Hepatitis

1. Question about increased bleeding potential
   a. If positive, require INR, platelet count, and platelet function tests
   b. Delay elective procedure if <50,000 platelets/mm^3
2. Question about PMN cell count
   a. Delay elective procedures if <500 cells/mm^3
3. Question about disease control and drug therapy
   a. Both prescription and OTC meds (herbs, etc.).
   b. Use analgesics recommended by MD, as needed
   c. Investigate drug side effects in drug reference; follow clinical recommendations
4. Follow established infection control and standard precautions.

(Reprinted with permission from DePaola, LG. Managing the care of patients infected with bloodborne diseases. *JADA.* 2003;134:350–358.)

---

minutes. The patient needs to understand this principle to promote compliance with antifungal drug therapy. Antiviral topical agents must be applied during the prodromal phase to be most effective.

The patient who understands the reasons for dosing instructions with the specific pharmacologic agent is more likely to be compliant with therapy. Dosing instructions should include the factors that can cause therapy to be ineffective. For these reasons the dental hygienist's role in therapy may involve ensuring that the patient has a complete understanding of dosing instructions and any factors that prohibit treating him or her during an active viral infection.

When antifungal or antiviral drugs are reported on the health history, a drug reference should be consulted with attention paid to side effects that can influence the dental hygiene treatment plan. In addition, the reason for taking the drug can be important to consider. Box 10-3 provides clinical implications for treating an individual with HIVD, and Box 10-4 provides clinical implications for the individual with hepatitis.[6] These recommendations should be considered when providing periodontal débridement for the individual with either of these infections.

CONCLUSION

Advances in medical and pharmacologic treatment have resulted in greater life expectancy for patients with malignant and metabolic disease, HIV infection, immune suppression, organ transplantation, and other systemic conditions that can predispose patients to oral and systemic mycoses and viral infections. The dental hygienist may be the oral health professional to identify a fungal or viral infection in an unsuspecting patient. Images of various clinical appearances of oral infections are found in this textbook's colored insert. Knowledge

CLINICAL APPLICATION EXERCISES

☐ **Exercise 1.** Describe dosing instructions for the various doseforms of nystatin, including giving drops to a 2-month-old infant, preparing and administering a nystatin popsicle for a 3-year-old child, and using a suspension, pastille, and cream for a denture patient.

☐ **Exercise 2.** A patient with recurrent herpes labialis receives a prescription for penciclovir cream. You are to tell the individual how to use the product. Describe dosing instructions for penciclovir cream.

of pharmacologic therapies and patient information related to these therapies will improve the provision of dental hygiene care for these infections.

References

1. Axell T, Samaranayake LP, Reichart PA, et al. A proposal for reclassification of oral candidosis. *Oral Surg Oral Med Oral Pathol Oral Radiol Endod.* 1997;84(2):111–112.
2. Fotos PG, Hellstein JW. Candida and candidosis. *Dent Clin North Am.* 1992;36(4):857–877.
3. Scott DA, Coulter WA, Lamey PJ. Oral shedding of herpes simplex virus type 1: A review. *J Oral Pathol Med.* 1997;26:441–447.
4. Boon R, Goodman JJ, Martinez J, et al. Penciclovir cream for the treatment of sunlight-induced herpes simplex labialis: A randomized, double-blind, placebo-controlled trial. *Clin Ther.* 2000;22:76–90.
5. DePaola, LG. Managing the care of patients infected with blood-borne diseases. *JADA.* 2003;134:350–358.
6. Pickett F, Terezhalmy G. *Dental Drug Reference with Clinical Implications.* Baltimore: Lippincott Williams & Wilkins; 2006:25–96.

11

Conscious Sedation and General Anesthesia

KEY TERMS

Conscious sedation: Light sedation to relax the patient who can respond to situations and questions

General anesthesia: Generalized, reversible depression of the central nervous system (CNS) characterized by loss of consciousness, amnesia, and immobility, but not necessarily complete anesthesia

Hematopoiesis: The formation of blood or blood cells in the living body (bone marrow)

N_2O/O_2: Nitrous oxide mixed with oxygen

The dental hygienist is generally not involved in **general anesthesia** procedures; however, many states allow dental hygienists to monitor and/or administer nitrous oxide gas for **conscious sedation**. As in past chapters, this chapter focuses on clinical applications that are relevant to dental hygiene practice. Consequently, more information on the pharmacology of nitrous oxide than that of general anesthesia is discussed.

USE OF NITROUS OXIDE IN THE ORAL HEALTH CARE SETTING

Conscious Sedation

Nitrous oxide is commonly used in combination with oxygen (**N_2O/O_2 combination**) for conscious sedation and analgesia, a situation in which the patient is conscious and pain sensation is diminished. The goal of conscious sedation is to have a lightly sedated and relaxed patient who can respond to situations and questions. Therefore, the four effects of N_2O/O_2 for conscious analgesia are

1. the patient remains conscious;
2. the protective reflexes are intact;
3. relief of anxiety;
4. analgesia.

The dose of the gas combination for conscious sedation is variable, according to the patient response. A 50% nitrous and 50% oxygen combination may be adequate, with a 60% nitrous and 40% oxygen level being the recommended maximum nitrous limitation. Vital signs are taken before the administration of nitrous oxide and monitored during the procedure. The procedure begins with 100% oxygen administration for 2 to 3 minutes, followed by adding nitrous oxide slowly in 10% increments. Onset of sedation occurs rapidly, within 3 to 5 minutes. The patient is told to notify the clinician when tingling or other sensations are felt. The addition of nitrous oxide is maintained at the level where the patient reports being relaxed and comfortable. At the end of the procedure, nitrous oxide is slowly reduced, and 100% oxygen is administered for 5 minutes. Recovery is rapid, with a full return to psychomotor capacity within a few minutes.

Diffusion Hypoxia

At the termination of nitrous oxide sedation, the rapid movement of large amounts of nitrous oxide from the circulation into the lungs may dilute the oxygen in the lungs. This dilution may result in a phenomenon known as *diffusion hypoxia*. To prevent this, the clinician would administer 100% oxygen for the amount of time needed to clear the nitrous oxide from the lungs. Termination of nitrous oxide effects is by *exhalation*.

Induction of General Anesthesia

Nitrous oxide/oxygen combination is often used with other drugs to induce general anesthesia. The next section describes the role of nitrous oxide in this procedure.

■ Self-Study Review

1. Is nitrous oxide used by itself or in combination with another agent? If so, which agent?
2. List four effects of N_2O/O_2 for conscious analgesia.
3. Identify the recommended dose of oxygen and that of nitrous oxide for conscious analgesia.
4. Describe the procedure for administering nitrous oxide for conscious sedation, including patient responses.
5. Describe the cause of *diffusion hypoxia* and how it is prevented.
6. How is the effect of nitrous oxide terminated?
7. List two uses for nitrous oxide.

GENERAL ANESTHESIA

Before the discovery of general anesthetics, pain and shock severely limited the possibilities of surgical intervention to treat disease. Surgery-related mortality dropped dramatically in 1846 following the introduction of diethyl ether. Since then, the induction and maintenance of anesthesia has become a distinct medical specialty. Today, anesthesiologists are responsible for all aspects of patient health during surgery.[1,2] As part of this process, anesthesiologists control not only the depth of anesthesia, but also maintain homeostatic equilibrium with a combination of inhaled and intravenous (IV) anesthetics, and a number of adjuvant drugs. General anesthetics induce a generalized, reversible depression of the CNS characterized by loss of consciousness, amnesia, and immobility (i.e., a lack of response to noxious stimuli), but not necessarily complete analgesia.

As mentioned earlier, the CNS is the primary site of action of anesthetics. Loss of consciousness and amnesia appear to result from supraspinal action (i.e., action in the brain stem, midbrain, and cerebral cortex), while immobility in response to noxious stimuli is caused by the depression of both supraspinal and spinal sensory and motor pathways. Based on observations of the effects of diethyl ether Arthur Guedel made in 1920, the deepening anesthetic state can be divided into four stages (Table 11-1).

As the patient progresses through the stages of anesthesia, it is recognized that different sites of the CNS are affected sequentially:

- Stage I—As induction begins, the initial signs include reduced sensation to pain (depending on the particular anesthetic agent), while consciousness is maintained so the patient can respond to commands; reflexes are present and respiration is regular; and some amnesia may be evident.
- Stage II—As anesthesia deepens, a period of excitation characterized by autonomic activity (coughing, salivation,

Table 11-1	Guedel's Stages of General Anesthesia
Stage I: Analgesia	Analgesia Amnesia Euphoria Consciousness
Stage II: Excitement	Excitement Delirium Combativeness
Stage III: Surgical anesthesia	Unconsciousness Regular respiration resumes Decreasing eye movement
Stage IV: Medullary depression	Respiratory arrest Cardiac depression and arrest No eye movement

hypertension), muscle twitching, vomiting, and incontinence can occur; the jaw muscles may tighten, and an attempt to insert an oral airway may stimulate gagging and laryngospasm; this stage is undesirable, and these responses are reduced or abolished as more anesthesia is given.
- Stage III—A decreasing loss of the eyelash reflex and the development of rhythmic respiration indicate the beginning of surgical anesthesia; muscles relax, and normal pulse rates are evident; most surgery is performed in stage III.
- Stage IV—Further deepening of anesthesia would lead to respiratory depression; cardiac arrest and death occurs later in stage IV. This stage is avoided.

Modern medicine has expanded the objectives of general anesthesia to include control over such physiologic variables as skeletal muscle contraction, autonomic responses, cardiovascular and respiratory dynamics, cognitive functions (including amnesia), and perioperative pain and anxiety.[1,2] There is no one drug that provides this wide variety of pharmacologic effects. To achieve these objectives, anesthesiologists today use a combination of agents to achieve surgical anesthesia, which may include volatile gaseous and IV anesthetics, nitrous oxide, analgesics, sedatives, antianxiety agents, and neuromuscular blocking agents in a sequential process known as induction (Table 11-2).[1,2] In clinical practice, this combination of agents is used to achieve

- rapid loss of consciousness;
- amnesia of surgical events;
- minimal amount of time in the excitement phase (stage II);
- stable plateau of surgical anesthesia;
- analgesia;
- appropriate levels of respiratory and cardiovascular responsiveness, and skeletal muscle relaxation.

■ Self-Study Review

8. Describe the effects of general anesthesia. What is the limitation?
9. What is the primary site of action for general anesthetic agents?
10. List and explain features of the four stages of anesthesia.

Table 11-2	Anesthetics and Adjuvant Drugs Used in the Induction of Anesthesia	
Drug Class	**Specific Agents**	**Clinical Uses**
Inhaled general anesthetics	Nitrous oxide	Fast induction of anesthesia Weak anesthetic Analgesic at subhypnotic concentrations Minimal cardiopulmonary depression General anesthesia
	Diethyl ether Desflurane Sevoflurane Enflurane Isoflurane Halothane	
IV general anesthetics	Thiopental Methohexital	Fast induction, movement through stage II and recovery
	Propofol	Fast induction and maintenance of anesthesia Antiemetic
	Etomidate	Fast induction and recovery
	Ketamine	Dissociative anesthesia and analgesia
Benzodiazepines	Diazepam Lorazepam Midazolam	Given 15 to 60 min before the induction of anesthesia to calm the patient and obliterate memory of the induction (amnesiac effect) Anticonvulsant
Opioids	Morphine Meperidine Fentanyl Remifentanil	Adjuvant analgesia
Neuromuscular blockers	Tubocurarine Pancuronium	Long duration adjuvant muscle relaxant
	Vecuronium Cis-atracurium	Intermediate duration adjuvant muscle relaxant
	Mivacurium	Short duration adjuvant muscle relaxant
	Succinylcholine	Very short duration adjuvant muscle relaxant

11. List the various types of drugs used to achieve general anesthesia.
12. List six goals of general anesthetic drugs.
13. Note the clinical uses for general anesthetic agents. What drugs provide an amnesiac effect?

Induction of Anesthesia

While inhalation anesthetics are useful for maintaining stable, long-term anesthesia, it is difficult to raise their blood concentrations rapidly enough to provide for rapid loss of consciousness and to minimize the time in the excitation phase. General anesthesia is therefore induced using highly lipid-soluble anesthetic agents, which can be injected directly into the circulation via IV administration and then maintained by inhalation anesthetics.

Intravenous General Anesthetics

Short-Acting Barbiturates

Short-acting barbiturates (thiopental, methohexital) are used to move the patient through stage II quickly. For those individuals who cannot tolerate barbiturates, there are other alternatives (Table 11-2). Thiopental and methohexital are both highly lipid-soluble barbiturates. Both drugs induce unconsciousness within about 20 seconds following an IV injection, mainly because of their very high lipid solubility, which allows rapid penetration into the CNS. Following the injection,

however, blood and brain levels decline rapidly as the drugs diffuse into tissues with a lower blood supply, mainly skeletal muscle. Skeletal muscle and adipose tissue act as a reservoir of the drug, resulting in a long hangover period in which the patient will remain drowsy and more susceptible to CNS depressant drugs. Like all barbiturates, these IV compounds can produce marked respiratory and cardiovascular depression.

Etomidate

Although clinically unrelated to barbiturates, the general anesthetic *etomidate* resembles these agents pharmacologically and provides for rapid induction and recovery. It is also metabolized rapidly in the liver, and the dangers associated with a long hangover are lessened. On the negative side, it can cause adrenal suppression after repeated exposures.

Propofol

Propofol is a rapidly acting IV general anesthetic agent used for induction, as an antiemetic, and for IV sedation. It can cause a burning sensation when administered, although patients are reported to recover from propofol more quickly than after any other anesthetic. It can also cause cardiovascular and respiratory depression. It is metabolized in the liver.

Ketamine

Ketamine resembles the hallucinogenic drug phencyclidine (PCP, or "angel dust"). Both produce a state of functional and electroencephalographic anesthesia, but with persistent eye and skeletal muscle movement. Patients may have their eyes open and be able to make some voluntary movement, but they appear unaware of (or, dissociated from) their surroundings. This state is known as *dissociative anesthesia*. It is accompanied by marked analgesia. Ketamine has some sympathomimetic properties and may cause cardiovascular stimulation. Ketamine is among the safest of general anesthetics, causing minimal cardiopulmonary depression. It is a valuable anesthetic when full hospital facilities are not available, such as at the site of major natural disasters. Ketamine is mainly used by oral surgeons, not by general dentists.

Inhalation Anesthetics

Inhalation anesthetics are gases or volatile liquids that are administered by inhalation in air or with oxygen at a sufficient gaseous partial pressure to achieve the appropriate concentrations in the brain.[3] There is a high correlation between the lipid solubility of anesthetic agents and their clinical efficiency in producing anesthesia. Anesthetics appear to interact with lipophilic (hydrophobic) sites on key cellular proteins mainly on the medullary reticular activating system involved with the regulation of sleep and wakefulness. Anesthetics also have marked inhibitory effects on the hippocampus of the brain, affecting the release of and sensitivity to acetylcholine. This may explain the effects of amnesia from anesthetics, characterized by difficulty recalling events associated with the induction and early recovery from anesthesia. With the exception of nitrous oxide and diethyl ether, the inhalation anesthetics are colorless, nonexplosive, volatile liquid halogenated hydrocarbons. While nitrous oxide is a good analgesic even in subhypnotic concentrations, it is only a weak anesthetic. Consequently, nitrous oxide provides for fast induction, but it is not an effective anesthetic unless combined with other analgesic agents, such as meperidine (Demerol).

Induction for General Anesthesia

Nitrous Oxide

Nitrous oxide provides for fast onset of action and rapid recovery because of its low solubility in blood. As mentioned earlier, it is a good analgesic even at subanesthetic concentrations, but the requirement to maintain an acceptable partial pressure of oxygen prevents achieving the concentrations of nitrous oxide required to reach full anesthesia. Other major concerns of nitrous use include hypoxia during recovery and the discovery that repeated use of nitrous oxide can disrupt methionine synthesis (necessary for vitamin-B synthesis), which can disturb DNA and protein synthesis and lead to severe anemia on prolonged exposure.

For nitrous oxide anesthesia, the recommended dosage for induction is 60% nitrous with 40% oxygen, and 30% nitrous with 70% oxygen for maintenance. During recovery the patient should be given oxygen by mask and encouraged to breathe deeply to promote ventilation. Nitrous oxide is often combined with other anesthetic agents to enhance its effects. It is excreted 100% unchanged through the lungs by exhalation. In the past an adverse event could occur in which too much nitrous was delivered to the client. This occurred when the hoses on the oxygen and nitrous oxide tanks were switched. A new equipment fitting design prevents this from occurring so that the fitting for the blue nitrous tank will not fit the green oxygen tank, and vice versa. The current practice of inducing general anesthesia with an IV-administered anesthetic before inhalation anesthesia promotes rapid transition from consciousness to surgical anesthesia, and the early stages of anesthesia are not seen. If the IV anesthetic is given slowly, however, usually all stages of anesthesia can be observed.

Side Effects and Contraindications

The most notable side effects of nitrous oxide are nausea, vomiting, or delirium, and it has no known drug interactions. A headache may result if 100% oxygen is not breathed for a full 5 minutes at the end of the procedure. Replacing the oxygen mask to allow better oxygenation will eliminate the headache. Nitrous oxide is contraindicated when the patient reports having recent ocular surgery for retinal detachment within the past 3 months. Modern techniques for ocular surgery often use intraocular gases as inflating agents. These gases persist in the eye for up to 3 months after surgery. During this period, using nitrous oxide for further anesthesia will cause the intraocular gas bubble to expand, which can result in high levels of intraocular pressure and irreversible blindness.[4]

As mentioned earlier, an extreme case of megaloblastic anemia may occur with repeated use (abuse) of nitrous oxide, and inhibition of methionine synthetase activity (the enzyme involved in the function of vitamin B_{12}) may occur during nitrous oxide sedation. This appears to cause no harm to the routine dental patient. The same exposure to nitrous oxide for dental purposes may be dangerous for the fetus, for the patient with severe infection, and the patient with impaired **hematopoiesis**. Because of reports of fetal abnormality, nitrous oxide should not be used during pregnancy. Nitrous oxide/oxygen can be safely administered to children who will tolerate having the mask placed over their noses. This requires a cooperative patient.

Occupational Hazard

An increased risk for fetal exposure to nitrous oxide and spontaneous abortion exists for pregnant oral health care workers who practice in locations where nitrous oxide is used. Room air must be monitored regularly to ensure the nitrous scavenging system is operating properly and that nitrous oxide concentrations in office air are at acceptable levels. Good ventilation (opening windows) is recommended, although this may not be allowable in offices with construction that allows no access to open windows.

Abuse of Nitrous Oxide

There are reports of using nitrous oxide for nonmedical purposes, and it may become a drug of abuse. Self-administering nitrous oxide on a regular basis can lead to numbness of the hands and legs (neuropathy). For dental personnel who rely on tactile sensitivity of fingers as a component of their work, this can significantly reduce the ability to perform skills necessary to their jobs. This is discussed more fully in Chapter 23.

New Induction Agents

Halothane

Halothane is a widely used general anesthetic in humans, although it is only a weak analgesic. It produces marked hypotension and cardiac depression and sensitizes the heart to catecholamines, leading to arrhythmias. Halothane is mainly eliminated through the lungs, although around 15% is metabolized in the liver. Rare hepatotoxicity has been reported with repeated use, due to reactive metabolites.

Enflurane and Isoflurane

These less-potent halogenated hydrocarbons resemble halothane in many respects. Most of the gas is eliminated from the body through exhalation, although about 2% of enflurane is metabolized in the liver with the production of fluoride ions and fluoridated metabolites, which are believed to account for a greater risk of renal toxicity.

Desflurane and Sevoflurane

These newer anesthetics are much more potent than nitrous oxide, but provide fast induction and similar recovery times. However, desflurane is a poor induction agent because of its pungent odor and may produce laryngospasm. Major side effects include cardiovascular and respiratory depression.

■ Self-Study Review

14. List drugs used to quickly move the patient through the excitement stage of general anesthesia.
15. Which is the safest of the general anesthetic agents?
16. Which of the drugs in the general anesthetic combination provides for effective analgesia during surgery?
17. Compare the recommended dose of nitrous for induction of general anesthesia versus the dose for conscious sedation. What is the concentration for maintenance?
18. List side effects or adverse drug effects of nitrous oxide. Which patients should not receive nitrous oxide?
19. Identify potential occupational hazards of having nitrous oxide in the dental office.

DENTAL HYGIENE APPLICATIONS

The primary clinical applications for the dental hygienist of general anesthetic agents are for administration of and/or monitoring of nitrous oxide in conscious sedation and analgesia. Parental (guardian) consent must be obtained when nitrous oxide is to be administered to individuals under 18 years of age. The medical history should be reviewed for evidence of conditions or previous medical procedures that would contraindicate the use of nitrous oxide. The equipment

---

> **BOX 11-1.** Technique for N_2O/O_2 Administration
>
> - Start the procedure by having the patient breathe 100% oxygen and slowly add small concentrations of nitrous in 5% to 10% increments (according to the equipment being used) until the sensation of "tingling" is felt in the patient's face and hands.
> - Talk with the patient to determine the degree of cognitive function as nitrous oxide is added to gaseous oxygen.
> - Question the patient to determine if adequate analgesia is achieved, not to exceed maximum concentrations (40% oxygen/60% nitrous).
> - Begin dental procedures when the patient reports being relaxed.
> - Monitor vital signs every few minutes during the procedure.
> - Provide 100% oxygen for at least 5 minutes at the end of the procedure to avoid diffusion hypoxia.
> - Provide postprocedure instructions related to potential adverse effects, such as headache, nausea, and vomiting.

must be checked before use to ensure proper function. Office safety protocol must include frequent monitoring of room air to assess levels of nitrous oxide. Box 11-1 includes proper techniques for N_2O/O_2 administration.

CONCLUSION

Dental hygienists are required to attend a training session approved by the state regulatory agency to gain certification and permission to monitor or administer nitrous oxide during clinical procedures. Although the training may not be included in the traditional dental hygiene education program, when the duty is permissible within the state, many practitioners will become certified to provide the procedure within the dental office. Safe practice requires the practitioner to be informed of warnings and safety precautions associated with all drugs the dental hygienist may administer or monitor. It is interesting to be familiar with this information because nitrous oxide may be offered to you as a dental patient.

References

1. Wiklund RA, Rosenbaum SH. Anesthesiology. *N Engl J Med.* 1997;337:1132–1141, 1215–1219.
2. Winter PM, Miller JN. Anesthesiology. *Sci Am.* 1985;252:124–131.
3. Campagna JA, Miller KW, Forman SA. The mechanisms of volatile anesthetic actions. *N Engl J Med.* 2003;348:2110–2124.
4. Yang YF, Herbert L, Ruschen H, et al. Nitrous oxide anaesthesia in the presence of intraocular gas can cause irreversible blindness. *BMJ.* 2002;312:532–533.

CLINICAL APPLICATION EXERCISES

◻ **Exercise 1.** A 15-year-old individual presents for periodontal services. The medical history is noncontributory but reveals that the patient has never had an oral prophylaxis because he is "afraid." The dentist advises using nitrous oxide for the ultrasonic débridement procedure and rescheduling for tissue evaluation and fine scaling in 4 weeks. Vital signs are 138/88, P 90 regular, R 19 shallow. Describe the administration technique you will use.

◻ **Exercise 2.** Interpret the vital signs as they relate to the above patient's characteristics.

◻ **Exercise 3.** In a child younger than 18 years of age, describe preliminary steps prior to the administration of nitrous oxide.

◻ **Exercise 4.** Illustrate the treatment record entry when nitrous oxide is administered for 30 minutes during periodontal débridement at a 50/50 nitrous to oxygen ratio.

12

Drugs for Medical Emergencies

A medical emergency can occur unexpectedly in the dental office. However, the vast majority of medical emergencies could be prevented if proper steps were taken based on information from the health history review. There is an old saying: "Never treat a stranger!" The best way to prevent a medical emergency is to take a good health history.[1] The health history process can be described as "good" when it involves

- interpreting the information provided on the history form thoroughly (with all questions answered);
- asking appropriate questions related to specific risks for the condition;
- evaluating the responses to those follow-up questions (again related to risks for a medical emergency);
- considering the drug history and indications for each drug;
- verifying the necessary medical consultations before initiating treatment.

Further evaluation of systemic health includes comparing vital sign values and qualities to those of normal limits.

DETERMINE THE RISK STATUS

Oral health care providers must be able to assess the physical and emotional ability of a patient to tolerate dental care,

identify high-risk patients who may experience medical emergencies, and know how to sustain life with their hands, their breaths, a few basic therapeutic agents, and a great deal of common sense. The risk for a medical emergency is based on the overall physical and emotional health of the patient. In situations that involve using patient-supplied medications, such as a bronchodilator inhaler or sublingual nitroglycerin tablets, those medications should be located so they can be easily retrieved by the patient or health care worker.

Know What to Look For

Be familiar with the signs and symptoms of various medical emergencies that may occur in the oral health care setting. If a medical emergency develops, initial observations of associated signs along with recollections of the health history may help to determine the probable cause of the emergency. **Basic life support**—assuring an open airway, breathing, and circulation (A-B-C)—is the first step in management. Assessing the level of consciousness and the need for cardiopulmonary support is essential; emergency medical service (EMS) may need to be called. Drugs in an office emergency kit can be used to keep the individual stable until EMS personnel arrive and take over patient care.[2,3]

Develop an Office Protocol for Emergency Management

Drugs in the emergency kit are only administered by the dentist; however, the dental staff should have specific duties described in the office procedures manual regarding everyone's specific roles in managing a medical emergency. The dental hygienist might be the staff member to assist the patient in retrieving personal medications or to bring oxygen to the area of the emergency, institute the flow of oxygen, and place the face mask over the patient's mouth and nose. This procedure is within the scope of dental hygiene practice in the management of medical emergencies. Vital signs must be monitored every 5 minutes to determine adequate respiration and circulation. Someone must be assigned the responsibility of bringing the emergency kit to the area of the emergency. If circulation and respiration have stopped, drugs will not be useful because, without circulation, there will be no way to distribute them in the body.

Check Emergency Equipment and Medications Regularly

At regular intervals, an assigned staff member must ensure that the equipment is functioning properly and that the emergency drugs are not past their expiration dates.[2] This information should be recorded in a dated log to verify the procedure was completed.

Maintenance of Basic Life Support

Oxygen, sublingually administered drugs, and injected drugs may be useful when the patient has adequate circulation and respiration. While awaiting the arrival of EMS personnel, procedures to maintain circulation and respiration (such as CPR) may be necessary. Upon the arrival of EMS personnel, a description of events that occurred before the emergency should be provided, and any related health history information (including recent hospitalization), vital sign information, and a description of resuscitative procedures and medications administered in the dental office should be given to EMS personnel (Box 12-1). Finally, the emergency event, precipitating factors, management procedures provided, vital sign values plus the amount of time between taking blood pressure, and how the emergency was resolved must be recorded in the treatment record.[1]

BOX 12-1. Information for EMS Personnel

- Description of signs and symptoms of the emergency situation
- Related health history information and recent hospitalizations (if any)
- Vital sign information
- Resuscitative procedures and medications administered in dental office

---

■ Self-Study Review

1. List five components of an adequate medical history review.
2. How are vital signs used to assess systemic health?
3. Define *basic life support* and consider its use in medical emergency management.
4. Describe the roles of each member of the team in the dental office emergency management protocol.
5. Identify situations that limit the effectiveness of an emergency drug.
6. Identify information to provide to EMS personnel.

MEDICAL EMERGENCY SITUATIONS

For the purposes of this chapter, a *medical emergency* is a situation in which the patient exhibits possible life-threatening symptoms that require some form of immediate action on the dental health care practitioner's part. Most medical emergencies in the dental office develop as part of the stress response. Fear, anxiety, and pain are common causes of stress-related medical emergencies. During the stress response, the blood pressure may drop to the point that **hypoxia** develops and consciousness is lost. This is especially true when the patient is seated in the upright position in the dental chair. Cardiovascular emergencies are often precipitated by stress. The heart rate may increase to the point that the supply of oxygenated blood is inadequate for the increased cardiac workload, a response that provokes anginal pain.

Autonomic Response in the Seated Position

During the stress response, blood pressure initially rises, and then vasodilation in the muscles causes blood to move from the thoracic area to the peripheral tissues (arms, legs) and to pool in the extremities. Blood pressure decreases due to the vasodilation. If the individual is standing, running away, or fighting (using leg muscles), blood is returned to the heart via the vena cava system. What goes in equals what comes out, so if adequate amounts of blood enter the heart, then adequate amounts of oxygenated blood will be pumped into the aorta and then into the circulatory system. If no muscle activity occurs, blood pools in the skeletal muscle and does not return quickly to the heart. The resulting decrease in circulating blood volume, blood pressure, and blood flow to the brain (**cerebral ischemia**) is responsible for the ultimate loss of consciousness. This scenario can be related to positioning in the dental chair where the patient is seated with the legs extended, and no muscles are moving. If acute stress occurs, blood is still shunted to the arms and legs, but without muscle movement to help blood return to the heart, less blood enters the heart, thus reducing the cardiac output. When this occurs, the regulatory system in the central nervous system (CNS) stimulates the heart to pump (trying to get more blood into the circulation), vasodilation occurs (trying to get blood into tissues), and blood pressure continues to drop. When the patient sits in the upright position of the dental chair, there is inadequate blood pressure to pump oxygenated blood to the brain, hypoxia develops, and the patient loses consciousness.[4] This explanation is simplistic, but it represents the general situation. The resolution to this situation is basically not pharmacologic, although moving the patient to a supine position and giving 100% oxygen may help oxygenate the blood. An ammonia capsule may be needed to stimulate respiration, but the problem is usually solved by lowering the patient's head so oxygenated blood can flow into the **cerebral** vasculature by gravity rather than by using blood pressure to carry the blood to the area. This situation is common enough that it sets the stage for discussing those situations in which emergency drugs would be used.

Primary Drugs in an Emergency Kit

An emergency kit with specific drugs used for the most common medical emergencies should be available in the dental office and kept updated to ensure drugs are not out of date. Table 12-1 lists primary emergency drugs, doses, and routes of administration. The basic kit should include[3]:

- E cylinder oxygen with face mask, nasal cannula, Ambu-Bag
- Epinephrine in 1:1,000 and 1:2,000 concentrations (preloaded syringe)
- Nitroglycerin (sublingual tabs or spray)
- Glucose tablets
- Epinephrine or albuterol inhaler
- Benzodiazepine (diazepam, midazolam) for intramuscular (IM) or intravenous (IV) injection
- Chewable aspirin
- Ammonia ampule (perle)

Accessories should include a pillow, a blanket, a portable light source, a glucometer to measure blood sugar levels, and a portable sphygmomanometer with large, average, and small cuffs.[3]

Medical Conditions

Hypoxia and Loss of Consciousness

Oxygen

The life-threatening condition for which oxygen is required is *cerebral hypoxia*, or a lack of adequate oxygen in the circulation for brain function. The common overt indication of hypoxia is syncope or loss of consciousness. If adequate oxygenated blood is not provided within 5 minutes, brain damage can result. Oxygen, administered as a gas, comes compressed under pressure in metal cylinders of various sizes. A portable E cylinder oxygen tank with clear face mask and nasal cannula should be present. The green-colored E cylinder tank should be secured to a rolling device to make it portable. Oxygen by face mask at 4 to 10 L/minute is used, when indicated, for most emergency situations. When the nasal cannula is used, delivery tubes are secured over the patient's ears and the cannula is placed just below the nostrils. When **apnea** develops, a positive pressure respiration device (AmbuBag) can be connected to the oxygen line and used to force oxygen into the lungs. Probably the only instance in which oxygen is **contraindicated** in resolving a medical emergency is hyperventilation. During hyperventilation, rapid expiration results in excessive loss of carbon dioxide and inspiration of adequate amounts of oxygen. Rebreathing carbon dioxide is the management procedure, rather than providing 100% oxygen by face mask.

Immediate Hypersensitivity Reaction (Anaphylaxis)

Anaphylaxis can develop within a matter of minutes following administration of an allergenic drug or substance. Dangerous signs include low blood pressure leading to cardiovascular collapse (shock) and constriction of the bronchioles (bronchospasm) leading to suffocation.

Epinephrine

If an acute allergic reaction involving **dyspnea** occurs following administration of a drug or exposure to latex

---

Table 12-1 Primary Drugs for an Emergency Kit

Drug	Route	Dose (Adult)	Formulation	Use
Oxygen	Inhalation	2 to 10 L/min	E cylinder	Hypoxia
Epinephrine	IM or SC (muscle or floor of mouth	0.2 to 0.5 mg	Preloaded syringe EpiPen: 1 mg/mL (1:1,000); EpiPen Jr: 0.5 mg/mL (1:2,000)	Anaphylaxis
Albuterol	Inhalation	1 to 2 puffs	Metered dose inhaler	Bronchospasm
Nitroglycerin	Sublingual	0.4 mg	Tablet or metered spray	Angina pectoris
Diazepam	IM or IV	5 to 10 mg	Solution (intensol): 5 mg/mL	Seizure
Ammonia	Inhalation	Crushable glass perles: 0.33 mL, 0.4 mL	Aromatic spirit inhalant	Syncope
Aspirin	Oral	325 mg	Tablet	MI
Glucagon	SC, IM, or IV	1 mg/mL	Solution	Hypoglycemia

IM, intramuscular; SC, subcutaneous; L/min, liters per minute; MI, heart attack.

products in the dental office, the proper drug to secure from the emergency kit is epinephrine. The adult doseform contains 1 mg/mL (1:1,000) epinephrine (EpiPen), and the child doseform contains 0.5 mg/mL (1:2,000) epinephrine (EpiPen Jr.). This is an epinephrine-only product with a much higher concentration of epinephrine than is contained in a dental cartridge. Epinephrine is the drug of choice for anaphylaxis because it increases blood pressure and dilates bronchiolar muscle. The patient with environmental allergies may carry the EpiPen at all times; however, one cannot expect this product to be carried by all patients at risk because anaphylaxis can occur unexpectedly. The dentist (or the patient who has brought an EpiPen to the appointment) will administer epinephrine IM and rub the area vigorously to aid absorption into the circulation. A video demonstrating the procedure can be viewed at http://www.epipen.com/howtouse.aspx. Effects from epinephrine administration with the injectable device last 15 to 20 minutes, which is generally enough time for the EMS personnel to arrive. However, an additional dose of epinephrine can be repeated in 20 minutes if necessary.[2] During anaphylaxis, the combination of poor circulation and inadequate breathing leads to hypoxic conditions and a lowering of the threshold for arrhythmia. Epinephrine is an arrhythmogenic agent in itself. Therefore, proper oxygenation of the patient is required whenever epinephrine is used to manage anaphylaxis.

■ Self-Study Review

7. Identify the source of most medical emergencies in the dental office.
8. Describe the relationship between stress, hypoxia, and altered consciousness as a response of the autonomic nervous system.
9. Describe the resolution of *hypoxia*.
10. List the primary emergency drugs and describe the use of each.
11. List accessory items in the emergency kit and identify the purpose of each.
12. Describe the equipment needed to reverse cerebral hypoxia.
13. Identify contraindications for use of oxygen.
14. What actions of epinephrine are useful in the management of anaphylaxis? What additional drug is also used, and why?

Anginal Pain

Angina is caused when cardiac muscle receives too little oxygenated blood. This can result from a blood clot obstructing a vessel or due to spasm of the blood vessel and constriction of the lumen. Increased cardiac workload in the presence of atherosclerosis narrowing the lumen of coronary blood vessels can also promote angina. For the individual who reports a history of anginal pain, pretreatment questioning must include identifying what precipitates the angina and how the patient manages the pain, as well as how often it occurs.[1]

Nitroglycerin

The drug of choice to manage angina is *nitroglycerin*, a drug with strong vasodilation effects. It is supplied in a spray form (shelf life: 3 years) or **adsorbed** to a tablet (shelf life: 3 to 6 months). Physicians prescribe nitroglycerin and instruct that it be carried at all times in case an anginal event is not relieved by rest. If the patient brings nitroglycerin to the appointment, this preparation should be used to manage angina if it occurs in the dental office. The patient should be instructed to bring this personal supply of nitroglycerin to all dental appointments. Examine the label on the prescription to ensure it is not past the expiration date. When the patient does not have nitroglycerin or the prescription is out of date (and likely inactive), the supply in the dental office emergency kit can be used. Oxygen at 4 L/minute will help oxygenate the patient and should be provided before each dose of sublingual (SL) nitroglycerin. The patient will self-administer nitroglycerin, or, if the office emergency kit supply is used, the dentist will administer SL nitroglycerin. Nitroglycerin placed sublingually (either one spray or one SL tablet) will cause vasodilation and facilitate getting oxygenated blood to cardiac muscle. The doseform should be administered every 5 minutes, with a maximum dose of three doses in a 10-minute period. The blood pressure must be monitored following each nitroglycerin dose because the vasodilation effect can cause blood pressure to fall. If systolic blood pressure is lowered to values <100, withhold giving more nitroglycerin to avoid excessive blood pressure reduction.[5] Following the administration of nitroglycerin, recovery is generally rapid (within 5 minutes), and the appointment can be continued (if the patient requests it) or rescheduled.[2] If pain is not relieved within 10 minutes following the last dose, the 911 system should be activated because the patient may be experiencing a myocardial infarction (MI; currently called acute coronary syndrome or heart attack). For patients with no history of angina, EMS should be called immediately, and nitroglycerin from the office emergency kit should be administered by the dentist while waiting for EMS to arrive.[1,5] Both angina and MI have the same signs of substernal pain and pressure. The event is initially treated as angina, but if the pain is not relieved by nitroglycerin, MI may be occurring.

Drug Interactions with Nitroglycerin

Patients who are diagnosed with coronary artery disease and require the periodic administration of nitroglycerin should avoid the use of drugs for erectile dysfunction (phosphodiesterase Type-5 inhibitors: sildenafil [Viagra], tadalafil [Cialis], and vardenafil hydrochloride [Levitra]). These drugs in combination with nitroglycerin may produce severe hypotension (additive vasodilating effect) and possibly lead to death. This potential drug–drug interaction will preclude physicians from prescribing drugs for erectile dysfunction to patients with significant coronary artery disease where the need for nitroglycerin is unpredictable. Sildenafil and vardenafil are removed from the body within 12 hours (terminal half-life is 4 to 5 hours), while tadalafil has a half-life of 17.5 hours and a 36-hour duration of action. Before administering nitroglycerin to a client experiencing acute angina pectoris, it should be determined if these drugs have been taken within the past 12 (sildenafil, vardenafil) or 48 hours (tadalafil). An additional consideration is the function of the client's kidneys and the liver, which if compromised could lead to a longer duration of the vasodilating effect. Erythromycin interferes with the metabolism of sildenafil and vardenafil and increases the blood levels of both drugs.

Myocardial Infarction

The American Heart Association recommends having the patient chew a 325-mg aspirin tablet after calling the EMS if the patient is suspected of having a heart attack. An MI is most often caused by a blood clot that occludes a blood vessel within the heart. Aspirin's antiplatelet effect (i.e., it keeps platelets from clumping together) may prevent the formation of a **thrombus** and thus prevent further vascular obstruction, which is the basis for the recommendation. Aspirin does not dissolve blood clots. Chewing the aspirin gets the drug into a liquid form so that it can bypass dissolving stages in the stomach, thereby resulting in rapid absorption into the blood. Oxygen is administered when chest pain is reported, as well as nitroglycerin. Nitroglycerin will not resolve chest pain from MI, although it can resolve anginal pain. A dental team member will ask the patient if he or she wants to chew the aspirin and provide the tablet to the patient as needed. Basic life support (A-B-C) should be provided and CPR initiated if respiration and circulation cease.

Hypoglycemia

When diabetes is reported on the health history, questioning *must* include when the last meal was eaten and when the last dose of insulin or antidiabetic medication was consumed. The most likely reason for **hypoglycemia** is taking insulin or antihyperglycemic medication and *not eating a meal*. The dose of the medication is based on projected blood sugar levels after the meal, so failure to eat makes the dose too high (overdose). This is the most common event preceding hypoglycemia associated with diabetes. Inquiring about the recent frequency of hypoglycemia may also identify the individual at an increased risk for the emergency.

Glucose

Glucose tablets will raise blood sugar levels quickly when allowed to dissolve in the mouth. In conscious individuals, drinking a beverage with sugar will also quickly reverse most cases of hypoglycemia. Most individuals with diabetes carry a sugar source to reverse signs of hypoglycemia.

Difficulty Breathing

Aerosolized bronchodilators are included in the emergency kit in order to resolve bronchoconstriction. The most likely cause would be an acute asthma attack, but the products are used with several respiratory diseases, including emphysema and chronic obstructive pulmonary disease (COPD). The most common cause of acute asthma is allergy to an environmental substance, but stress-induced asthma may occur in the dental office. When a history of respiratory disease is reported on the health history, the individual should be required to bring the personal bronchodilator inhaler to all dental appointments. Should breathing difficulty develop, raise

the patient's chair back to the upright position so the bronchodilator inhaler can be used. In the individual with COPD who develops difficulty breathing, 100% oxygen administered at 2 L/minute can be used with albuterol inhalation or another short-acting β_2-agonist.[2] While the administration of oxygen to COPD patients is not contraindicated, the low infusion rate is dictated by the fact that in such patients, the rate of respiration is controlled by the partial pressure of oxygen. A higher infusion rate may lead to severe respiratory depression.

Albuterol

The rescue inhaler may include albuterol or pirbuterol, agonists for beta-2 receptors in bronchiolar muscle. Beta-2 receptors produce bronchodilation. Some patients may use aerosolized epinephrine to manage emerging asthma attacks. It is sold over the counter (Primatene Mist and others) and is used in the same manner as prescription bronchodilators. Generally two inhalations taken over a 4- to 5-minute period will open airways and resolve bronchoconstriction. This can be followed with 100% oxygen at 2 to 4 L/minute by nasal cannula as needed.[2]

Seizure

The most serious seizure to result in a management emergency is the generalized *tonic-clonic convulsive seizure*, or grand mal seizure. In most instances management is to refrain from intervening and allow the seizure to resolve. Dental equipment that may harm the individual should be moved out of the way while the seizure is occurring. Those patients who can identify impending seizures can be moved from the dental chair to the operatory floor if there is time before seizure activity develops. Benzodiazepines (diazepam) have strong anticonvulsant and indirect muscle-relaxant effects and may be used to stop uncontrolled or severe seizures. In this state, the diaphragm and intercostal muscles are in spasm, and the patient may stop breathing. Similarly, IM or IV diazepam is appropriate for the management of continuous seizures (**status epilepticus**). Uncontrolled seizure can result from a variety of situations (such as local anesthetic overdose, prolonged syncope, stroke, alcohol withdrawal, and hypoglycemia), and a benzodiazepine is the appropriate drug to stop seizure activity in these situations.

Benzodiazepines

Diazepam, administered by the dentist IM with vigorous massage of the site, is the drug of choice to halt uncontrolled seizure. Oxygen, 4 to 6 L/minute by nasal cannula, should be given when seizures cease.

Ammonia Ampule (Crushable Glass Perles)

If the return to consciousness following unconsciousness is delayed, a stimulant, such as an ammonia perle or ampule, can be broken or crushed and quickly passed under the nostril openings. The active agent is ammonia gas or vapor that breaks down in air when the cartridge is crushed. Ammonia irritates the reflexogenic zones in the nasopharyngeal wall, which carries afferent impulses to the respiratory and vaso-motor centers. Aromatic spirits of ammonia are respiratory and cardiovascular stimulants, and if the patient is breathing, noxious stimulation of the respiratory passages will promote the return to consciousness. The patient will turn the head away to avoid the pungent odor. This also may force the patient to take a deep breath and may increase the blood pressure. One usually only has to use it once to get the intended result! Management includes administration of 100% oxygen when consciousness returns, as needed.

Accessory Equipment

The pillow is placed under the right hip of a pregnant woman who is receiving oral health services. This rotates the weight of the fetus to the left, away from compressing the vena cava and blocking return of blood to the heart. When an emergency occurs in the hallway of the office or in any area where blood pressure equipment is not available, a portable sphyg-momanometer must be taken to the location of the individual and used to monitor blood pressure. Similarly, an E cylinder oxygen tank on a rolling stand is essential equipment.

■ Self-Study Review

15. Describe the action of nitroglycerin in the management of angina. What patient instruction is essential for the patient who uses nitroglycerin? What are precautions when it is used for anginal pain?
16. When anginal pain occurs in an individual with no history of cardiovascular disease, how is the management procedure changed?
17. Describe the number of doses of nitroglycerin and the timing of dose administration for angina.
18. Identify drugs that interact with nitroglycerin. How does this affect emergency care?
19. How is *angina* differentiated from *MI*?
20. Identify the most likely behavior preceding hypoglycemia in the patient with diabetes.
21. List situations that can lead to breathing difficulties during dental hygiene care. What patient instruction is recommended for the individual with respiratory disease?
22. Describe management of an acute asthma attack.
23. Identify the type of seizure that causes a medical emergency during oral health care.
24. What type of seizure is managed with a drug? What is the drug of choice to stop uncontrolled convulsive seizures?
25. Identify possible causes for uncontrolled seizures.

Secondary Emergency Drugs
Naloxone

If the dental practitioner uses opioid analgesics by any route or for any purpose in the dental office, then naloxone (Nar-

can), a specific opioid antagonist, must be available in the emergency kit. In the case of life-threatening opioid-induced respiratory depression, naloxone is injected by the dentist by IV, IM, or subcutaneously (SC) in a dose of 0.4 mg every 3 minutes or as the clinical monitoring of respiration dictates. The EMS system must be activated, and the patient's vital signs must be monitored and recorded until EMS personnel arrive.

Flumazenil

The antagonist to reverse the actions of benzodiazepines is flumazenil (Romazicon). When an IV benzodiazepine (diazepam, midazolam, and others) is administered as a sedative in the dental office, flumazenil should be included in the emergency kit in case of a benzodiazepine overdose. Signs of overdose include bizarre behavior, hyperexcitable reactions with irrational behavior, and the patient's trying to leave the dental office. The usual adult dose is 0.2 mg IV, administered over 30 seconds. Consciousness should return in 30 seconds following administration. Further doses may be administered at 1-minute intervals as needed. Although this emergency is not life threatening, the individual should be treated to regain a stable emotional state.

DENTAL HYGIENE APPLICATIONS

The role of the dental hygienist is determined by the dental office emergency protocol. Box 12-2 lists steps to follow in managing most emergencies. When dental patients bring rescue medication to the dental appointment, those agents should be placed within easy reach for the patient. Monitoring vital signs, finding drugs in the kit that the dentist requests,

---

BOX 12-2.   Management Procedures for a Medical Emergency

1. Recognize the emergency or most likely cause of the emergency.
2. Position the patient (loss of consciousness, lie flat; difficulty breathing, upright position) to open the airway.
3. Assess the airway, breathing, and circulation.
4. Activate the 911 system, if needed, and note the time called.
5. Notify the dentist of the emergency.
6. Assist the patient in securing personal emergency medications.
7. Bring the emergency kit to the emergency area.
8. Monitor vital signs (blood pressure, pulse, respiration) and record the time between measurements.
9. Provide 100% oxygen (except in hyperventilation).

CLINICAL APPLICATION EXERCISES

☐ **Exercise 1.** Secure the emergency kit in your dental hygiene clinic. List each item in the kit and describe what it is used for, how it is administered, and what monitoring procedures are necessary following the use of each agent.

☐ **Exercise 2.** Examine the clinic's oxygen tank. Make sure you know how to turn the oxygen on, how to set the regulator at 10 L/minute, and how to place the face mask and nasal cannula on the patient.

☐ **Exercise 3.** A 17-year-old patient with a history of asthma presents for oral prophylaxis. Vital signs are normal, except breathing is "raspy," and the pulse rate is

106 and thready. What precautionary procedure should be completed? As the periodontal procedure is initiated, the patient begins to cough and shows signs of breathing difficulty. Describe how management of an emergency involving an acute asthma attack should be recorded in the treatment record. Include signs of the event, precipitating factors (if known), management procedures provided, and resolution of the event.

☐ **Exercise 4.** WEB ACTIVITY: Watch the video at http://www.epipen.com/howtouse.aspx that illustrates how to use the injectable epinephrine device. The client or the dentist will inject the epinephrine to relieve an acute allergic reaction.

providing 100% oxygen via the face mask or nasal cannula and regulating the flow rate, using ammonia, helping the patient retrieve personal emergency drugs, providing a source of glucose when hypoglycemia is suspected, and assisting if CPR is needed are all functions in the dental hygienist's scope of practice. The dental hygienist is prepared to evaluate information on the health history and determine the clinical relevance of vital sign values. Should a medical emergency develop during dental hygiene care, emergency management begins with the hygienist, according to the dental office protocol for emergency management.

Self-Study Review

26. Identify two antagonists used in emergency management and specify when each is used.
27. Describe duties that could be delegated to the dental hygienist in the emergency management protocol.

CONCLUSION

What knowledge is needed to determine the risk for an acute medical emergency? Asking the right questions to identify the degree of risk for an emergency situation *before providing treatment* is important. One must recognize the specific

emergency that is occurring and initiate immediate procedures to resolve the situation while maintaining an open airway and helping restore oxygenation and circulation. Dental personnel must make good judgments regarding whether to call EMS immediately or to determine if management procedures in the dental office can restore function. Knowledge of the signs associated with systemic pathology and the relationship of the medical history information is essential. Knowledge of the drugs contained in the office emergency kit and an understanding of when and for what purpose each is used is important. Finally, the office protocol for procedures to follow during emergency management must be practiced so that the clinician can remain calm as those procedures are completed.

References

1. Pickett F, Gurenlian J. *The Medical History: Clinical Implications and Emergency Prevention in Dental Settings.* Baltimore: Lippincott Williams & Wilkins; 2005:2, 20–25.
2. Terezhalmy G. Management of medical emergencies in the oral health care setting. In: Pickett F, Terezhalmy G, eds. *Dental Drug Reference with Clinical Implications.* Baltimore: Lippincott Williams & Wilkins; 2006:140–160.
3. American Dental Association Council on Scientific Affairs. Office emergencies and emergency kits. *J Am Dent Assoc.* 2002; 133:364–365.
4. Blakey G. Syncope. In: Bennett JD, Rosenberg MB, eds. *Medical Emergencies in Dentistry.* Philadelphia: WB Saunders; 2002: 184.
5. Malamed S. *Medical Emergencies in the Dental Office.* 5th ed. St. Louis: Mosby; 2000:23, 449, 462.

13

Pharmacologic Management of Selected Oral Conditions

The dental hygienist may be the first oral health care worker to observe an oral lesion. Patients not only want to know what caused the lesion, but also what to do about it. Oral pathology courses inform the dental hygienist about identifying lesions from their clinical appearance, in conjunction with questioning about historical information. The dentist makes a diagnosis and prescription for therapy using clinical, microbiologic/histopathologic and/or historical information. This chapter provides information to assist the practitioner in explaining possible therapies for a wide variety of oral lesions. An emphasis on patient instructions for applying topical products and warnings for potential side effects of systemic therapy is included.

Although most oral conditions are self-limiting (i.e., they heal on their own), they often produce enough discomfort to prompt the patient to seek attention in a dental facility. There is always the concern that the lesion is malignant, and this influences the decision to possibly follow a "wait and see" approach with biopsy and histopathologic diagnosis. In some

cases, treatment is directed toward minimizing the likelihood that the patient will transmit an infection to others. The purpose of this chapter is to discuss common orally related primary and secondary conditions and their management protocols. One group of drugs (topical corticosteroids) is discussed fully in Chapter 14, but it is mentioned here to illustrate the variety of oral situations in which topical steroids are used.

ACUTE ODONTOGENIC PAIN

The most common complaint causing a person to seek the services of an oral health care provider is pain. Proper management of pain requires an accurate diagnosis of the causative factors and selection of therapies to eliminate those factors. The most common presentation involves pulp infection through dental caries or trauma to the tooth. Most patients can attain satisfactory relief of acute odontogenic pain through an approach that incorporates primary dental care (débridement of the infection, cleaning the area) in conjunction with local anesthesia and administration of analgesics.

Pharmacologic Therapies

A variety of agents are used when managing acute odontogenic pain. These include topical and injectable local anesthetic agents and analgesics. Following treatment with primary dental care, over-the-counter (OTC) COX-inhibitor preparations (aspirin, ibuprofen, naproxen, acetaminophen [APAP]) are the drugs of choice for mild odontogenic pain. For situations in which mild analgesics are ineffective, hydrocodone with APAP, 5 mg/500 mg (two tablets qid for 3 days), is recommended. Management of severe pain requires stronger agents. Oxycodone in combination with a COX-inhibitor is the primary drug for the management of severe odontogenic pain. Chapter 9 describes management of odontogenic infection, which is a primary cause of acute odontogenic pain.

ORAL MUCOSAL CONDITIONS

Oral Lichen Planus

The exact etiology of *lichen planus* is not known, but it is believed to be an autoimmune disease with a genetic predisposition. It is the most common dermatologic disease with oral manifestations. An estimated 65% of patients with dermal lichen planus also experience oral lichen planus (OLP), with the buccal mucosa the most commonly affected site. Trauma, viral and bacterial infections, emotional stress, and drug therapy have all been implicated as precipitating factors. A possible association between OLP and oral squamous cell carcinoma mandates that all cases of OLP be followed closely. A simple classification system recognizes three forms of OLP: Reticular, atrophic, and erosive. Common sites of occurrence include the tongue, lips, floor of the mouth, palate, and gingiva.

Pharmacologic Management

There is no cure for OLP, and oral lesions tend to be more persistent and recalcitrant to therapy than dermal lesions. Strate-gies are aimed at relieving symptoms and reducing exacerbations and progression. Asymptomatic reticular OLP only requires routine follow-up for changes in lesion appearance, while symptomatic cases usually require some form of drug therapy.

Primary Therapy

For patients with mild to moderately symptomatic OLP, topical corticosteroids are usually prescribed. Therapy is empiric, and the agent chosen depends largely on the lesion presentation, patient preference, and practitioner experience. **Ointments** or gels work well for localized lesions, whereas **elixirs** are better suited for more widespread presentations. Ointments may also be mixed with an oral paste, such as Orabase, to improve adhesion of the steroid to the mucosa. When effective, improvement should be apparent within 2 weeks. Once improvement is noted, the dosing is titrated down to the lowest dose required to maintain patient comfort. Measures to reduce the predictable risk of developing secondary candidiasis should be undertaken.

Intermediate-Potency Topical Steroids

Table 13-1 lists available topical corticosteroid agents according to potency. Triamcinolone acetonide (Kenalog), a topical cream, is applied after meals and at bedtime. Patients are instructed not to eat or drink for 30 minutes following use to ensure the cream is not removed. When ointments are used, such as betamethasone valerate (Betatrex) and fluocinonide (Lidex), they are applied with the same instructions. The ultrapotent ointment clobetasol propionate (Temovate) can be used in the same manner.

Secondary Therapy

For moderate to severe OLP, or for cases unresponsive to topical corticosteroids, a systemic steroid should be used. Localized lesions may respond favorably to the local injection of such an agent as triamcinolone acetonide. The most commonly used systemic corticosteroid is prednisone. The approach is to prescribe a high-dose (40 to 80 mg/day), short-course (no more than 10 days) regimen to maximize the therapeutic effect while minimizing long-term side effects, such as hypothalamic-pituitary-adrenal axis suppression. However, other possible adverse effects, such as insomnia,

Table 13-1	Topical Corticosteroids for Oral Use	
Potency	**Drug**	**Formulation**
Very high	Clobetasol propionate	0.05% cream, ointment
High	Betamethasone valerate	0.1% ointment, 0.2% cream
	Fluocinolone acetonide	0.05% cream, ointment, gel
	Fluocinonide	0.5% cream, ointment
	Triamcinolone acetonide	0.1% paste
Medium	Betamethasone benzoate	0.025% cream, gel
	Fluocinolone acetonide	0.025% cream, ointment
	Fluticasone propionate	0.05% cream, 0.005% ointment
	Triamcinolone acetonide	0.025%, 0.1% cream, ointment
Low	Dexamethasone	Oral solution, elixir 0.5 mg/5 mL

mood swings, nervousness, diarrhea, fluid retention, muscle weakness, and hypertension, may occur. Patients who respond favorably to a short-course systemic regimen should be placed on a topical agent with the goal of reducing acute exacerbations of OLP.

Tertiary Therapy

For patients unresponsive to the secondary line of therapy or for those who quickly relapse after cessation of short-term steroid therapy, a more aggressive approach is necessary. Long-term corticosteroid regimens with or without additional agents, such as immunosuppressants (methotrexate) or immunomodulating agents (azathioprine), may be beneficial for such patients. However, the side-effect liability is such that these medications should only be prescribed by or in close collaboration with the patient's physician.

Recurrent Aphthous Stomatitis/Ulceration

Recurrent aphthous stomatitis (RAS) is recognized as the most common oral mucosal disease to affect humans. For most individuals, RAS proves to be a localized self-limiting episodic annoyance. However, for others, RAS may be so severe as to interfere with eating and drinking and/or be associated with an underlying, often serious, systemic condition. The specific etiology of RAS is unknown, but it likely involves an alteration in the cell-mediated immune system. Possible causes include local factors (trauma, toothpaste allergy, or sensitivity), nutritional deficiencies (iron, folic acid, zinc, B_1, B_2, B_6, or B_{12}), absorptive disorders (gluten-sensitive enteropathy, celiac sprue), food allergies, and other systemic conditions manifesting ulcerations (Behçet disease, Crohn disease, systemic lupus erythematosus [SLE], cyclic neutropenia, HIV, Reiter syndrome).

Pharmacologic Management

A primary goal in the management of RAS is to identify and eliminate or manage any contributory factors or conditions associated with the RAS. An appropriate medical consultation or referral is warranted for RAS associated with systemic conditions such as nutritional deficiencies, Behçet disease, and HIV. Targeted lesion therapy is aimed at providing palliation, promoting healing, and reducing recurrence.

Primary Therapy

There are numerous prescription and OTC topical gels, creams, ointments, and rinses marketed for the treatment of RAS (Table 13-1). Commonly found ingredients include corticosteroids, covering agents, antiseptics, oxygenating agents, anti-inflammatory agents, cauterizing agents, and topical anesthetics. No validated studies exist to demonstrate the clinical superiority of any formulation over another. Problems related to the consistent application and retention of these agents over the lesion often limit their effectiveness.

Topical Steroid Preparations
Topical steroid ointments may be compounded with a mucosal adherent (e.g., Orabase) to improve and prolong retention. A rinse formulation of a steroid may be more effective to treat widespread or hard-to-reach lesions. Topical corticosteroids predispose to oral candidiasis, and prolonged use may lead to thinning of the mucosa or mucosal atrophy. Topical creams should be applied four to five times/day, after meals or toothbrushing, and at bedtime. A thin coat of the preparation is applied with a cotton-tipped applicator. Topical steroids can be used up to 2 weeks, or until the ulcer heals. Preparations include the ointments fluocinonide (Lidex) and triamcinolone (Kenalog). Dexamethasone (Decadron), a steroid elixir, can be used as a rinse (1 tsp rinsed for 2 minutes, four times/day, and expectorated).

Nonsteroid Preparations
Amlexanox (Aphthasol) is a paste applied to the lesion up to four times daily following meals, toothbrushing, and at bedtime. A small dab of paste can be applied to the ulceration. It can be used up to 10 days or until the lesion heals. The mechanism of action of amlexanox is unknown, but the drug accelerates healing, possibly by inhibiting the release of inflammatory mediators (histamine, leukotrienes). Agents to cover ulcerated mucosa (Orabase Soothe-N-Seal) have no pharmacologic action, but provide a barrier between nerve endings within the lesion and outside irritants. Products of this type are to be applied according to the manufacturer's directions, as needed to relieve pain. Several barrier agents are available, and all are equal in efficacy.

Secondary Line of Treatment

The secondary line of therapy entails the use of a systemic corticosteroid and is indicated for patients whose symptoms are not relieved by primary therapy or for patients whose initial presentation warrants a more aggressive treatment approach. Prednisone, the most commonly chosen systemic corticosteroid for use, is discussed fully in Chapter 14. The development of secondary candidiasis is predictable; thus, concurrent antifungal therapy is indicated. The therapeutic response of RAS is usually rapid and dramatic. However, recurrence is likely. For some patients, the prompt application of a topical agent when the lesions recur will be all that is necessary to manage their RAS. Others will require occasional repeat, high-dose, short-term corticosteroids to control acute exacerbations.

Tertiary Line of Therapy

A more aggressive therapeutic protocol is indicated for patients whose RAS is recalcitrant to secondary lines of therapy. Tertiary lines of therapy include chronic systemic corticosteroid regimens, chronic systemic corticosteroid regimens with steroid sparing agents, or thalidomide. All of these protocols are associated with potentially serious side effects and should only be undertaken in close cooperation with the patient's physician.

Erythema Multiforme

Erythema multiforme (EM) is the general term applied to a spectrum of acute mucocutaneous vesiculobullous erosive disorders. Typically a self-limiting process, the severity of EM varies from mild (EM minor and oral EM) to moderate

(EM major) to potentially fatal (Stevens-Johnson syndrome [SJS] and toxic epidermal necrolysis [TEN]). The pathophysiology of EM has not been clearly established, although it likely represents a genetically predisposed allergic-host response to antigenic challenge. Most cases of oral EM, EM minor, and EM major are related to an infectious agent, usually the herpes simplex virus (HSV). In contrast, most cases of SJS and TEN are related to pharmacologic agents, most frequently sulfonamides, anticonvulsive drugs, and nonsteroidal anti-inflammatory drugs (NSAIDs). In addition, EM has been reported to develop following immunizations or radiotherapy, while other reports associate it with Crohn disease, Addison disease, lupus erythematosus, pregnancy, sarcoidosis, and malignancies, such as Hodgkin disease, multiple myeloma, and others. In many cases a causative agent is not identified.

Pharmacologic Management

Most cases of EM are self-limiting, with resolution occurring in 1 to 6 weeks. For such cases, treatment is generally directed toward reducing symptoms. The withdrawal of any suspected causative medications should be undertaken and a careful history obtained to identify any other possible underlying causes.

Primary Therapy

Topical anesthetic/antihistamine products, such as diphenhydramine (Children's Benadryl) or viscous lidocaine, may be prescribed for oral pain. Such agents may be mixed with a covering agent (Kaopectate or Maalox) to improve local retention. Box 13-1 illustrates compounding information to include in a prescription for the compounding pharmacist. A small amount (5 mL) is rinsed to coat oral ulcerations and expectorated. Adequate hydration and nutrition are mandatory. Nutritional supplements (Ensure) may be prescribed to ensure the maintenance of adequate nutritional intake. The use of systemic corticosteroids (prednisone) for the treatment of EM, particularly the more severe forms, remains controversial and has not been validated in clinical trials. Any potential value of corticosteroid therapy is likely predicated on its prompt administration to a patient who presents at the earliest onset of the EM.

BOX 13-1. Compounding Information for Prescription

Rx*
Diphenhydramine (Children's Benadryl) elixir,
    12.5 mg/5 mL [OTC] 4 oz, mixed with
    Kaopectate or Maalox [OTC] 4 oz (50% mixture
    by volume)
Disp: 8 oz
Sig: Rinse with 1 tsp every 2 hours and spit out

---

*By interacting with H_1-receptors on peripheral afferent fibers, where it acts as a neurotransmitter, diphenhydramine has a small anesthetic effect; at times, lidocaine viscous is added to the mixture.

Secondary Therapy

Referral to a physician is warranted for all cases of EM that are unresponsive to primary therapy, or for any suspected case of SJS or TEN. These cases often require a multidiscipline approach to management, in a manner similar to that of a patient with extensive burns.

Prevention

For cases of EM associated with HSV infection, prophylactic antiviral therapy often proves beneficial. Acyclovir or valacyclovir, oral antiviral drugs, are used for the prevention of virally induced EM. In those cases of EM attributed to side effects from a specific drug, strict avoidance of the suspect drug and all drugs with crossreactive potential is mandatory to prevent recurrence. For cases in which the cause is unknown, patient education concerning the possibility of recurrence and the necessity to ensure prompt medical intervention is recommended.

Cicatricial Pemphigoid

Cicatricial pemphigoid (CP), also known as mucous membrane pemphigoid, is a rare chronic mucocutaneous bullous condition. It is a heterogeneous autoimmune disease, characterized by the production of autoantibodies against basement membrane zone (BMZ) antigens. The mean age of onset of CP is 62 years, and it appears to have a 2:1 predilection for women, without racial or geographic bias. Oral CP is most commonly found on the buccal and labial aspects of the attached gingiva, followed by the buccal or labial mucosa, palate, tongue, and pharynx. Gingival lesions may be characterized as desquamative (having a **positive Nikolsky sign**), erythematous, painful, and, at times, hemorrhagic. The primary oral mucosal lesions of CP are vesiculobullous and tend to rupture within hours, resulting in painful erosions or ulcerations with smooth borders. Although oral mucosal lesions usually heal slowly without scarring, scarring as a result of submucosal fibrosis is a key feature of disease progression in other sites, such as the conjunctiva of the eye and larynx.

Pharmacologic Management

The extent of the dentist's involvement in managing CP depends on the presentation. For cases of CP restricted to the oral cavity, the dentist should be prepared to deliver initial therapeutic interventions. However, cases of CP manifesting extraoral involvement require a multidisciplinary approach to therapy, usually coordinated by a dermatologist. In all cases, oral care includes familiarity with immunopharmacologic strategies intended to minimize morbidity or induce remission; participation in monitoring the patient's response to therapy; and anticipation, recognition, and reporting of treatment-related adverse drug events to the primary caregiver.

Primary Therapy

For mild cases of CP limited to the oral cavity, a regularly applied topical high-potency or ultrapotency corticosteroid ointment or gel may be all that is necessary to successfully manage the patient. Ointments may also be mixed with a non-water-soluble oral paste to improve adhesion (Kenalog with Orabase). For lesions restricted to the gingiva, custom trays may be fabricated to improve the delivery of steroids to the affected tissues. The frequency of application should be titrated down to the minimum required to maintain lesion control and patient comfort. Measures to reduce the predictable risk of developing secondary candidiasis should be undertaken. In addition, the patient should be educated to reduce the risk of intraoral trauma and to maintain excellent oral hygiene. All teeth and restorations should be smooth and free of jagged edges.

Secondary Therapy

In the management of recalcitrant cases, a regimen of dapsone tablets (75 to 150 mg/day) may be prescribed by the dentist and added to the first line of therapy. Dapsone, a sulfone antimicrobial agent, is a competitive antagonist of para-aminobenzoic acid (PABA) and prevents the normal use of PABA in the synthesis of folic acid. It also inhibits the chemotaxis of polymorphonuclear leukocytes (PMNs) and directly diminishes tissue inflammation. Dapsone is associated with several potentially serious side effects, such as headache, hemolytic anemia, methemoglobinemia, bone marrow suppression, and liver toxicity. Its use is contraindicated in patients with glucose-6-phosphate dehydrogenase deficiency. The patient's complete blood count, with white cell differential, should be established at baseline and monitored every 2 weeks during therapy. The development of serious adverse drug effects (ADEs), such as agranulocytosis, warrants immediate drug cessation and prompt medical evaluation. To reduce the side effect risk, a small initial dose is prescribed, with subsequent doses gradually tapered up to reach therapeutic levels. Once control is obtained, the dosage is gradually reduced to the minimum required for maintenance. Partial or complete remission may be observed after 2 to 12 weeks of dapsone treatment.

Tertiary Therapy

For cases of oral CP not controlled by topical steroids and dapsone and for cases of CP manifesting extraoral involvement, more aggressive therapeutic measures are prescribed. Initially, a regimen of long-term systemic corticosteroid and dapsone may induce disease remission. However, severe unresponsive cases of CP often require more aggressive immunosuppressive therapies with such agents as azathioprine, methotrexate, mycophenolate mofetil, cyclophosphamide, tacrolimus, or mitomycin C. The side effect liability of all tertiary lines of therapy is such that they should only be prescribed by, or in close collaboration with, the patient's physician.

Actinic Cheilosis

Actinic cheilosis (AC) is the labial equivalent of actinic keratosis and, as such, represents the early clinical manifestation of a condition that may ultimately progress to squamous cell carcinoma. The cause of AC is chronic exposure to sunlight, especially from an early age. Although ultraviolet-B (UVB)

radiation is principally responsible, ultraviolet-A (UVA) radiation adds to the risk. Other risk factors include a fair complexion, an outdoor occupation, and immunosuppression. Men are affected more often than women, and, although most cases occur in men after the age of 40, the condition is increasingly being diagnosed in younger men. The potentially progressive nature of AC to squamous cell carcinoma emphasizes the need for early recognition and implementation of preventive and therapeutic strategies. Any time a lesion exhibits induration, ulceration, bleeding, rapid growth, or pain, an immediate biopsy is indicated.

Pharmacologic Management

When the dental hygienist observes sun-damaged skin in the extraoral examination, a recommendation to wear sunscreen routinely when in the sun should be an important part of the oral health education program, as well as general lifestyle recommendations related to avoiding harmful rays of the sun. The American Cancer Society recommends avoiding sun exposure when UV rays are strongest (10:00 AM to 4:00 PM); covering exposed skin with long sleeves; wearing a hat that shades the neck, face, and ears; wearing sunglasses; and using a sunscreen with a minimum sun protection factor (SPF) of 15. The SPF ratings apply only to UVB rays. Studies over the years have shown that sunscreen with an SPF of 30 blocks about 97% of ultraviolet rays. A rating of 15 SPF means 93% of UV rays are blocked, and an SPF >30 remains in the 97% or 98% range. In 1999, the Food and Drug Administration (FDA) recommended that sunscreens with an SPF >30 be labeled "30(PLUS)," mostly to prevent people from developing a false sense of security that might lead them to spend more time in the sun. A recent study found that applying <2 oz over the entire body at one time can leave an individual with an SPF protection far lower than what is identified on the bottle.[1] Other studies found that typically users apply less than the amount recommended on the product label. The patient *who already has* sun-damaged skin should consistently use a broad-spectrum sunscreen product (protecting against both UVB and UVA rays) with a minimum SPF of 30. This is different from recommendations to prevent sun damage by wearing sunscreen with an SPF of 15 or higher. Ideally, the product chosen should block both UVB and UVA (such as formulations containing zinc oxide, avobenzone, or ecamsule [Athelios SX]) and be specifically formulated for use on the lips. Sunscreen should be applied liberally 15 to 30 minutes before anticipated exposure and reapplied liberally after any vigorous activity that may wash or rub the sunscreen away.

Primary Therapy

OTC products include Blistex Clear Advantage, Burnout SPF 32, and Zinc Stick SPF 30+.

■ Self-Study Review

1. Describe the role of the RDH in pharmacologic management of common oral conditions.

2. Identify the recommended therapies to resolve acute odontogenic pain.
3. List the drugs of choice for mild odontogenic pain.
4. Describe recommendations to relieve pain from RAS, OLP, oral EM, and oral CP. List secondary therapies also.
5. Identify potential ADEs associated with the above therapies.
6. Describe oral health education topics and application instructions for each condition or agent identified in no. 4.
7. Identify dermatologic conditions with oral lesions. Which one is the most common?

Herpetic Infection

Herpetic infections are caused by either HSV type 1 (HSV-1) or HSV type 2 (HSV-2). A unique feature of these viruses is their ability to establish latency following primary infection, thus creating the potential for recurrence. An estimated 500,000 cases of primary oral infection and 100 million cases of recurrent oral infection occur annually in the United States. The diagnosis of herpetic infections is based on history and clinical findings. Laboratory tests such as Tzanck smear, serology, and culturing are rarely necessary, but they can assist in the diagnosis of atypical cases.

Primary Herpetic Infection

Most primary infections are asymptomatic or mildly symptomatic and typically occur between 2 to 3 years of age. Symptomatic primary infection, although less common, usually presents as a painful herpetic gingivostomatitis. Nonspecific prodromal signs and symptoms include fever, malaise, irritability, headache, and cervical lymphadenopathy. These prodromal signs typically occur 1 to 3 days before the development of painful, widespread vesicular eruptions and gingival inflammation. All oral soft tissues may be affected. Within a few days, the vesicles coalesce, rupture, and form large, irregularly shaped erosions or ulcerations. The lesions heal without scarring in 1 to 2 weeks. In some cases, the pain may be intense and interfere with eating and drinking, placing the patient at risk for dehydration and malnutrition. Conditions that predispose to systemic dissemination include immunologic immaturity, malignancy, malnutrition, pregnancy, and therapeutic or acquired immunosuppression.

Recurrent Herpetic Infection

Following primary infection, many of those affected experience recurrence, most commonly recurrent herpes labialis (RHL). Patients usually report prodromal sensations of tingling, itching, burning, or pain before the eruption of the characteristic focal vesicular lesions affecting the lip vermilion or other perioral sites, such as the skin or ala of the nose. The vesicles rapidly rupture and crust, with ultimate uneventful healing occurring within 2 weeks. Viral shedding precedes the prodromal period and continues into convalescence; during these times, the patient should be considered infectious. This can lead both to autoinoculation and crossinfection. Less

frequently observed are intraoral recurrent herpetic eruptions. Intraoral lesions appear as small clusters of pinpoint ulcers, usually restricted to the keratinized mucosa. Numerous trigger factors, such as ultraviolet radiation, trauma, menstruation, fever, and immunosuppression, have been implicated. In immunocompromised patients, the lesions are usually more severe and recovery is lengthy.

Pharmacologic Management

No cure exists for HSV and its establishment of latency. Therapy is tailored to the individual patient, taking into account the severity of the infection and the patient's overall health. Most cases resolve in 7 to 10 days; however, some topical agents can shorten the outbreak by increasing healing time.

Primary Herpetic Infection

Because the primary infection can present as multiple painful ulcerations, strategies are targeted to ensure adequate hydration and nutrition and to provide palliation. A topical anesthetic agent, such as diphenhydramine hydrochloride (Children's Benadryl syrup) or lidocaine viscous, and, if necessary, a systemic analgesic should be recommended. When topical anesthetics are used, the patient should be warned that these agents may increase the risk of self-induced trauma, may interfere with the pharyngeal phase of swallowing, and may lead to aspiration. Systemic analgesics, such as acetaminophen and, in rare instances, an acetaminophen/codeine formulation, may be needed. Aspirin should be avoided for children younger than 18 years of age because of the risk of Reye (also called Reye's) syndrome. Nutritional liquid supplements (Ensure) are recommended when the patient cannot eat comfortably. Patients with primary herpetic infections who are immunocompromised, manifest immunologic immaturity, or present with evidence of systemic dissemination should be promptly referred for medical evaluation and management. Possible signs and symptoms of dissemination include the presence of extraoral lesions, conjunctivitis, ocular pain, visual impairment, lethargy, **dysphagia**, **hemiparesis**, or seizure.

Recurrent Herpetic Infection

There are two forms of recurrent herpetic infection, including intraoral lesions and lesions on the lips and skin. While often painful and at times unsightly, recurrent herpes lesions are self-limiting and often require no treatment. All patients should be advised to avoid touching the lesion and practice good hygiene (e.g., wash hands) to reduce the risk of autoinoculation. A wide variety of OTC topical agents are marketed to provide palliation and promote the healing of RHL. However, docosanol (Abreva) is the only OTC formulation specifically approved by the FDA for the treatment of RHL. Docosanol cream is approved for individuals ages ≥12 and should be applied at the first prodromal sign. It can be reapplied using a cotton-tipped applicator five times per day until the lesion is healed. It shortens the healing time and duration of symptoms and is to be used on the skin or lips (not intraorally). For patients who manifest frequent recurrent episodes or who otherwise desire antiviral therapy, the FDA

BOX 13-2. Agents for Recurrent Herpetic Lesions

- Docosanol: 1% cream; apply to lips and skin at first prodromal sign; use five times/day until healed
- Acyclovir: 5% cream; apply at first prodromal sign; use five times daily until healed
- Penciclovir: 1% cream; apply at first prodromal sign; use every 2 hours until healed
- Valacyclovir: 1,000-mg tab; take two tabs bid for 1 day

---

has approved three prescription antiviral agents. Penciclovir (Denavir), a 1% cream, is an antiviral agent to be applied every 2 hours until lesions heal. Acyclovir (Zovirax), a 5% cream, is to be applied five times per day until lesions heal. An oral antiviral, valacyclovir (Valtrex), 1,000-mg tablet, is a 1-day therapy, with two tablets taken twice daily (Box 13-2). Regardless of the agent chosen, therapy is most effective when initiated during the prodromal phase. Finally, in those individuals for whom sunlight precipitates an outbreak, recommending an SPF 15 or higher lip balm may prevent future RHL.

Recurrent intraoral herpetic lesions typically occur as an isolated event associated with an antecedent traumatic event, such as may occur with dental manipulation. Such cases only require recognition, reassurance, and, if necessary, palliation with the application of a topical anesthetic. Unlike docosanol, acyclovir or penciclovir can be used for intraoral lesions.

Candidiasis

Candidiasis is the most frequently occurring opportunistic fungal infection that affects humans. Whereas most cases are caused by *Candida albicans*, other species have been implicated, especially in immunosuppressed patients. *C. albicans* has the ability to exist in a commensal state in such areas as the skin and the gastrointestinal and genitourinary tracts. The shift from a state of commensalism to a pathogenic infection is almost always associated with an underlying predisposing factor. Established predisposing factors include immunosuppression, immunologic immaturity, certain medications, salivary changes, malignancies, numerous endocrinopathies, epithelial alterations, nutritional deficiencies, high-carbohydrate diet, poor oral hygiene, dental prostheses, advanced age, and smoking. Oral candidiasis may manifest a variety of clinical presentations, including pseudomembranous, atrophic, and hyperplastic lesions, as well as median rhomboid glossitis and some cases of angular cheilitis.

Pharmacologic Management

Essential to any management strategy is a thorough review of the patient's medical and dental histories to identify predisposing factors. Acute cases attributed to short-term antibiotic therapy are usually easily managed, while chronic or recurrent cases attributed to a poorly controlled systemic disease

may be more problematic and require medical referral. In all cases, the goals of therapy are to remove predisposing factors when possible, to prevent further spread or dissemination, to provide symptomatic relief, and, when appropriate, to provide patient education to reduce the risk of recurrence.

Primary Therapy

The use of a topical antifungal agent, such as nystatin, clotrimazole, or ketoconazole, is usually effective for mild localized lesions. Nystatin is supplied as a rinse and a pastille. The rinse (5 mL) is swished for 5 minutes and swallowed or expectorated. It is used five times per day. The pastille is allowed to slowly dissolve in the mouth; it is used four to five times per day. Therapy may take up to 4 weeks for lesions to resolve. The pastille is not to be chewed or swallowed. Clotrimazole troche is dissolved slowly in the mouth five times per day for 14 days. Saliva should be retained (not swallowed) to increase the contact time with the antifungal agent. The troche should not be chewed or swallowed. Ketoconazole cream 2% should be applied to the affected area once daily for 2 to 4 weeks.

Improvement should be noted within a week, at which time the topical therapy should be continued for another 3 to 5 days. In resistant cases, therapy may need to be extended for up to 4 weeks. The efficacy of topical formulations is largely dependent on prolonged contact time with the affected tissues. Thus, patients must be instructed on the appropriate use of topical therapies. Both nystatin solution and clotrimazole troches contain sucrose, which may limit their use in patients with diabetes and those who are at high risk for caries. Topical fluoride agents and xylitol products should be used during prolonged therapy to reduce caries risk. In cases of candidiasis associated with a dental prosthesis, it is important to also treat the prosthesis. Specifically, the prosthesis should not be worn during sleep, but instead should be soaked in an antifungal solution. These instructions should be included in the oral health care plan to promote the most efficacious use of an antifungal agent. Most commercial denture solutions exhibit antifungal properties, as do nystatin solution, chlorhexidine gluconate, and diluted sodium hypochlorite.

Secondary Therapy

For patients unresponsive to topical therapy or noncompliant or intolerant with its use, a systemic oral antifungal agent is often effective. Available drugs include ketoconazole, fluconazole, and itraconazole. Fluconazole is usually the drug of choice, because it is readily absorbed and exhibits a better safety profile than ketoconazole. Itraconazole is usually reserved for treating candidiasis resistant to fluconazole.

■ Self-Study Review

8. Differentiate between the clinical appearances of *herpes labialis* and *intraoral recurrent herpetic infection*.
9. Differentiate between treatments for *primary* versus *recurrent* herpetic infection.

10. How efficacious are preparations for treating recurrent HSV infection?
11. Describe oral health instructions related to the presence of RHL and warnings when topical anesthetic agents are recommended for recurrent herpetic lesions.
12. List products for the treatment of herpetic infection and describe instructions for their use.
13. List products for candida infection and describe patient instructions for their use.

Xerostomia

Xerostomia, or dry mouth, is not a specific disease entity, but it may occur in conjunction with a number of significant local and systemic factors. A reduction in salivary flow has been attributed to such factors as heavy smoking and alcohol intake, altered psychic states, and idiopathic conditions. Specific local factors may include the rare congenital absence, or *aplasia*, of one or more of the major salivary glands or ducts; glandular hyperplasia associated with mumps, sialolithiasis, and sialoadenitis; and neoplasias, which usually affect an isolated gland (although there may be infiltration of multiple glands in leukemia and lymphoma). Systemic conditions associated with xerostomia include uncontrolled diabetes mellitus and Sjögren syndrome. Sjögren syndrome is a relatively common condition that typically affects women between the ages of 40 to 60 and is characterized clinically by parotid enlargement and, histologically, by lymphocytic infiltration and displacement of the acinar cells in salivary glands. Xerostomia may also be associated with other connective tissue disorders, such as systemic lupus erythematosus, scleroderma, and mixed connective tissue disease. The major classes of drugs capable of inducing xerostomia include anticholinergics, antidepressants, antihypertensives, antipsychotics, diuretics, gastrointestinals, antihistamines, antineoplastics, central nervous system (CNS) stimulants, systemic bronchodilators, and a small number of cancer chemotherapeutic agents. Probably the most problematic and profound form of xerostomia is seen secondary to external irradiation of the head and neck. Finally, it is quite common for the patient to have more than one factor contributing to xerostomia.

The diagnosis of xerostomia is usually made upon clinical examination. Characteristic clinical findings include a noticeable lack of wetness to the mucosal tissues and teeth; saliva that is thick and ropey; absence of saliva pooling in the floor of the mouth; red, dry, and atrophic mucosa; an atrophic and fissured tongue; incisal and smooth surface caries, especially at the cervical margins; and candidiasis. When used as a retractor, the dental mirror will often stick to the xerostomic patient's buccal mucosa. Once the clinical diagnosis of a dry mouth is made, a careful and exhaustive review of the patient's medical history must be obtained to identify any predisposing factors.

Pharmacologic Management

Depending on the etiology, treatment strategies for xerostomia may be either targeted or palliative and supportive, or both.

Primary Therapy

Efforts to remove or reduce identified predisposing factors should be undertaken whenever possible. Underlying systemic disorders that predispose to xerostomia should be addressed by the patient's physician. The dentist may consult with the patient's physician to attempt to discontinue, reduce, or change any medications that predispose to xerostomia. Patient education to reduce exposure to OTC medications that predispose to xerostomia should be provided. A drug reference would identify potential side effects for OTC drugs being used. Patients should be advised to maintain hydration throughout the day; use a fluoride dentifrice twice a day and 0.05% sodium fluoride rinses daily, and remove and clean prostheses at night; avoid products that irritate the mucosa (alcohol, tobacco, acidic or spicy food, and fruits and vegetables with high acid content); reduce dietary sugar intake; and use xylitol-containing or sugar-free gums or candies to stimulate salivation. Alcohol-containing mouth rinses should be avoided if burning on the mucosa is reported.

A variety of salivary substitutes are available (OralBalance, Optimoist, Salivart). However, these agents represent poor imitators of natural saliva, and patient acceptance is notoriously poor. A new linseed-extract product (Numoisyn) has favorable patient acceptance. The liquid formulation contains linseed extract and mucins that have a superior viscosity and reduced friction compared with water or carboxymethylcellulose (an ingredient of most artificial saliva products). It is available in lozenge and liquid doseforms and requires a prescription. For chapped lips, a lip balm that contains vitamin E may be helpful.

For patients with residual salivary function, a sialagogue (tablet) may prove beneficial. Pilocarpine (Salagen) is approved for the treatment of xerostomia associated with head and neck radiotherapy and Sjögren syndrome; cevimeline (Evoxac) is approved for the treatment of xerostomia associated with Sjögren syndrome. Either drug may be prescribed on a trial basis to improve salivary flow in all patients with xerostomia. They should be used with caution in patients with significant cardiovascular disease, asthma, chronic bronchitis, chronic obstructive pulmonary disease (COPD), biliary tract disease, and kidney disease. Common side effects include sweating, headache, nausea, gastrointestinal upset, urinary frequency, rhinitis, and flushing. Either drug may be started at a low dose and titrated upward to maximize effects while minimizing side effects.

Caries Control

An alcohol-free formulation of chlorhexidine gluconate rinse (Chlorhexidine Gluconate Oral Rinse) and supplemental topical fluoride should be prescribed to reduce caries development. The additional application of a fluoride varnish on a regular basis may be beneficial. Xylitol products (gums, mints) help to stimulate salivation and have an anticaries effect. Studies suggest a range of 6 to 10 g xylitol divided into at least three consumption periods per day is necessary for xylitol to be effective for a cariostatic effect with chewing gum as the delivery system.[2] It is interesting to note that a dental hygienist is part of a team at the University of Washington investigating the efficacy of various xylitol products in caries control.[3] Lastly, patients with xerostomia should be placed on an accelerated recall schedule, typically every 3 months.

Pericoronitis

Pericoronitis, seen most commonly in young adults, is a localized gingivitis associated with a partially erupted tooth. While it may be associated with any deciduous or succedaneous tooth, it most often affects the permanent third molars. Bacterial plaque and food debris accumulate beneath the operculum, providing an ideal milieu for rapid bacterial growth. The ensuing bacterial infection consists of a predominately anaerobic flora mainly comprised of α-hemolytic streptococci, *Veillonella*, *Prevotella*, *Bacteroides*, *Capnocytophaga*, *Campylobacter*, and *Actinomyces*. Contributing factors include lowered systemic resistance, decreased flow of saliva, poor eating habits, lack of sleep, and inadequate oral hygiene.

The diagnosis of pericoronitis is usually straightforward. Mild or early cases present with pain or discomfort associated with gingival inflammation around the offending tooth. Frequently, occlusal trauma from an opposing (often supraerupted) tooth acts to aggravate or occasionally initiate the process. Palpation of the inflamed gingival tissue may elicit a purulent exudate. More advanced cases may manifest malaise; fever; lymphadenopathy; foul taste; pain in the ear, throat, and floor of the mouth; tonsillar and pharyngeal inflammation; cellulitis; and loss of masticatory function.

Pharmacologic Management

Mild cases of pericoronitis usually respond promptly to therapies that establish drainage, remove sources of trauma, improve oral hygiene, and relieve pain. Drainage (the first step in management) can often be established by simply inserting a curet or periodontal probe under the operculum.

Primary Therapy

Following establishment of drainage, the area should be thoroughly irrigated with saline or an antiseptic rinse, such as 3% hydrogen peroxide diluted to half strength with either saline or 0.12% chlorhexidine gluconate. A wick of iodoform gauze may be temporarily inserted under the operculum to allow for continuous drainage. The patient is further instructed to rinse with warm salt water for 2 minutes every waking hour.

For cases in which the opposing tooth is traumatizing the operculum, the opposing tooth should either be extracted or undergo an odontoplasty to reduce the traumatic insult. Some experts caution that extracting teeth in the presence of pericoronitis increases the risk of developing septicemia, cavernous sinus thrombosis, or mediastinal abscess. They recommend extraction of the offending tooth once the infection associated with pericoronitis has been appropriately managed.[4] Patients should be advised to rest; avoid drinking alcoholic beverages and smoking cigarettes; maintain hydration; and eat a soft, balanced diet. The importance of removing bacteria at the area of pericoronitis must be stressed and its relationship to pericoronitis discussed. For patients with mild-to-moderate pain, a COX-inhibitor or an opioid combination may be prescribed.

Secondary Line of Therapy

For patients manifesting systemic signs of infection (fever, lymphadenopathy, and malaise), an antimicrobial regimen should be prescribed following débridement to remove exudate. Penicillin remains the initial drug of choice. If significant improvement is not noted with penicillin VK in 48 to 72 hours, the empirical addition of 7 days of metronidazole (to kill the anaerobic component of infection) is reasonable because it is beta-lactamase resistant.

Alveolar Osteitis

Alveolar osteitis (AO), or dry socket, is a relatively common postextraction complication that affects mandibular third-molar sites ten times more frequently than other sites. It is postulated that surgical trauma or the presence of existing inflammation leads to the release of bioactive substances from the alveolar bone or adjacent tissues that convert plasminogen in the clot to the fibrinolytic agent plasmin. Plasmin acts to dissolve the clot, which leads to the release of kinins. Numerous predisposing factors have been associated with AO, including smoking, contraception use, gender, surgical trauma, practitioner inexperience, pre-existing infections, inadequate infection control, increased patient age, and insufficient irrigation during surgery. AO is a transient phenomenon that will resolve itself in about 7 to 10 days, although it can result in significant discomfort during the postoperative time.

The diagnosis of AO is usually easily made and is based on the presence of an empty extraction site 2 to 3 days postprocedure, severe (often radiating) pain in and around the extraction site, and halitosis. It is unlikely to occur within the first 24 hours postextraction. Occasionally, fever, trismus, and lymphadenopathy may be present, but such findings may also indicate the presence of infection. Other conditions to consider in the differential diagnosis include retained tooth or bony fragments, foreign debris, or jaw fracture.

Pharmacologic Management

Unfortunately, no universally accepted or validated protocols exist to prevent or manage AO. Almost all proposed protocols incur additional office visits with substantial extra costs and may induce adverse drug reactions. If an adverse reaction were to occur, defending the use of an unproven product may prove difficult. However, in spite of all the apparent contradictions in the literature, some prudent recommendations can be offered.

Primary Therapy

A chlorhexidine rinse should be administered immediately before tooth extraction and for 1 week (twice daily) postoperatively. An atraumatic surgical technique should be used with attention to irrigate the extraction site with saline, ensure the removal of any bone or tooth fragments, and verify the formation of a viable clot. Verbal and written postoperative instructions should be provided to emphasize the need to avoid

- smoking;
- sucking through a straw;
- drinking carbonated beverages;
- vigorous rinsing for 48 hours.

A nutritious soft diet is recommended, and the use of gentle toothbrushing for oral hygiene should be prescribed. For pain relief, 7.5 mg of hydrocodone and 200 mg of ibuprofen (Vicoprofen) can be recommended. While eugenol gauze provides for a certain degree of comfort when placed in the socket, it must be noted that AO heals by secondary intention; anything placed in the socket will delay the healing process.

Treatment

The goal in treating AO is to reduce discomfort and promote healing. Currently, there are no products available that completely meet both of these goals. Conservative therapy consists of the following:

1. Remove any sutures to allow easy access to the extraction site, which often requires local anesthesia.
2. Thoroughly irrigate the site with warm saline to loosen any debris and carefully suction the site.
3. There is no need to curette the site to incur bleeding (once AO occurs, healing will occur through secondary intention).
4. Provide and instruct the patient on the appropriate use of a curved tip plastic syringe to keep the socket site clean by irrigating with either chlorhexidine gluconate or saline.
5. The dental surgeon will prescribe an analgesic; reassure and educate the patient on the process and the therapeutic goals.

Stomatitis

Stomatitis is an encompassing term used to refer to any inflammatory condition affecting the mucosal tissues of the mouth. As such, many of the conditions addressed in this chapter qualify as forms of stomatitis. The degree of mucosal involvement in stomatitis varies greatly, depending on the predisposing and etiologic factors involved. Typically, stomatitis is associated with mild-to-moderate pain and a potential for secondary bacterial and fungal infections.

The diagnosis of stomatitis is usually easily made based on the patient's presenting complaint and findings of the clinical examination. However, a careful and thorough discernment of the patient's history is often required to identify possible etiologies and determine the most likely cause of the inflammation. The differential diagnosis can include mucosal burns (chemical, physical, thermal), chemotherapy and radiation-induced ulcerations, immunologic-based ulcerations, and traumatic injury.

Oral Health Education

Misguided patients must be advised that the topical application of medicaments such as aspirin (designed for systemic use) is ill advised. The adverse mucosal effects caused by tobacco use afford the practitioner a tangible opportunity to discuss and promote tobacco cessation. Oral lesions associated with accidental mucosal exposure to gasoline and other chemicals generally are not severe, although they may require supportive treatment, and complete healing usually occurs within 7 days. The treatment of stomatitis caused by ill-fitting or poorly maintained removable dental prostheses may require only minor denture adjustment or cleaning or complete refabrication of the prostheses. Patients should be educated on the need to not wear the prostheses 24 hours per day. The importance of meticulous oral hygiene cannot be overemphasized as an effective preventive and therapeutic modality in the management of stomatitis.

Pharmacologic Management

Depending on the etiology and severity, the management strategies to address stomatitis will vary. For many cases, simple recognition along with patient education and reassurance is all that is necessary. For others, more aggressive therapies may be required.

Primary Therapy

There are numerous prescription and OTC topical gels, creams, ointments, and rinses marketed for the treatment of mouth sores (see the section on RAS). However, clinicians are reminded that no validated studies exist to demonstrate the clinical superiority of any formulation over another. For cases of stomatitis thought to be caused by a medication, the patient should be advised to cease using the medication if self-prescribed. For cases possibly caused by a prescription medication, a medical consultation with the physician is warranted to consider the use of an alternative agent. Palliative relief may be provided by topical corticosteroid products.

Secondary Therapy

For more severe cases, such as may occur with radiation therapy and/or chemotherapy, strategies to provide palliation and prevent secondary infection are indicated. Patients should be instructed to carefully remove plaque, either with a soft toothbrush or with a foam toothette, to minimize trauma; to avoid products irritating to oral soft tissues (such as alcohol and tobacco; hot, spicy, and coarse foods; and fruits and beverages with a high acid content); to refrain from wearing removable prostheses; to eat a dental soft diet; and to frequently rinse with alkaline saline (sodium bicarbonate) solution. A topical anesthetic agent, such as lidocaine viscous or diphenhydramine hydrochloride, and, if necessary, a systemic analgesic may be prescribed. When topical anesthetics are used, the patient should be warned that these agents reduce the feeling in tissues and can increase the risk of self-induced trauma, interfere with the pharyngeal phase of swallowing, and can lead to aspiration. An alkaline saline mouth rinse can be recommended and is formulated by mixing 1/2 tsp each of salt and baking soda in 16 oz of water.

Necrotizing Ulcerative Gingivitis

Necrotizing ulcerative gingivitis (NUG) is a unique, painful bacterial infection affecting the interdental and marginal gingival tissue. Consistently implicated microorganisms include *Prevotella intermedia*, *Fusobacterium fusiforme*, *Bacteroides melaninogenicus*, *Treponema*, and *Selenomonas*. The positive clinical response to antibiotics tends to support the role of these organisms as etiologic agents. Although bacteria underlie the etiology, NUG is not considered to be a communicable disease. There seems to be a direct relationship between the occurrence of NUG and reduced host resistance. Other established predisposing factors include malnutrition, smoking, psychologic stress, preexisting gingivitis, and trauma. In some cases, particularly in those with an immunosuppressive disorder, (such as AIDS, NUG) may progress to affect the deeper periodontal ligament and osseous tissues, resulting in necrotizing ulcerative periodontitis (NUP).

Pharmacologic Management

Reinforcement of personal plaque control combined with professional débridement is undertaken to reduce the bacterial mass. While ultrasonic instrumentation with copious amounts of water represents an excellent choice for débridement, judicious and gentle hand scaling with copious irrigation will also suffice. The goal is to perform a simple débridement, not a thorough fine scale.

Oral Health Information

Patients should be instructed on how to gently brush their teeth using a soft-bristle toothbrush. In addition, instructions should include rinsing with a 3% hydrogen peroxide diluted solution (4 oz of peroxide mixed with 12 oz of water) or with chlorhexidine gluconate. Patients should be advised to rest, avoid smoking cigarettes and drinking alcoholic beverages, eat a soft nutritious diet, and maintain adequate hydration. Prompt clinical improvement is the rule, and the patient should be seen on a daily basis until the acute phase is eliminated.

Primary Therapy

A 3% hydrogen peroxide solution or chlorhexidine gluconate rinse is the chosen therapy in most cases. Close follow-up is mandatory to verify adequate resolution of NUG. Unresponsive patients should undergo further medical evaluation to rule out conditions such as leukemia, severe malnutrition, or HIV infection. A high degree of suspicion for the presence of an underlying immunosuppressive disorder is warranted for the patient who initially presents with necrotizing ulcerative periodontitis (NUP). For all patients, additional periodontal surgical interventions may be necessary to address any residual soft tissue deformities that reduce oral hygiene efficacy.

Secondary Therapy

The use of a systemic antimicrobial regimen should be considered for the patient who does not promptly respond to the primary line of therapy, who initially presents with constitutional signs such as lymphadenopathy and/or fever, or who initially manifests NUP. Either penicillin or metronidazole may be used, and improvement should be prompt.

Burning Mouth Disorder

Burning mouth disorder (BMD) is a chronic, painful condition that manifests as a burning sensation affecting the oral mucosa, particularly the mucosa of the anterior tongue and lips. When limited to the tongue, BMD is often referred to as **glossodynia**. The etiology of BMD is unknown, but there is a predilection to afflict women (6:1). An estimated 50% of cases are associated with oral dryness and dysgeusia. The clinical examination is usually unremarkable for obvious abnormalities, causing frustration for both the patient and the clinician. Numerous conditions, such as hormonal changes in women (especially in the perimenopausal or postmenopausal periods); iron, folic acid, or B_{12} deficiency; diabetes mellitus–associated neuropathy; candidiasis; and neurotic glossodynia may cause burning sensations of the oral mucosa. Appropriate medical consultations may be necessary to rule out suspected comorbid factors before establishing a diagnosis of BMD.

Pharmacologic Management

The treatment of burning mucosal sensation associated with an identifiable cause is cared for primarily by managing the underlying cause. BMD, being a diagnosis of exclusion, is managed with neuroleptic agents, such as clonazepam. Such medications should be prescribed in close collaboration with the patient's physician. The recommendations below are provided for completeness with the acknowledgment that many general dental practitioners will choose to refer such off-label therapies to the patient's physician.

Primary Therapy

Clonazepam taken at bedtime may be effective in relieving BMD. The initial dose is low and slowly titrated up every 3 to 7 days until a therapeutic effect is observed or the maximum recommended dose is attained. For clonazepam, the maximum daily dose is 4 mg. Alternatively, a benzodiazepine such as chlordiazepoxide (Librium) may be prescribed.

Secondary Therapy

For patients unresponsive to primary therapies, the use of a tricyclic antidepressant, such as desipramine, may prove effective. Desipramine is preferred over amitriptyline because it induces less oral drying. The initial dose of 10 mg is increased by 10 mg weekly until therapeutic relief is attained. For patients refractory to the above therapies, the use of the anticonvulsant gabapentin may be effective. Gabapentin is approved for the treatment of postherpetic neuralgia. The initial dose of 300 mg/day is steadily increased to 300 to 600 mg three times per day until relief is attained.

■ Self-Study Review

14. Describe clinical signs of *xerostomia* and agents for managing it.
15. Identify situations in which sialagogues are recommended. In what disease conditions should these drugs be used with caution?
16. Describe management of *pericoronitis*. Write out instructions for an alkaline saline mouth rinse.
17. Describe management of *dry socket*.

Table 13-2 | Dental Hygiene Applications for Topical Agents

Topical Agents	Application Instructions	Adverse Effects, Comments
Steroids	Cream or gel: Apply thin coat with cotton-tipped applicator, use 4 to 5 times per day after meals or toothbrushing and at bedtime. Use until lesion heals or up to 2 weeks. Elixir: Rinse for 2 min and expectorate; use up to 4 times per day until lesion heals.	Warn to report signs of candidiasis to dentist. Monitor for mucosal atrophy at maintenance appointment.
Nonsteroids	Paste: Apply in same manner as steroid cream, using small dab of paste. Use up to 10 days or until lesion heals. Barrier: Apply product over dry mucosa to enhance attachment. Reapply as needed. Mouth rinse: Small amount is swished in mouth to cover ulceration, then expectorated. Use every 2 h or as needed to reduce symptoms. Sunscreen SPF 30: Apply product 15 to 30 min before sun exposure. Reapply after any activity that removes product.	None reported.
Anti-infectives	Antiviral cream: Apply small amount at first sign of prodrome. Reapply every 2 h, up to 5 times/day, using cotton-tipped applicator. Antifungal cream: Apply with cotton-tipped applicator once daily for 2 to 4 wk. Antifungal rinse: Swish 5 mL for 5 min and swallow or expectorate; use 5 times per day. Antifungal pastille: Slowly dissolve 1 to 2 pastilles in mouth; use 5 times per day for 14 days. Hold saliva in mouth 5 min. Do not swallow pastille. Antifungal troche: Slowly dissolve 1 troche in mouth; use 5 times per day for 14 days. Hold saliva in mouth 5 min. Do not chew or swallow troche.	Stinging, burning. Stinging, burning; instruct that removable prostheses should be treated with antifungal agent at night. Caries is possible; use anticaries agents to diminish caries process. Caries is possible; use anticaries agents to diminish caries process.

18. Describe oral health information in management of *stomatitis*.
19. Describe management of *NUG*.
20. Describe management of *burning mouth syndrome*.

DENTAL HYGIENE APPLICATIONS

Dental hygienists are often asked by patients about pharmacologic products to assist in relieving oral conditions. Knowledge of products that are effective, along with how to use the products, is necessary in order to provide helpful information to the patient. Recognizing clinical manifestations of common ADEs is essential in order to facilitate medical intervention and pharmacologic changes. Dental hygiene education prepares the practitioner to recognize common oral conditions; however, the dentist is the legal and professional member of the dental team to make a diagnosis of oral pathology. Following the definitive diagnosis and prescription of topical agents, the dental hygienist may play a role in explaining application instructions, warnings, and potential ADEs of therapeutic agents (Table 13-2). For mouth rinses that can be mixed at home, the amounts of each ingredient must be provided along with instructions for use. Some conditions should be monitored frequently, so the maintenance schedule should accommodate this need. For conditions related to skin damage from sun exposure, the oral health education plan should include appropriate warnings to avoid sun exposure and, if sun exposure is unavoidable, to use products with an effective SPF sunscreen (SPF 30). As well, the dental hygienist should be familiar with administration instructions

CLINICAL APPLICATION EXERCISES

■ **Exercise 1.** As you perform the pretreatment intraoral exam, you notice a large ulceration in the vestibule of the labial mucosa, adjacent to tooth 27. Upon questioning, the patient says it is painful, and similar ulcerations seem to develop several times a year. The lesions seem to appear during stressful events or sometimes following the menstrual period. This recurrent aphthous lesion is so painful that it keeps the patient from being able to eat, and she requests the dental hygienist to avoid procedures in that area. What is the most likely topical agent the dentist will prescribe, and what are the application recommendations?

■ **Exercise 2.** Write out OTC agents and application instructions for the patient who spends a day at the beach and comes to the dental hygiene appointment with initial lesions of RHL.

■ **Exercise 3.** WEB ACTIVITY: Find out the newest FDA consumer warning regarding sunscreens at http://www.fda.gov/consumer/updates/sunscreen082307.pdf.

of agents prescribed following various dental treatments, because patients often ask for clarification when the hygiene appointment follows recent dental care.

CONCLUSION

The clinical manifestations of many diseases, either local or systemic, appear typically on certain areas of the face, lips, areas of oral mucosa, or gingivae. Knowledge of the more common sites of involvement of a disease assists in its diagnosis. Definitive diagnosis is often complicated. Therefore, the evaluation and integration of the clinical appearance and characteristics of a lesion, along with its history of development and other appropriate diagnostic findings, should always determine the final diagnosis and therapeutic approach.

References

1. Faurschou A, Wulf HC. The relation between sun protection factor and amount of sunscreen applied in vivo. *BDJ*. 2007;156(4): 716–719.
2. Kiet AL, Milgrom P, Rothen M. Xylitol, sweeteners, and dental caries. *Pediatr Dent*. 2006;28:154–163.
3. Rothen M. The wonder of xylitol. *Dimen Den Hyg*. 2005;3(10): 18–20.
4. Ohshima A, Ariji Y, Goto M, et al. Anatomical considerations for the spread of odontogenic infection originating from the pericoronitis of impacted mandibular third molar; computed tomographic analyses. *Oral Surg Oral Med Oral Pathol Oral Radiol Endod*. 2004;98:589–597.

Part 3

Drugs Used to Control Systemic Disorders

14

Drugs of the Endocrine System and Metabolic Agents

This chapter provides a basic overview of selected drugs that affect the endocrine system as well as hormones used as drugs. Only those hormonal agents likely to be reported on a medical history are included in order to make the chapter information clinically relevant to dental hygiene practice. Dental hygienists do not use these drugs, but some agents, such as topical steroids, are prescribed by dentists for the treatment of oral lesions, and the dental hygienist may provide patient instruction for application of topical agents. When endocrine-related drugs are reported on the health history, both the drug effects and an assessment of disease control for the specific hormonal disorder should be considered. Dental hygiene functions also include providing information to the patient related to the effects of dental hygiene treatment, specific drugs, and dental implications for potential adverse drug effects (ADEs).

THE ENDOCRINE SYSTEM

Endocrine glands are those that secrete humoral substances internally, primarily into the systemic circulation (Box 14-1). The primary function of the endocrine system is to regulate cellular metabolism and maintain homeostasis. Consequently, hormones secreted by the various endocrine glands seldom, if ever, act in isolation. The effect of one hormone can be seen in a series of complex interactions with others, and a functional abnormality in one endocrine gland will produce a number of compensatory reactions in other glands. Endocrine hormones released into the bloodstream or portal systems are delivered indiscriminately to target and nontarget tissues. Target cells for a particular hormone contain specialized molecules or receptors that bind the hormone and cause cellular activity.

Pituitary Gland

The *pituitary gland*, called "the master gland" because it secretes many hormones that regulate numerous vital processes, is illustrated in Figure 14-1. Endocrine drugs are natural or synthetic hormones that mimic effects of the hormones produced by the pituitary. In humans, the pituitary gland rests in a cavity of the sphenoid bone, referred to as the *sella turcica*. The gland has two parts, an anterior portion and a posterior portion. The posterior pituitary gland is nourished by branches of the inferior hypophysial arteries. The vascular supply of the anterior pituitary gland is provided by the superior hypophysial arteries derived from each internal carotid.

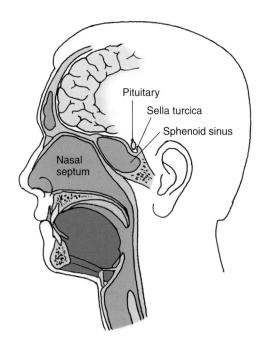

Figure 14-1 Location of Pituitary Gland. (From Roach SS. *Introductory Clinical Pharmacology*. 7th ed. Baltimore: Lippincott Williams & Wilkins; 2004 with permission.)

Anterior Pituitary

Hormones of the *anterior* pituitary gland regulate virtually every peripheral endocrine organ. Figure 14-2 identifies hormones secreted by the anterior portion of the pituitary and the tissues and organs they affect. One can see from this illustration that the effects have a wide range.

Anterior pituitary drugs are used therapeutically to control the function of the thyroid and adrenal glands and the ovaries and testes. Most are administered by injection because they are destroyed in the gastrointestinal (GI) tract. **Humoral substances** that either stimulate or inhibit the anterior pituitary originate in the hypothalamus and are transported to anterior pituitary cells via the portal vessels of the pituitary stalk; hence, they are carried in the bloodstream.

Posterior Pituitary

The *posterior* pituitary gland stores and releases vasopressin and oxytocin believed to be synthesized in the ganglionic cells of the hypothalamus. Vasopressin regulates reabsorption of water by the kidneys. The major physiologic action of vasopressin is antidiuresis, hence its designation as antidiuretic hormone (ADH). The posterior pituitary secretes vasopressin when body fluids must be conserved. For example, when severe vomiting and diarrhea occurs with little to no fluid intake, vasopressin is released and water in the kidneys is reabsorbed into the circulation (conserved). This results in urine's becoming concentrated. In the absence of ADH, there is a failure to concentrate the urine despite an increased solute concentration of the plasma. This endocrine deficiency state is known as (neurogenic) diabetes insipidus. The clinical manifestation of diabetes insipidus is associated with polyuria and polydipsia, which usually begin abruptly. Synthetic vasopressin is provided as the drug desmopressin acetate (Octostim, DDAVP). This drug is used to treat diabetes insipidus and certain clotting disorders (such as hemophilia A and von Willebrand disease). It is available as a nasal solution. Oxytocin induces contractions in the gravid uterus and promotes postpartum lactation. It is supplied by injection or intranasally. These drugs are unlikely to be reported on the medical history, so a complete discussion is not included in this chapter.

Adrenal Hormones

The *adrenal glands* are located on the kidneys and are composed of a cortex and a medulla. The adrenal cortex secretes glucocorticoids (also called glucocorticosteroids) and mineralocorticoids. The synthesis and secretion of glucocorticoids are under the control of the adrenocorticotropic hormone (ACTH). Glucocorticoids have a variety of actions or drug effects. The main glucocorticoid hormone is cortisol. The renin–angiotensin pathway controls mineralocorticoid secretion. Mineralocorticoids regulate sodium retention in the distal convoluted tubule of the kidney. The main mineralocorticoid is aldosterone, which regulates salt and water balance. Of these hormones, glucocorticosteroids are the most commonly prescribed agents, so this discussion is limited to them.

Pituitary Gland

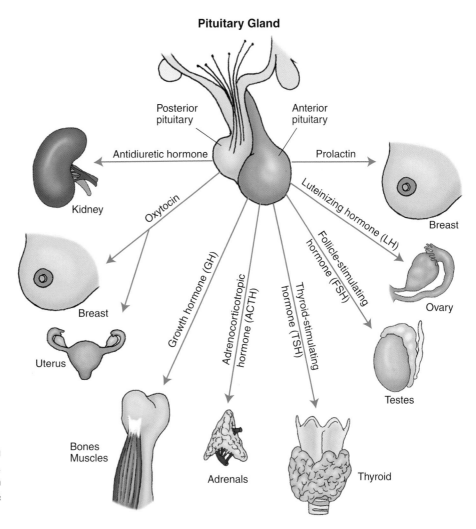

Figure 14-2 Hormones from Anterior Pituitary. (From Roach SS. *Introductory Clinical Pharmacology*. 7th ed. Baltimore: Lippincott Williams & Wilkins; 2004 with permission.)

Cortisol

Cortisol exerts its effect on target tissues by regulating cell metabolism. It stimulates peripheral fat and protein catabolism to serve as substrates for the hepatic production of glucose. Cortisol induces pronounced anti-inflammatory and immunomodulatory effects by preventing leukocyte migration from the circulation into the extravascular space, reducing the accumulation of monocytes and granulocytes at inflammatory sites, and suppressing the production of numerous cytokines and other proinflammatory mediators. Cortisol also acts in a permissive role to allow other hormones, such as catecholamines and angiotensin II, to modulate cardiac contractility, vascular tone, and blood pressure. Finally, cortisol provides negative feedback to the hypothalamus and the anterior pituitary in regulating corticotropin-releasing hormone (CRH) and ACTH secretion.

Glucocorticosteroids

Glucocorticosteroids regulate cell metabolism, promote gluconeogenesis (carbohydrate metabolism), and have pronounced anti-inflammatory and immunomodulatory effects. It is likely the dental hygienist will see one of these products

listed on a health history drug section, because several formulations are among the 200 most commonly prescribed drugs (Box 14-2). Topical formulations of steroids are often used for the treatment of oral inflammatory lesions (denture sores, aphthous ulcers, and so forth) to reduce signs and symptoms of inflammation. However, because corticosteroids have pronounced anti-inflammatory and immunomodulatory effects, they should never be used for the treatment of mucocutaneous viral infections. An exception to this rule may be the coadministration of prednisone and an antiviral agent in the management of severe herpes (varicella) zoster infections.

Mechanism of Action

Glucocorticoids, also referred to as *steroids*, decrease inflammation by suppressing the migration of polymorphonuclear leukocytes and reducing capillary permeability. They also suppress the immune system by reducing activity of the lymphoid cells. These actions make them ideal agents for conditions that involve inflammation. The downside, however, is that these actions may result in delayed wound healing and possible infection.

BOX 14-2. Glucocorticosteroids in the Top 200

- Prednisone (Deltasone)
- Methylprednisolone (Methylprednisolone)
- Triamcinolone (Triamcinolone acetonide, Nasacort AQ)
- Mometasone (Nasonex)
- Fluticasone (Flonase)
- Fluticasone propionate (Flovent)
- Budesonide (Rhinocort Aqua)

Indications

Addison Disease

Systemic glucocorticoids are prescribed when endogenous cortisol hyposecretion develops, a condition called adrenocortical insufficiency, or *Addison disease*. Affected patients have very low to undetectable levels of aldosterone and cortisol in blood, and cortisol levels do not increase in response to stress and ACTH. Cortisol deficiency is manifested by lethargy, anorexia, nausea, weight loss, **hypoglycemia**, and the loss of sodium, which leads to decreased cardiac output with hypotension, hyperkalemia, cardiac arrhythmias, and muscular weakness. There may be patchy brown to blackish pigmentation of the skin, buccal mucosa, and tongue, and less frequently of the lips and gingivae. The treatment of Addison disease includes the daily administration of an oral glucocorticoid and a mineralocorticoid. When stressful events are anticipated, patients may need to supplement daily doses to accommodate for additional cortisol needs. In the past some authors have suggested using the "Rule of Twos" (a guideline based on situations in which 20 mg of hydrocortisone or equivalent were taken for more than 2 weeks within the past 2 years) to identify the patient at risk for adrenal crisis. This rule is no longer used, because available evidence no longer supports routine recommendations for corticosteroid supplementation for all dental procedures. Adrenal crisis is an extremely rare event in dentistry, and most routine dental procedures can be performed without glucocorticoid supplementation.[1] This recommendation against giving supplemental steroids also takes into consideration potential risks associated with the administration of additional glucocorticosteroids, such as fluid retention, hypertension, hyperglycemia, increased risk of infection, impaired wound healing, GI bleeding, and psychiatric disturbances.

Inflammatory Conditions

Glucocorticosteroids (also called corticosteroids or steroids) are prescribed for their anti-inflammatory effects in a variety of medical conditions that stimulate inflammation, including allergic rhinitis, asthma, and autoimmune diseases (systemic lupus erythematosus, rheumatoid arthritis, and others). *Prednisone* is the most common corticosteroid used for oral administration. Corticosteroids are used for this effect in immunosuppressive therapy, such as in combination with the va-riety of medications to prevent rejection of organ transplants. Spinal cord injury is often treated with prednisone. Corticosteroids may be prescribed as part of lymphocytic leukemia chemotherapy. Large doses are sometimes administered to manage symptoms of various conditions and are referred to as **supraphysiologic** doses. When supraphysiologic doses are used for prolonged periods of time, Cushing syndrome may develop. Depending on the condition being treated, corticosteroids in medicine generally are administered at target doses equal to or greater than the normal daily output of cortisol. Secretory rates of ACTH and cortisol are high in the early morning, but low in the late evening, ranging from a high of ~20 μg/dL an hour before rising in the morning and a low of ~5 μg/dL around midnight; therefore, measurement of blood cortisol is meaningful only when expressed in terms of the time in the cycle at which the measurements are made.[2] Levels of physiologic cortisol secretion are often described as 15 to 20 mg/day.[2] Examples include hydrocortisone, which has the equivalent anti-inflammatory potency of cortisol, usually given at 20 mg/day; prednisone and prednisolone, which have four times the anti-inflammatory potency of cortisol, usually given at 5 mg/day; and dexamethasone, which has 25 times the anti-inflammatory potency of cortisol, given at 0.75 mg/day.[1] When an oral glucocorticoid, such as methylprednisolone (Medrol), is prescribed, the administration includes a stepped-down approach whereby the total daily dose of the drug is reduced incrementally over several days. This allows for the adrenal gland to recover from suppression and regain its functional capacity by the time the dose-pack is completed.

Dental Uses

Glucocorticoids are frequently used in the management of a variety of oral conditions involving inflammation. Topical steroid elixirs, creams, or gels are used for the treatment of autoimmune oral conditions (aphthous stomatitis, lichen planus, erythema multiforme, cicatricial pemphigoid), but, as noted earlier, not for the management of viral infections. These agents alter the immune response and reduce inflammation and, consequently, pain. Steroids (e.g., Triamcinolone hexacetonide, intra-articular, 20 mg/mL suspension) may be injected into the temporomandibular joint (TMJ) space to relieve acute inflammation. In oral maxillofacial procedures, systemic glucocorticoids (e.g., Methylprednisolone sodium succinate, intramuscular (IM) or intravenous (IV), 40 mg/mL) are often used to reduce perioperative vascular congestion and edema (Box 14-3).

In all cases, topical agents or short-term burst therapy with systemic agents are most often used, so the risk of cortisol suppression is negligible, and aldosterone suppression does not occur. Topical products include such agents as triamcinolone (Kenalog), clobetasol (Temovate), and fluocinonide (Lidex). They are usually applied three to four times per day after meals and at bedtime. The application procedure includes application of small amounts on the lesion using a cotton-tipped applicator. These agents are sometimes formulated with non-water-soluble products with **adsorptive** qualities (gelatin, pectin, methylcellulose) to keep the active ingredient localized to the area of concern (e.g., Kenalog in Orabase).

> BOX 14-3. Dental Uses of Glucocorticoids
>
> • Topical: Mucosal injury, aphthous ulcers, ulcerations from lichen planus, erythema multiforme, pemphigus, pemphigoid
> • Injection: TMJ pain and swelling
> • Oral: Perioperative and postoperative vascular congestion, edema

Doseforms

Glucocorticoids are supplied as tablets, elixirs, sprays, pastes, creams, or gels. Oral doseforms (tablets) have greater potential to produce ADEs. Topical and inhalational doseforms can result in minor ADEs because less of the steroid is absorbed into the circulation.

Adverse Drug Effects

Potential ADEs associated with oral glucocorticoid therapy that can affect dental hygiene management include masked symptoms of infection, candidiasis, nervousness, **hyperglycemia**, vision disturbances, edema, hypertension, peptic ulceration, osteoporosis, and Cushing syndrome. Most cases of Cushing syndrome develop as a consequence of the chronic administration of supraphysiologic doses of glucocorticoid for their anti-inflammatory and immunomodulatory effects. Topically administered agents rarely result in these effects. When high doses of oral glucocorticoids are taken for a long duration, signs and symptoms of Cushing syndrome may be observed, such as a round face (moon face), fat distribution on the shoulders (buffalo hump), and truncal obesity. Increased blood sugar over a prolonged time may predispose to signs of diabetes mellitus (DM). The most likely side effects impacting dental hygiene practice are related to the masking of signs of infection and opportunistic infections, such as candidiasis. For patients who report using a steroid spray for respiratory disease, oral tissues should be monitored for evidence of yeast infection, and positive findings should be reported to the dentist. Rinsing the mouth following use of a steroid spray is recommended to reduce the risk for candidiasis. Topical intraoral steroid gels are used for short-term therapy and are unlikely to result in yeast infection. Periodontal health is assessed using probe-depth information because the clinical appearance is not reliable due to the possibility of masked infection.

Potential Drug–Drug Interactions in the Dental Setting

Although dental hygienists do not prescribe drugs, they need to anticipate potential drug interactions with systemic therapeutic agents prescribed by the dentist. Potential drug–drug interactions and the clinical relevance include

• possible methylprednisolone toxicity when macrolide antibiotics are taken (avoid concurrent use);

• decreased metronidazole effect when corticosteroids are taken concurrently (avoid concurrent use);
• increased risk of peptic ulcers with cyclooxygenase-1 (COX-1) inhibitors (monitor clinical status).

Potential Medical Emergencies

The most significant acute adverse outcome of adrenal insufficiency (AI) is an Addisonian crisis (acute adrenal insufficiency). This event is most likely to develop in stressful surgical procedures when Addison disease is reported. A search of the literature discovered only four purported cases of dental treatment-related adrenal crises published between 1972 and 1999.[1] In reviewing the reports, the authors noted that in three cases the crises were poorly defined, and other conditions that may have been responsible for the crises (e.g., hypovolemia, hemorrhage, infection, or hypoglycemia) were not excluded. The fourth case appeared to document a hypotensive–hypoglycemic event. Hypertensive syndrome is a more likely emergency situation when systemic steroids are taken. Follow-up questioning involving the individual's ability to respond to stressful situations, as well as the history of blood pressure fluctuations, should be investigated, and blood pressure should be monitored during each appointment. This potential emergency situation is mostly related to stressful dental treatment, such as oral surgery. However, in the individual with dental phobia, even dental hygiene procedures may provoke extreme stress and blood pressure fluctuations.

Clinical Considerations

When investigating ADEs during the patient interview, the clinician will make extraoral observations, examine for candidiasis, correlate probe depths with the clinical appearance of periodontal tissues, and examine bone anatomy in radiographs. Vital signs should be monitored at each dental appointment, with attention paid to blood pressure values. When values are $\geq 180/110$, treatment should be delayed and the patient should be referred for medical evaluation. Questioning related to other side effects of steroids may provide additional relevant information. Examples include vision disturbances, which may influence oral hygiene demonstrations and require questioning to assure that demonstrated procedures can be seen and performed. As well, peptic ulcers can develop following long-term oral steroid therapy, resulting in gastric hemorrhages and/or intestinal perforation. In this situation, COX-1 inhibitors (ibuprofen, naproxen) should not be recommended for dental pain. Osteoporosis may influence dental procedures (tooth extraction), but it has little relevance to dental hygiene procedures. Rinsing following use of inhaled steroid formulations should be recommended to reduce the risk of candidiasis (Color Plate 17). These are summarized in Table 14-1.

■ **Self-Study Review**

1. List hormones secreted by the anterior portion of the pituitary gland and the organs they supply. How are they administered exogenously, and why?

Table 14-1	Clinical Considerations for Systemic Corticosteroid Administration

ADE	Clinical Procedure
Chronic, high dosing	Extraoral exam
Masked infection	Comprehensive periodontal assessment
Opportunistic infection	Intraoral exam for candidiasis
Hypertension	Monitor blood pressure
Miscellaneous	Assess vision capabilities Acetaminophen for postop analgesia If oral steroid spray is used, recommend rinsing after use

2. Explain the action of *vasopressin* and name the deficiency state. What is the synthetic drug for vasopressin? How is it administered, and why?
3. List hormones secreted by the adrenal cortex. Which glucocorticoid is the most commonly prescribed?
4. Describe the various actions of glucocorticoids.
5. List examples of steroid agents and their uses in medicine and oral health care.
6. Are supplemental steroids needed for dental hygiene procedures when the patient takes supraphysiologic doses of a steroid?
7. Compare the potency of prednisone and dexamethasone with that of cortisol; list their usual doses per day.
8. List topical corticosteroids used in dentistry and describe the application instructions.
9. Why is Orabase added to triamcinolone paste?
10. Which steroid doseforms are most likely to produce ADEs?
11. Describe the oral health recommendation when steroid sprays are used.
12. Describe clinical considerations for the patient who takes a glucocorticosteroid.

Hormones of Reproduction

The hypothalamic luteinizing hormone (LH) releasing factor stimulates the release of both LH and follicle-stimulating hormone (FSH) from the anterior pituitary gland. LH induces development of ovarian follicles, causes ovulation, brings forth corpus luteum formation, and forms ovarian steroids in females and androgen in males. FSH induces development of ovarian follicles, promotes formation of ovarian steroids, and maintains spermatogenesis. The activities of LH and FSH are in turn regulated by feedback inhibition. Estrogens and progesterones are drugs taken, when needed, for supplementation. Oral contraceptives contain various hormones. Some contain estrogen only, some contain progesterone only, and some contraceptives are combinations of both estrogens and progesterones. These are the drugs most likely to be reported on the health history and, for that reason, are discussed in this chapter.

Estrogens

Estrogen is synthesized mainly in the ovaries, the placenta, and the adrenal glands. A minute amount is synthesized in

---

BOX 14-4. Estrogens in the Top 200

Relief of Menopausal Symptoms
- Conjugated estrogens (Premarin, Menest, Cenestin, Enjuvia)
- Estradiol (Climara, Estrace, Vivelle, EvaMist, and others)
- Conjugated estrogens/medroxyprogesterone (Prempro)

Oral Contraception Combination Products
- Estradiol/medroxyprogesterone (Lunelle)
- Norethindrone/ethinyl estradiol (Ortho-Novum, Microgestin Fe, Necon)
- Norgestimate/ethinyl estradiol (Ortho Tri-Cyclen, Ortho-Cyclen)
- Levonorgestrel/ethinyl estradiol (Trivora-28, Aviana)
- Desogestrel/ethinyl estradiol (Apri)

---

the testes and from stored fat deposits. During menopause, fat is the main source of estrogen in women, but this does not compensate for the loss of follicular estrogen. Estrogen dramatically influences the growth and development of female reproductive organs by inducing the synthesis of specific proteins via intracellular receptors. As menopause approaches, the secretion of estrogen diminishes, and supplemental hormones may be prescribed to relieve hot flashes or other symptoms associated with diminished estrogen and progesterones. Products for these indications are among the top-200-most-prescribed drugs (Box 14-4). Some are used to treat symptoms associated with menopause, and others are combined with progestins and used for oral contraception. Doseforms include tablets, patches, injections, and creams.

Mechanism of Action

Estrogens inhibit the release of gonadotropin-releasing hormones from the hypothalamus and reduce the release of FSH and LH from the pituitary. It is this action that permits the use of estrogen in contraception. Estrogen reduces thinning of mucosal tissues of the vaginal area and prevents vasomotor symptoms (hot flashes). Estrogen inhibits osteoclastic action in bone and reduces bone loss associated with osteoporosis.

Therapeutic Indications

The effects of estrogen allow its use in the resolution of symptoms associated with menopause, removal of the ovaries, or any condition that reduces secretion of estrogen. It is prescribed prophylactically to reduce fertility in women and to reduce bone loss associated with osteoporosis in both men and women. Box 14-5 illustrates conditions for which estrogen is prescribed therapeutically.

Oral Contraceptives

Oral contraceptives may involve both estrogen and progesterone. They suppress ovulation by inhibiting feedback at the

> **BOX 14-5.** Therapeutic Indications for Estrogen
>
> - Atrophic vaginitis
> - Hypogonadism
> - Primary ovarian failure
> - Menopausal symptoms
> - Prostatic carcinoma
> - Prevention of osteoporosis

hypothalamus and the anterior pituitary. In addition, they produce cervical mucosal thickening and impede implantation of the fertilized ovum should fertilization take place. Oral contraceptives are taken for 21 days of a 28-day cycle. In some products, placebos or iron pills are taken the remaining 7 days to maintain a regimen of one pill per day. Monophasic preparations have a fixed dose of progestin through the cycle. Biphasic preparations have low-dose progestin for 10 days, followed by a higher dose for 11 days. In triphasic preparations, the concentration of progestin begins low and then increases for 7 days through the 21-day cycle. Triphasic formulations more closely resemble normal physiologic concentrations of progestin and appear to be as effective as monophasic or biphasic preparations. A recent study found that oral contraceptive users had poorer periodontal health than nonusers.[3] Those women who used oral contraceptives had deeper probing depths than nonusers and more severe attachment loss.

Indications

Oral contraceptive products are used for a variety of reasons, including prevention of pregnancy (including emergency contraception), prevention of acne (Ortho Tri-Cyclen), and treatment of hypermenorrhea, endometriosis, and female hypogonadism.

Pharmacokinetics

Estrogens are well absorbed after oral administration but tend to be extensively metabolized by the liver during first pass. Active metabolites that survive the first-pass effect include glucuronide and sulfide conjugates of estradiol, estrone, and estriol. They are eliminated by the kidneys.

Adverse Drug Effects

Potential ADEs associated with estrogen therapy that can affect dental hygiene management include candidiasis, peripheral edema, hypertension, thromboembolism, stroke, and myocardial infarction (MI). Smoking tobacco increases the risk for formation of intravascular blood clots, leading to an increased risk for thromboembolism, stroke, and MI.

Potential Medical Emergencies

Emergency situations include hypertensive syndrome and conditions involving intravascular blood clot formation (angina pectoris, MI, stroke). Questioning should include determination of a previous history of these conditions, and blood pressure values should be analyzed for normal limits.

Potential Drug–Drug Interactions in the Dental Setting

There are no documented interactions between estrogen and drugs used in the dental office. However, when oral contraceptives are taken, there are potential drug interactions that should be communicated to the patient when acetaminophen or antibiotics are prescribed by the dentist. These include

- possible decreased analgesic effect of acetaminophen when oral contraceptives are taken (mechanism unclear);
- decreased contraceptive effect with fluconazole, ketoconazole, systemic tetracyclines (not locally applied products), cephalosporins, macrolides, metronidazole, and penicillins (mechanism unknown);
- variable psychomotor impairment with single doses of oral diazepam, and possibly other benzodiazepines, when oral contraceptives are taken (mechanism unclear).

Clinical Considerations

ADEs associated with estrogen may lead to clinical management issues. Hypertension is associated with oral contraceptive use, more so than with estrogen for menopause. However, blood pressure should be monitored when estrogen is taken (for any reason) to determine if hypertension has developed. If estrogen has been taken for months to years and blood pressure is within normal limits (WNL), this means that the possible side effect is not expressed in the patient. After determining a normal blood pressure limit, dental management includes monitoring blood pressure annually, according to the policy of the American Dental Association (ADA).[4] When values are above normal limits for three different appointments, the patient should be referred to the prescribing physician for evaluation. Females who smoke should be encouraged to enroll in a smoking cessation program and informed of the increased risk of thromboembolytic disease.

Antibacterial Agents and Oral Contraceptives

There are no pharmacokinetic data at this time to support the contention that antibacterial agents reduce the efficacy of oral contraceptives, except for rifampin, an antituberculin drug. In a recent decision, the United States District Court for the Northern District of California also concluded, "scientific evidence regarding the alleged interaction between antibacterial agents and oral contraceptives did not satisfy the '*Daubert* standard' of causality."[5] However, according to the American Medical Association (AMA), such interactions cannot be completely discounted. The AMA recommends that women be informed of the possibility of such interactions (see "Web Resources," at the end of the chapter). Similarly, the ADA Council on Scientific Affairs recommends that patients be advised of the potential risk, that patients consider alternative contraception during periods of antibacterial chemotherapy, and that patients be advised of the importance of compliance with their oral contraceptive regimen.[6]

| Table 14-2 | Drugs Used to Treat Hypothyroidism | | |

Drug	Mechanism of Action	Indication	ADEs
Levothyroxine (Levoxyl, Levothroid, Synthroid)	T_4 and T_3 replacement (T_4 is converted to T_3 in plasma)	Drug of choice	No ADEs at therapeutic dosages, but hyperthyroidism at overdose
Liothyronine (Cytomel, Triostat)	T_3 replacement	Used when levothyroxine is not absorbed adequately	
Liotrix (Thyrolar)	T_4 and T_3 replacement	Used when the conversion of levothyroxine from T_4 to T_3 is abnormal	

Patients may be under treatment for cancer, so the indication for taking estrogen should be investigated. Consider dental implications for the specific indication.

■ Self-Study Review

13. List the actions of estrogen in the body.
14. List ADEs associated with estrogen use and their relationship to smoking tobacco.
15. Describe clinical considerations for the dental hygiene treatment plan when estrogen products are reported by the patient.

THYROID HORMONES

The thyroid gland is located in the neck in front of the trachea. This gland manufactures and secretes two hormones, thyroxine and tri-iodothyronine. Iodine is essential for the manufacture of both of these hormones. Patients with thyroid dysfunction may be characterized as **euthyroid**, hypothyroid, and hyperthyroid to reflect normal, inadequate, and excessive circulating hormone levels, respectively. Some thyroid disorders manifest a disorder whereby initial glandular hypersecretion evolves into a state of hyposecretion. Many of the more commonly encountered thyroid disorders (Graves disease, Hashimoto thyroiditis, postpartum thyroid dysfunction, and painless sporadic thyroiditis) represent autoimmune phenomena. Myxedema is a severe hypothyroidism manifested by lethargy, apathy, memory impairment, emotional changes, cold intolerance, and other signs and symptoms. The activity of the thyroid gland is regulated by thyroid-stimulating hormones (TSH). TSH is produced in the anterior pituitary gland. When the level of circulating thyroid hormones decreases, the anterior pituitary secretes TSH, which then activates cells of the thyroid to release stored thyroid hormones. Circulating concentrations of tri-iodothyronine (T_3) and thyroxine (T_4) are maintained at physiologic levels by the interaction of the secretions of the hypothalamus, pituitary, and thyroid glands. The thyroid hormones are involved in the regulation of growth and development, thermoregulation, and the metabolism of carbohydrates, proteins, and lipids. The exact mechanisms by which thyroid hormones exert their influence on body or-gans and tissues are not well understood. They are used as hormone replacement therapy in hypothyroidism.

Thyroid Drugs in the Top 200

- Levothyroxine (Synthroid, Levoxyl, Levothroid)

Table 14-2 illustrates the variety of drugs used to manage hypothyroidism. There are no ADEs at therapeutic doses. ADEs generally are a result of excessive hormone dose levels.

Mechanism of Action

Thyroid hormones exert their metabolic effects by promoting oxygen consumption by tissues and increasing the basal metabolic rate and metabolism of carbohydrates, lipids, and proteins. Thyroid hormones act synergistically with epinephrine to stimulate **glycogenolysis** (resulting in hyperglycemia) and enhance tissue sensitivity to catecholamines.

Indications

Thyroid hormones are prescribed to control the effects of hypothyroidism and return the individual to a euthyroid state. They are also used in the treatment or prevention of various types of euthyroid goiters (enlarged thyroid gland) and in the management of thyroid cancer.

Adverse Drug Effects

Nervousness, palpitations, dysrhythmias, hypertension, angina, and shortness of breath are ADEs that could affect the dental hygiene treatment plan. It is interesting to note that these ADEs reflect increased hormone doses that cause a hyperthyroid condition. Hormone therapy at excessive doses is generally responsible. Cardiovascular side effects (hypertension, increased pulse rate) can be determined by monitoring vital signs and qualities. Other possible side effects can be discovered through the patient interview.

Potential Drug–Drug Interactions in the Dental Setting

A review of the literature reveals no ADEs associated with vasoconstrictors in patients with hypothyroidism without significant cardiovascular disease (CVD).[7] Well-controlled, medically supervised patients on thyroid replacement and patients with mild to moderate symptoms of hypothyroidism may safely undergo routine dental care under local anesthesia. Epinephrine interaction with *increased levels* of thyroid hormones is possible, however. Because dental hygienists can administer local anesthetics in many states, they should administer local anesthetic agents containing vasoconstrictors with caution, using an aspirating technique and low concentrations of vasoconstrictor (1:100,000 or 1:200,000). Low concentrations of vasoconstrictor can be defined as using no more than two cartridges of 1:100,000 or four cartridges of 1:200,000. Patients with *uncontrolled* hypothyroidism are hyperreactive to central nervous system (CNS) depressants (opioid analgesics, anxiolytic agents), which should be administered judiciously.

Antithyroid Hormones

Hyperthyroidism

Hyperthyroidism is a clinical disease state produced by the effect of excessive thyroid hormone on peripheral tissues. Diffuse toxic goiter, toxic multinodular goiter, toxic uninodular goiter, lymphocytic thyroiditis, and thyrotoxicosis secondary to excessive intake of thyroid hormone (overdose) given for thyroid suppression or replacement therapy account for 98% to 99% of all cases of hyperthyroidism. The severity of the illness caused by thyrotoxicosis is related to the severity and duration of the hormone excess, the age of the patient, and the presence or absence of other disease. Therapeutic strategies include reducing the dose of thyroid hormone (if patient is being treated for hypothyroidism) or controlling hyperthyroidism with antithyroid drugs for 1 year, followed by partial resection of the thyroid gland if needed to bring a hyperactive thyroid to the euthyroid state. Antithyroid drugs are the cornerstones in the management of hyperthyroidism (Table 14-3). They may be used as primary treatment for hyperthyroidism or as preparative therapy before surgery or radioiodine therapy. Antithyroid drugs are usually stopped or tapered after 12 to 18 months of therapy. Lifelong follow-up is required for patients in remission, because spontaneous hypothyroidism may develop decades later. Beta-adrenergic antagonists may be used to suppress some of the symptoms of hyperthyroidism, such as tremor, anxiety, and tachycardia.

Propylthiouracil (PTU), methimazole (Tapazole), and carbimazole exert their effects by inhibiting iodide and the synthesis of thyroid hormones. Iodides (potassium iodide, Lugol solution containing 5% iodine and 10% potassium iodide) exert their beneficial effects by inhibiting the release of thyroid hormones and decreasing the size and vascularity of the thyroid gland, hence preparing the patient for surgery. Radioactive iodine, given orally in the treatment of older patients with thyrotoxicosis, accumulates in the storage follicles and emits beta rays with a half-life of 5 days. The iodides and radioactive iodine are different compounds.

Potential Medical Emergencies

Hypertensive crisis, angina pectoris, and cardiac arrhythmia (thyroid storm) leading to acute coronary syndrome are potential emergencies for the individual taking excessive doses of thyroid hormones or when hyperthyroidism is uncontrolled. Thyroid storm is the extreme manifestation of hyperthyroidism. It is characterized by an elevated temperature, tachycardia, and high blood pressure. Blood pressure $\geq 180/110$ mm Hg represents a hypertensive crisis. An "at-rest" pulse rate <60 or >100 beats/min in adults, if symptomatic (sweating, weakness, dyspnea, and/or chest pain), should be considered a cardiac risk in association with noncardiac procedures. Respiratory rates <10 (or >20) breaths/min may indicate respiratory distress.

Drug Interactions

Evidence reveals the cardiovascular responses of thyroid hormones to epinephrine or norepinephrine are not significantly altered in most patients with controlled hyperthyroidism.[7] In most cases, careful administration of small doses of vasoconstrictors coupled with monitoring of vital signs will result in little to no risk for a cardiac-related emergency. However, the use of a local anesthetic agent containing a vasoconstrictor in patients with high concentrations of T_4 and T_3 (uncontrolled disease) is an area of concern. Thyroid hormones appear to act synergistically with epinephrine by increasing tissue sensitivity to catecholamines and by possibly up-regulating adrenergic receptors. An additional problem associated with the use of local anesthetic agents containing epinephrine is related to the management of cardiovascular symptoms from hyperthyroidism with a nonselective beta-adrenergic antagonist to reduce the heart rate and cardiac workload. However, these concerns must be balanced against the value of a vasoconstrictor in inducing profound local anesthesia, which is essential

Table 14-3	Drugs Used to Treat Hyperthyroidism		
Drug	**Mechanism of Action**	**Indication**	**ADEs**
Methimazole (Tapazole)	Inhibits the transformation of inorganic iodine to organic iodine	Long-term thyroxin suppression or in preparation for surgery or ^{131}I therapy	Agranulocytosis, hepatotoxicity, urticarial or macular reactions, arthralgia, sialadenitis (rarely) with methimazole
Propylthiouracil	Inhibits the transformation of inorganic iodine to organic iodine and blocks the conversion of T_4 to T_3	Same as above	Same as above
Iodine or iodide	Short-term inhibition of thyroxin release	Adjunctive therapy to the drugs above and in preparation for surgery	None

Table 14-4	Management of a Patient Taking Thyroid Hormones
Hypothyroid Drug	**Hyperthyroid Antithyroid Drug**
• Monitor vital signs for normal limits. • Question about occurrence of side effects and adjust procedures as needed. • Determine functional capacity: If it is ≥4 METs, dental hygiene procedures can be performed; if it is <4 METs, delay treatment until functional capacity is improved to the 4-MET level. • Observe for signs of excessive thyroid hormone. • Use vasoconstrictor in low concentrations if evidence of overdose is noted.	• Monitor vital signs for normal limits. • Observe for signs of excessive thyroid hormone. • Determine functional capacity: If it is ≥4 METs, dental hygiene procedures can be performed; if it is <4 METs, delay treatment until functional capacity is improved to the 4-MET level. • If blood pressure is ≥180/110, refer for medical evaluation and reschedule the appointment. • Question about occurrence of side effects and adjust procedures as needed. • Use vasoconstrictor in low concentrations (1:100,000 or 1:200,000) with aspirating technique.

in reducing the physiologic stress associated with pain. For the patient with overt evidence of uncontrolled hyperthyroidism, the use of vasoconstrictors in local anesthesia should be avoided. For all other scenarios, the cautious use of vasoconstrictors based on the patient's functional capacity should be considered. For those patients whose functional capacity is ≥4 **metabolic equivalent** functions (METs), 4.5 mL of a local anesthetic agent with epinephrine 1:100,000 (or equivalent) can be administered safely (Chapter 6).[8] Four METs is approximately equivalent to the workload produced by climbing a flight of stairs, walking 4.8 km/hour, doing light yard work (raking leaves, weeding, or pushing a power mower), painting, or doing light carpentry work. Furthermore, combination analgesics containing acetylsalicylic acid (ASA) are contraindicated in patients with hyperthyroidism, because ASA interferes with the protein binding of T_4 and T_3 (increasing their free form) and leads to thyrotoxicosis.

Clinical Considerations

When treating patients with thyroid dysfunction in the oral health care setting, the goals are to develop and implement timely preventive and therapeutic strategies compatible with the patient's physical and emotional ability to undergo and respond to dental care. When thyroid disease is controlled, treatment risks are low. Uncontrolled hyperthyroidism represents the greatest risk for an emergency during dental hygiene procedures.

Functional Capacity

Because T_4 and T_3 exert direct inotropic and chronotropic effects on cardiac muscle and appear to act synergistically with epinephrine, questions in the health history should also seek to determine the patient's functional capacity. *Functional capacity*, which is expressed in terms of metabolic equivalents (METs), is a measure of an individual's ability to perform a spectrum of common daily tasks (physical stressors).[8] Cardiac risk in association with noncardiac procedures is increased in patients unable to meet a 4-MET demand during normal daily activities. The **hemodynamic** effects of 4 METs are equivalent to those produced by 0.045 mg of epinephrine. The most important physical assessment to determine the cardiovascular effects of thyroid hormones is to monitor vital signs at each appointment. In the hypothyroid

individual, the dose of thyroid hormones is very low and must be regulated on a frequent basis, and the potential for overdose is high. Because of this risk, it is not unusual for signs of hyperthyroidism to develop. Older texts caution the dental professional to be suspicious of the individual with thyroid disease who complains of being very hot. This is a sign of hyperthyroidism or an overdose of thyroid hormone medication. Although there is no contraindication for using vasoconstrictors with hypothyroidism, because of the possibility of the dose-related initiation of *hyperthyroidism*, a vasoconstrictor in low concentrations (1:100,000 or 1:200,000) would be the safest formulation to use. Use of an aspirating syringe can prevent inadvertent injection into the circulation. Table 14-4 includes clinical considerations for management of the patient with thyroid disease.

■ Self-Study Review

16. When ADEs are noted in a hypothyroid individual, what is the most likely cause?
17. Identify the risk factors of an interaction between *vasoconstrictors* and *thyroid hormones*.
18. Identify drugs used to manage symptoms of hyperthyroidism.
19. What factors increase the risk for thyroid storm? What are the signs and symptoms?
20. Identify potential drug interactions in the hyperthyroid individual.
21. Discuss clinical considerations when treating a patient with thyroid disease.

PARATHYROID HORMONES

One recombinant human parathyroid hormone is used to treat postmenopausal women with osteoporosis who are a high risk for fracture and men with osteoporosis who need to increase bone mass. *Parathyroid hormone* is the primary regulator of calcium and phosphate metabolism in bones and kidneys and in intestinal calcium absorption. The drug teriparatide (Forteo) is administered as a subcutaneous injection once daily into the thigh or abdomen. It stimulates bone formation on trabecular and cortical bone surfaces. It is approved for 2 years of therapy, because the safety and efficacy has not been evaluated for more than 2 years. Teriparatide carries a warning of an increase in the incidence of osteosarcoma, a malignant bone tumor, in rats that was dependent on a high dose and long duration of therapy. It is in pregnancy category C and should not be used in lactating females. Forteo (teriparatide) is not the most common drug used to treat postmenopausal osteoporosis. The bisphosphonate (BIS) class of agents is the most commonly used and is discussed below.

Adverse Drug Effects

The most common side effects of teriparatide are dizziness and leg cramps. There are no interactions with drugs used in dentistry.

Clinical Implications

Osteoporosis is associated with a potential for periodontal attachment loss. Management should include a periodontal evaluation and taking care to avoid putting excessive pressure on the jaw, such as in tooth extraction. Dental hygiene procedures would be unlikely to incite a problem when this drug is taken.

Bisphosphonate Derivatives

Calcium is normally absorbed from and endogenously secreted into the gut. It is filtered by and reabsorbed from the kidneys, and it may be reabsorbed from or deposited into bones. These movements are under the overall regulation of the parathyroid hormone (which increases osteoclastic and osteoblastic activity), vitamin D and its metabolites (which increase osteoclastic activity), and calcitonin (which decreases osteoclastic activity). BIS lead to osteoclast apoptosis (cell death).

Drugs in the Top 200

Box 14-6 includes the various BIS available to prevent or treat osteoporosis and Paget disease of the bone, and those used in cancer chemotherapy. Two of the agents are in the top-200 drug list:

- alendronate (Fosamax)
- risedronate (Actonel)

The Food and Drug Administration (FDA) approved ibandronate (Boniva) in 2005 in an oral doseform to prevent or treat osteoporosis in postmenopausal women. In 2006, an IV doseform of ibandronate was approved to treat postmenopausal osteoporosis. The oral doseform was approved for once monthly dosing and was shown to be as efficacious as the once weekly doseform of alendronate. Ibandronate will likely be commonly prescribed due to its once-monthly use versus a daily or weekly administration. All three of the drugs above are nitrogen-containing BIS formulations. There are two other nitrogen-containing formulations administered by IV, pamidronate (Aredia) and zoledronate (Zometa, Reclast).

> **BOX 14-6.** Bisphosphonates and Indications
>
> **Treatment or prevention of osteoporosis**
> - alendronate (Fosamax)
> - risedronate (Actonel)
> - ibandronate (Boniva)
> - zoledronate (Reclast)
>
> **Treatment of Paget disease**
> - tiludronate (Skelid)
> - etidronate (Didronel)
> - zoledronate (Reclast)
>
> **Cancer chemotherapy**
> - zoledronate (Zometa)
> - pamidronate (Aredia)

Older non-nitrogen-containing formulations of oral BIS used mainly in the treatment of Paget disease of the bone include tiludronate (Skelid) and etidronate (Didronel).

Mechanism of Action

BIS inhibit bone resorption via a suppressive action on osteoclasts or on osteoclast precursors and indirectly decrease bone formation.

Indications

The oral doseforms of BIS are most often used to prevent or treat osteoporosis. They are indicated at a higher dose level for treatment of Paget disease of the bone. The FDA recently approved an IV formulation of the BIS zoledronate (Reclast) for a once-yearly administration to treat osteoporosis and Paget disease of the bone. The IV formulation of ibandronate (Boniva) used to treat osteoporosis is administered every 3 months. The IV formulations of zoledronate (Zometa) and pamidronate (Aredia) are commonly used as part of chemotherapy for malignancies in which bone loss develops or when hypercalcemia occurs.

Adverse Drug Effects

The most important ADE of these drugs for dental implications is osteonecrosis of the jaw (ONJ). This ADE has occurred most often when IV formulations of nitrogenous BIS have been given, but there are rare reports of ONJ with oral doseforms. The mechanism for ONJ from BIS is unclear but is related to the suppression of osteoclast action and increased **apoptosis**. At this time it is only associated with the nitrogen-containing formulations. It is impossible to identify what makes a patient at risk for necrosis of the bone, but many reports of the condition have occurred in those taking BIS medication following oral surgery or who have dental or periodontal infection.[9] Some individuals developed ONJ spontaneously, with no previous dental inflammation or dental treatment. The typical lesion develops as a desquamation of mucosa, revealing exposed bone in the jaw; pain and purulent exudate may be present. The condition can develop in either jaw, but the mandible is most often affected. The lingual area along the mylohyoid ridge is frequently affected. Gastroesophageal reflux disease and dysphagia are additional potential ADEs with BIS that may affect the dental hygiene treatment plan.

Clinical Considerations

The ADA has published a patient information sheet to be provided to all dental patients who have taken a BIS drug.[10] The ADA published recommendations of an expert panel for dental management of patients receiving oral BIS therapy.[11] It refers the dental practitioner to the management recommendations by the American Academy of Oral Medicine (AAOM).[9] The implications for the oral health education plan are explained in the next section of this chapter.

Additional clinical considerations include the effects of osteoporosis in dental hygiene management. Osteoporosis may render patients susceptible to pathologic fractures. The relationship of this to jaw pressure during instrumentation is unclear and may have no relationship at all.

Prevention of ONJ from Bisphosphonate Therapy

Dental hygienists play a role in the AAOM recommendations for individuals who have taken a BIS. These guidelines include recommendations for prevention, as well as recommendations for managing the necrotic lesion of the jaw. The dental hygienist is involved in patient information directed to prevention of ONJ. These preventive procedures are summarized in Table 14-5.

Before Taking a Bisphosphonate
The preventive regimen begins when the physician decides to prescribe a BIS.[12] The patient should be referred by the physician for a dental evaluation prior to taking the BIS. At the dental appointment, the ADA patient information sheet[10] should

be discussed with the patient, and consideration should be given to the rare, but possible development of ONJ. Instructions on the early signs of ONJ should be described so the patient may be able to recognize the condition should it develop. This is an essential component of the preventive program and one in which the dental hygienist can play a major role. Dental therapy to remove disease or inflammation (restorative therapy, periodontal therapy) should be provided before the drug is taken and the risk of developing ONJ increases. Extraction of teeth should be completed as soon as possible to allow for healing (2 to 3 months) prior to initiating BIS therapy. An evaluation of third-molar areas should be completed to determine if the teeth should be removed. Periodontal health should be evaluated and treated to remove inflammation and infection, and a recommendation should be made for periodic maintenance visits to reinforce the importance of plaque control and to examine the jaw areas for lesions. Plaque control education to prevent recurrence of periodontal inflammation should be provided. Prosthodontic appliances may not be appropriate for some patients, and any appliances should be evaluated for fit, stability, and occlusion, with adjustments made as needed.

While Taking a Bisphosphonate
When the health history includes taking a BIS, or when a malignancy is reported and follow-up questioning reveals a BIS was taken as part of cancer chemotherapy or treatment of Paget disease, the dental hygienist should discuss information from the ADA patient information handout with the individual. Signs and symptoms of ONJ should be explained, and the individual should be told to return to the dental office if they develop. A dental examination should involve a complete dental evaluation, including full series radiographs. The patient should be warned to maintain a regular maintenance schedule (3 to 6 months) to ensure dental disease does not develop in the bone surrounding the tooth. Endodontic therapy rather than tooth extraction is recommended for pulp disease.

Table 14-5 Prevention of Bisphosphonate-Associated Osteonecrosis of the Jaw	
Physician refers prior to initiating a BIS	• Discuss the ADA patient information sheet • Describe signs and symptoms of ONJ • Perform oral exam to identify disease or inflammation • Remove dental/periodontal disease • Place on 3- to 6-month maintenance schedule • Evaluate fit of removable and fixed appliances and third molars • Instruct in biofilm removal to prevent periodontal inflammation
Patient reports taking a BIS	• All of the above procedures • Many dentists and oral surgeons will not remove teeth • Endodontic therapy may be the safest procedure if pulpal inflammation is found

Source: Migliorati CA, Casiglia J, Epstein J, et al. Managing the care of patients with bisphosphonate-associated osteonecrosis. *J Am Dent Assoc.* 2005;136(12);1658–1668.

Potential Medical Emergencies

None are anticipated in a dental setting.

Potential Drug–Drug Interactions in the Dental Setting

None have been documented.

■ Self-Study Review

22. Identify the ADE associated with BIS medications.
23. Describe the role of the registered dental hygienist in providing oral health information when a BIS is reported or will be used in the future.

PANCREATIC HORMONES

Two pancreatic hormones, glucagon and insulin, are synthesized by pancreatic (alpha and beta) cells, respectively. Glucagon and insulin have opposing effects on circulating glucose levels. *Insulin* stimulates cellular glucose uptake and is a hypoglycemic agent. *Glucose* is an optional fuel for such tissues as muscle, fat, and liver because they can also use fatty acids and other substances to satisfy their energy needs. However, glucose is an essential fuel for the CNS. Impairment or destruction of pancreatic production of insulin leads to either type 1 or type 2 diabetes mellitus (DM). When sig-

nificant hyperglycemia is chronically present (blood sugar values >250 mm/dL), healing can be compromised.

Medical Management

The goals of therapy for the individual patient in the management of DM are to reduce fasting blood glucose to levels <120 mg/dL and Hb A1c levels (also referred to as A1C) to <6%.[13] These recommendations are based on evidence that improved glycemic control is associated with sustained decreased rates of retinopathy, nephropathy, and neuropathy and the potential of intensive glycemic control to reduce CVD.

Insulin and Oral Hypoglycemic Agents

Type 1 DM is characterized by an absolute deficiency of insulin; patients are treated with short-, intermediate-, and/or long-acting *injectable* insulin preparations and *inhaled* insulin. *Type 2* DM is due to a decreased release of insulin and/or decreased number of insulin receptors. Patients with type 2 DM are initially treated with an *orally administered* hypoglycemic agent, but they may progress to insulin dependency.

Insulins and Antidiabetic Drugs in the Top 200

The treatment of type 1 DM may include short-, intermediate-, or long-acting insulin preparations. The goal of insulin therapy is to provide adequate glucose control through each 24-hour period while minimizing the number of injections required to achieve control. Most regimens today combine short-acting insulin with an intermediate- or a long-acting agent. Table 14-6 identifies the antidiabetic drugs

Table 14-6 Drugs Used to Control Diabetes Mellitus

Antidiabetic Drugs	Classification	Clinical Consideration	Emergency Drug
Insulins Human insulin NPH (Humulin N) Human insulin 70/30 (Humulin 70/30) Insulin lispro (Humalog)	Hormone	Hypoglycemia is possible—ensure meal has been eaten following insulin injection Monitor control of disease—A1C ≤6 is goal Ultra-short-acting insulin, less risk for hypoglycemia	Glucose—tablet, liquid Monitor for recent history of hypoglycemia and management used Indicated for type 1 or type 2 DM
Oral antidiabetics Glyburide (Micronase) Glipizide (Glucotrol XL) Glimepiride (Amaryl)	Sulfonylurea	High risk for hypoglycemia Monitor control of disease—A1C ≤6 is goal	Glucose—tablet, liquid Monitor for recent history of hypoglycemia and management used
Metformin (Glucophage, Glucophage XR)	Biguanide	Hypoglycemia is uncommon, unless sulfonylurea is used	
Pioglitazone (Actos) Rosiglitazone (Avandia)	Thiazolidinedione	Hypoglycemia is uncommon, unless sulfonylurea is used	
Acarbose (Precose)	Alpha-glucosidase inhibitor	Hypoglycemia is uncommon, unless sulfonylurea is used	
Other agents Exenatide	Incretin mimetic	SC injection only, no risk for hypoglycemia unless used with sulfonylurea or insulin	
Glyburide/metformin (Glucovance)	Combination product	Monitor control of disease—A1C ≤6 is goal	

SC, subcutaneous.

(insulins and various oral agents) in the top-200 list and the classification of each. Inhaled insulin preparations were recently discontinued by the manufacturer. Clinical considerations for antidiabetic agents include consideration of the risk for ADEs, such as hypoglycemia, and monitoring for disease control. Hypoglycemia is most likely to occur when the insulin is at the peak effect. Patients should preferentially be treated in the morning, after having taken their normal insulin or oral hypoglycemic agent and after having eaten a normal breakfast. This timing of the appointment will place the patient in the oral health care setting before the peak activity of the therapeutic agents is reached (i.e., a time of high-glucose and low-insulin or oral hypoglycemic agent activity).

The Hb A1c lab test (A1C) that determines long-term control is usually completed at quarterly medical appointments. The goal is ≤6, according to the current guidelines on diabetes management.[13] Older drugs used less often for diabetes control are first-generation sulfonylureas (acetohexamide, chlorpropamide, tolazamide, or tolbutamide). Newer agents used less often include two agents in the meglitinide classification (repaglinide, nateglinide). Companies are providing combination products with second-generation sulfonylureas and metformin (glyburide/metformin, glipizide/metformin), with glitazones and metformin (rosiglitazone/metformin, pioglitazone/metformin), and with glitazones and sulfonylureas (rosiglitazone/glimepiride). A combination agent containing a sulfonylurea increases the risk for hypoglycemia. This increase is due to the hypoglycemic effects of the sulfonylurea.

Mechanism of Action

Insulin is a hormone secreted by the beta cells in the pancreas to stimulate cellular glucose uptake. Insulin binds to receptors on cell surfaces to allow glucose to leave the blood and enter the muscle or various other cell types. Oral antidiabetic agents have various actions, according to the type of drug. These include

- stimulating insulin release from pancreatic beta cells (sulfonylureas);
- reducing glucose output from the liver (biguanides);
- increasing sensitivity of peripheral target cells to insulin (thiazolidinediones).

Either insulin or the oral sulfonylurea agents are the most likely antidiabetic agents to cause hypoglycemia to develop. The risk is negligible with the other classes of antidiabetic drugs.

Indications

Insulin hormone is indicated for type 1 DM; type 2 DM is managed with either insulin, oral antidiabetic agents, or a combination of both. Often the form of DM can be determined by analyzing the drug used for blood sugar control.

Adverse Drug Effects

Headaches, heartburn, nausea, vomiting, hypoglycemia, and blood dyscrasias are possible with insulin and oral sulfonylurea agents, but each antidiabetic drug can have a differ-

ent ADE profile and should be investigated in a drug reference. Thiazolidinediones (pioglitazone [Actos], rosiglitazone [Avandia]) have been implicated as having a risk for increased cardiovascular events; however, a meta-analysis of randomized trials found that pioglitazone was associated with a significantly lower risk of heart attack, stroke, or death among those with type 2 DM who took the drug.[14] A risk for congestive heart failure requiring hospitalization was increased with pioglitazone therapy, although without an associated increase in mortality. As with any drug, questioning should attempt to determine if the patient has experienced any ADE that has a relationship to the oral health care appointment. Hypoglycemia is managed with a glucose source, and the patient at risk often carries a personal supply.

Pain Management

Treatment strategies should also include an effective postoperative pain management. Opioid-based analgesics effectively block not only pain, but, importantly, they tend to contribute to cardiovascular stability. A possible increased hypoglycemic effect with large doses of salicylates has been reported in patients on insulin, and increased hypoglycemia with large doses of salicylates has been reported in combination with chlorpropamide, a sulfonylurea. However, usual therapeutic doses of ASA have little effect. These potential drug–drug interactions are not an absolute contraindication to the use of an opioid/ASA formulation for pain management in the dental setting, but rather provide another indication to monitor blood glucose levels in the postoperative period. Because many patients with DM are taking ASA as primary or secondary therapy to prevent cardiovascular events, an opioid/ASA formulation is more appropriate than an opioid/ibuprofen formulation, which may interfere with the antiplatelet effect of ASA. While acetaminophen (APAP) has not been implicated in these drug–drug interactions, APAP is not an anti-inflammatory agent. Because pain of dental origin is predictably associated with inflammation, an opioid/APAP formulation should, in general, be considered a secondary therapeutic agent in the management of dental pain.

Potential Medical Emergencies

Hypoglycemia is the most common medical emergency in diabetes. Hyperglycemic crisis (diabetic coma) occurs rarely in the dental office, but in uncontrolled individuals, infection and stress can promote the development of diabetic coma.[15]

Potential Drug–Drug Interactions in the Dental Setting

Hypoglycemic coma has occurred when glipizide and fluconazole are taken together; therefore, the dentist should consider another antifungal agent (such as nystatin) for oral mycotic disease management. Epinephrine can raise blood glucose levels, but the small amount of epinephrine included in local anesthetic formulations will not appreciably raise blood glucose levels.

There are two drugs not prescribed by the dentist that can influence development of hypoglycemia. ACE inhibitors may increase the sensitivity of peripheral target cells to insulin and produce severe recurrent hypoglycemia in susceptible patients. β_1-adrenergic-receptor antagonists may mask signs and symptoms of hypoglycemia.

Clinical Considerations

There is a variety of drugs to manage DM, and the clinician should consider the type of DM as well as side effects of the specific drug therapy used. Oral health care providers can best judge glycemic control by assessing the results of the patient's self-monitored blood glucose level, performed on the day of the dental appointment, and the patient's most current A1C result.

Pharmacologic therapy may reveal individuals at increased risk for hypoglycemia. Individuals with type 1 DM are at increased risk because they take insulin; however, those with type 2 DM who take sulfonylureas are also at risk. When these drugs are taken, anticipate hypoglycemic symptoms: Weakness, dizziness, hunger, sweating, tachycardia, tremor, headaches, visual disturbances, impaired consciousness, and loss of concentration. Patients with hypoglycemia often have a history of taking the hypoglycemic drug and failing to eat a meal. This, in effect, produces an overdose of the medication because the dose is calculated on the assumption that food will be consumed. Question about hypoglycemic drug therapy and if a meal was consumed. Patients should be seen soon after breakfast for dental hygiene therapy when blood sugar levels are high. Drug interactions that predispose to hypoglycemia should be considered when signs of hypoglycemia are observed.

Individuals with DM often develop hypertension. For this reason, vital signs should be monitored at each appointment.

Prophylactic Antibacterial Agents

The reciprocal relationship between increased infection and poor glycemic control has led some to advocate the administration of antimicrobial prophylaxis prior to dental therapy, particularly in the poorly controlled diabetic patient. However, there are no studies directly supporting this recommendation. Any infection in the diabetic patient, including periodontal disease, must be managed promptly and aggressively. Most of these infections can be resolved satisfactorily through an approach that incorporates appropriate, early débridement (primary dental care) in conjunction with local anesthesia. There is no evidence that antibiotic therapy decreases the infection or increases healing. When a patient with DM presents with significant oral infection, the primary physician should be consulted promptly, because the patient's therapeutic antidiabetic regimen may have to be adjusted to ensure adequate glycemic control. In addition, the patient must be instructed to practice meticulous oral hygiene and should be recalled at regular intervals to monitor resolution of the infection and compliance with recommended preventive measures.

■ Self-Study Review

24. Identify goals of therapy in the management of DM.
25. Differentiate between the fasting blood sugar test and other tests to determine control of DM.

26. Identify antidiabetic drugs associated with hypoglycemia.
27. Describe the signs of hypoglycemia.
28. Describe clinical considerations when treating a patient with DM.

DENTAL HYGIENE APPLICATIONS

Endocrine diseases are generally chronic conditions that are not *cured* with drugs, but rather *managed* with drugs. The individual with an endocrine disease usually will take drugs to control symptoms and hormone irregularities for the lifetime. The dental hygienist must consider the effects of the disease, as well as the potential ADEs when planning treatment. When the cardiovascular system is affected by the disease, vital sign values may reveal significant information related to whether the appointment should proceed. Attention should be paid to potential emergency situations, and plans should be made to prevent the emergency or to manage the emergency quickly.

Patients Taking Oral Glucocorticosteroids

Dental hygiene management of patients who are taking oral glucocorticosteroids includes inquiring about the reason the steroid is being taken and considering the pathophysiology of the disease and its relationship to dental hygiene procedures (Box 14-7). ADEs can be identified by performing an extraoral examination (round face, fat distribution, edema), evaluating blood pressure values, and asking the patient about the presence of side effects. When blood pressure

---

BOX 14-7. Management of the Patient Who Is Taking or Has Taken Corticosteroids

- Consider indication and clinical effects
- Investigate drug effects, including side effects
- Monitor vital signs (blood pressure and pulse) for increased values (blood pressure $\geq 180/110$ should be referred for medical evaluation, and treatment should be delayed)
- Perform extraoral and oral exam for evidence of disease
- Ensure that vision is adequate for oral hygiene skill instruction
- Steroid spray user should be instructed to rinse mouth after use

When the Dentist Prescribes a Topical Steroid
- Patient instruction should include placing a small amount on a cotton-tipped applicator for application to the ulcer or lesion
- Instruct to notify the dentist if the area worsens and to stop using the drug

values are ≥180/110, treatment should be delayed and the patient should be referred for medical evaluation. Osteoporosis may influence dental procedures (tooth extraction), but it has little relevance to dental hygiene procedures. A multi-year study in healthy postmenopausal women revealed there was not a statistically significant correlation between clinical attachment level and bone mineral density.[16] Nervousness and vision loss can affect oral hygiene education. When steroid sprays are used, intraoral examination for opportunistic infection is important, and patient instruction should include a recommendation to rinse the mouth after the spray is used. Acetaminophen is appropriate when analgesia is anticipated.

Dentist-Prescribed Topical Steroids

The dental hygienist may be asked to instruct on the proper use of a steroid gel. Small amounts placed on the ulceration with a cotton-tipped applicator should be advised. The patient should be told to stop applying the agent and to notify the dentist if pain, itching, or ulceration develops in the area, because these are signs of allergy.

Patients Taking Thyroid Hormone or Antithyroid Drugs

Dental hygiene management includes questioning about the reason the drug is being taken and consideration of the pathophysiology of the disease and its relationship to dental hygiene procedure. These drugs include hormone replacement in hypothyroidism (levothyroxine [Synthroid]) or drugs to suppress the function of the thyroid in hyperthyroid disease. Because thyroid hormone dose level needs can fluctuate, blood pressure and pulse values may be an indication of overdose. Hypothyroidism is associated with hypotension, and hyperthyroidism results in hypertension and increased pulse rates. Side effects of thyroid hormone may mimic excess thyroid hormone levels. This requires that ADEs be investigated. The functional capacity of the individual needs to be assessed; the patient should be able to complete daily activities equal to 4 METs, or the risk for a cardiovascular event is raised. Thyroid storm is a potential medical emergency of excess thyroid hormone levels and is characterized by excessive blood pressure and body temperature. If vital sign values are elevated (≥180/110), the patient should be referred for medical evaluation. Table 14-4 summarizes dental hygiene management procedures for the individual with thyroid disease.

Patients Taking Bisphosphonates

When a patient has been given a prescription by a medical provider, referral for a dental examination is recommended. Generally the patient will report to the dentist and say, "My physician is prescribing (Fosamax, Actonel, Boniva) for me and told me to see my dentist before I start taking the drug." The dental professional should provide the ADA patient information sheet for patients taking BIS and explain each item.[10] Dental pathology should be treated, and the importance of semiannual dental visits in identifying dental dis-

---

BOX 14-8. Dental Hygiene Management of the Patient Who Is Taking or Has Taken a Bisphosphonate Drug

- Provide and explain the ADA patient information sheet
- Examine for evidence of dental disease or areas likely to be chronically irritated
- Recommend treatment of existing dental disease
- Place on an appropriate maintenance schedule
- Describe the signs and symptoms of ONJ

---

ease early should be explained. Signs and symptoms of ONJ should be explained so it can be identified early, should it develop.

For those individuals who are taking or have taken a BIS, the same ADA patient information sheet should be provided and explained. An oral exam for evidence of ONJ or for oral disease that may predispose to ONJ should be completed and signs and symptoms of the condition explained so that early management can be initiated if the condition develops. Dentists are urged not to perform tooth extraction or oral surgery in these patients. It would be the physician's decision whether to advise the patient to stop taking the drug, but this might be a consideration if ONJ develops. There is a report that the condition improved in several patients when the IV formulation of the BIS was withdrawn (although this did not help all patients in the study who stopped taking the BIS).[17] Box 14-8 summarizes dental hygiene management procedures for the client currently taking or who has taken a BIS.

Patients Taking Antidiabetic Agents

Before periodontal therapy is initiated, the degree of control over DM disease should be assessed by asking about recent

---

BOX 14-9. Management of the Patient Who Is Taking Antidiabetic Agents

- Inquire about the most recent blood sugar level and A1C level
- Schedule a morning appointment following medication and breakfast
- Ensure a meal was eaten prior to the appointment when hypoglycemic drugs (insulin, sulfonylureas) are taken
- Have a glucose source available chairside in case of hypoglycemia
- Monitor vital signs because hypertension is common in DM
- Encourage frequent maintenance appointments for poorly controlled DM

CLINICAL APPLICATION EXERCISES

☐ **Exercise 1.** Describe patient information indicated for the oral health education plan when Fosamax is listed on the medical history.

☐ **Exercise 2.** Identify questions that should be asked during the medical history review related to the patient with DM who takes insulin, and identify the clinical considerations to which the questions relate.

☐ **Exercise 3.** WEB ACTIVITY: Access the Web site of the American Association of Oral and Maxillofacial Surgeons. Utilize information in this source when identifying dental procedures that can and cannot be provided when a patient has taken an oral BIS for 3 or more years or an IV BIS for 6 months or longer in treatment for any condition. [http://www.aaoms.org/docs/position_papers/osteonecrosis.pdf]

blood sugar measurements and A1C test results. Although it is uncommon, diabetic ketoacidosis has been reported to occur in the dental office in individuals with very high blood sugar and dental infection. Poorly controlled patients may also have poor healing following therapy. The most likely medical emergency is hypoglycemia, so a source of glucose should quickly be available chairside to manage the situation. It is essential to inquire if a meal was eaten following the administration of insulin or a sulfonylurea, because those medications can lead to hypoglycemia. For poorly controlled individuals, the risk of periodontal inflammation and infection is increased. These patients may need a frequent periodontal maintenance schedule. Box 14-9 summarizes dental hygiene management considerations for the client with DM.

CONCLUSION

Endocrine disorders can affect an individual in various ways. Uncontrolled disease poses the greatest risk for a medical emergency during oral health care procedures. ADEs may affect the care plan and should be followed up when disease control is determined.

References

1. Miller CS, Little JW, Falace DA. Supplemental corticosteroids for dental patients with adrenal insufficiency: Reconsideration of the problem. *J Am Dent Assoc.* 2001;132:1570–1579.
2. Guyton AC, Hall JE. *Textbook of Medical Physiology.* 10th ed. Philadelphia: WB Saunders; 2000:872, 880.
3. Mullally BH, Coulter WA, Hutchinson JD, et al. Current oral contraceptive status and periodontitis in young adults. *J Periodontol.* 2007;78:1031–1036.
4. American Dental Association (ADA) Council on Dental Health and Health Planning and Bureau of Health Education and Audiovisual Services. Breaking the silence on hypertension: A dental perspective. *J Am Dent Assoc.* 1985;10:781.
5. LaCasa C. California court denies wrongful birth claim. *J Law Med Ethics.* 1996;24:273–274.
6. ADA Council on Scientific Affairs. Antibiotic interference with oral contraceptives. *J Am Dent Assoc.* 2002;133:880.
7. Yagiela JA. Adverse drug interactions in dental practice: Interactions associated with vasoconstrictors. *J Am Dent Assoc.* 1999;130:701–708.
8. Niwa H, Satoh Y, Matsuura H. Cardiovascular responses to epinephrine-containing local anesthetics for dental use: A comparison of hemodynamic responses to infiltration anesthesia and ergometric-stress testing. *Oral Surg Oral Med Oral Pathol Oral Radiol Endod.* 2000;90:171–181.
9. Migliorati CA, Casiglia J, Epstein J, et al. Managing the care of patients with bisphosphonate-associated osteonecrosis: An American Academy of Oral Medicine position paper. *J Am Dent Assoc.* 2005;136:1658–1668.
10. ADA Division of Communications and ADA Council on Scientific Affairs. Bisphosphonate medications and your oral health. *J Am Dent Assoc.* 2006;137:1048.
11. ADA Council on Scientific Affairs. Dental management of patients receiving oral bisphosphonate therapy. *J Am Dent Assoc.* 2006;137:1144–1150.
12. Pickett F. Bisphosphonate-associated osteonecrosis of the jaw: A literature review and clinical practice guidelines. *J Dent Hyg.* 2006;80(3):1–12.
13. American Diabetes Association Professional Practice Committee. Summary of revisions for the 2006 clinical practice recommendations. *Diabetes Care.* 2006;29(Suppl 1):S3.
14. Lincoff AM, Wolski K, Nicholls SJ, et al. Pioglitazone and risk of cardiovascular events in patients with type 2 diabetes mellitus: A meta-analysis of randomized trials. *JAMA.* 2007;298(10):1180–1188.
15. Chandu A, MacIsaac RJ, Smith ACH, et al. Diabetic ketoacidosis secondary to dentoalveolar infection. *Int J Oral Maxillofac Surg.* 2002;31:57–59.
16. Pilgram TK. Relationships between clinical attachment level and spine and hip bone mineral density: Data from healthy postmenopausal women. *J Periodontol.* 2002;73:298–301.
17. Dimitrakopoulos I, Magopoulos C, Karakasis D. Bisphosphonate-induced avascular osteonecrosis of the jaws; a clinical report of 11 cases. *Int J Oral Maxillofac Surg.* 2006;35:588–593.

Web Resources

American Medical Association (AMA) Council on Scientific Affairs. Drug interactions between antibiotics and oral contraceptives. Available at: www.ama-assn.org/ama/pub/article/2036-2927.html. Accessed March 1, 2007.

American Association of Oral and Maxillofacial Surgeons. Position paper on bisphosphonate-related osteonecrosis of the jaws. September 25, 2006. Available at: http://www.aaoms.org/docs/position_papers/osteonecrosis.pdf. Accessed September 1, 2007.

15

Gastrointestinal System Drugs

Disease-induced changes of the gastrointestinal (GI) tract and liver can influence body homeostasis. Moderate dysfunction leads to illness, and extreme dysfunction leads to death. In addition, the GI tract is a primary route for drug administration and absorption, and biotransformation/detoxification of drugs and toxins also occur in the liver. Many patients in a health care setting require drug therapy that may be altered by GI and hepatic structural and functional abnormalities and related pharmacotherapy. Consequently, oral health care providers must have a basic understanding of principles of medical management for GI and hepatic dysfunction and the influence these factors may have on the dental management of affected patients. At least 7 of the top-50 drugs prescribed in the United States are agents used for the management of GI problems, and some of these formulations are also available over the counter (OTC). Given this statistic, it would not be unusual to find one of the agents listed on the health history. The dental hygienist must consider both the drug effects and the medical condition the drug is intended to manage when formulating the plan for care. For example, the clinician must anticipate potential drug–disease interactions (e.g., nonsteroidal anti-inflammatory drugs [NSAIDs] are contraindicated in peptic ulcer disease [PUD]) when analgesic therapy is considered. Some GI conditions, such as gastroesophageal reflux disease (GERD), are exacerbated by the

supine position, and a semisupine chair position may need to be provided. When medical conditions are reported that are likely to be managed with OTC agents, questioning should determine if those drugs were reported on the health history. It cannot be overemphasized that patients often fail to report the intake of OTC drugs unless specifically questioned by the clinician. Acid-reduction drugs can alter the normal pH of the GI tract and interfere with the absorption of some antimicrobial agents the dentist might prescribe.

GASTROESOPHAGEAL REFLUX DISEASE

The squamous epithelium of the esophagus is not designed to resist the digestive action of acidic gastric juice, and it frequently becomes inflamed and eroded in patients with GERD. The primary determinant of GERD appears to be a transient relaxation of the lower esophageal sphincter not induced by a swallow. Episodes of transient relaxation are more common after meals. Slow gastric emptying and increases in intra-abdominal pressure may induce reflux. A hiatal hernia can serve as a reservoir for gastric contents, and transient relaxation of the lower esophageal sphincter is more likely to be followed by an episode of reflux when there is a hiatal pouch with retained gastric acid. GERD is further exacerbated by obesity and smoking (nicotine relaxes the lower esophageal sphincter).

Symptoms of GERD

The typical symptom associated with GERD is substernal burning pain radiating up to the neck (relieved immediately by antacids) brought on by positions that encourage gastroesophageal reflux, such as lying flat, being placed in a supine position prior to oral health care, or stooping after a meal. Esophageal pain may sometimes mimic cardiac pain. Complications of GERD include peptic strictures due to scarring of inflamed tissue, asthma, hoarseness, and dental erosions. Additionally, prolonged acid injury may lead to metaplastic transformation of the esophageal squamous epithelium (Barrett esophagus) with a potential for esophageal cancer. These patients usually sleep propped up with pillows to prevent reflux and may require a semisupine chair position for dental hygiene services. Teeth may be affected by chemical erosion.

Medical Treatment

Medical treatment for GERD consists of neutralizing stomach contents or reducing gastric acid secretion. If endoscopic examination reveals no evidence of esophagitis H_2-receptor blocking agents (ranitidine [Zantac]), proton pump inhibitors (PPIs; omeprazole magnesium [Prilosec] and others), sucralfate, or cisapride are all equally effective.[1] The drugs used to manage GERD and PUD are similar and are listed in Box 15-1. For maintenance treatment of reflux esophagitis, omeprazole alone or in combination with cisapride is more effective than an H_2-receptor blocker alone or cisapride alone, and the combination of omeprazole and cisapride is more effective than an H_2-receptor blocker plus cisapride. Cisapride was removed from the market due to several dangerous drug interactions; however, it is available for selected individuals with GERD on a compassionate basis.

H_2-Receptor Blocking Agents

Mechanism of Action

H_2-receptor antagonists are antihistamines that block receptors in the GI tract. They inhibit the action of histamine at H_2-receptors of **parietal cells**, decreasing both basal- and food-stimulated acid secretions. Most of the agents in this class are equally effective in reducing the secretion of acid in the GI tract. Examples of these drugs are represented in Box 15-2 and include cimetidine, nizatidine, ranitidine, and famotidine. These agents are sold OTC.

Adverse Drug Effects

Adverse drug effects (ADEs) include headache, lethargy, confusion, depression, and hallucinations. Rarely, these agents have been associated with hepatitis or hematologic toxicity. Narcotic analgesic toxicity (e.g., respiratory depression) may be increased with cimetidine due to decreased metabolism of the analgesic. Overall, however, H_2-receptor antagonists have very good safety records.

BOX 15-1. Drugs for the Treatment of GERD and PUD

Antibiotics and bacteriostatics
• Bismuth subsalicylate (Pepto-Bismol)
• Tetracycline hydrochloride (Achromycin V)
• Metronidazole (Flagyl)
• Amoxicillin (Amoxil)
• Clarithromycin (Biaxin)

Antacids
• Magnesium hydroxide
• Aluminum hydroxide
• Calcium carbonate
• Sodium bicarbonate

H_2-receptor antagonists
• Cimetidine (Tagamet)
• Ranitidine (Zantac)
• Famotidine (Pepcid)
• Nizatidine (Axid)

PPIs
• Omeprazole magnesium (Prilosec)
• Lansoprazole (Prevacid)
• Esomeprazole magnesium (Nexium)
• Pantoprazole (Protonix)
• Rabeprazole (AcipHex)

Cytoprotective agents
• Sucralfate (Carafate)

Anticholinergic Drugs
• Propantheline (Pro-Banthine)

Prostaglandin Analogs
• Misoprostol (Cytotec)

Prokinetic Drugs
• Metoclopramide (Reglan)

Drug Interactions

Cimetidine inhibits the activity of hepatic cytochrome P450 enzymes and may interfere with the hepatic metabolism of many drugs. Ranitidine may result in decreased absorption of diazepam and reduce its pharmacologic effects. Pharmacologic effects of ketoconazole, fluconazole, and tetracyclines

---

BOX 15-2. H_2-Receptor Antagonists

• Cimetidine (Tagamet)
• Nizatidine (Axid)
• Ranitidine (Zantac)
• Famotidine (Pepcid)

may be decreased by cimetidine due to decreased absorption. Staggering administration times, such as taking doses 2 hours apart, may avoid this interaction. Bupivacaine and benzodiazepine toxicity is possible with ranitidine because of decreased metabolism of those agents. Concurrent use should be avoided.

Proton Pump Inhibitors

Mechanism of Action

Omeprazole is the prototype drug in the PPI classification and illustrates the drug action. The drug binds to the proton pump of parietal cells lining the wall of the intestines and inhibits the final step in the secretion of hydrogen ions into the gastric lumen, thus preventing the ions' release. Hydrogen provides for gastric acidity. Omeprazole is also approved for the short-term treatment of peptic ulcers. Omeprazole and newer agents, such as lansoprazole (Prevacid), pantoprazole (Protonix), esomeprazole magnesium (Nexium), and rabeprazole (AcipHex), are the most effective available compounds for acid suppression. All are equally effective in therapeutic doses. Box 15-3 contains currently available PPIs. There is some concern about long-term use and a carcinogenic potential because of the occurrence of carcinoid tumors in rats receiving high doses during experimental studies.

Drug Interactions

PPIs may decrease the blood levels of some azole antifungals (itraconazole, ketoconazole) due to a possible reduction in tablet dissolution in the presence of a high gastric pH. Concomitant administration should be avoided, and drugs should be taken 2 hours apart. As well, PPIs may cause enteric-coated salicylates to dissolve rapidly, increasing gastric side effects. Omeprazole and esomeprazole inhibit the activity of some hepatic P450 enzymes, decreasing the clearance of drugs inactivated by this isoenzyme in the liver (e.g., benzodiazepines). Dental drug interactions include a possible diazepam, flurazepam, and triazolam toxicity with omeprazole or esomeprazole. Concurrent use between these drugs should be avoided. Other potential interactions include a decrease in the effects of prednisone when taken with omeprazole; and possible black tongue, glossitis, and stomatitis when lansoprazole (Prevacid) and macrolides are taken together. Clinical status should be monitored when these drugs are used together.

BOX 15-3. PPI Drugs

- Omeprazole magnesium (Prilosec)
- Lansoprazole (Prevacid)
- Pantoprazole (Protonix)
- Esomeprazole magnesium (Nexium)
- Rabeprazole (AcipHex)

Cytoprotective Agents

Sucralfate

Sucralfate is an aluminum hydroxide complex of sucrose. Its effectiveness in healing peptic ulcers and the prevention of relapse is related to a topical (local) effect via its negatively charged sulfate groups, which bind electrostatically to positively charged proteins in ulcerated GI mucosal tissue, possibly retarding acidic and proteolytic damage. Only a small amount of sucralfate is absorbed from the GI tract, and the drug has no known serious adverse effects but may decrease the absorption of other drugs.

Cisapride

Cisapride, a prokinetic agent, was removed from the market due to several dangerous drug interactions, but it is available for compassionate use in special circumstances. Because it is unlikely to be used, it is not included in this chapter.

■ **Self-Study Review**

1. Describe situations in which the client with GERD is most likely to experience reflux. How do these affect dental hygiene care?
2. List factors associated with GERD.
3. Describe the symptoms of GERD.
4. Are there oral signs related to GERD?
5. Describe the medical treatment of GERD. Which therapy is most effective for esophagitis?
6. Describe the mechanism of action of H_2-receptor blockers and their effects.
7. Describe the strategy for reducing the drug–drug interaction when one drug affects the absorption of another.
8. Describe the mechanism of action of PPIs and their effects.
9. Why should enteric-coated aspirin be avoided if PPIs are taken?
10. List potential drug interactions or oral effects of interactions with PPIs.
11. Describe the mechanisms of action and kinetics of the cytoprotective agents.

PEPTIC ULCER DISEASE

PUD is characterized by erosion of the gastric or duodenal mucosa by acid and pepsin. It is exacerbated by stress, alcohol, cigarette smoking, NSAIDs, *Helicobacter pylori* infection, and genetic factors.[2] The two main causes of PUD are infection with *H. pylori* and chronic ingestion of NSAID drugs. *H. pylori* has been found in more than 95% of patients with duodenal ulcers and in 75% of the patients with gastric ulcers.[3] When patients with ulcers induced by NSAIDs are excluded, the prevalence of infection with *H. pylori* in patients with gastric ulcers is around 96%.

Physiologic Protective Effects

The normal gastroduodenal mucosa resists injury from acid and pepsin in the gastric juice by three homeostatic defense mechanisms. Surface epithelial cells secrete mucus and bicarbonate, creating a pH gradient in the mucous layer from the highly acidic gastric lumen to the nearly neutral surface of the mucosa. Gastric mucosal cells have a specialized surface membrane that resists the diffusion of acid back into the cells. In addition, to maintain mucosal integrity, surface epithelial cells continually slough, and mucosal injury is rapidly repaired by proliferating cells. Prostaglandins also enhance the resistance of mucosal cells to injury, perhaps by maintaining mucosal blood flow (which may remove the acid that has diffused across the compromised mucosa) and/or by stimulating the secretion of mucus and bicarbonate. Two major factors, NSAIDs and *H. pylori* infection, appear to disrupt mucosal resistance to injury. *H. pylori* infection is associated with an inflammatory response that disrupts mucosal architecture.

Drug–Disease Interactions

The ulcerogenic effects associated with NSAIDs are most likely attributable to systemic inhibition of prostaglandin synthesis in mucosal cells of the GI tract, diminishing their protective effects. Several epidemiologic studies also indicate that treatment with NSAIDs considerably increases the risk of such ulcer complications as GI bleeding and perforation. PUD associated with NSAIDs is usually due to gastric irritation.

Prostaglandin Analogs

Misoprostol can prevent gastric ulcers in patients on chronic NSAID therapy (usually due to arthritic pain and inflammation) by increasing mucin and bicarbonate release. Prostaglandins are effective in the prevention of NSAID-related erosive disease, but they are not recommended in the therapy of ulcer disease. Dose-related diarrhea is the most common adverse effect.

Symptoms of Peptic Ulcer Disease

The principal symptom of uncontrolled PUD is pain. The patient often has a history of remissions, with complete freedom from symptoms for weeks or months. Vomiting may occur with uncontrolled PUD, and the patient is predisposed to hemorrhage, perforation, and pyloric stenosis. Hemorrhage may vary from slight bleeding to massive hemorrhage. The patient may vomit large quantities of blood. If the blood enters the intestines, large amounts of altered blood in the stools makes them black and tarry (melena). The medical history review should include questions related to a recent history of vomiting.

Medical Treatment

The medical management of PUD primarily consists of antibacterial chemotherapy, the administration of H_2-receptor blocking agents to reduce gastric acid secretion, and antacids to neutralize stomach contents. Other strategies include agents for increasing the rate of gastric emptying, inhibiting the proton pump of gastric parietal cells, and providing for a preventive coating in the stomach; anticholinergic drug therapy; and the use of endogenous prostaglandins to promote the release of mucin and bicarbonate in the GI tract.

Antibacterial Chemotherapy

Because most cases of PUD not caused by NSAIDs are now thought to be associated with infection of the gastric mucosa by *H. pylori*, eradication of this bacterium with various antibacterial combinations has led to rapid healing of active peptic ulcers and low recurrence rates. The antibacterial agents used most often include combination therapy with tetracycline, metronidazole, amoxicillin, and clarithromycin. Two or three of these antibacterial agents are usually given in combination with an H_2-receptor blocker or omeprazole and a coating agent, such as bismuth subsalicylate (Pepto-Bismol).

Antacids

Antacids consisting of mixtures of magnesium hydroxide (milk of magnesia), aluminum hydroxide, calcium carbonate (Tums), and sodium bicarbonate compounds can be effective in promoting the healing of duodenal ulcers. Their efficacy is based on their inherent ability to react with and neutralize gastric acid. Sodium bicarbonate has the potential risk of causing systemic alkalosis and sodium overload. Calcium salts may cause hypercalcemia, which may be detrimental in patients with impaired renal function. Aluminum salts may cause constipation, and magnesium hydroxide has a laxative effect. Antacids are rarely used alone in the treatment of PUD because of the advent of potent acid-suppressing agents that are effective with one daily dose.

Drug Interactions

Antacids may interfere with drugs in three ways:

1. Increasing the gastric pH that may alter tablet dissolution, ionization, and gastric emptying time. Absorption of weakly acidic drugs is decreased. Weekly basic drug absorption is increased, possibly resulting in toxicity or adverse effects.
2. Adsorbing or binding drugs to their surface, resulting in decreased drug absorption or effect (tetracycline is an example).
3. Increasing urinary pH, affecting the rate of drug elimination. Excretion of basic drugs is decreased, and acidic drug excretion is enhanced.

H_2-Receptor Antagonists

Drugs in this class are discussed in the GERD section. The drugs in this class approved for treatment of peptic ulcers are equally effective.

Anticholinergic Drugs

Vagal impulses release acetylcholine at the parietal cells and at gastric mucosal cells containing gastrin, a peptide hormone. Both the directly released acetylcholine and the indirectly released gastrin stimulate parietal cells to secrete acidic hydrogen ions into the gastric lumen. The most useful anticholinergic drug is propantheline (Pro-Banthine). Propantheline may be used as adjunctive therapy in combination with antacids, but not as a single agent. The timing of medication is critical in ulcer therapy. Anticholinergic drugs should be given about 30 minutes *before* meals, and antacids should be taken about 1 hour *after* meals. The side effects and contraindications for propantheline are prostatic hypertrophy, urinary retention, glaucoma, and cardiac arrhythmias. Today, anticholinergic agents are rarely used in the treatment of PUD because of their low efficacy and their undesirable side effects.

Mechanism of Action

GI anticholinergics inhibit the muscarinic actions of acetylcholine at postganglionic parasympathetic neuroeffector sites, including smooth muscle, secretory glands, and central nervous system (CNS) sites. Anticholinergic responses are dose related. Very large doses are required to inhibit gastric acid secretion.

■ Self-Study Review

12. Describe features, signs, and symptoms of PUD. How can this information be used in the medical history follow-up?
13. List two factors associated with the development of PUD.
14. Describe the drug–disease interaction of NSAIDs and PUD.
15. Identify a drug that prevents ulcers when NSAIDs are needed on a chronic basis.
16. Describe the medical treatment for PUD.
17. List the agents used for the management of PUD, and describe the mechanism of action for each agent.
18. List antacids used in the management of PUD.
19. What is a dental drug class that contraindicates the concomitant use of antacids?
20. Describe the effect of vagal impulses on gastric acidity.
21. Identify anticholinergic agents used for PUD, and describe the mechanism of action for each agent.

CONSTIPATION

Constipation may be defined as the passage of excessively dry stool, infrequent stool, or stool of insufficient size. It involves the subjective sensations of incomplete emptying of the rectum, bloating, passage of **flatus**, lower abdominal discomfort, anorexia, malaise, headache, weakness, and giddiness. Constipation may be of brief duration (e.g., fol-

---

> **BOX 15-4.** Laxatives and Cathartics
>
> Bulk-forming and saline laxatives
> - Inorganic salts
>   - Magnesium salts (milk of magnesia)
>   - Sodium salts
> - Organic hydrophilic agents
>   - Methylcellulose (Cologel)
>   - Calcium polycarbophil (Mitrolan)
>   - Psyllium (Metamucil)
>
> Irritants
> - Danthron (Goldline)
> - Castor oil (Neoloid)
> - Senna (Senokot)
> - Phenolphthalein (Prulet, Ex-Lax)
>
> Lubricants
> - Mineral oil
> - Docusate (Colace)
> - Glycerin
> - Lactulose (Chronulac)

lowing an abrupt change of one's living habits and diet), or it may be a lifelong problem. Major causes of constipation include functional abnormalities, colonic disease, rectal problems, neurologic diseases, and metabolic conditions. In addition, the administration of many drugs can lead to constipation. Constipation in most nonhospitalized patients can be resolved by increasing the fiber content of their diets or by supplementing the diet with bulk-forming agents. In addition, the medical management of patients may include the administration of irritants and lubricants (Box 15-4).

Medical Treatment

Bulk-Forming Agents and Saline Laxatives

Bulk-forming agents and saline laxatives may be classified into inorganic salts (magnesium sulfate, magnesium citrate, milk of magnesia, sodium sulfate, sodium phosphate) and organic hydrophilic colloids (methylcellulose, calcium polycarbophil, psyllium, bran, and fruits). The onset of action of inorganic salts is relatively fast (2 to 6 hours). They are poorly absorbed and draw water into the lumen. Magnesium citrate is commonly used to prepare for colonoscopy and enhances the cleaning of the GI tract over a 12-hour period when used as directed. Organic hydrophilic colloids exert their effects by absorbing and retaining water and increasing the bulk of desiccated fecal material in 1 to 3 days. These agents are more effective when administered with water.

Irritants

Irritants include danthron, castor oil, senna, bisacodyl, and phenolphthalein. Most of these agents (except castor oil) are slow in their onset of action (24 hours). Castor oil becomes hydrolyzed to ricinoleic acid, a **surfactant** that decreases water and electrolyte absorption and increases motility. It has an onset of action of 2 to 6 hours. Phenolphthalein, senna, danthron, and bisacodyl are thought to exert their effects by inhibiting the movement of water and sodium from the colon into the circulation, stimulating mucous secretion, and increasing intestinal motility. The misuse of any of these agents has been shown to cause hypokalemia, dehydration, and severe diarrhea. Phenolphthalein-containing products may cause alkaline urine to turn red. Because these agents affect the environment in the GI tract, they may produce systemic problems by the resulting effect on electrolyte and water balance.

Lubricants

Lubricants include mineral oil, docusate, glycerin, and lactulose. Docusate improves penetration of dietary water and fat into feces. Mineral oil lubricates feces and prevents absorption of water from feces. Both agents are taken orally. Mineral oil, when used chronically, may interfere with absorption of fat-soluble vitamins and other essential nutrients. Docusate may cause diarrhea and abdominal cramps. Glycerin and lactulose produce hyperosmolarity and draw water into the colon.

DIARRHEA

Diarrhea and associated fecal urgency and incontinence may be defined as passage of liquefied stool with increased frequency. Acute diarrhea is usually caused by infection, toxins, or drugs. Diarrhea may result from the inhibition of ion transport or from stimulation of ion secretion in the intestine (secretory diarrhea). Osmotic diarrhea occurs when poorly absorbable solutes are present in the intestine. Diarrhea may also result from increased intestinal motility, such as a side effect of some drugs or foods. Chronic diarrhea may be due to laxative abuse, lactose intolerance, inflammatory bowel disease, malabsorption syndromes, endocrine disorders, and irritable bowel syndrome (IBS).

Medical Treatment

Viral- or bacterial-induced diarrhea is usually transient and requires only a clear liquid diet and increased fluid intake. Opioids, such as the combination of diphenoxylate (a derivative of meperidine) and atropine (Lomotil), work to reverse diarrhea due to the side effect of constipation. Anticholinergic agents act by blocking the cholinergic response of defecation. Diarrhea resulting from antimicrobial therapy may be indicated by the presence of blood in the stool (pseudomembranous colitis). Intravenous fluids may be required if dehydration occurs. Drug- or toxin-induced diarrhea is best treated by discontinuing the causative agent when possible. Treatment of chronic diarrhea should be aimed at correcting the cause of diarrhea rather than alleviating the symptoms. Glucocorticoids may be used for diarrhea associated with inflammatory bowel disease. These agents are usually taken on a short-term basis and ADEs are minimal. Box 15-5 lists the variety of agents used to manage diarrhea.

BOX 15-5. Antidiarrheal Agents

Opiates/Anticholinergics
- Diphenoxylate and atropine (Lomotil)
- Loperamide (Imodium)

Absorbents
- Bismuth salicylate (Pepto-Bismol)
- Kapectolin Attapulgite (Kaopectate)

Hypolipoproteinemia agents
- Cholestyramine (Questran)

Anti-inflammatory agents
- Corticosteroids

Irritable Bowel Syndrome

IBS is a condition that results in either diarrhea or constipation. It is explained in this section because it commonly involves diarrhea. It is a motility disorder involving the entire GI tract, causing recurrent abdominal pain and bloating, diarrhea, and/or constipation. The cause of IBS is unknown. No anatomical causes can be found. Emotional factors, diet, drugs, or hormones may precipitate or aggravate GI motility. Therapy is palliative and supportive.

Medical Management

Increased dietary fibers can help patients with constipation in combination with anticholinergic drugs (hyoscyamine). In patients with diarrhea, diphenoxylate or loperamide may be given before meals. Antidepressants may help in either type of IBS. Tegaserod maleate (Zelnorm), a serotonin 5-HT$_4$ receptor agonist, was approved for short-term treatment of women with IBS whose primary bowel symptom is constipation. It stimulates serotonin receptors in the GI tract and normalizes peristalsis, relieving abdominal pain and discomfort. It was removed from the market in March 2007, because a safety analysis found a higher chance of heart attack, stroke, and unstable angina (heart/chest pain) in patients treated with Zelnorm compared with treatment with an inactive substance (placebo). However, in July 2007, the Food and Drug Administration (FDA) announced that it was permitting the restricted use of Zelnorm under a treatment investigational new drug (IND) protocol to treat IBS with constipation (IBS-C) and chronic idiopathic constipation (CIC) in women younger than 55 who meet specific guidelines (*http://www.fda.gov/bbs/topics/NEWS/2007/NEW01673.html*). The safety and efficacy of tegaserod in men with IBS-C have not been established.

■ Self-Study Review

22. Identify agents used in the medical management of constipation.

23. Identify an agent in this group that is used to prepare for colonoscopy.
24. List irritants used to manage constipation.
25. List agents used to manage symptoms associated with diarrhea and IBS.

NAUSEA AND VOMITING

The physiologic purpose of nausea is to prevent food intake; that of vomiting is to expel food or other toxic substances present in the upper part of the GI tract. The vomiting center, located in the lateral reticular formation of the medulla, is the origin of the final common pathway along which different impulses induce **emesis**. The second important medullary site is the chemoreceptor trigger zone in the medulla of the brain. The chemoreceptor trigger zone is outside the blood–brain barrier and, thus, it is accessible to humoral stimuli (chemicals, toxins, viruses, ions) circulating either in the blood or in the cerebrospinal fluid. However, the chemoreceptor trigger zone cannot initiate emesis independently, but only through stimulation of the vomiting center. The vomiting center may also be activated by impulses that originate from the pharynx, the GI tract, and the cerebral cortex. As well, emotional trauma and unpleasant olfactory and visual stimuli may cause nausea and vomiting. Finally, stimulation of the vestibular apparatus (movements of the head, neck, and eye muscles) may cause nausea and vomiting by stimulating the vomiting center. Protracted vomiting may cause electrolyte imbalance, dehydration, and malnutrition syndrome; it may result in mucosal laceration and upper GI hemorrhage.

Antiemetic Agents

Mechanism of Action

These agents block dopaminergic receptors in the chemoreceptor trigger zone of the medulla and abolish the emetic response caused by a variety of stimulants. They are mainly used for vomiting, motion sickness, and anxiety-induced emesis. The most common agents used to reduce vomiting include promethazine (Phenergan) and metoclopramide (Reglan). Box 15-6 includes available antiemetic agents. Selected agents most likely to be reported on the medical history are included in the discussion.

Medical Treatment

Nausea and emesis are adverse effects of a variety of drugs used in cancer chemotherapy and general anesthesia. Other drugs have ADEs that may result in emesis. These effects are reduced with antiemetic drugs.

Phenothiazines

Phenothiazines block dopamine (D_2) receptors in the chemoreceptor trigger zone and have been shown to effectively abolish the emetic response due to some cancer chemotherapeutic agents, general anesthetic and other agents, and radiotherapy. Postoperative nausea and vomiting is di-

---

BOX 15-6.   Antiemetic Agents

Dopamine (D_2) antagonists
  Phenothiazines
      Prochlorperazine (Compazine)
      Chlorpromazine (Thorazine)
      Thiethylperazine (Torecan)
      Perphenazine (Trilafon)
      Promethazine (Phenergan)
      Triflupromazine (Vesprin)
      Fluphenazine (Prolixin, Permitil)
      Promazine (Sparine)
  Butyrophenones
      Droperidol (Inapsine)
      Haloperidol (Haldol)
      Domperidone (Motilium)
  Substituted benzamides
      Metoclopramide (Reglan)
      Trimethobenzamide (Tigan)
      Cisapride (Propulsid)
  Serotonin (5-HT$_3$) antagonists
      Ondansetron (Zofran)
      Granisetron (Kytril)
  Cannabinoids
      Dronabinol (Marinol)
      Nabilone (Cesamet)
  Corticosteroids
      Dexamethasone (Decadron)
      Methylprednisolone (Medrol)
  Antihistamines
      Diphenhydramine (Benadryl)
      Dimenhydrinate (Dramamine)
      Meclizine (Antivert)
  Benzodiazepines
      Lorazepam (Ativan)
      Alprazolam (Xanax)
  Anticholinergic drugs
      Scopolamine (Transderm-Scop)

---

rectly related to the type and dose of the general anesthetic used. It has been shown that the use of a muscle relaxant, which substantially reduces the amount of anesthetic needed, lessens the incidence of postoperative nausea and vomiting. In addition, phenothiazines (especially promethazine) may also be used to control anesthesia-induced emesis. The antiemetic activity of phenothiazines is dose dependent. However, because of their dopaminergic–antagonist actions, higher doses of phenothiazines can induce extrapyramidal activity (smacking lips, tardive dyskinesia), sedation, hypotension, and restlessness. Extrapyramidal effects can complicate intraoral procedures, especially radiographic procedures.

Substituted Benzamides

Substituted benzamides, such as metoclopramide, are both D_2- and 5-HT$_3$-receptor antagonists that at higher doses reduce cisplatin-induced emesis (common cancer chemotherapy agent). The use of higher doses is limited by their antidopaminergic side effects, which include extrapyramidal activity, anxiety, and depression.

Cannabinoids

Recent studies have confirmed that naturally occurring and synthetic cannabinoids (dronabinol [Marinol]) are also effective in patients receiving moderately emetogenic chemotherapy when administered prior to the infusion of chemotherapeutic agents. Cannabinoids also increase the appetite, produce euphoria, and have analgesic properties. These properties are useful in patients in terminal stages of cancer and as an appetite stimulant in HIV disease. Dronabinol (Marinol), available as a gel cap, is administered by mouth. CNS side effects, such as dizziness, drowsiness, and poor concentration, are the main ADEs. It is in the controlled-substance schedule III, Canada N. Drug interactions with agents used in dentistry include additive or synergistic CNS effects (drowsiness, sedation, confusion, dizziness) with sedatives. Also, clearance of barbiturates may be decreased, possibly because of inhibition of metabolism.

Antihistamines

Although histaminergic (H$_1$) receptors are found in the vomiting center, antihistamines have only a weak antiemetic action. However, they are often administered in combination with high-dose metoclopramide to reduce the incidence of extrapyramidal reactions of the latter drug. Common examples are cetirizine (Zyrtec), chlorpheniramine maleate (Chlor-Trimeton), loratadine (Claritin), desloratadine (Clarinex), and diphenhydramine hydrochloride (Benadryl). H$_1$ antagonists have also proved useful in treating emesis associated with motion sickness. Cetirizine, chlorpheniramine, loratadine, and diphenhydramine are in pregnancy category B, but safety for use during pregnancy has not been established. They should be used only when absolutely necessary, but they are the drugs of choice for the treatment of nausea and vomiting associated with the first trimester of pregnancy. They are contraindicated for use during the third trimester of pregnancy, because newborn and premature infants may have severe reactions (convulsions) to some antihistamines.[4] Common side effects include drowsiness and xerostomia.

Anticholinergics

Antagonists to acetylcholine have proven useful in treating emesis associated with motion sickness. Scopolamine (Transderm-Scop), administered as a patch, and propantheline bromide (Pro-Banthine), administered as a tablet, are examples. The addition of transdermal scopolamine to a regimen of metoclopramide and dexamethasone was recently reported to have increased the antiemetic efficacy of the regimen. Common side effects include drowsiness and xerostomia. Short-term therapy (1 to 3 days) may result in drowsiness and xerostomia. Longer therapy (>3 days) may result in candidiasis.

URINARY ANTISPASMOTICS

Agents in this category are prescribed for urinary incontinence, also referred to as overactive bladder. The main agents used are anticholinergics, including tolterodine (Detrol LA) and oxybutynin (Ditropan). An agent approved in 2004 is darifenacin (Enablex). These drugs are available in tablet, extended-release tablet (Enablex), capsule (extended-release Detrol LA), syrup, and transdermal system doseforms. Potential ADEs associated with these drugs include xerostomia (60%), dry eyes, tachycardia, dyspepsia, constipation, headache, cognitive impairment, and urinary retention. Heat prostration (fever, heat stroke) is possible in high environmental temperatures because of decreased sweating.

Mechanism of Action
Oxybutynin Chloride

Oxybutynin exerts a direct antispasmodic effect on smooth muscle and inhibits the muscarinic action of acetylcholine on smooth muscle. This diminishes frequency of contractions of the detrusor muscle and delays the initial desire to void, urgency, and the frequency of incontinent episodes and voluntary urination. Oxybutynin has about 20% of the anticholinergic activity of atropine but up to ten times the antispasmodic activity. It does not block nicotinic receptors. There are no drug interactions with drugs used in dentistry.

Tolterodine Tartrate and Darifenacin

Tolterodine tartrate and darifenacin are competitive muscarinic receptor antagonists that inhibit urinary bladder contractions and salivation via the blocking effect on cholinergic muscarinic receptors. Patients receiving cytochrome P450 3A4 inhibitors (erythromycin, clarithromycin, azole antifungal agents) require a dose reduction of these anticholinergic agents because the anticholinergics use this pathway (P450 3A4) for drug metabolism.

■ Self-Study Review

26. Identify the area of the brain that controls vomiting.
27. List common agents used for emesis and motion sickness.
28. Describe the mechanism of action of phenothiazines.
29. Identify ADEs with long-term use of phenothiazines that may affect the dental hygiene appointment.
30. List a cannabinoid used in emesis management. Is it a scheduled drug?
31. Identify a drug of choice for first-trimester nausea associated with pregnancy.
32. List examples of agents used to prevent motion sickness.
33. Identify ADEs associated with drugs used for urinary incontinence and their dental hygiene implications.

34. Describe dental hygiene clinical considerations for each GI disorder.

DENTAL HYGIENE APPLICATIONS

Gastroesophageal disorders can present clinical management problems related to chair positioning and oral disorders, such as caries, chemical erosion (especially on the lingual surfaces), and xerostomia. Oral health education programs should include therapies to minimize tooth destruction that may result from either the GI disorder or from ADEs. The dental hygienist must assess the control of the GI disorder and anticipate alterations in the treatment plan to make the patient comfortable. A semisupine chair position may be needed for the client. Each therapeutic agent should be investigated for side effects, and the treatment plan should be modified as needed.

Gastroesophageal Reflux Disease

The clinical implications for GERD relate to disorder control. Questioning to determine how GERD may affect treatment procedures will assist in patient management. Patient positioning issues should be investigated. For situations in which chemical erosion or dental caries is present, oral health education should include how to minimize tooth destruction and recommendation of anticaries products.

Peptic Ulcer Disease

Questioning related to PUD control (absence of GI pain) and a recent history of vomiting should be completed. Be aware of the potential for an episode of emesis. If poor disease control is reported, the semisupine chair position is recommended.

Constipation

Narcotic analgesics are drugs used in dentistry that can cause constipation. When these drugs are prescribed by the dentist, ensure that the patient is informed of the potential for this ADE. For the client taking medications to manage symptoms of constipation, questioning related to comfort in positioning may be indicated. A semisupine position may be needed.

Diarrhea

An individual experiencing uncontrolled diarrhea would be unlikely to present for an oral care appointment. In the event that an antidiarrheal agent is reported on the health history, questioning related to why the drug is being taken and any reservations concerning the need for a restroom break should be discussed.

Emesis

Clinical considerations involve the condition of emesis and the difficulty of providing dental hygiene care for an individual uncontrolled by the drug therapy. Other considerations involve potential ADEs associated with the agents, namely drowsiness, dysrhythmia, orthostatic hypotension, xerostomia, and tardive dyskinesia. The dental hygienist must anticipate orthostatic hypotension, leading to unconsciousness following supine positioning. Patients should be allowed to sit upright for several minutes at the end of the appointment before dismissal. With the exception of dronabinol, there are no drug interactions with these agents and drugs used in dentistry.

Incontinence

Management involves allowing the incontinent patient to use restroom facilities before the appointment. The patient may also need to use restroom facilities during the appointment. Xerostomia can be pronounced and sialogogues may need to be prescribed. The dental hygienist should examine the oral cavity for conditions associated with chronic dry mouth. Home-applied fluoride therapy and xylitol gum should be recommended for their anticaries and salivary stimulatory effects.

CONCLUSION

The GI system is both structurally and functionally adapted for the mixing, digestion, and absorption of food and other agents, and the elimination of catabolic residue. Pathophysiologic disruption may lead to reduced metabolic function, malnutrition, electrolyte imbalance, bleeding diatheses, and compromised immune function. Health care providers must recognize that patients with GI disease may require multidisciplinary treatment and coordination of care. Many of the agents in this group of drugs are widely prescribed, and several are sold OTC to relieve gastric disorders. Dental hygienists will treat patients with GI disease and must be aware of the relationships to provision of dental hygiene services.

References

1. Vigneri S, Termini R, Leandro G, et al. A comparison of five maintenance therapies for reflux esophagitis. *N Engl J Med.* 1995;333:1106–1110.
2. Hentschel E, Branstatter G, Dragosics B, et al. Effect of ranitidine and amoxicillin plus metronidazole on the eradication of *Helicobacter pylori* and the recurrence of duodenal ulcer. *N Engl J Med.* 1993;328(5):308–312.
3. Blaser MJ. Gastric *Campylobacter*-like organisms, gastritis, and peptic ulcer disease. *Gastroenterology.* 1987;93:371–383.
4. *Drug Facts & Comparisons.* St. Louis: Wolters-Kluwer Health; 2007:699a.

CLINICAL APPLICATION EXERCISES

☐ **Exercise 1.** A new patient reports for oral prophylaxis. The medical history reveals GERD, which is managed with Prevacid and Pepto-Bismol or Tums. Recently the patient experienced a bacterial upper-respiratory tract infection and took clarithromycin, although it is no longer being taken. Vital signs are within normal limits, and the patient's chief complaint is that "my teeth are sensitive and my tongue is discolored." What elements of the health history are related to the chief complaint?

☐ **Exercise 2.** Describe potential alterations to the dental hygiene treatment plan for the patient whose medical history reports experiencing GERD. What oral effects will you look for as you examine the oral cavity? Describe oral health recommendations for when toothbrushing should occur following an episode of reflux.

☐ **Exercise 3.** A client presents for periodontal débridement and has severe periodontitis. The medical history reveals a history of PUD, managed with lansoprazole and antacids as needed. Use a dental drug reference and look up the drug lansoprazole, a drug for PUD. List the clinical considerations. If an analgesic is needed following periodontal débridement, which product is indicated?

16

Respiratory System Drugs

Respiratory disease can take a variety of forms, including transmissible infection (viral cold, tuberculosis) as well as reduced respiratory function. When respiratory disease is reported, the dental hygienist should question the patient to learn the type of disorder and determine what pharmacologic agents are being used to manage symptoms of the condition. Just as important is the determination of efficacy of the drugs in improving respiratory function. This is usually accomplished by assessing the patient's respiratory rate and qualities (noiseless? labored?) and observing the facial color for cyanosis. Extraoral examination can be important to identify individuals with breathing difficulties. For example, the upper chest may be enlarged (chronic obstructive pulmonary disease [COPD], asthma) due to hyperinflation of the lungs secondary to an increase in functional residual capacity. This chapter highlights the clinical relevance of respiratory disease and the effects of drugs used to open airways, reduce inflammation in the respiratory system, improve breathing, and treat infections. Potential adverse drug effects (ADEs) of the various agents must be investigated, because some may impact the dental hygiene treatment plan.

THE RESPIRATORY SYSTEM

The respiratory tract is divided into two parts, upper and lower. The upper respiratory tract is comprised of the nasal cavity, nasopharynx, and larynx. The trachea, bronchi, and lungs constitute the lower respiratory tract (LRT). The lungs, containing millions of alveoli, are connected with the nose and oral cavity by the bronchioles and the trachea. With each inspiration the alveoli expand, and air is forced out during expiration. Thus, there is a continuous renewal of air in the alveoli whereby oxygen is supplied to and carbon dioxide is removed from the tissues. A serious result of most respiratory diseases is **hypoxia**, which reduces the availability of oxygen to the various cells of the body.

Types of Hypoxia

In *hypoxic hypoxia* oxygen fails to reach the blood of the lungs. The obvious causes are (a) too little oxygen in the atmosphere, (b) obstruction of the respiratory passages,

(c) thickening of the pulmonary membrane, and (d) loss of functional pulmonary tissue. *Stagnant hypoxia* means there is failure to transport adequate oxygen to the tissues because of too little blood flow. The most common cause of stagnant hypoxia is low cardiac output as a result of heart failure. *Anemic hypoxia* means there is too little hemoglobin in the blood to transport oxygen to the tissues. In this situation the person may have adequate hemoglobin in the cells, but the oxygen-carrying capacity of hemoglobin is compromised by carbon monoxide or some other poison. *Histotoxic hypoxia* means there is failure of the tissues to utilize oxygen even though adequate quantities are transported to them. The classic cause of histotoxic hypoxia is cyanide poisoning and vitamin deficiencies resulting in diminished quantities of oxidative enzymes in cells. **Dyspnea** means there is air hunger as a result of some respiratory abnormality, causing the blood to be hypoxic or, even more often, when too much carbon dioxide collects in the body fluids. An occasional person develops psychic dyspnea because of neurosis.

Diseases of the Upper Respiratory Tract

Common Cold

The common cold is a self-limiting, inflammatory viral infection of the upper respiratory tract. It is spread by direct person-to-person contact as the viruses from infected persons become airborne in droplet nuclei, which are emitted during respiration, talking, sneezing, and coughing. The main anatomical location of infection is the muscular, membranous area behind the nasal cavity and above the nasopharynx. Because the nasopharynx is continuous with the oral cavity and the larynx, the site of infection may involve any or all of these areas and give rise to the terms rhinitis, nasopharyngitis, pharyngitis, and laryngitis. The viruses have an incubation period of 1 to 4 days before symptoms begin to appear. Actual shedding of the virus usually precedes the onset of clinical symptoms by 1 to 2 days, but the peak viral excretion occurs during the symptomatic phase. The clinical implication of this is that an individual is contagious during viral shedding periods and before the onset of symptoms. A properly fitted face mask worn by the clinician during treatment, as well as gloves, can reduce the risk of crossinfection.

The frequency of upper respiratory tract infections in many patients is probably due to the large number of different, potentially pathogenic organisms. Age, seasonal factors, general state of health, nutrition, fatigue, emotional disturbances, allergic disorders, and noxious fumes may all play parts in facilitating infection. The diagnosis is made almost entirely on the basis of the history and symptoms (nasal discharge, sneezing, headache, fever, malaise, dryness, soreness, hoarseness, tickling of the throat). As the illness progresses, coughing may appear as an increasingly prominent symptom and may persist for 1 or 2 weeks. Smell and taste are also frequently impaired. Complications primarily result from secondary bacterial infections. In general, they are infrequent and consist of suppuration in the nasopharynx with involvement, by direct extension from the nose, to the accessory sinuses, ears, mastoids, throat, larynx, bronchi, and lungs.

Medical Treatment

At present there are no antiviral agents that are effective against the viruses responsible for the common cold in humans. General measures consist of rest, sufficient fluids to prevent dehydration, and a light, palatable, well-balanced diet. An analgesic/antipyretic agent may be given for the relief of headache, fever, and associated muscular aches and pains. Cough may be reduced by (a) steam inhalation, (b) antitussive syrups containing codeine, or (c) an expectorant, such as guaifenesin (Mucinex).

Antitussive Syrups

Codeine is the most commonly used opioid antitussive and is safe and effective when used as directed. Because codeine can inhibit respiration, it is not recommended when chronic pulmonary disease is present. Another commonly used agent is *dextromethorphan*, the active ingredient in most over-the-counter (OTC) antitussive syrups. It is safe and effective to reduce cough.

Guaifenesin

Guaifenesin enhances the output of respiratory tract fluid by reducing adhesiveness and surface tension of respiratory secretions. Consequently, it facilitates the removal of viscous mucus and promotes productive and more frequent coughing. The drug provides relief of cough associated with respiratory tract infections and related conditions (sinusitis, pharyngitis, laryngitis, bronchitis, and asthma) when these conditions manifest tenacious mucus (or mucous plugs) and congestion. There are no documented drug–drug interactions associated with agents used in dentistry.

Allergic Rhinitis

Allergic rhinitis (IgE-mediated rhinitis) may be seasonal or perennial. The seasonal type is usually caused by pollens from trees, grasses, or flowers. It lasts several weeks, disappears, and then returns the following pollenating season. Perennial rhinitis is due to sensitivity to a variety of allergens, such as house dust, and may occur throughout the year. Large numbers of eosinophils are found in the nasal secretions. The usual symptoms of allergic rhinitis include nasal congestion, sneezing, profuse watery nasal discharge, pruritus, and often conjunctivitis and pharyngitis.

Medical Treatment

The best management strategy for allergic rhinitis is to eliminate the responsible allergen. When this is not possible, a course of desensitization injections is often helpful. This therapy is often effective in the seasonal type of allergy, but not in the perennial type. Pharmacologic strategies include inhibition of the effect of histamine at receptor sites (H_1-receptor antagonists, or antihistamines), reduction of watery secretions (anticholinergics, decongestants), the resolution of allergic inflammation (nasal corticosteroids), and interruption of the release of histamine from IgE-sensitized cells (mast-cell stabilizing drugs). Leukotriene-receptor antagonists (LRAs) are effective in relieving nasal symptoms in

Table 16-1	Pharmacologic Strategies for the Treatment of Allergic Rhinitis		
Drugs	**Mechanisms of Action**	**Therapeutic Effects**	**Major Side Effects**
Fexofenadine (Allegra) Cetirizine (Zyrtec) Loratadine (Claritin, Alavert) Desloratadine (Clarinex) Azelastine Astelin	Second-generation oral and intranasal (azelastine) antihistamines, block H_1-receptors	Reduce sneezing, ocular and nasopharyngeal itching, and rhinorrhea	Mild sedation and dry mouth when amount taken exceeds recommended doses
Pseudoephedrine (Sudafed)	Alpha-adrenergic agonist, acts as a vasoconstrictor	Relieves nasal decongestion	Arrhythmias, hypertension, nervousness
Beclomethasone (Beconase) Budesonide (Rhinocort) Fluticasone propionate (Flonase) Mometasone (Nasonex) Flunisolide (Nasalide) Triamcinolone (Nasacort)	Nasal corticosteroids, inhibit influx of inflammatory cells	Reduce sneezing, ocular and nasopharyngeal itching, rhinorrhea, and nasal congestion	Nosebleeds, nasal septal perforation, potential for systemic corticosteroid effects is low
Cromolyn sodium (NasalCrom)	Mast-cell stabilizer, inhibits histamine release	Reduces symptoms of allergic rhinitis	Sneezing, nasal irritation, nosebleeds
Ipratropium (Atrovent Nasal)	Anticholinergic agent, blocks acetylcholine receptors	Reduces watery rhinorrhea	Headache, nosebleeds
Montelukast (Singulair)	LRA, blocks leukotriene receptors	Reduces nasal inflammation	Elevated levels of AST*, ALT*, and bilirubin

*AST – aspartate aminotransferase, serum
ALT – alanine aminotransferase, serum

patients with allergic rhinitis; however, in comparison to nasal corticosteroids, LRAs are relatively weak as a monotherapy.

Antihistamines

All antihistamines are effective H_1-receptor antagonists, but patients may vary in their responses to individual agents and in their susceptibilities to potential adverse effects. Antihistamines may conveniently be classified as either first- or second-generation agents. Both first- and second-generation oral antihistamines substantially reduce symptoms of nasal itching and watery eyes and have moderate effects on reducing rhinorrhea and sneezing. However, they have minimal effects on the symptoms of nasal congestion. Table 16-1 includes the various agents used.

FIRST-GENERATION ANTIHISTAMINES. The clinical use of first-generation antihistamines (diphenhydramine hydrochloride [Benadryl] and others) is limited because of their anticholinergic and sedative effects. The most common ADEs of first-generation antihistamines are sedation (drowsiness, dizziness), dry mouth, and gastrointestinal symptoms, such as nausea, constipation, and abdominal pain. Even without subjective symptoms of sedation, many antihistamines may impair psychomotor performance.

SECOND-GENERATION ANTIHISTAMINES. Second-generation antihistamines are the first line of therapy for the treatment of mild allergic rhinitis because they lack substantial anticholinergic and sedative properties. Loratadine (Claritin) has virtually no sedative or anticholinergic effects, but it may rarely cause cardiac arrhythmias in the presence of liver disease, overdose, or the concurrent use of erythromycin, ketoconazole (Nizoral), and possibly other drugs that inhibit

hepatic metabolism. All second-generation antihistamines have similar clinical efficacy in equivalent therapeutic doses.

USES. Some experts recommend a combination of a first-generation OTC antihistamine (all of which can cause sleepiness) at bedtime and a second-generation antihistamine during the day. However, next-day sedation has been observed with such regimens. Nasal antihistamines are considered to be similar in efficacy to oral antihistamines. Ophthalmic formulations of antihistamines significantly reduce symptoms of itching, redness, and watery eyes associated with allergic conjunctivitis.

ACTION. The H_1-receptor antagonists act by blocking histamine in target tissues, thereby reducing such histaminic effects as nasal itching, sneezing, and rhinorrhea, but not nasal congestion. To relieve nasal congestion, an alpha-adrenergic agonist such as pseudoephedrine (Sudafed), with significant vasoconstrictive properties, is the decongestant usually recommended. Some products contain a combination of an antihistamine and a decongestant.

Decongestants (Alpha-Adrenergic Receptor Agonists)

As mentioned earlier, antihistamines have minimal effects on symptoms of nasal congestion. To reduce nasal congestion, the coadministration of an oral decongestant with an antihistamine is recommended for a period of no more than 10 days. Pseudoephedrine, an alpha-adrenergic receptor agonist, counters histamine-induced vascular engorgement of the turbinates and improves nasal air flow. Pseudoephedrine in combination with an antihistamine has been shown to be more effective than either drug alone and at least as effective as the nasal corticosteroid beclomethasone in the treatment of nasal symptoms. It is superior for the short-term relief of ocular symptoms of allergy. However, alpha-adrenergic agonists can cause arrhythmias, hypertension, and nervousness in susceptible patients. Patients with coronary artery disease, hypertension, diabetes mellitus, or hyperthyroidism, and those receiving monoamine oxidase inhibitors should be cautioned about the concurrent use of pseudoephedrine. The drug may also aggravate narrow-angle glaucoma and cause symptoms of bladder obstruction because of smooth muscle contraction.

Corticosteroids

Nasal corticosteroid sprays are recommended as the first line of treatment for moderate to severe allergic rhinitis. They are clinically and statistically better than oral or nasal antihistamines in the treatment of nasal congestion and sneezing. However, there is no significant difference between nasal corticosteroids and oral or nasal antihistamines in relieving ocular symptoms. Because antihistamines and nasal corticosteroids influence different physiologic mechanisms, combination therapy is often used for patients who do not respond adequately to a single agent. ADEs with nasal corticosteroids are uncommon and are less likely than with the higher steroid doses used for oral inhalation in asthma. The most common effect is **epistaxis**, noted in about 10% of patients. Rarely, patients with severe symptoms who do not respond to or are intolerant of other medications may be treated with daily or alternate-day oral or preseasonal injected corticosteroids. The well-recognized risks associated with the prolonged use of a systemic corticosteroid make other therapies preferable to manage symptoms of allergic rhinitis.

Mast-Cell Stabilizers

A nasal spray formulation of cromolyn sodium (NasalCrom) is available OTC. It inhibits histamine release and appears to be more effective when administered just before exposure to an allergen. Ophthalmic preparations (cromolyn, nedocromil, lodoxamide) significantly reduce ocular symptoms associated with allergic conjunctivitis.

Anticholinergic Agents

Nasal ipratropium, a quaternary ammonium compound related to atropine, blocks acetylcholine receptors and relieves rhinorrhea in patients with allergic rhinitis, with effects similar to those of nasal corticosteroids.

Nonsteroidal Anti-Inflammatory Agents

Ketorolac (Toradol), an ophthalmic formulation of a nonsteroidal anti-inflammatory agent (NSAID), significantly reduces ocular symptoms of itching associated with allergic conjunctivitis.

Leukotriene-Receptor Antagonists

The first LRA was zafirlukast (Accolate), a tablet taken twice daily, and it was followed by once-daily montelukast (Singulair). Both are effective in relieving nasal symptoms in patients with allergic rhinitis. Generally, the LRA is used empirically as an adjunct to an antihistamine, a nasal corticosteroid, or both. These drugs are well tolerated, with side effects similar in occurrence to the placebo.

DRUG INTERACTIONS. There is a possible decreased efficacy (increased metabolism) when LRAs are taken with erythromycin, and increased toxicity (reduced metabolism) with aspirin has been reported. There is a possible increased risk of edema when montelukast and prednisone are taken together (mechanism not established).

Vasomotor Rhinitis

Some patients complain of chronic nasal obstruction or stuffiness that is not due to allergy. It is characterized by intermittent vascular engorgement of the nasal mucous membrane, sneezing, and a watery rhinorrhea. In some cases, this is the result of overuse of nasal decongestant sprays; they initially improve symptoms, but "rebound congestion" develops when they are used excessively. In this situation, there is compensatory relaxation of the blood vessels of the turbinates, and further stuffiness develops.

Another anatomical cause of nasal obstruction is deviation of the nasal septum. This is resolved by surgical correction of the deviated septum, and symptoms may disappear after surgery. Frequently patients with vasomotor rhinitis have underlying emotional problems that make treatment difficult.

Medical Treatment

The treatment of vasomotor rhinitis is empirical, and the outcome is unpredictable. Some patients may benefit from humidified air, such as that obtained by placing a vaporizer in the workroom or bedroom. Systemic sympathomimetic drugs, such as pseudoephedrine, may relieve symptoms, but they are not recommended for long-term use. Topical vasoconstrictors are not recommended because they cause the nasal blood vessels to lose their sensitivity to other vasoconstrictive stimuli, such as humidity and the temperature of inspired air. Sprays can result in taste disturbances.

Acute Laryngitis

Acute laryngitis may occur during the course of a common cold or as an isolated infection. The throat becomes sore and irritated, and the voice sounds hoarse. Later, the patient may lose the voice altogether. A nonproductive cough is usually present. Small children may have a brassy cough with associated swelling of the mucous membrane, which can cause obstruction of the airway passages. The patient with acute laryngitis does not always have an elevated temperature.

Medical Treatment

The patient is advised not to talk or smoke to avoid irritating the larynx. Steam inhalations, hot gargles, and drinks give relief. An expectorant, such as guaifenesin, is administered to remove viscous mucus, making a nonproductive cough more productive and less frequent.

Chronic Laryngitis

Chronic laryngitis is more common in occupations for which the voice is used constantly, such as singers and public speakers. Excessive use of tobacco and alcohol are often predisposing factors. Chronic sinusitis may also make the patient susceptible to chronic laryngitis. Hoarseness is the chief symptom, and the patient usually coughs frequently. Pain is absent or minimal. Examination of the larynx shows the vocal cords to be thickened and red. Medical examination of the larynx in patients with persistent hoarseness that has been present for more than 3 weeks is essential to exclude papilloma, carcinoma, cord paralysis, or, more rarely, tuberculosis or syphilis.

Medical Treatment

Pharmacologic therapy is usually not indicated. Resolution generally occurs when the voice is rested, and smoking and alcohol use is stopped. Steam inhalations are of value. Gargling with warm salt water may have a palliative result. In cases resistant to therapy, biopsy of the cords may be necessary to distinguish between laryngitis and neoplasm.

Tuberculosis

Tuberculosis (TB) is a major health problem throughout the world. TB is recognized worldwide as the leading cause of death from an infectious disease, responsible for approximately two million deaths annually. In the United States, a total of 14,093 cases (4.8 cases/100,000) of TB were reported in 2005, representing a 3.8% decline in the rate from 2004. The rate of TB in foreign-born persons is 8.7 times that of those born in the United States. In addition, Hispanics, blacks, and Asians had TB rates 7.3, 8.3, and 19.6 times higher than whites, respectively. Moreover, the number of multidrug-resistant (MDR) cases of TB increased by 13.3% compared to 2003 (the most recent year for which complete drug-susceptibility data are available). The disparity of TB rates between whites and racial/ethnic minorities and the increased incidence of MDR cases of TB all threaten progress toward the goal of eliminating TB in the United States.

Tuberculosis is an infectious disease caused by *Mycobacterium tuberculosis* (MTB), a bacillus. The disease is transmitted from one person to another by droplet infection when an infected person coughs or sneezes. These droplet nuclei are between 1 and 5 microns in size, can remain suspended in air for hours, and can be carried in normal air currents throughout a room or building. When expelled from the lungs, droplet nuclei are released into the air and inhaled by noninfected persons. The probability that a person who is exposed to MTB will become infected depends on the concentration of infectious droplet nuclei in the air and the duration of the exposure to a person with infectious TB disease. Individuals living in crowded conditions, those with compromised immune systems (HIVD), and individuals with debilitating conditions are susceptible to TB. Although TB primarily affects the lungs, other organs may also be affected. When the quantity or virulence of the TB bacilli is such that they overwhelm the immune response, the bacilli may disseminate throughout the body by lymphatic and hematogenous spread. For example, if a person's immune system is poor, then the infection can spread from the lungs to other organs of the body. *Extrapulmonary* (outside the lungs) TB is the term to describe an infection from the bacillus that affects tissues outside the lungs. Organs that can be affected include the liver,

kidneys, spleen, uterus, and bones. People with AIDS are at increased risk for TB because of their compromised immune systems. TB is treated with long-term administration of two or more anti-TB drugs. For situations in which a person is at risk of being infected with TB (living in home with someone who has TB, living in crowded conditions where TB may be present, etc.) one anti-TB drug is administered as a preventive therapy. The drugs used to treat TB render the patient noninfectious to others, unless the patient has drug-resistant TB.

Medical Treatment

Early diagnosis of infection with MTB is important because of the infectious nature of the disease. The tuberculin skin test (TST, or Mantoux test) is commonly used for screening groups of people for latent TB infection. The antigen is injected intracutaneously into the forearm. In patients infected with the bacillus, the TST evokes a delayed hypersensitivity reaction to the antigen mediated by T-lymphocytes and produces an indurated area of redness and swelling. The test is read at 48 to 72 hours. Erythema is disregarded in the determination of a positive reaction, and the diameter of the induration is measured to determine a positive test. Definitive diagnosis of TB usually requires the demonstration of MTB in the patient's secretions.[1] Bacteriologic examination of sputum smears examined microscopically may provide the first bacteriologic clue to TB disease. However, due to the fact that not all acid-fast bacilli are tubercle bacilli, a positive bacteriologic culture for MTB is essential to confirm the diagnosis. DNA probes specific for the genus *Mycobacterium* now are used routinely to identify specific mycobacterium. When the presence of MTB has been confirmed, it is then necessary to perform drug susceptibility testing on positive cultures to determine the most effective pharmacologic therapy.

Anti-TB drugs are classified as primary (first-line) and second-line drugs (Table 16-2). Primary (first-line) drugs provide the foundation for treatment. Second-line drugs are less effective, and usually more toxic than primary agents. Drugs are used in combination to treat TB. Sensitivity and culture testing is completed to identify the most effective combination treatment, especially in areas where multi-drug-resistant TB is present. To reduce the risk of bacterial resistance, the Centers for Disease Control and Prevention (CDC) recommend the use of three or more drugs in initial therapy (~2 months), followed by a reduction of therapeutic agents when cultures verify the drugs are effectively controlling the infection (4 to 6 months). Common regimens include initial therapy with three or more of the following drugs: Isoniazid (INH), rifampin, and pyrazinamide, along with either ethambutol or streptomycin for 2 months, followed by rifampin and INH for 4 months in areas with a low incidence of TB. In areas of high incidence of TB, the CDC recommends the addition of streptomycin or ethambutol for the first 2 months.

Bactericidal Agents

INH is bactericidal, with rifampin and streptomycin having some bactericidal activity. INH is used as a single drug therapy to *prevent* TB and is combined with other agents for *treatment* of an established TB infection. When a family member of an infected individual is given INH prophylactically, it is

Table 16-2 Anti-TB Agents

Drug	Mechanism of Action	ADEs
First-line Drugs		
Ethambutol	Inhibits arabinosyl transferase	Optic neuritis Loss of visual acuity
Pyrazinamide	Inhibits fatty acid synthetase	Morbilliform rash Arthralgias Hyperuricemia
Izoniazid (INH)	Inhibits fatty acid synthetase	Hepatitis Peripheral neuropathy Inhibits CYP450 enzymes

Rifamycins
  Rifampin
  Rifabutin
  Rifapentine
	Bind to RNA polymerase and inhibit transcription	Hepatitis
		Flulike symptoms
		Morbilliform rash
		GI disturbances
		Induce CYP450 enzymes

Second-line Drugs		
Cycloserine	Inhibits monomer synthesis	Psychosis Seizures Peripheral neuropathy
Ethionamide	Inhibits fatty acid synthetase	Hepatitis Hypothyroidism

Aminoglycosides
  Streptomycin
  Capreomycin
  Kanamycin
  Amikacin
	Bind to the 30S ribosomal subunit and inhibit translation	Ototoxicity
		Nephrotoxicity
		Neuromuscular blockade

Fluoroquinolones
  Ciprofloxacin
  Ofloxacin
  Gatifloxacin
  Levofloxacin
  Moxifloxacin
	Inhibit topoisomerase II (DNA gyrase), thereby releasing DNA with staggered double-stranded breaks	Nausea
		Abdominal pain
		Restlessness
		Confusion

Aminosalicylic acid	Competitive para-aminobenzoic acid antagonist	GI disturbances
Combination Drugs		
Rifamate	INH + rifampin	
Rifater	INH + rifampin + pyrazinamide	

GI, gastrointestinal.

taken for 6 months to 1 year. ADEs of anti-TB drugs are identified in Table 16-2.

Bacteriostatic Agents

Most anti-TB drugs are bacteriostatic and slow down the growth and multiplication of the TB infection. Combination therapy of these drugs must be taken on a regular schedule every day or several times weekly to reduce the development of drug resistance and to resolve the active infection. Some communities require a directly observed treatment approach, whereby a public health official delivers the drugs daily or three times weekly and observes to ensure the drugs are taken. Most are taken by mouth, but streptomycin is usually given daily as a single intramuscular injection.

Implications for Dental Hygiene Care

In 2005, the CDC published new guidelines for preventing the transmission of MTB in health care facilities.[1] These guide-lines replace all previous CDC guidelines for TB infection control in health care settings and apply to all settings in which health care workers (HCWs) might either share air space with persons with infectious TB disease or have contact with clinical specimens that contain MTB. The magnitude of the risk varies by setting, occupational group, prevalence of TB in the community, patient population served in the setting, procedures performed, and effectiveness of TB-infection-control measures. However, in every setting where oral health care is provided to persons who have suspected or confirmed TB disease, a TB-infection-control plan must be established. The 2005 guidelines explicitly identify oral health care facilities as outpatient settings in which patients with suspected or confirmed infectious TB disease are expected to be encountered. As well, the probable transmission of MTB from patients to two oral health care workers (OHCWs) has been documented, and there is evidence of TB transmission from an oral surgeon to 15 patients following extractions.[2,3] Standard precautions provide the basis for strategies to prevent or reduce the risk of exposure to blood-borne pathogens and other potentially infectious material. However, standard precautions are inadequate to prevent the spread of organisms through droplet nuclei 1 to 5 microns in diameter, and additional measures are necessary to prevent the spread of MTB. Therefore, oral health care settings must have a written TB-infection-control program based on the prevalence of the disease in the local community or surrounding area. The most important part of this program is the implementation of administrative controls. Administrative controls are intended to reduce the risk of exposure to persons who might have infectious TB.

A client with signs and symptoms of active TB should not be seen in a dental facility. The CDC has advised dental offices to add screening questions for TB to the health history (administrative control), and if any of the signs and symptoms of TB are reported the health care professional is advised to refer the patient to have a medical evaluation before a dental appointment is provided. Signs include persistent cough for more than 3 weeks, blood in sputum, night sweats, unexplained weight loss, and close association with someone who has had TB. Patients with suspected or confirmed TB disease requiring urgent dental care must be promptly referred to an oral health care facility that meets the requirements for an airborne infection isolation area and provides adequate respirator-protection equipment for dental personnel. Another administrative control is to screen OHCWs annually using the tuberculin skin test and implement medical care for those who test positive to eliminate the risk for crossinfection among HCWs. Personnel with TB disease (pulmonary or laryngeal) should be excluded from the workplace until documentation is provided from their health care providers to show that (a) they are receiving adequate therapy, (b) their cough has resolved, and (c) they have had three consecutive sputum smears collected on different days with negative results for MTB.[1]

Anti-TB drugs are taken for a long time. Patients are monitored medically to determine when they are no longer infectious. For clients with a history of TB infection, a medical consultation must be secured that verifies the client is not contagious to dental office personnel.

■ Self-Study Review

1. Describe the method for determining efficacy of pharmacologic treatment for a respiratory disorder.
2. What anatomical structures differentiate the upper respiratory tract from the LRT?
3. Differentiate between the types of *hypoxia*. What is a serious problem of hypoxia?
4. Describe the clinical implications for the common cold.
5. Identify actions of each drug therapy for the common cold.
6. Identify the best management for allergic rhinitis.
7. Identify actions of drugs used to manage allergic rhinitis. What are side effects of these agents?
8. What is the benefit of the second-generation antihistamines?
9. List dental drug interactions with antihistamines.
10. Identify the actions of drugs used for vasomotor rhinitis, and name a common adverse effect.
11. Identify medical treatment to manage symptoms of laryngitis.
12. Differentiate between drug therapies used to prevent TB from those used to treat the infection. Discuss the clinical implications of this disease to receiving oral procedures.

Diseases of the Lower Respiratory Tract

LRT disorders involve a variety of conditions (asthma, bronchitis, emphysema, COPD); however, they are all managed with one or more of the following agents: Corticosteroids to reduce inflammation, beta-2 bronchodilators to open airways and improve ventilation, mast-cell stabilizers to inhibit mucus formation, anticholinergic agents to promote bronchodilation and to reduce airway secretions, and LRAs to reduce secretions. Table 16-3 includes the variety of agents used for the disorders of the LRT.

Asthma is a chronic respiratory disease characterized by periods of remission and acute exacerbation in response to a variety of inflammatory stimuli. It manifests as exaggerated bronchoconstriction resulting in a reversible airway obstruction. *Chronic bronchitis* results in excess mucous production in response to smoking and exposure to allergens, chemicals, and pollutants; and it is complicated by recurrent respiratory infections. *Emphysema* is characterized by irreversible destruction of the alveoli, which become filled with trapped air. *COPD* is a syndrome of progressive airflow limitation and irreversible airway obstruction caused by chronic inflammation of the airways and lung parenchyma. A clinical overlap between asthma, chronic bronchitis, emphysema, and COPD can occur in patients who smoke.[4] The diagnosis of asthma and chronic bronchitis is clinical, made by history. The diagnosis of emphysema is based on histologic examination of lung tissue. The diagnosis of COPD is based on physiologic pulmonary function.

Bronchial Asthma

Bronchial asthma is a respiratory disease characterized by reversible airway obstruction from bronchial smooth muscle spasms, hypersecretion of cells, collection of mucus on the bronchiole lining, and inflammation of alveolar epithelium. *Extrinsic asthma*, which is associated with allergy, usually occurs in younger age groups. The individual may give a history of such allergic problems as rhinitis, urticaria, or eczema, in which case the patient may be said to be "atopic." There is frequently a family history of such atopy. *Intrinsic asthma* tends to occur in older age groups for whom the asthma attack is more severe. Immunologic mechanisms leading to development of intrinsic asthma are unclear. Asthma is a major cause of chronic airflow limitation. Exhalation is reduced more than inhalation. Airflow limitation, however, is usually reversible, either spontaneously or after treatment with an inhaled β_2-adrenergic agonist.

Table 16-3	Drugs for Respiratory Disease and Bronchospasm

Anti-inflammatory Drugs	Bronchodilators
Corticosteroids	Beta$_2$-Selective Adrenergic Agents
Beclomethasone dipropionate (Beclovent, Vanceril, Qvar) Budesonide (Pulmicort) Flunisolide (AeroBid, Aerospan) Fluticasone propionate (Flovent) Mometasone furoate (Asmanex Twisthaler) Triamcinolone acetonide (Azmacort) Prednisone or prednisolone	Albuterol (Proventil, Ventolin, and others) Bitolterol mesylate (Tornalate) Pirbuterol (Maxair) Terbutaline (Brethine, Brethaire, and others)
Mast-Cell Stabilizers	Anticholinergics
Cromolyn (Intal)	Ipratropium bromide (Atrovent)
Nedocromil (Tilade)	Tiotropium bromide (Spiriva)
LRAs	
Zafirlukast (Accolate) Montelukast sodium (Singulair)	
Others	
Theophylline (Theo-Dur and others) Aminophylline	

Respiratory viruses appear to be responsible for most asthmatic attacks, particularly in children, and there may be an associated bacterial infection of the respiratory tract. Asthma may also be provoked by cold weather and exercise, which is also common in younger individuals. About 10% of intrinsic asthmatics have a triad of aspirin-induced asthma, nasal polyps, and sinusitis. Emotional stress is also a common provoking cause of asthma. Coughing or shortness of breath during exercise may be the first signs of early asthma. In a moderate to severe attack, wheezing occurs due to spasm of the bronchial tubes. In severe cases, the individual may use the accessory muscles of respiration (sternocleidomastoid, trapezius, and scalenus) to assist breathing. They may be observed sitting down or leaning forward against a support in order to fix the shoulder muscles so these accessory muscles may obtain better leverage on the chest wall. Asthma is characterized by wheezing; however, in the most severe cases, the bronchospasm is such that wheezing may not be heard at all due to the extremely small amount of air that is able to pass into the lungs.

Medical Treatment

Most experts now consider asthma to be an inflammatory disorder of the airway, with inflammation caused by allergy or other stimuli leading to bronchial hypersecretion and obstruction of airflow. The new therapeutic emphasis, therefore, is on the use of anti-inflammatory drugs, such as inhalational steroids. The first-line therapy for asthma is a corticosteroid spray to reduce inflammation in the bronchioles. Other agents used to manage symptoms are bronchodilators (aerosols or tablets), mast-cell stabilizers, and LRAs (Table 16-3). The goal is for patients to control disease to the extent that the sprays are used no more than twice daily. Aerosol medications can dry oral tissues and increase plaque and calculus levels.

Inhaled Corticosteroids

Regular, continuous use of inhaled corticosteroids suppresses inflammation, decreases bronchial hypersecretions, and decreases symptoms in patients with chronic asthma. Inhaled corticosteroids appear to be more effective than regular use of β_2-selective adrenergic drugs and tend to decrease the dosage of systemic steroids needed for patients with severe asthma. In adults, inhaled corticosteroids have generally been free of serious toxicity. Inhaled corticosteroids can suppress the hypothalamic–pituitary–adrenal axis, but they rarely cause clinical adrenal insufficiency. Dental procedures have not been shown to produce a level of stress that might mandate perioperative steroid supplementation.[5,6] **Dysphonia** and oral or esophageal candidiasis can occur due to local deposition of the drug on tissues. All patients who use inhaled steroids should be counseled to rinse following use of the agent to reduce the risks for candidiasis. In children, continuous daily use of inhaled corticosteroids can slow growth.

Systemic Corticosteroids

Oral or injected corticosteroids are the most effective drugs available for acute exacerbations of asthma uncontrolled by bronchodilators. Even when an acute exacerbation responds to bronchodilators, many clinicians treat recovering patients for 8 to 10 days with oral corticosteroids to decrease symptoms and prevent relapse. Prolonged daily use of oral corticosteroids can cause glucose intolerance, weight gain, increased blood pressure, bone demineralization, cataracts, immunosuppression, and retarded growth in children.

Mast-Cell Stabilizers

Cromolyn sodium (Intal) and nedocromil (Tilade) stabilize mast cells (and may perform other anti-inflammatory activities) to inhibit mucous formation and decrease airway hyperresponsiveness in some patients with asthma. Mucous collections can reduce the airway space and block alveoli in the lungs. Coughing may dislodge the mucous plug and improve breathing temporarily; however, another goal of therapy is to reduce the formation of mucus and other secretions associated with inflammation. Pretreatment with these agents can also prevent bronchospasm induced by exercise or cold.

Beta-2 Agonists

Inhaled β_2-selective adrenergic agonists have no anti-inflammatory activity, but they are the most effective drugs available for the treatment of acute bronchospasm and for the prevention of exercise-induced asthma. Albuterol, terbutaline, pirbuterol, and bitolterol are β_2-selective aerosols that produce bronchodilation by their effects on beta-2 receptors in the bronchioles. They produce more bronchodilation with fewer cardiovascular effects than the older adrenergic aerosols, such as epinephrine (Primatene Mist), isoproterenol, or metaproterenol. Nevertheless, tachycardia, palpitations, increased blood pressure, and tremors can occur. Monitoring the blood pressure perioperatively is prudent, especially if vasoconstrictors are used.

Other Bronchodilators

Oral theophylline (Theo-Dur and others), dyphylline, and aminophylline are less effective bronchodilators than inhaled beta-2 agonists and have a slower onset of action. Although it has limited usefulness for the treatment of acute symptoms, theophylline can decrease the frequency and severity of symptoms in patients with chronic asthma and can decrease oral steroid requirements in corticosteroid dependent patients. It is supplied in tablet, capsule, and liquid doseforms. In addition to adverse side effects of vomiting, headache, tachycardia, cardiac arrhythmias, and seizures, theophylline can cause a variety of adverse drug interactions. Drug interactions of interest to dentistry include increased myopia with pilocarpine (Salagen), a drug used to stimulate salivation, and possible theophylline toxicity with macrolide antibacterial agents (decreased metabolism).

Anticholinergic agents that produce bronchodilation and are used as maintenance treatment for bronchospasm include ipratropium bromide (Atrovent) and tiotropium bromide (Spiriva). These drugs are atropine derivatives also used for inhalation treatment of COPD. Ipratropium is a relatively weak bronchodilator with no serious adverse effects. It has been used to supplement beta-2 agonists or theophylline in a limited number of patients with asthma.

Leukotriene-Receptor Antagonists

Leukotrienes promote chemotaxis of inflammatory cells and production of mucus, and they can cause bronchoconstriction. Zafirlukast and montelukast have been shown to be as effective as low-dose inhaled corticosteroids in some patients with mild to moderate persistent asthma.

Bronchitis

Bronchitis is inflammation of the mucous membrane lining the bronchi and may be either acute or chronic in nature.

Acute Bronchitis

Acute bronchitis is most commonly a complication of colds, influenza, measles, and whooping cough. The condition causes soreness behind the sternum and a dry, painful cough. Both the bronchioles and the trachea can be affected. When the infection involves the bronchi, the patient wheezes and has difficulty breathing. If secondary bacterial infection occurs, a thick, purulent sputum is produced. The condition produces a variable degree of malaise, being more serious in young children and older, debilitated patients.

Chronic Bronchitis

Chronic bronchitis is an abnormality of varied etiology accompanied by increased secretion and chronic inflammation of the alveolar epithelium. It is seen most commonly in smokers 35 years or older. Severe, recurrent respiratory infections as a child and air pollution may also be contributory. The patient with chronic bronchitis is usually heavyset and relates a history of coughing and sputum production for at least 3 months in each of 2 consecutive years. Hypoxic hypoxemia, carbon dioxide retention, respiratory acidosis, and right heart failure may occur early. Chronic hypoxia leads to polycythemia and right heart failure. Because of reduced ventilation, arterial partial pressure of carbon dioxide is chronically increased to the range of >45 mmHg (normal range 35 to 45 mmHg), and the patient appears cyanotic. Because of the cyanosis and the edema secondary to heart failure, these patients are referred to as "blue bloaters."[7] The course of the disease is gradual until heart failure occurs. Some patients with chronic bronchitis may develop chronic airflow limitation, and the presence of chronic mucus hypersecretion is an indicator of a poor prognosis in patients with COPD.

Medical Treatment

In mild cases of acute bronchitis, steam inhalation and a cough suppressant will suffice. In young children and the elderly who may have suppressed immune systems, antibiotics are indicated. Chronic bronchitis is a more difficult condition to manage. Repeated respiratory tract infections and respiratory failure may be reversed by antibiotics and bronchodilators (tablet or aerosol). The role of corticosteroids and the use of oxygen therapy in the treatment of chronic bronchitis are not clearly defined.

Emphysema

Emphysema is characterized as an irreversible obstructive disease of the lungs with dilation and destruction of the walls of the terminal bronchioles without fibrosis. The destruction leads to irregular enlargement of respiratory spaces. The total surface area of the pulmonary membrane becomes greatly diminished, which in turn contributes to diminished aeration of the blood. Most cases of emphysema include a history of smoking tobacco, and, predictably, it usually is preceded by chronic bronchitis. Other cases may be due to a hereditary defect (α_1-antitrypsin deficiency) that allows for proteinase digestion of pulmonary elastic tissue. As the disease advances, air is trapped in the lungs, and the diaphragm is flattened;

there is noticeable use of the accessory muscles of respiration; and hyperinflation of the lungs occurs. In advanced cases, there is right heart failure, peripheral edema, and hepatomegaly. The patient is usually thin, leans slightly forward to facilitate breathing, and is "barrel chested." In patients with emphysema, the arterial partial pressure of oxygen is often ~75 mmHg (normal range 80 to 100 mmHg), while the partial pressure of carbon dioxide is low or normal. Because hemoglobin is almost fully saturated at a partial pressure of oxygen of 60 mmHg, these patients have been referred to as "pink puffers."[4]

Medical Treatment

At present, little can be done to treat patients with pulmonary emphysema, although low-flow oxygen therapy may be useful. In this treatment, an oxygen tank is carried and a nasal cannula is placed under the nose. This allows the individual to be mobile and travel in the community. The immediate goal of therapy is to raise oxygen saturation without reducing the drive to breathe. Low levels of oxygen stimulate the drive to breathe, so raising oxygen saturation can have toxic effects. These patients often use bronchodilators (albuterol and others) to open airways and drugs to reduce secretions. A newly approved anticholinergic agent, tiotropium bromide inhalation powder (Spiriva HandiHaler), relaxes muscarinic receptors in the bronchioles to produce bronchodilation. It is approved for COPD, emphysema, and chronic bronchitis to assist ventilation. Another anticholinergic bronchodilator is ipratropium bromide (Atrovent), which produces bronchodilation and reduces airway secretions.

Chronic Obstructive Pulmonary Disease

The primary physiologic abnormality in COPD is an accelerated decline in the forced expiratory volume in one second (FEV_1) from the normal rate in adults over 30 years of age of approximately 30 mL/year to nearly 60 mL/year.[4] The respiratory disorder is characterized by an initial asymptomatic phase in which lung function deteriorates without associated clinical symptoms. The subsequent symptomatic phase usually occurs when the FEV_1 has fallen to approximately 50% of the predicted normal value. Clinically, COPD is characterized by respiratory symptoms: Dyspnea, sputum production, and coughing. It is also known to contribute to cardiovascular dysfunction, lung cancer, metabolic syndrome, osteoporosis, and depression. Risk factors include exposure to a wide variety of inhaled particles and gases, but in the western world, inhaled cigarette smoke is *the most important causative factor*. Other risk factors, which account for far fewer cases, include α_1-antitrypsin deficiency, airway hyperresponsiveness, and indoor air pollution.

Medical Treatment

The major goals of therapy include smoking cessation, symptom relief, and improvement of respiratory function. Drug therapy includes inhaled bronchodilators (albuterol, ipratropium, formoterol, salmeterol, and tiotropium), theophylline, and inhaled and oral corticosteroids.

■ Self-Study Review

13. List diseases that affect the LRT, and describe the pathophysiology of those conditions.
14. Describe the symptoms of each condition and compare with other diseases of the LRT. What is a blue bloater? What is a pink puffer?
15. Identify the actions of the four classes of drugs used to manage disorders of the LRT.
16. Describe the medical management for LRT disorders.

DENTAL HYGIENE APPLICATIONS

Respiratory disease can complicate dental hygiene treatment that usually is completed in the supine position. The affected

> **BOX 16-1.** Dental Hygiene Considerations for the Patient with Respiratory Disease
>
> 1. Examine medical history to identify signs or a history of infectious respiratory disease.
> 2. Determine degree of infectiousness:
>   - Measure temperature, monitor cough. For history of tuberculosis, question to determine that medical evaluation has determined noninfectiousness. Medical consultation may be necessary to verify information if signs of respiratory disease are present.
> 3. Determine airway patency for evidence of obstruction:
>   - Congestion may require semisupine position; client may request semisupine position.
>   - Evaluate quality of breathing, congestion. Be aware that obstruction of the airway can develop during the appointment, posing a medical emergency situation.
> 4. Note drug therapies reported on the medical history:
>   - Monitor frequency of use of aerosol drugs to determine disease control.
>   - Aerosol bronchodilators should be brought to each appointment.
>   - Aerosol corticosteroid spray use should be followed by rinsing the mouth.
>   - Aerosol medications can dry oral tissues and promote plaque accumulation and calculus. Monitor self-care efficiency.
> 5. Examine oral cavity for ADEs associated with caries, candidiasis, xerostomia:
>   - Preventive therapies may include home fluoride; salivary stimulants, such as xylitol gum; or antifungal therapy.

CLINICAL APPLICATION EXERCISES

◻ **Exercise 1.** Describe the clinical considerations for the patient who reports for dental hygiene care who is recovering from a respiratory infection/cold and is taking decongestants.

◻ **Exercise 2.** Develop a treatment plan for the patient with chronic asthma who reports taking Singulair once daily, plus Flonase and Maxair Autohaler as needed, usually once daily. Identify oral health information related to the drugs above and patient instructions for future appointments.

◻ **Exercise 3.** WEB ACTIVITY: The Food and Drug Administration ordered manufacturers to discontinue marketing of some albuterol CFC inhalers by December 2008. See the rule at http://www.fda.gov/cder/mdi/mdifaqs.htm. What was the reason for the discontinuation of this popular drug doseform?

◻ **Exercise 4.** WEB ACTIVITY: Log on to the CDC Web site (http://www.cdc.gov) and search for the reference on tuberculosis in the dental workplace (MMWR 2005:54,No. RR-17).

client may prefer a semisupine chair position, or respiratory obstruction may require it. In addition the clinician must ensure the patient is not infectious and able to transmit a respiratory infection. For chronic respiratory disease, it is essential to assess disease control before continuing with treatment. Questioning the patient about positioning, measuring body temperature and evaluating respiration and the qualities of breathing are all procedures that must be completed to determine whether to modify the treatment plan or to continue with the treatment. Bronchodilators and aerosolized corticosteroids are commonly used for several respiratory conditions. When they are reported on the medical history, the patient should be instructed to bring them to each appointment. Questioning to determine the frequency of use may identify uncontrolled respiratory disease. Adverse effects of medications can include chronic xerostomia, candidiasis, drying of the mucosa, and thick plaque. Preventive recommendations related to rinsing the mouth after using aerosol agents should be made. Oral tissues should be examined for evidence of disease or increased plaque and calculus accumulation associated with chronic dry mouth. Preventive and therapeutic management specific to these situations should be considered (Box 16-1).

CONCLUSION

Respiratory diseases are common, and individuals who report for oral health care may present with signs and symptoms of respiratory congestion or obstruction. Specific management activities are indicated, such as determination of infectious-

ness or degree of disease control, adjustment of the chair position to enhance breathing, assurance that bronchodilating "rescue inhalers" are brought to the appointment, and monitoring the oral cavity for xerostomia and candidiasis. Vital sign measurements can identify other drug side effects, such as increased blood pressure and tachycardia. Assessment of the patient for disease control provides guidance for continuing with the dental hygiene appointment.

References

1. Centers for Disease Control and Prevention (CDC). Guidelines for preventing the transmission of Mycobacterium tuberculosis in health care settings, 2005. *MMWR Morb Mortal Wkly Rep.* 2005;54(No. RR-17):1–141.
2. Smith WHR, Mason KD, Davis D, et al. Intraoral and pulmonary tuberculosis following dental treatment. *Lancet.* 1982;8276:842–844.
3. Cleveland JL, Kent J, Gooch BF, et al. Multidrug-resistant *Mycobacterium* tuberculosis in an HIV dental clinic. *Infect Control Hosp Epidemiol.* 1995;16:7–11.
4. Pauwels RA, Rabe KF. Burden and clinical features of chronic obstructive pulmonary disease (COPD). *Lancet.* 2004;364:613–620.
5. Lipworth BJ. Systemic adverse effects of inhaled corticosteroid therapy: A systemic review and meta-analysis. *Arch Intern Med.* 1999;159:941–955.
6. Huber MA, Terezhalmy GT. Risk stratification and dental management of patients with adrenal dysfunction. *Quintessence Int.* 2007;38:325–338.
7. Ingram RH. Chronic bronchitis, emphysema, and airway obstruction. In: Wilson JD, et al., eds. *Harrison's Principles of Internal Medicine.* 12th ed. New York: McGraw-Hill; 1991:1075–1082.

17

Cardiovascular System Drugs

The client with cardiovascular disease (CVD) poses a risk for cardiovascular complications, such as myocardial infarction (MI) and stroke, during oral health care procedures. Many textbooks emphasize that CVD renders an individual less able to respond to stressful situations. In some anxious individuals, stressful situations could include dental hygiene treatment. Elevation in blood pressure has been described in older patients prior to initiation of dental treatment or in the midst of treatment unassociated with administration of local anesthetics. This suggests that endogenous epinephrine precipitates elevated blood pressure and that stress reduction procedures are indicated. This chapter emphasizes the clinical implications when providing dental hygiene care to an individual with CVD. Discussion of adverse drug effects (ADEs) of various CVD drugs includes those side effects relevant to dental hygiene procedures. There are many actions associated with the wide variety of CVD agents, but this chapter focuses on those effects that could influence the treatment plan and those signs that indicate exacerbation of a possible medical emergency while the patient receives dental hygiene care. Pharmacologic effects of CVD agents in relation to local anesthesia administration are highlighted, because many states allow dental hygienists to use local anesthetics, and most include vasoconstrictors.

In the 2005 list of common drugs prescribed in the United States, six cardiovascular agents were in the top 20, indicating that CVD drugs will frequently be reported on the medical history. To provide care to patients with CVD, oral health care providers must understand the disease, the drugs used in medical treatment, and the impact the disease or treatment may have on the patient's ability to undergo and respond to dental care.

CARDIOVASCULAR DISEASE

CVD refers to diseases of the heart and blood vessels. The heart pumps blood through a system of blood vessels under the control of an electric conduction system to deliver oxygen to all cells of the body. When the conduction system malfunctions, arrhythmias occur, and the heart is unable to pump blood through the vascular system at a regular rate and rhythm. When the blood volume becomes greater than the

BOX 17-1. Cardiovascular Diseases

Arrhythmia	Myocardial infarction
Hypertension	Congestive heart failure
Coronary artery disease (angina pectoris)	Thromboembolic disorders
Atherosclerosis/ hyperlipidemia disorders	

BOX 17-2. Activities for Various Levels of Metabolic Equivalents[1]

≥ 1 MET
- Dress, eat, or use the toilet
- Walk indoors around house
- Complete light housework (dusting, washing dishes)
- Walk a block on level ground at 2 to 3 mph

≥ 4 METs
- Climb a flight of stairs, walk up a hill
- Walk on level ground at 4 mph
- Run a short distance
- Complete heavy housework (scrubbing floors, moving heavy furniture)
- Participate in moderate recreational activities (golf, bowling, dancing)

≥ 10 METs
- Strenuous sports (swimming, singles tennis, basketball, skiing)

[1] ACC/American Heart Association (AHA). Guideline update for perioperative cardiovascular evaluation for noncardiac surgery. *J Am Coll Cardiol.* 2002;39(3):542–553.

limited volume capacity of the vascular system, the patient develops hypertension. When the myocardium does not get enough oxygen because of narrowing of or blockage in the coronary arteries, the patient will experience angina pectoris. If oxygen deprivation to the myocardium persists, usually due to blockage by a blood clot, the patient may develop damage to cardiac muscle or MI. When the heart is no longer able to pump enough blood to meet the body's metabolic demands for oxygen, the patient is said to have developed heart failure. Diabetes is a powerful promoter of heart disease, and chronic hyperglycemia is likely to result in atherosclerosis, leading to hypertension, heart attack, stroke, heart failure, and other cardiovascular conditions. Therefore, when diabetes is reported on the health history, the risk for CVD should be considered. In addition, many of the above conditions can lead to **thromboembolic** complications. These CVDs are the leading causes of morbidity and mortality in the United States and in most western countries (Box 17-1). In the United States alone, more than a million annual direct deaths and as many as three times that number of serious consequences can be attributed to these conditions.

Dental Implications of Cardiovascular Disease

The goal of treatment is to develop and implement timely preventive and therapeutic strategies compatible with the patient's physical and emotional ability to undergo and respond to dental care.

Patient Assessment

Clinicians must assess the status of the cardiovascular system within the patient's overall health. Associated conditions (such as hyperlipidemia) can heighten cardiovascular risk during dental care. Consequently, an initial medical history must be obtained from all patients, and it should be reviewed with the patient at each appointment to identify such serious cardiac conditions as hypertension, coronary artery disease (CAD; angina pectoris, recent or past MI), symptomatic arrhythmias, heart failure, cardiomyopathies, and any recent change in signs and symptoms of these disorders. The clinician should also note treatment for dyslipidemia, peripheral vascular disease, cerebrovascular disease, renal dysfunction, chronic pulmonary disease, orthostatic intolerance, diabetes mellitus, and anemia. It should be determined if the patient has a pacemaker or an implanted cardio defibrillator (ICD).

Although antibiotic prophylaxis is not an issue, in this situation certain electrical dental equipment may require special considerations. Epinephrine or other vasoconstrictors should be used with caution in patients with pacemakers and ICDs. An accurate record of current medications taken by the patient is imperative, and the use of tobacco products, alcohol, and over-the-counter and recreational drugs should also be documented. Cardiovascular risk (nonfatal MI, heart failure, and sudden death) in association with noncardiac procedures has been established by multivariate analysis.[1] Cardiac risks in association with noncardiac procedures, such as dental treatment, are increased in patients unable to meet a 4-metabolic-equivalent (MET) demand (e.g., they cannot climb flights of stairs, cannot walk 2 blocks at 4 miles/hour, cannot run short distances; Box 17-2) during normal daily activities.[1] Minor clinical predictors include a history of advanced age, atrial fibrillation, low functional capacity, stroke, and uncontrolled hypertension (>180/110 mm/Hg). Intermediate clinical predictors include stable angina, previous MI (>30 days), compensated heart failure, diabetes mellitus, and renal insufficiency. Major clinical predictors include unstable angina, decompensated heart failure, severe valvular disease, and significant arrhythmias.

Functional Capacity

In the past it was thought that an individual with a history of a recent MI should not have dental treatment for 3 to 6 months following the MI. Recently this recommendation was changed by the American College of Cardiology (ACC) in coordination with the American Heart Association (AHA) Task Force on Practice Guidelines.[1] The revised guidelines recommend the determination of the patient's functional capacity as a reliable indicator of reduced risk in treatment. An individual's capacity to perform a spectrum of common daily tasks has been shown to correlate well with maximum oxygen uptake by treadmill testing. Functional capacity can be expressed in terms of METs. The oxygen consumption of a 70-kg, 40-year-old man in a resting state is 3.5 mL/kg/minute and is defined as 1 MET. Functional capacity can be classified as excellent (>10 METs), good (7 to 10 METs), moderate (4 to 7 METs), and poor (<4 METs).[1] Cardiac risks in association with noncardiac procedures, such as dental treatment, are increased in patients unable to meet a 4-MET demand (for example, they cannot climb flights of stairs, cannot walk 2 blocks at 4 miles/hour, or cannot run a short distance) during normal daily activities.[1] This method represents an important aspect of evaluating the overall cardiac risk for oral health care procedures and, by extension, provides a reasonable approach to assess a patient's physical and emotional ability to undergo comprehensive dental hygiene care. If one or more of the activities in the 4-MET level cannot be accomplished, the patient should be referred for medical evaluation prior to receiving elective oral health care services. A patient who is classified as high risk because of known cardiovascular risk factors but who is asymptomatic, has blood pressure <180/110, and walks at 4 mph for 30 minutes daily may need no further evaluation before initiating dental hygiene procedures. In contrast, a patient with a sedentary lifestyle who has not been diagnosed with CVD but has clinical signs and symptoms (fatigue, dyspnea, and chest pain upon exertion) that suggest cardiac risk may benefit from a preoperative medical consultation. Such a preoperative evaluation may provide the first opportunity for a careful cardiovascular assessment for the patient in years.

Blood Pressure and Pulse

Determination of the blood pressure provides a useful clue from the physical examination that will either confirm or rule out significant CVD. It should be recorded for all new patients at the time of their initial appointments. In clients with histories of any CVD, it should be measured on every appointment. Blood pressure values ≥180/110 contraindicate elective procedures, and the patient should be referred for medical evaluation.

Pulse Rate and Rhythm

The pulse pressure, which closely correlates with the systolic pressure, is a reliable factor that will provide further evidence to either confirm or rule out significant CVD. The "hammering" effect of the pulse pressure damages arterial walls, contributes to arteriosclerosis, and leads to target organ damage. The pulse rate and rhythm should be recorded for all new patients at their initial appointments and at all subsequent appointments for patients with histories of CVDs. The presence of arrhythmia in the preoperative setting should provoke a medical consultation to search for underlying myocardial ischemia or infarction, drug toxicity, or metabolic disorders. In addition, premature ventricular contractions (PVCs), characterized by a pronounced pause in an otherwise normal rhythm, in patients with hypertension, coronary heart disease, congestive heart failure, and valvular disease are significant findings.

The incidence of PVCs can increase with age, fatigue, emotional stress, and the use of coffee and tobacco. They can also be occasional, insignificant findings in healthy adults.

Cardiovascular Disease and Periodontal Disease

It has been documented that patients with CAD tend to suffer from poorer oral health when compared to controls matched by age, gender, and socioeconomic status. It has also been noted that the classic risk factors (hypertension, diabetes mellitus, obesity, smoking, dyslipidemia) associated with coronary disease and stroke account for only one half to two thirds of the cases. Several observational studies suggest a possible link between periodontal disease and CAD. While there is little evidence to suggest that treatment of oral infections reduces ischemic heart disease, current research does suggest that periodontal disease may play a role in the thromboembolic aspect of coronary heart disease. Oral bacteria, such as *S. sanguis* and *P. gingivalis*, may increase the risk of a thromboembolic event via platelet aggregation.

Atherosclerotic changes in coronary arteries produce *ischemic heart disease*, which is the leading cause of sudden death in the United States. Ischemic heart disease predisposes the patient to atrial fibrillation, angina pectoris, and MI. Atherosclerosis may represent a response to injury to the blood vessel walls by mechanical, biochemical, or bacterial insult, including chlamydial infection and severe generalized periodontal disease.

Implications for Oral Health Care

Most individuals with CVD can be treated in the dental office and receive local anesthetic agents. However, a recent diagnosis of CVD or evidence of uncontrolled disease should prompt a physician consultation, with a medical clearance document identifying the procedures to be performed and whether vasoconstrictors are planned for use. There are some CVD conditions that are contraindicated for elective procedures, such as dental hygiene care. These include severe hypertension (blood pressure ≥180/110), a recent history of MI (less than one month) or uncontrolled congestive heart failure resulting in low functional capacity with the individual unable to meet a 4-MET demand, and unstable angina pectoris.

■ Self-Study Review

1. Describe how the medical history is used to assess the status of cardiovascular health. What are major predictors of increased risk in dental hygiene treatment?
2. Describe how to determine the functional capacity of a patient with a history of CVD. What is a *MET*? What is the relevance of 4 METs?
3. How often should blood pressure and pulse be evaluated in a patient with a history of CVD?
4. Identify cardiovascular situations that contraindicate receiving elective oral health care.

Hypertension

Fluid homeostasis is chiefly controlled by the renin–angiotensin–aldosterone system in the kidneys. The juxtaglomerular apparatus in the kidney senses low salt load and low blood pressure. In response, renin is released into the vascular compartment, where it reacts with an enzyme, angiotensinogen, converting it to angiotensin I. Angiotensin I, a weak vasoconstrictor, is then converted to angiotensin II when it combines with the angiotensin-converting enzyme (ACE) that is found naturally in body fluids. Angiotensin II, a powerful vasoconstrictor, also acts on the adrenal cortex to stimulate the production of aldosterone. Aldosterone, in turn, promotes increased uptake of sodium and water and, thus, the volume expansion necessary to restore blood pressure. When homeostatic mechanisms fail and the blood volume becomes greater than the limited volume capacity of the vascular system, the patient develops high blood pressure. The most common form of hypertension is *essential hypertension*. Essential hypertension is relatively common in the United States, and for this reason the American Dental Association recommends that all dental patients have an annual blood pressure measurement at recall appointments as a screening measure to identify hypertensive individuals.[2]

Medical Management of Hypertension

The goals of prevention and management of hypertension are to reduce morbidity and mortality by maintaining systolic blood pressure <140 mm Hg and diastolic pressure <90 mm Hg. Treatment to achieve lower levels may be useful, particularly to prevent stroke, to preserve kidney function, and to prevent or slow the progression to heart failure. While the mainstay of treatment for hypertension is pharmacologic, adoption of a healthy lifestyle is critical for the prevention of high blood pressure, and it is an indispensable part of the management of those with hypertension. Major lifestyle modifications shown to lower blood pressure include aerobic exercise for 30 to 45 minutes, three to five times a week; weight reduction (in overweight and obese individuals); adoption of a diet rich in fruits, vegetables, and low-fat dairy products that are rich in potassium and calcium; reduction of dietary sodium; and moderation of alcohol consumption.[3]

Therapeutic goals and pharmacologic strategies include (a) reducing volume overload, (b) blocking adrenergic receptors in the heart, (c) dilating peripheral blood vessels, and (d) reducing sympathetic outflow from the central nervous system (CNS; Table 17-1). Clinical trial outcome data prove that thiazide-type diuretics, β_1-adrenergic blocking agents, ACE inhibitors, angiotensin II-receptor blocking agents, and calcium channel blocking agents (CCBs) all reduce the complications of hypertension. In 2002, the Antihypertensive and Lipid-lowering Treatment to Prevent Heart Attack Trial (ALLHAT) showed that an inexpensive thiazide diuretic (chlorthalidone) was at least as good at lowering blood pressure and reducing the risk for heart attack and heart-related death as two newer, more expensive drugs (amlodipine, lisinopril).[4] Thiazide diuretics are the initial drugs of choice for most patients with hypertension. If the initial drug at full dose has no effect on the blood pressure or causes troublesome side effects, substituting a drug from a different

Table 17-1	Therapeutic Goals and Pharmacologic Strategies
Therapeutic Goal	**Pharmacologic Strategies**
Reduce volume overload	Diuretics
Block β_1-adrenergic receptors to decrease heart rate and cardiac output	β_1-adrenergic receptor antagonists
Dilate blood vessels	ACE inhibitors Angiotensin II-receptor antagonists Calcium-channel blocking agents Peripheral vasodilators (hydralazine)
Reduce sympathetic outflow from the CNS by blocking or reducing the effect of α_1-receptors	α_1-adrenergic receptor antagonists α_2-adrenergic receptor agonists

class is recommended. If the initial drug produces only a partial response but is well tolerated, adding another drug from a different class is indicated. Most patients with hypertension will require two or more antihypertensive agents to achieve their target blood pressure, especially if the blood pressure is 20/10 mm Hg above goal.[5]

Agents to Lower Blood Pressure

Dozens of drugs are available for lowering blood pressure. Their mechanisms of action are different, but ultimately most have the same effect of causing blood vessels to dilate. Dilation of blood vessels results in lower systolic and diastolic blood pressure. Some also reduce cardiac workload by preventing tachycardia. Table 17-2 illustrates the main classes of antihypertension medications, their mechanisms of action, and some commonly prescribed brands. There are agents used only for hypertension that are not controlled with the more common agents in Table 17-2. These include hydralazine, minoxidil, guanethidine, and reserpine. They are used rarely, but they frequently result in orthostatic hypotension, a complication following supine positioning used in oral health care.

Diuretics

There are three main types of diuretics: (a) thiazide, (b) loop, and (c) potassium sparing.

THIAZIDE DIURETICS. The prototype *thiazide* diuretic is hydrochlorothiazide (HCTZ). Thiazides are among the most common agents used for hypertension, and some individuals can control blood pressure with a thiazide alone, although most people with hypertension must use more than one drug to gain control. The mechanism of action is to interfere with sodium reabsorption in the distal tubule of the kidney and promote diuresis. The most common adverse reaction is *hypokalemia*, or loss of too much potassium. Patients may take potassium supplements (K-Dur) to counteract this effect. Another potential ADE of thiazides is *postural hypotension*. The most significant drug interaction associated with dentistry is that COX-inhibitor (COX-I) analgesics can reduce the antihypertensive effect of thiazides.

Table 17-2	Selected Common Antihypertensive Drugs

Class of Drug	Mechanism	Common Products
Diuretics	Cause body to eliminate excess fluids and sodium through urination	**Thiazides** Chlorothiazide (Diuril) Chlorthalidone (Hygroton) Hydrochlorothiazide **Loop** Furosemide (Lasix) **Potassium-sparing** Spironolactone (Aldactone) Triamterene (Dyrenium) **Combination product** Triamterene/ hydrochlorothiazide (Dyazide, Maxzide)
Beta-blockers (the olols)	Decrease the heart rate and output of blood from the heart by blocking beta-sympathetic stimulation in the heart	**Selective** Atenolol (Tenormin) Bisoprolol (Zebeta) Metoprolol (Lopressor, Toprol-XL) **Nonselective** Nadolol (Corgard) Propranolol (Inderal) **Both alpha- and beta-** Labetalol (Normodyne)
ACE inhibitors (the prils)	Expand blood vessels (vasodilation) and decrease resistance to blood flow	Captopril (Capoten) Enalapril (Vasotec) Lisinopril (Prinivil, Zestril) Ramipril (Altace) Trandolapril (Mavik)
Calcium-channel blockers (the pines)	Interrupt the movement of calcium into the cells of the heart and blood vessels to produce vasodilation	Diltiazem (Cardizem LA, Tiazac) Verapamil (Calan, Isoptin) **Dihydropyridines** Amlodipine (Norvasc, Lotrel) Isradipine (DynaCirc CR) Nifedipine (Adalat, Procardia) Nisoldipine (Sular)
Angiotensin-receptor blockers	Inhibit vasoconstriction by blocking angiotensin binding, resulting in vasodilation	Candesartan (Atacand) Eprosartan (Teveten) Irbesartan (Avapro) Losartan (Cozaar) Valsartan (Diovan)
Alpha-blockers	Prevent sympathetic innervation to alpha-receptors, thereby blocking vasoconstriction and tachycardia	Doxazosin mesylate (Cardura XL) Terazosin (Hytrin) Prazosin hydrochloride (Minipress) **Combination product** Prazosin and polythiazide (Minizide)

LOOP DIURETICS. The most commonly used *loop* diuretic is furosemide (Lasix). Loop diuretics act on the ascending limb of the loop of Henle (hence the name of the class) to inhibit the reabsorption of sodium and promote diuresis. As with thiazides, potassium is often lost and must be replaced with potassium replacement therapy. The most significant ADE is *hyperkalemia*. Furosemide is often used to reduce fluids associated with congestive heart failure. Interaction with COX-I analgesics, as with thiazides, can reduce the antihypertensive effect.

POTASSIUM-SPARING DIURETICS. These are two main drugs in the *potassium-sparing* class, spironolactone and triamterene. This drug group acts at a different site in the kidney than other diuretics. They interfere with the potassium/sodium exchange in the collecting tubules and collecting duct to conserve potassium that is reabsorbed at the expense of sodium in the ex-

change system. Potassium-sparing diuretic/thiazide combination therapy is common, with the most frequently used agent including triamterene and HCTZ (Dyazide, Maxzide).

Beta-Blocking Agents

There are three types of agents in this class: (a) nonselective beta-blockers that block both β_1- and β_2-adrenergic receptors, (b) selective agents that block beta-1 receptors more than beta-2 receptors, and (c) agents that block both alpha- and beta-receptors (labetalol). They are often referred to as the *olols* because most drug names in this category end with that suffix. Nonselective agents cause an increased risk of hypertension when vasoconstrictors are used in local anesthesia. Box 17-3 differentiates the nonselective agents from the selective agents. Selective beta-blockers and alpha-/beta-blockers have less risk with vasoconstrictors. Side effects of drugs in this class include bradycardia, dizziness, fatigue,

BOX 17-3. Beta-blocking Drugs

Selective	Nonselective
Acebutolol	Carteolol
Atenolol	Carvedilol
Betaxolol	Nadolol
Bisoprolol	Pindolol
Esmolol	Propranolol
Metoprolol	Timolol

nausea, and mild xerostomia. COX-I analgesics can antagonize antihypertensive effects.

NONSELECTIVE BETA-BLOCKERS.   The prototype nonselective beta-blocker is *propranolol* (Inderal). When nonselective beta-blockers are reported on the medical history, vasoconstrictors should be used in low concentrations with an aspirating technique, taking care to avoid intravascular injection of the local anesthetic.

SELECTIVE BETA-BLOCKERS.   Because these drugs block beta-1 receptors less than beta-2 receptors (found principally in the bronchioles, and they dilate the bronchioles), they have some advantages. They are the agent of choice for individuals with conditions of bronchospasm (asthma). Also, there is less risk of causing hypertension when vasoconstrictors are used. When doses of a selective beta-blocker are increased, the advantage of safety with vasoconstrictors reduces. The selective beta-blocker should be investigated in a drug reference that identifies the recommended dose. If the patient's dose regimen is higher than that recommended by the manufacturer, the hypertensive risk with a vasoconstrictor remains an issue for consideration.

ALPHA- AND BETA-ADRENERGIC BLOCKING AGENTS.   Labetalol (Normodyne) is a nonselective beta-adrenergic blocking agent that also blocks alpha-receptors. It has the same effects as propranolol with less peripheral resistance via the alpha-blocking action. It may be prescribed in combination with a diuretic. Side effects are similar to those of the beta-blocking class of drugs.

Calcium Channel Blockers

When calcium movement required for contraction of cardiac and vascular smooth muscle is inhibited, vasodilation results. This property makes this class of drugs effective for hypertension, arrhythmia, and angina pectoris management. Some CCBs increase coronary vasodilation to increase blood flow to cardiac muscle, whereas others decrease myocardial contractility, which reduces cardiac output. The choice of the specific CCB depends on the specific disease being managed. One type of CCB is derived from a dihydropyridine structure, and the names of these agents end with the suffix *-pine*. These are the most recent CCBs developed and are the agents most commonly used in this class. Several CCBs, especially nifedipine (Procardia), can cause gingival

hyperplasia, xerostomia, and **dysgeusia**. Amlodipine and isradipine are reported to be less likely to produce gingival hyperplasia, and dentists are encouraged to consult with patients' cardiologists to determine if a medication change to one of these agents can be made when gingival enlargement compromises periodontal health. When gingival enlargement is observed and a CCB is being used, the oral health education plan should include information on effective biofilm removal to reduce the rate of gingival enlargement, and the maintenance schedule should be quarterly rather than twice a year. Teeth should be monitored for caries, and home care should include caries preventive agents. Other side effects are often extensions of the class's pharmacologic effects, including postural hypotension, bradycardia, a "flushing" effect from vasodilation, shortness of breath from pulmonary edema, nausea, and inhibition of platelet function, which increases the tendency to bleed. CCBs are one of the few drug types used to manage hypertension that do not interact with COX-I analgesics, so these drugs can be used to manage pain in the patient taking a CCB.

Angiotensin Inhibitors

Two classes of drugs affect angiotensin receptors to reduce blood pressure. Angiotensin-converting enzyme inhibitors (ACEIs) prevent the formation of angiotensin II (which is a strong vasoconstrictor) by blocking the release of the enzyme responsible for converting angiotensin I to angiotensin II. The other group of agents includes angiotensin-II receptor antagonists, which do not disturb the enzyme levels but block angiotensin-II receptors, preventing vasoconstriction. The angiotensin-II receptor antagonists are considered to be more selective agents with fewer side effects. These agents are commonly prescribed with a diuretic or with an agent from another class of antihypertensives to reduce blood pressure. COX-I can antagonize the antihypertensive effects of this group of agents.

ANGIOTENSIN-CONVERTING ENZYME INHIBITORS.   The names of drugs in this group end with the suffix *-pril*. By blocking vasoconstriction, peripheral resistance and fluid retention, blood pressure is reduced. Cardiac output and heart rate are not affected. ACEIs retard the progression of nephropathy in diabetes and are often the agent of choice for management of hypertension in diabetic patients. Side effects associated with these drugs are similar to other antihypertensives, except ACEIs can produce a dry, hacking cough that worsens in the supine position. This is thought to occur from activation of bradykinin (which produces signs of allergy, including cough), which is usually inactivated by the ACE.

ANGIOTENSIN-II RECEPTOR INHIBITORS.   The prototype angiotensin-II antagonist is *losartan* (Cozaar). When vasoconstriction is blocked, aldosterone secretion is also inhibited. These effects produce lower blood pressure. Side effects are minimal with this group, but they are not to be used during pregnancy (category D, second and third trimester).

Other Antihypertensives

There are several drugs used when the agents discussed above are not successful (alone or in combination therapy). These include α_1-adrenergic blockers (doxazosin, terazosin), agents that reduce blood pressure by a CNS-mediated action (clonidine, guanethidine, and reserpine), and hydralazine. The side effects relevant to dental hygiene practice include postural hypotension, taste disturbance, and xerostomia. These agents are often used in combination therapy.

ALPHA-ADRENERGIC BLOCKERS.   There is a potential drug interaction with epinephrine (which activates both alpha- and beta-receptors) that increases the antihypertensive effects. When alpha-receptors are blocked, this prevents vasoconstriction by epinephrine, reducing duration of local anesthesia. This also allows beta stimulation to prevail (peripheral vasodilation), which can cause severe postural hypotension and, less frequently, reflex tachycardia. COX-I can reduce the antihypertensive effect of alpha-blocking agents.

HYDRALAZINE.   *Hydralazine* acts on arterioles to produce vasodilation. There are few side effects with hydralazine, and it is the drug of choice for hypertension associated with pregnancy. Side effects that influence the dental hygiene treatment plan include orthostatic hypotension and cardiac palpitation. Blood pressure should be monitored at each appointment, and the protocol to prevent orthostatic hypotension should be followed at the end of the appointment.

Adverse Drug Effects

Common side effects include frequent urination with diuretics, fatigue with beta-blockers, chronic dry cough with ACEIs, gingival hyperplasia with some CCBs, and postural hypotension and xerostomia with several classes. Each drug should be investigated in a drug reference for its specific side effects. When multiple agents are included in one formulation, each agent may need to be investigated. Some drug references include combination products in one drug monograph.[6]

Gingival Hyperplasia

CCBs are used extensively for the management of CVD. Nifedipine was the first such drug to be associated with gingival hyperplasia. Subsequent reports have confirmed the association and implicated most other CCBs. Gingival enlargement is usually noted within 1 to 2 months after the initiation of therapy and appears to affect primarily the labial/facial interdental papillae. While the enlarged tissue may be firm and painless, it is often associated with erythematous and edematous chronic inflammation. The patient may report pain, gingival bleeding, and difficulty with mastication due to the hyperplastic tissue. A frequent maintenance schedule and plaque removal via oral hygiene procedures is recommended to reduce the overgrowth of tissue; however, plaque control will not prevent gingival hyperplasia.

Interactions with Drugs Used in Dentistry

Each drug should be investigated in a drug reference for specific drug interactions, but COX-1 inhibitor analgesics can reduce the efficacy of most antihypertensive agents and lead to hypertension. Similarly, a decreased antihypertensive effect of beta-adrenergic blockers (resulting in increased blood pressure) may be anticipated with sympathomimetic amines (epinephrine) because of pharmacologic antagonism.

Nonselective beta-blockers and the concomitant administration of epinephrine may lead to a hypertensive reaction because of unopposed alpha-adrenergic stimulation. When nonselective beta-blocking agents are reported on the health history, the vasoconstrictor in local anesthesia should be in low concentrations (1:100,000 or 1:200,000) with careful monitoring of blood pressure during treatment. Some sources refer to a "cardiac dose" of vasoconstrictor, which is described as no more than two cartridges of 1:100,000 epinephrine or four cartridges of 1:200,000. Conversely, alpha-blockers can result in excessive hypotension if epinephrine is introduced into the vascular system. Pilocarpine (Salagen), used in dentistry to stimulate salivation, may have an additive effect with antihypertensive agents and lead to hypotension.

■ Self-Study Review

5. List four goals in the medical management of hypertension, and identify drugs used to meet each goal.
6. What is the initial drug class of choice to treat hypertension?
7. List three types of diuretics, give examples of drugs in each group and the prototypes, and describe side effects and dental drug interactions for each.
8. List three types of beta-blocking agents, give examples of drugs in each group and the prototypes, and describe side effects and dental drug interactions for each.
9. Identify examples of CCBs, and describe side effects relevant to dental hygiene procedures and dental drug interactions for each.
10. Identify examples of ACEIs, and describe side effects relevant to dental hygiene procedures and dental drug interactions for each.
11. Identify examples of angiotensin-II blocking agents and the prototypes for this class, and describe side effects relevant to dental hygiene procedures and dental drug interactions for each.
12. Identify side effects relevant to dental hygiene procedures for other antihypertensives.
13. Which agent is best for hypertension associated with pregnancy?

Coronary Artery Disease

The heart is a muscle referred to as the *myocardium*. Atherosclerosis, a complication of dyslipidemia and hypertension, causes CAD. CAD impedes the supply of oxygenated blood when there is an increased demand for oxygen in cardiac muscle. The factors that increase the oxygen demand of the heart are heart rate, vascular wall tension, and contractile state. The faster the heart rate, the more oxygen it utilizes. The larger the heart, the more oxygen it requires for

Table 17-3	Therapeutic Goals and Pharmacologic Strategies

Therapeutic Goal	Pharmacologic Strategies

Inhibit progression of atherosclerosis	Lipid-lowering agents
	   HMG-Co-A reductase inhibitors
	   Bile acid sequestrants
	   Niacin, others

Improve circulation in coronary arteries	Nitrates Calcium channel blocking agents
Reduce workload	β_1-adrenergic receptor antagonists
Prevent thrombus formation	Antithrombotic agents
Prevent coagulation (Warfarin)	Anticoagulants (Warfarin)

BOX 17-4. HMG CoA Inhibitor Drugs

- Atorvastatin (Lipitor)
- Fluvastatin (Lescol)
- Lovastatin (Mevacor)
- Pravastatin (Pravachol)
- Rosuvastatin (Crestor)
- Simvastatin (Zocor)

contraction. The greater the force of myocardial contraction, the greater the amount of oxygen consumed. Myocardial hypoxia or anoxia is due primarily to narrowing of the coronary arteries due to atherosclerosis. If there is a temporary deficiency of oxygen (ischemia) to a portion of the myocardium, painful coronary insufficiency occurs. This event is described as an *attack of angina pectoris*. When the deficient supply of oxygen to a portion of the myocardium is permanent, necrosis develops and MI occurs.

Medical Management of Coronary Artery Disease

While the mainstay of treatment for ischemic heart disease is pharmacologic with vasodilating agents, such lifestyle modifications as smoking cessation, dietary control, and increased exercise are also important. The goals of pharmacologic intervention in the management of CAD (Table 17-3) are to control symptoms and reduce mortality by preventing formation, slowing progression, and causing regression of atherosclerotic lesions; improve coronary circulation; reduce the workload of the heart; and prevent thromboembolic episodes.[7–9] The dental hygienist should consider that the patient taking drugs for CAD is at an increased risk for cardiovascular emergencies and should follow a protocol to reduce stress associated with oral health care procedures. Limiting the dose of epinephrine to 0.04 mg (one cartridge 1:50,000, two cartridges 1:100,000, etc.) may be warranted in some clients.

Lipid-Lowering Agents

Elevated levels of cholesterol, low-density lipoproteins (LDLs), and triglycerides are considered to be significant risk factors for CAD, leading to stroke, MI, and hypertension. Lowering cholesterol levels can arrest or reverse atherosclerosis in vascular beds and can significantly decrease the morbidity and mortality associated with atherosclerosis.[8] Excessive levels over time promotes *atherosclerosis*, the formation of fatty deposits within the blood vessel walls. Both cholesterol and triglycerides play a role in this plaque formation, and most cholesterol-reducing agents also reduce triglyceride levels. The cholesterol content of the liver is derived mainly from three sources: It can synthesize cholesterol, take up cholesterol from the lipoproteins in circulating blood, or take up

cholesterol absorbed by the small intestine. Intestinal cholesterol is derived primarily from cholesterol in bile and from dietary cholesterol. The current recommendation is to have total cholesterol levels <200 mg/dL, and to reduce LDL levels to <130. Individuals with established CVD should have a goal to reduce their LDL levels to <100. Protective high-density lipoprotein (HDL) levels should be ≥35 mg/dL. There are several agents that lower cholesterol levels, and each has a different mechanism of action.

HMG CoA Reductase Inhibitors

HMG CoA reductase inhibitors are the most widely used class of anticholesterol drugs. They are commonly referred to as *statins*. This class contains such drugs as atorvastatin (Lipitor), lovastatin (Mevacor), pravastatin (Pravachol), simvastatin (Zocor), rosuvastatin (Crestor), and fluvastatin (Lescol). In 2006, Lipitor was the most commonly prescribed drug in the United States. Agents in this class lower cholesterol levels by interfering with cholesterol synthesis in the liver. Box 17-4 illustrates agents in this popular class of drugs. Some of the drugs in this class can interact with azole antifungals (lovastatin) and macrolide antibacterials (erythromycin, clarithromycin), which reduce the metabolism of the anticholesterol agent and increase blood levels and ADEs, such as myopathy. If azole antifungals are needed, consultation with the physician to reduce the cholesterol-lowering agent is recommended. The dentist should avoid prescribing macrolide antibiotics. The side effect profile for each agent varies, and a drug reference should be used to investigate a specific drug. These agents are generally well tolerated, and ADEs are usually mild and do not affect the dental hygiene treatment plan.

Bile Acid Sequestrants

Agents in the *bile acid sequestrant* class include cholestyramine (Questran, Prevalite), colesevelam (WelChol), and colestipol (Colestid). Bile acids contain high levels of cholesterol. These agents bond with bile in the intestine to form an insoluble complex (not absorbed into the systemic circulation) that is excreted in the feces. They are sometimes used in conjunction with HMG CoA reductase inhibitors. There are no interactions with drugs used in dentistry, but these agents may delay or reduce the absorption of other oral medications (such as COX-1 inhibitors, penicillins, tetracyclines, or corticosteroids); when the dentist prescribes any of these oral agents, the patient should be instructed to take the drug 1 hour before or 4 to 6 hours after a bile acid sequestrant. The side effect profile is similar to that of the placebo in trials.

Fibric Acid Derivatives

Agents in the *fibric acid derivative* class are used to lower both cholesterol and triglycerides and to increase HDL levels; they include gemfibrozil (Lopid) and fenofibrate (TriCor). They inhibit synthesis and increase clearance of LDL cholesterol and reduce triglyceride levels by decreasing hepatic extraction of free fatty acids. The mechanism for increased HDL levels is unknown. There are no interactions with drugs used in dentistry, and the side effect profile is mild, mainly involving dyspepsia, abdominal pain, and diarrhea.

Niacin

Nicotinic acid (Niacor) produces a 10% to 20% reduction in total and LDL cholesterol, a 30% to 70% reduction in triglycerides, and an average 20% to 35% increase in HDL cholesterol. The mechanism by which nicotinic acid exerts these effects is unclear, but it may involve several actions, including decreased esterification of hepatic triglycerides. It is formulated in an extended release product (Niaspan) and is included in a combination product with lovastatin (Advicor). The product is to be taken with meals to avoid gastrointestinal (GI) upset. It can cause orthostatic hypotension, which should be considered following dental hygiene care performed in a supine position, because there is a warning to avoid a sudden change in posture. There are no drug interactions with drugs used in dentistry.

Other Agents

Ezetimibe (Zetia), a new agent, was approved by the Food and Drug Administration (FDA) in 2002. It reduces blood cholesterol by inhibiting the absorption of cholesterol from the small intestine. It does not inhibit cholesterol synthesis in the liver or increase bile acid excretion. Instead, it appears to act at the surface of the small intestines to inhibit absorption of cholesterol, leading to a decrease in plasma cholesterol and delivery of cholesterol to the liver, thereby reducing stored cholesterol. Ezetimibe has no clinically meaningful effect on plasma concentrations of fat-soluble vitamins (A, D, E). This drug is complementary to the action of the statin class of anticholesterol agents. A new product (Vytorin) is a combination of ezetimibe and simvastatin. The side effect profile is similar to that of the placebo, and there are no reported drug interactions with drugs used in dentistry.

Plant stanol esters are found as additives in various food products (Benecol and others) and are effective in reducing cholesterol levels; however, they are less efficacious than prescription products.

Vasodilating Agents

Anginal pain is most commonly due to a narrowing of a major coronary artery by atherosclerosis or a blood clot. Spasm of the coronary arteries can produce a variant angina. When a history of angina pectoris is reported, the patient should be questioned to determine the medical therapy and control of the disorder. There are two fast-acting agents (amyl nitrite, nitroglycerin) for the immediate relief of angina pectoris, and other longer-acting formulations are used for the prevention and treatment of angina pectoris (isosorbide dinitrate, isosorbide mononitrate, CCBs). The fast-acting products are discussed more fully in Chapter 12.

Nitroglycerin

Nitroglycerin is a common vasodilator used to manage anginal pain. Patients with a history of angina pectoris are usually prescribed a sublingual (SL) formulation (spray [Nitrolingual] or tablet [Nitrostat, NitroTab]) to carry with them at all times. A transdermal ointment formulation is used to prevent angina. An intravenous formulation is available for hospital use. Therapeutic doses may reduce systolic, diastolic, and mean arterial blood pressure. Heart rate is usually slightly increased as a compensatory response to the fall in blood pressure. Should an emergency develop during oral health care, it is advisable to use the patient's prescription. Headache and hypotension are the most common ADEs, but there are a wide variety of possible side effects. During the drug review process, those side effects that may impact the dental hygiene appointment should be investigated (such as cardiovascular, CNS, GI, or xerostomia).

Isosorbide Mononitrate or Dinitrate

Isosorbide mononitrate and *isosorbide dinitrate* are used to prevent and treat angina caused by CAD; however, because the onset of action is significantly slower than that of SL nitroglycerin, neither is the first drug of choice for acute angina. These are supplied as capsules, extended-release tablets, or SL tablets. There are no interactions with drugs used in dentistry, but blood pressure should be monitored when general anesthetics are used due to additive hypotensive effects.

Dental Hygiene Considerations

Patients with CAD can receive dental hygiene care if a 4-MET level of functional capacity is met. Appointments should be kept short and minimally stressful. Endogenous adrenalin levels peak during morning hours, and the majority of sudden cardiac arrests occur in the morning. Consequently, early afternoon appointments are recommended. Profound local anesthesia should eliminate pain and reduce stress-related cardiac events. However, if angina occurs during dental treatment, the procedure should be terminated and the patient placed in a semisupine position, with 100% oxygen provided and sublingual nitroglycerin administered. Pain that persists after SL nitroglycerin and a 10-minute time period (or if diaphoresis, nausea, vomiting, syncope, or hypertension develops) is an indication of sudden cardiac insufficiency or MI. The emergency medical service should be contacted for immediate transportation of the patient to the hospital. Oxygen should be administered to the patient during the entire management procedure, and a 325-mg aspirin should be chewed. If the heart stops beating, application of automatic external cardio-defibrillation equipment should be used, followed by CPR as needed.

■ Self-Study Review

14. Describe the role of CAD in reduced cardiac function and ischemia.
15. Identify classes of drugs used to lower lipids and reduce atherosclerosis. Give examples of drugs in each class.

16. Identify recommended cholesterol levels.
17. List dental drug interactions with anticholesterol drugs, and describe patient recommendations when bile acid sequestrants are used and penicillin is prescribed.
18. What is an ADE with niacin relevant to dental hygiene procedures?
19. Identify long-acting vasodilators used to prevent angina and their relevance to the treatment plan.
20. Identify dental hygiene considerations for managing the patient with CAD.

Cardiac Arrhythmia

The primary pacemaker of the heart is the *sinoatrial* (SA) node. Under the influence of the autonomic nervous system, the SA node generates electrical impulses at regular intervals to control heart rate with a frequency of 60 to 100 beats/minute. The impulses spread rapidly through the atria and enter the *atrioventricular* (AV) node. After a brief delay at the AV node, the impulses propagate over the His-Purkinje system as depolarization progresses over the ventricles. Interruption of this system from arrhythmia compromises tissue oxygenation and may lead to death. Cardiovascular causes include myocardial ischemia, bradycardia, hypertensive heart disease, valvar heart disease, increased sympathetic activity, and congestive heart failure. It is well known that the initial sign preceding MI is arrhythmia. Abnormal impulse generation or abnormal impulse conduction can lead to arrhythmia, also called *dysrhythmia*. A disturbance in the rhythm of the heart may manifest as bradyarrhythmia (or bradycardia, slow rhythm) or tachyarrhythmia (or tachycardia, rapid rhythm).[10]

Medical Management of Arrhythmia

The goals for treatment of the various cardiac arrhythmias are to restore synchronous myocardial contraction and to prevent thromboembolic episodes (Table 17-4). A variety of different agents are used to achieve these goals.

Antiarrhythmic Agents

Antiarrhythmic agents are divided into four classes, with a miscellaneous class. Box 17-5 illustrates the available drugs in this group. Many of these antiarrhythmic drugs are used to treat other CVDs. Therefore, the dental hygienist should question the patient to determine why the specific agent is being taken. Agents used to prevent clot formation are also effective in preventing cardiac arrhythmia.

Adverse Drug Events
The drugs used to manage cardiac arrhythmias may also induce ADEs. The ADEs are related to specific drugs; however, xerostomia, gingival enlargement, and blood dyscrasias are possible.

Drug Interactions
Increased CNS effects (such as dizziness and anxiety) are possible when local anesthetics (lidocaine-additive CNS de-

Table 17-4	Therapeutic Goals and Pharmacologic Strategies

Therapeutic Goal	Pharmacologic Strategies
Restore synchronous myocardial contraction	Class I antiarrhythmic agents Make cardiac cell membrane less permeable to the influx of sodium ion, and slow depolarization and repolarization. Class II antiarrhythmic agents Block β_2-adrenergic receptors and slow depolarization, lengthen AV conduction, reduce cardiac contractility, and slow the heart rate. Class III antiarrhythmic agents Inhibit potassium and sodium channels and prolong both repolarization and the refractory period. Class IV antiarrhythmic agents Slow influx of calcium ions and slow depolarization, repolarization, and AV conduction. Unclassified Decrease conduction velocity primarily at the AV node.
Prevent thrombus formation	Antithrombotic agents
Prevent coagulation	Anticoagulants

pression) are used in the individual taking propafenone. Use of the lowest dose necessary is advised. Vasoconstrictors may adversely interact with digoxin and nonselective beta-adrenergic blocking drugs. Most studies indicate that local anesthetics containing vasoconstrictors are desirable to obtain profound anesthesia and reduce bleeding, but quantities should be limited. With careful adherence to safety principles, local anesthetics with vasoconstrictors can be given when arrhythmia is reported on the medical history. Most patients can safely tolerate epinephrine, but patient response can be widely variable and careful monitoring is indicated. Epinephrine or other vasoconstrictors are contraindicated in intractable arrhythmias and should be used with caution in patients with pacemakers and ICDs.[11,12]

Dental Hygiene Considerations

Patients with normal pulse pressure rate and rhythm can undergo oral health care procedures and receive vasoconstrictors. During vital sign assessment, the regularity and rate of the pulse should be evaluated for disease control. Local anesthetics with vasoconstrictors can be used in low concentrations (1:100,000 or 1:200,000). Recurrent supraventricular and ventricular tachyarrhythmias are being managed by implantation of automatic cardioverter defibrillators, often in combination with single- or dual-chamber pacemakers.[11] The AHA does not recommend antibiotic prophylaxis coverage for these devices. Because agents come from a variety of drug classifications, the specific drug should be investigated for side effects and the patient questioned to determine if there is a relevance to the dental hygiene appointment.

BOX 17-5. Antiarrhythmic Drugs

Class I	Disopyramide (Norpace)	Mexiletine (Mexitil)
	Procainamide (Pronestyl)	Flecainide (Tambocor)
	Quinidine (Quinaglute)	Moricizine (Ethmozine)
	Lidocaine (Xylocaine)	Propafenone (Rythmol)
	Tocainide (Tonocard)	Phenytoin (Phenytek, Dilantin)
Class II	Propranolol (Inderal)	
	Esmolol (Brevibloc)	
	Acebutolol (Sectral)	
Class III	Amiodarone (Cordarone)	
	Bretylium (generic)	
	Sotalol (Betapace)	
Class IV	Verapamil (Calan)	
Miscellaneous	Digoxin (Lanoxin)	
	Adenosine (Adenoscan)	

Table 17-5 Therapeutic Goals and Pharmacologic Strategies

Therapeutic Goal	Pharmacologic Strategies
Prevent thrombus formation	Antithrombotic agents Aspirin Clopidogrel (Plavix)
Prevent coagulation	Anticoagulants Warfarin (Coumadin) Heparin

As with most cardiovascular drugs, blood pressure and pulse changes plus postural hypotension are possible. Functional capacity should be assessed and dental hygiene care provided if the client can meet a 4-MET demand.

Thromboembolytic Complications of Cardiovascular Disease

Coagulation is the normal process when an event disrupts the integrity of a blood vessel. This protective process is called *hemostasis* and is designed to prevent blood loss due to breakage of blood vessel integrity. When the clotting mechanism overacts, a clot may form within the vessel, impairing blood flow to tissues. A blood clot, or *thrombus*, that forms in a blood vessel or heart chamber may be either arterial or venous in origin. The formation of an arterial thrombus begins when platelets aggregate (clump together) and become surrounded by fibrin and erythrocytes. Eventually, arterial thrombi, like atherosclerotic plaques, can occlude blood vessels and cause tissue ischemia. Venous thrombi develop in areas of slow blood flow. The clot forms rapidly and lacks the organization of the arterial thrombus. Although venous occlusion does occur, a far greater concern is the tendency of small emboli to detach from venous thrombi (often in the legs), move through the large vessels of the cardiovascular system, and wedge into small pulmonary arteries, preventing deoxygenated blood from entering that portion of the lung.

Arterial thrombi contribute to a variety of complications:

- transient ischemic attacks and stroke
- occlusion of coronary artery grafts
- coronary artery rethrombosis after treatment to remove clots

- MI and death in unstable angina
- increased incidence of periprocedural MI in patients who are undergoing coronary angioplasty
- mural thrombosis (blood clot in the heart wall) after MI
- recurrent MI

Arterial thrombi can also contribute to systemic embolism in patients with prosthetic heart valves, or atrial fibrillation and death in patients with valvular heart disease. Venous thrombi are responsible for venous thrombosis and pulmonary embolism, whereas arterial thrombi are responsible for blood clots in the brain (stroke).

Anticoagulant therapy is frequently administered for patients with prosthetic cardiac valves as well as thromboembolic disease.

Medical Management

The goals of treatment are to reduce morbidity and mortality from thromboembolic events (Table 17-5). Antithrombotic agents are generally effective for this goal. Oral anticoagulants, such as warfarin (Coumadin), are effective in the primary and secondary prevention of venous thromboembolism; in the prevention of systemic embolism in patients with prosthetic heart valves or atrial fibrillation; and in the prevention of stroke, recurrent infarction, and death in patients with valvular heart disease. Heparin is effective in the prevention and treatment of venous thrombosis and pulmonary embolism, in the prevention of thrombosis after MI, in the treatment of patients with unstable angina and a history of acute MI, and in the prevention of recurrent thrombosis in coronary arteries.

Antithrombotic Agents

The two main drugs used to reduce intravascular clotting are aspirin and clopidogrel (Plavix). Aspirin is used in the low-dose formulation (81 mg), or one 325-mg tablet is sometimes used (cheaper, but no more efficacious). Clopidogrel (75 mg once daily) is an antiplatelet agent that acts similar to aspirin in that it affects the ability of the platelets to clump together. It is prescribed for those who cannot tolerate aspirin. Both aspirin and clopidogrel increase the bleeding time but do not alter the prothrombin time (PT) or the international normalized ratio (INR). There is no contraindication for dental hygiene treatment when aspirin or clopidogrel is taken, and no medical consultation is recommended; however, during any procedure that causes bleeding in the oral cavity, the area should be monitored to ensure formation of a clot and to identify excessive bleeding.

Clopidogrel

Clopidogrel is an antiplatelet agent that inhibits platelet aggregation induced by adenosine diphosphate, thereby reducing ischemic events. Clopidogrel, in combination with aspirin, produces an additive effect, prevents a range of ischemic coronary events (such as severe refractory ischemia, MI, and heart failure), and creates a trend toward fewer ischemic strokes. The use of clopidogrel in addition to aspirin was associated with an increased risk of bleeding; however, there were not significantly more patients with episodes of life-threatening bleeding or hemorrhagic strokes. There is no reliable test to monitor bleeding when clopidogrel is taken.

Anticoagulants

This group of agents includes two main drug groups: Heparin, given by injection, and warfarin (Coumadin), administered by mouth (tablet). Heparin is used in hospitals, but there is a group of low-molecular-weight heparins (LMWHs; Box 17-6) recently introduced for use by the patient at home (subcutaneous injection in abdomen) following joint replacement surgery or abdominal surgery. The indication is to reduce deep vein thrombosis leading to pulmonary embolism. These low-molecular-weight products would be the most likely heparins reported on the medical history, so they are discussed in this chapter. Warfarin is commonly prescribed, alone or in combination with clopidogrel.

Low-Molecular-Weight Heparin

There are three LMWH products available; however, two main agents are available for home use (dalteparin and enoxaparin). These products work by inhibiting Factor X_a and thrombin activity so that fibrinogen cannot be converted to fibrin. The main ADE is excessive bleeding, but the risk is minimal. The effect of heparin is monitored by the laboratory test of activated partial thromboplastin time (aPTT). ADEs are medically monitored by complete blood count (CBC) and platelet count (to identify development of thrombocytopenia). The dental hygienist should monitor for excessive bleeding during treatment and, if suspected, apply digital pressure over the area affected. When the area stops bleeding, treatment can resume. Drugs that affect hemostasis (such as aspirin, ibuprofen, naproxen, or ketorolac) should not be taken when LMWHs are used due to the increased risk of bleeding. Acetaminophen is a safer alternative.

BOX 17-6.   Low-Molecular-Weight Heparins

- Dalteparin sodium (Fragmin)
- Enoxaparin sodium (Lovenox)
- Tinzaparin sodium (Innohep)

Warfarin

Warfarin works differently from heparin. It resembles vitamin K in its structure and acts to interfere with the synthesis of several vitamin-K-clotting factors, including thrombin (factors II, VII, IX, and X) in the liver. The most serious ADE is excessive bleeding. Serum levels of clotting factors are monitored via a corrected prothrombin time, called the INR. Normal INR value is 1, while therapeutic doses of warfarin sustain the INR between 2 and 3.5. When warfarin therapy is initiated, it takes 12 to 36 hours for the effect to develop to therapeutic levels. Conversely, when periodontal débridement/deep scaling is planned and the physician decides to reduce the warfarin dosage to levels at which excessive bleeding would not occur, it takes 3 days for the clotting factors to develop. It has been determined that subgingival scaling/débridement can safely be performed when the INR is ≤ 3.5.[13]

Therefore, oral procedures involving bleeding should be scheduled 3 days following the dose reduction (if determined by the physician), and the INR lab test should be completed immediately prior to the oral procedure. Therapeutic INR levels are often kept at levels resulting in no contraindication for dental hygiene procedures; however, a patient taking warfarin should be encouraged to bring his or her latest INR value when an appointment is scheduled. When the INR is not recent or is unavailable, the patient should be asked if the dose was lowered at the last laboratory assessment. If the dose was reduced, the dental hygiene procedure should be scheduled several days to a week after the dose reduction because of the latent time to drug effect and recovery of clotting levels. The information related to this investigation should be recorded in the treatment record as verification of the follow-up and decision to provide treatment.

DRUG INTERACTIONS.   Drugs used in dentistry that can increase the INR level when warfarin is taken include COX-1 inhibitors and some antibiotics. Phenobarbital can increase warfarin metabolism and reduce the anticoagulant effect. Short-term acetaminophen or opioid analgesics without aspirin can be used when analgesia is indicated.

Other Anticoagulants

The drug dipyridamole (Persantine) is used in individuals following replacement of prosthetic heart valves. It inhibits platelet adhesion and prolongs the life of platelets that can be damaged due to mechanical destruction when platelets contact the mechanical valve. It does not add additional reduction in clotting when aspirin or warfarin is being taken, so it does not affect bleeding related to dental hygiene treatment. Dipyridamole is combined with 25 mg of aspirin (Aggrenox) to reduce the risk of stroke in patients who have had transient ischemia of the brain or ischemic stroke due to thrombosis.

Dental Hygiene Considerations

Agents that affect platelet adhesiveness, such as clopidogrel, will not result in excessive bleeding requiring blood tests prior to dental hygiene care. Warfarin users should be monitored for INR levels ≥ 3.5 for dental hygiene procedures. If uncontrolled bleeding develops, digital pressure, augmented with local hemostatic measures as needed, can be used to induce clotting. Application of topical clotting agents, such as

Gelfoam, oxidized cellulose, thrombin, or synthetic collagen, can be used. Oral rinsing with tranexamic acid can promote postsurgical hemostasis when warfarin is taken, although it is costly and is not a usual drug in the dental emergency kit. Aspirin is often used in combination with anticoagulant therapy. Aspirin in doses of 81 to 325 mg/day will not significantly alter bleeding time and are unlikely to cause prolonged bleeding. Patients taking higher doses are at risk for prolonged postoperative bleeding following periodontal therapy, and bleeding should be monitored. Discontinuing aspirin therapy for 1 to 2 weeks prior to periodontal procedures will allow normal platelet aggregation. This strategy should be advised only after consultation with the physician, unless the patient is self-administering aspirin.

■ Self-Study Review

21. Identify drugs used in the medical management of *arrhythmia*.
22. List dental drugs that interact with antiarrhythmics, and describe their interactions.
23. Identify complications of *arterial* thrombi and of *venous* thrombi.
24. Identify drugs used to manage intravascular thrombosis and describe their mechanisms of action.
25. Identify the analgesic that should be recommended when LMWHs are used.
26. Which lab test should be obtained when warfarin is taken? What is the safe level for dental hygiene procedures?
27. Identify the action and use of *dipyridamole*.

Heart Failure

Cardiac muscle contraction is under the regulatory control of the autonomic nervous system. On a cellular level, the combination of a catecholamine with its membrane-bound β_1-adrenergic receptor activates the enzyme adenylate cyclase. The resulting cascade of events promotes increased myocardial contraction by facilitating transmembrane calcium flux. In cardiac muscle, the β_1-adrenergic pathway can therefore be characterized as a series of events that begins with the combination of a beta-1 agonist with a receptor and concludes with an increase in muscle contraction. Consequently, in patients with normal heart function, the pumping action of the left and right sides of the heart complement each other and produce a continuous flow of oxygenated blood to the tissues. When the heart is no longer able to pump an adequate supply of blood to meet the metabolic needs of tissues, heart failure (HF; a state of circulatory stasis) follows. HF is also referred to as congestive heart failure (CHF) or, more specifically, *right-sided* CHF and *left-sided* CHF. Edema in the lower legs is a classic sign of right-sided CHF. **Orthopnea** is a sign of left-sided CHF. *Orthopnea* refers to edema that develops in the lungs. This occurs as a complication of inefficient contraction of the chambers of the left side of the heart, leaving blood in the left ventricle and "backing up"

blood flow into the left atrium coming from the pulmonary tissues. The resulting "congestion" in the lungs gives rise to the term *congestive heart failure*. Most of those affected develop both right- and left-sided CHF.

Medical Management

While the mainstay of treatment for HF is pharmacologic, an essential part of management involves lifestyle modifications. These include avoiding excessive fluid intake, avoiding ethyl alcohol intake, and using spices and herbs instead of sodium chloride (salt) to flavor food. Patients should also avoid exposure to heavy air pollution. Air-conditioning is essential for patients with HF who live in a hot and humid environment. Regular physical activity, such as walking or dancing, should be encouraged in patients with mild to moderate HF to improve functional capacity and to decrease symptoms.

The pharmacologic management of HF is aimed at the identification and correction of both the underlying disorder and the precipitating factors. Specific goals include a reduction of cardiac workload and myocardial oxygen consumption, improvement in cardiac muscle contractility, control of sodium and fluid retention, increased peripheral tissue perfusion and oxygenation, and prevention of thromboembolic episodes (Table 17-6).

Agents Used for the Treatment of Heart Failure

All of the agents used to treat HF have been discussed except for cardiac glycosides, found in plants (foxglove) and on the skin of the common toad. *Cardiac glycosides* increase the force of cardiac muscle contraction (inotropic effect) to improve cardiac output and the amount of blood leaving the left ventricle. Agents in this class include digitalis, digitoxin, and digoxin. The most commonly used agent of the group is digoxin (Lanoxin). The improved force of myocardial contraction allows the heart to work more efficiently as a pump. Heart size decreases, and systemic circulation improves tissue perfusion and reduces edema. In 2005, the FDA approved the only combination drug specifically for African American individuals with heart failure, a combination of isosorbide dinitrate and hydralazine hydrochloride (BiDil).

Table 17-6	Therapeutic Goals and Pharmacologic Strategies

Therapeutic Goal	Pharmacologic Strategies
Reduce workload	Diuretics ACE inhibitors β_1-adrenergic receptor antagonists Vasodilators
Improve myocardial contractility	Cardiac glycosides
Prevent thrombus formation	Antithrombotic agents
Prevent coagulation	Anticoagulants

Digoxin

There is a variety of ADEs with digoxin, and it has generally been replaced with safer drugs, such as carvedilol (Coreg), a beta-adrenergic blocking agent. The ADEs occur as a result of the very narrow margin of safety of the drug. Blood levels are monitored frequently to reduce the possibility of overdose (toxicity). Toxicity can develop due to changes in dose level, metabolism, or absorption of digoxin. Digitalis toxicity is relatively common, and the dental hygiene clinician should be alert for evidence of toxicity. GI effects (nausea, vomiting, gagging, increased salivation, or anorexia) are usually the first sign of toxicity; other signs include fatigue, dizziness, and altered cardiac rhythm.[11] Dose reduction resolves these effects.

DRUG INTERACTIONS. Drugs used in dentistry that may increase digoxin serum levels include benzodiazepines, itraconazole, erythromycin, clarithromycin, and tetracyclines. Concurrent use of sympathomimetics with digoxin can increase the risk of cardiac arrhythmia; therefore, use of a 1:200,000 vasoconstrictor formulation is advised.

Dental Hygiene Considerations

Heart failure is associated with pulmonary congestion and venous hypertension. Patients have various levels of functional capacity that must be assessed before providing treatment. The presence of increasing dyspnea at rest indicates poor functional capacity. Elective treatment for patients with poor functional capacity should be delayed until their conditions have been stabilized with medical treatment. Medical consultation is indicated prior to treatment in those with pulmonary congestion and dyspnea. Placing the patient in a supine position may allow peripheral blood to return to the central circulation and overwhelm the decompensated myocardium, resulting in orthopnea.[11] Because GI effects can also occur in some individuals with therapeutic levels of digoxin, semiupright chair positioning should be implemented for dental hygiene care. Appointments should be kept short, and the dental chair kept in a semisupine or erect position according to the patient's needs. Appropriate sedatives should be considered for the anxious patient, and supplemental oxygen should be readily available.

Cardiac Risk During Dental Procedures

There are no adequately controlled or randomized clinical trials that help define the process of stratifying cardiac risk for various dental procedures. However, a recent study provides some evidence that dental procedures in general are comparable in cardiac risk stratification to a spectrum of medical procedures (dermatology, neurology, obstetrics and gynecology, occupational medicine, ophthalmology, otolaryngology, physical therapy and rehabilitation, radiology, psychiatry, surgical specialties, and urology) provided in an ambulatory setting.[14] According to this study, in Seattle and King counties, Washington, with a combined population of 1.5 million (based on the 1990 census), over a period of 7 years (1990–1996), six cardiac arrests were documented in 9,707 community-based dental practices for an annual incidence of <0.002 cardiac arrests/dental practice/year (note: per dental *practice*, not per *dentist*). Based on this evidence,

it can be concluded that dental procedures generally have low or very low cardiac risks.

Local Anesthesia with a Vasoconstrictor

The selection of a local anesthetic agent and the type and concentration of the vasoconstrictor, particularly in the management of patients with CVDs, is a topic of considerable debate. To resolve some of the controversy related to the use of local anesthetic agents containing a vasoconstrictor, investigators in a recent study started with the proven premise that functional capacity is a simple and reliable index to estimate cardiac function.[15] They evaluated the cardiovascular effects of infiltration anesthesia compared with those produced by ergometric exercising. The hemodynamic effects of infiltration anesthesia with 0.045 mg of epinephrine were found to be less than those produced by ergometric-stress testing at 25 watts in young patients and at 15 watts in older subjects. Based on this report, 4.5 cc of a local dental anesthetic agent with epinephrine 1:100,000 (approximately two cartridges) can be administered safely to patients whose functional capacity is ≥4 METs. In this study, there were no differences in hemodynamic responses (evaluated by echocardiography) between normotensive and hypertensive patients. This observation is useful, because elevated blood pressure is a common marker for CAD, and structural coronary arterial abnormalities, their consequences, and hypertension-induced hypertrophic cardiomyopathy are the cause of 90% to 95% of arrhythmias that lead to sudden death.

■ Self-Study Review

28. Describe the drugs used to manage signs of HF and their actions.
29. Describe the ADEs of *digoxin*.
30. Identify the local anesthetic/vasoconstrictor recommendation when digoxin is taken.
31. Describe the cardiac risk during oral health care procedures.
32. Discuss the limitations of local anesthetics with vasoconstrictors in patients with CVD.

DENTAL HYGIENE APPLICATIONS

Because stress is a factor in cardiovascular emergencies during oral health care, the dental hygienist must employ procedures to reduce stress (such as pain reduction, establishing trust and rapport, not making the client wait excessively in the waiting room). The patient's functional capacity should meet a 4-MET level of ability before elective procedures are provided. Blood pressure should be measured at each appointment when CVD is reported to assess disease control. Local anesthetics with low concentrations of vasoconstrictors are useful to reduce pain associated with oral health care procedures and can be used in most individuals with CVD. Vasoconstrictors are contraindicated in patients with some arrhythmias, excessive blood pressure (≥180/110), and

BOX 17-7. Dental Hygiene Implications for Cardiovascular Disease

1. Take care to reduce stress levels and pain associated with treatment.
2. Plan afternoon appointments when blood pressure is lowest.
3. Monitor vital signs at each appointment to assess disease control.
4. Assess functional capacity; the patient must meet a 4-MET level to receive treatment.
5. Investigate drug effects and monitor accordingly (postural hypotension, gingival hyperplasia, excessive salivation, gagging, degree of anticoagulation, etc.).
6. Local anesthesia with vasoconstrictors can be used in low concentrations using an aspirating syringe, except with blood pressures ≥180/110, serious arrhythmias, or unstable angina.
7. Inform the patient about the value of periodontal health when CVD exists.

unstable angina pectoris. They should be used in low concentrations and with careful monitoring of pulse qualities when pacemakers and ICDs are reported. Drug effects and side effects that affect the oral cavity should be considered. For example, most CCBs cause gingival hyperplasia; digitalis toxicity is common and can result in excessive salivation, gagging, and arrhythmia; and ACEIs commonly cause a cough, which can impact oral procedures. The report of HF should prompt the clinician to use a semiupright chair position. Before using agents that affect coagulation, the patient should be questioned about INR levels. If uncontrolled bleeding develops, digital pressure or local hemostatic agents can be used to initiate a clot. Past research has shown an association between periodontal disease and CVD. Periodontal health is important for the reduction of inflammatory chemicals in the circulation, the risk for intravascular clotting, and bacteremia levels; this information should be communicated to the client (Box 17-7).

CONCLUSION

Successful and safe management of the patient with CVD is predicated on obtaining a thorough medical history and physical examination. The examination should include identification of any physical signs and symptoms of cardiac dysfunction and evaluation of vital signs, including blood pressure, pulse rate/rhythm, and respiratory function. Medical consultation should be sought when indicated. In view of the available data suggesting that cardiac risk for dental procedures appears to be low or very low, once the need for dental intervention has been established, the assessment of patient-specific factors provides the best information for coronary risk stratification.

References

1. Eagle KA, Berger PB, Calkins H, et al. ACC/AHA guideline update for perioperative cardiovascular evaluation for noncardiac surgery. *J Am Coll Cardiol.* 2002;39(3):542–553.
2. American Dental Association Council on Dental Health and Health Planning and Bureau of Health Education and Audiovisual Services. Breaking the silence on hypertension: A dental perspective. *J Am Dent Assoc.* 1985;10:781–782.
3. MacMahon S, Rodgers A. Blood pressure, antihypertensive treatment and stroke. *J Hypertens Suppl.* 1994;12:S5–S14.
4. Furberg CD, Wright JT, Davis BR, et al. The antihypertensive and lipid-lowering treatment to prevent heart attack trial (ALLHAT): Major outcomes in high-risk hypertensive patients randomized to angiotensin-converting enzyme inhibitor or calcium channel blocker vs. diuretic. *JAMA.* 2002;288(23):2981–2997.
5. Chobanian AV, Bakris GL, Black HR, et al. The seventh report of the Joint National Committee on Prevention, Detection, Evaluation, and Treatment of High Blood Pressure. *JAMA.* 2003; 289:2560–2578.
6. Pickett FA, Terezhalmy GT. *Lippincott Williams & Wilkins' Dental Drug Reference with Clinical Implications.* Baltimore: Lippincott Williams & Wilkins; 2006.
7. Abramowicz M, ed. Drugs for lipid disorders. In: *Drugs of Choice.* 15th ed. New York: The Medical Letter; 2003:153–174.
8. *Facts & Comparisons.* St. Louis: Wolters Kluwer; 2007:532.
9. Wahedra AJ, Timmis AD. Management of stable angina. *Postgrad Med J.* 2003;79:332–336.

CLINICAL APPLICATION EXERCISES

☐ **Exercise 1.** A new patient reports for examination and oral prophylaxis. The medical history reveals a history of angina pectoris 3 years ago. What procedures should be completed or questions asked before deciding to provide an oral prophylaxis?

☐ **Exercise 2.** A new patient reports for examination and oral prophylaxis. The medical history reveals a history of transient ischemic attack 5 months ago, and the patient is taking warfarin for anticlotting prophylaxis. The patient reports monthly for laboratory tests to monitor the INR but is unsure of her last lab value. What procedures should be completed or questions asked before deciding to provide an oral prophylaxis?

☐ **Exercise 3.** WEB ACTIVITY: Log on to the FDA Web site and read the updated prescribing information on warfarin, the second-most-common drug that brings patients to the emergency room (http://www.fda.gov/bbs/topics/NEWS/2007/NEW01684.html).

10. Hand H. Common cardiac arrhythmias. *Nurs Stand.* 2002;16: 43–58.

11. American Academy of Periodontology Research, Science and Therapy Committee. Periodontal management of patients with cardiovascular diseases. *J Periodontol.* 2002;73(8):954–968.

12. Perusse R, Goulet JP, Turcotte JY. Contraindications to vaso-constrictors in dentistry: Part 1. *Oral Surg Oral Med Oral Pathol.* 1992;74:679–686.

13. Herman WW, Konzelman JL, Sutley SH. Current perspectives on dental patients receiving coumarin anticoagulant therapy. *J Am Dent Assoc.* 1997;128(3):327–335.

14. Becker L, Eisenberg M, Fahrenbruch C, et al. Cardiac arrest in medical and dental practices: Implications for automated external defibrillators. *Arch Intern Med.* 2001;161:1509–1512.

15. Kenney WL, ed. *ACSM's Guidelines for Exercise Testing and Prescription.* 5th ed. Baltimore: Lippincott Williams & Wilkins; 1995:93–94.

Clinical Implications for Central Nervous System Drugs

KEY TERMS

Akinesia: Absence or loss of the power of voluntary movement
Anterograde amnesia: A condition in which no memory extends forward from a particular point in time
Anxiolytic: Having to do with the relief of anxiety

Bradykinesia: A decrease in spontaneity of movement
Dysgeusia: Taste disturbance or perversion
Psychotropic: Capable of affecting the mind, emotions, and behavior

KEY ACRONYMS

AA: Atypical antidepressant
ARAS: Ascending reticular activating system
GABA: Gamma-aminobutyric acid
MAOI: Monoamine-oxidase inhibitor
MDD: Major depressive disorder

NREM: Nonrapid eye movement
PD: Parkinson disease
REM: Rapid eye movement
SSRI: Selective serotonin reuptake inhibitor
TCA: Tricyclic antidepressant

The dental hygienist is very likely to treat a patient who is taking drugs that stimulate or depress the central nervous system (CNS), because several are among the top-20 most commonly prescribed drugs. Questioning to determine why the agent is being used will help to identify potential patient management issues. Drugs included in this chapter that affect the CNS are antianxiety agents, antidepressants, antipsychotic agents, and drugs to manage symptoms of Parkinson disease (PD). Some agents are used for a variety of indications; for example, some antidepressants are administered for panic disorder. Dentists prescribe antianxiety and antidepressant agents for a variety of reasons, such as dental phobia, relaxation of temporomandibular joint (TMJ) musculature, and treatment of status epilepticus. This chapter focuses on the conditions for which these drugs are used, effects of these agents that may impact the oral health care appointment, and principles of dental management.

ANXIETY

Anxiety is the distressing experience of dread and foreboding, with a wide spectrum of symptoms that can adversely affect the dental client (Table 18-1). Fear of dental treatment is a barrier to receiving dental care, and subjects with high degrees of anxiety are very likely to avoid seeking oral health care procedures.[1,2,3] For individuals with a history of stress-related events occurring during a dental appointment, the question of whether or not to prescribe an **anxiolytic** agent must be answered. Individuals who have experienced anxiety about receiving oral-related therapy in the past are likely to experience the same feeling again. The therapeutic benefits obtained from anxiolytic agents are a matter of controversy when weighed against the potential adverse drug

Table 18-1	Physical Signs and Symptoms of Anxiety

- Anorexia
- "Butterflies" in stomach
- Chest pain or tightness
- Decreased pain threshold
- Diaphoresis
- Diarrhea
- Dizziness
- Dyspnea
- Dry mouth
- Fainting
- Flushing
- Headache
- Hyperventilation
- Lightheadedness
- Muscle tension
- Nausea
- Pallor
- Palpitations
- Paresthesias
- Sexual dysfunction
- Shortness of breath
- Stomach pain
- Tachycardia
- Tremulousness
- Urinary frequency
- Vomiting

effects (ADEs). However, viewed in the context of symptoms or illnesses for which they are prescribed, rigorous and extensive surveys have concluded that reckless overprescription is rare and that the **psychotropic** drugs are relatively safe with rational use.

Medical Illness

A significant number of those presenting with symptoms of anxiety may have underlying, undiagnosed medical or physical illnesses that are responsible for their distress. Given the variety of autonomic symptoms associated with anxiety, the possible medical diagnoses are numerous (Table 18-2). Many clients, however, will be able to give the medical reason for taking a specific antianxiety drug. For the otherwise apparently healthy patient, particular attention should be paid to symptoms commonly associated with anxiety (such as arrhythmias, excessive ingestion of caffeine or other stimulants, drug or alcohol withdrawal, thyroid abnormalities, and hypoglycemia). In a patient with a known medical illness, that ailment (including its possible symptoms, complications, and treatment) should be considered in terms of its effects on oral health.

Psychiatric Illness

Vague uneasiness extending to severe anxiety, with such clinical features as auditory hallucinations or bizarre thinking, may be an early or persistent symptom of a psychotic episode. Patients with depressive syndromes often present with complaints of frequent anxiety in addition to impairment of mood, sleep, appetite, energy, and concentration. A more common syndrome in the general patient population is *panic disorder*. These patients have panic-level anxiety that last seconds or minutes with impressive autonomic symptoms, including tachycardia, dyspnea, tremulousness, dizziness, and diaphoresis, accompanied by a desire to flee. Panic attacks often include a mild persistent anticipatory anxiety, as well as phobias and depressive symptoms. In some instances, a recent onset of symptoms attributable to anxiety may reflect emotional upheaval in a patient's life. Compassionate inquiry by the oral health professional may elicit a history of psychotherapy, marital turmoil, or other interpersonal problems,

Psychologic Anxiety

The essential feature of *psychologic anxiety* is a persistent and irrational fear of a specific object (such as dental instruments),

Table 18-2	Physical Causes of Anxietylike Symptoms

Type of Cause	Specific Cause
Cardiovascular	Angina pectoris, arrhythmias, congestive heart failure, hypertension, hypovolemia, myocardial infarction, syncope (of multiple causes), valvular disease, vascular collapse (shock)
Dietary	Caffeinism, diarrhea, intestinal gas, vitamin deficiency
Drug-related	Akathisia (secondary to antipsychotic drugs), anticholinergic toxicity, digitalis toxicity, hallucinogens, hypotensive agents, stimulants (amphetamines, cocaine, and related drugs), withdrawal syndromes (alcohol or sedative hypnotics)
Hematologic	Anemias
Immunologic	Anaphylaxis, systemic lupus erythematosus
Metabolic	Hyperadrenalism (Cushing disease), hyperkalemia, hyperthermia, hyperthyroidism, hypocalcemia, hypoglycemia, hyponatremia, hypothyroidism, menopause, porphyria (acute intermittent)
Neurologic	Encephalopathies (infectious, metabolic, and toxic), essential tremor, intracranial mass lesions, postconcussion syndrome, seizure disorders (especially of the temporal lobe), vertigo
Respiratory	Asthma, chronic obstructive pulmonary disease, pneumonia, pneumothorax, pulmonary edema, pulmonary embolism

activity, or situations that result in a compelling desire to avoid the dreaded object, activity, or situation (such as the dental phobic stimulus). Patients may experience simple phobias characterized by overwhelming fear with symptoms identical to those of a panic attack when they are exposed to the phobic stimulus (a dental appointment). These patients will often try to gain a great deal of information before entering the situation in which the phobic stimulus will be encountered. They frequently fail to appear for dental appointments and often have significant oral disease when they do appear due to unresolved pain. The physical signs and symptoms of anxiety (Table 18-1) may be noted during the initial patient interview. Antianxiety drug therapy may enhance the patient's ability to cope and reduce avoidance behavior.

Antianxiety Agents

Agents used to manage anxiety include benzodiazepines, barbiturates, and nonbarbiturate sedative hypnotics.

Benzodiazepines

Benzodiazepines are generally considered to be the mainstay of anxiolytic pharmacotherapy. When compared with other sedative and hypnotic agents, which are general depressants of the CNS, benzodiazepines are more selectively anxiolytic, with fewer ADEs and less risk for acute withdrawal. The ability of these agents to relieve anxiety corresponds to their affinity for certain neuronal receptors. Examples of available products and their onset times are included in Table 18-3. They are in the controlled substance schedule IV.

Benzodiazepine receptors have been isolated in the brain and in other organs, although their density is highest in the CNS. The net therapeutic effects of the interaction of benzodiazepines with their receptors are to reduce anxiety, induce skeletal muscle relaxation, and exert an anticonvulsant effect. They reduce anxiety by enhancing the inhibitory properties of the neurotransmitter gamma-aminobutyric acid (GABA) found naturally in the CNS. Benzodiazepines are also thought to exert an anxiolytic effect by selectively depressing the hyperactivity of neuronal circuits in the limbic system. By facilitating GABA-induced neuronal inhibition in the spinal cord, benzodiazepines may promote some degree of skeletal muscle relaxation. By facilitating GABA-induced neuronal stabilization, benzodiazepines (diazepam [Valium]) also possess anticonvulsant activity and are used for medical emer-

gencies involving uncontrolled seizure (such as overdose of local anesthetics or status epilepticus). Diazepam is specifically approved for the treatment of muscle spasm or musculoskeletal disorders and is used to manage symptoms of TMJ dysfunction. The efficacy of diazepam in situations that exacerbate pain and muscle spasm may be due primarily to its anxiolytic effects, because patients with muscle spasm commonly experience anxiety or agitation. Benzodiazepines are also used for the reduction of morbidity and mortality associated with alcohol-withdrawal syndrome because of their efficacy and relatively low incidence of cardiovascular and respiratory depression.

Adverse Drug Effects

Anterograde Amnesia
An important and unique side effect of benzodiazepines is the induction of **anterograde amnesia**. This is a beneficial side effect of benzodiazepines used with intravenous (IV) administration for conscious sedation during oral surgery or other selected dental procedures, because patients will not usually remember what occurred during the drug therapy, though their memory prior to the administration of the drug will be left intact.

Sedation and Impairment of Performance
Active metabolites of long-acting benzodiazepines accumulate for days, but profound sedation does not usually occur, allowing the individual to work or be active in society. This is thought to occur because patients rapidly acquire tolerance to the sedative effects of these agents. The effects may, however, diminish alertness and eye–hand coordination, impair the ability to drive an automobile, and cause personality changes. Benzodiazepine-induced CNS depression manifested as fatigue, drowsiness, muscle weakness, and ataxia has been reported. "Paradoxical" reaction of increased hostility and aggression in certain impulsive patients and geriatric individuals may be observed.

Oral Side Effects
Benzodiazepines may reduce salivary secretion through an anticholinergic mechanism. Both xerostomia and increased salivation have been reported, as well as taste disturbance or metallic taste.

Potential for Abuse

Evidence of drug abuse with most benzodiazepines is generally lacking, and there is no consistent evidence that appropriate antianxiety therapy impairs the incentive to seek more definitive anxiety-relieving solutions. Because physiologic dependence is more likely to occur with longer drug exposure, minimizing the duration of continuous treatment is recommended. Diazepam is a more commonly abused benzodiazepine because of its fast onset of action, which can give a transient "high."

Withdrawal
Symptoms consistent with withdrawal may include tremors, sweating, sensitivity to light and sound, difficulty in sleeping, abdominal pain, and systolic hypertension. Serious

Table 18-3	Benzodiazepines

Long-Acting	Short-Acting
Chlordiazepoxide (Librium)	Alprazolam (Xanax)
Clorazepate (Tranxene)	Estazolam (ProSom)
Diazepam (Valium)	Lorazepam (Ativan)
Flurazepam (Dalmane)	Oxazepam (Serax)
Halazepam (Paxipam)	Temazepam (Restoril)
Prazepam (Centrax)	Triazolam (Halcion)
Quazepam (Doral)	Midazolam (Versed)

withdrawal syndromes, such as depression, psychosis, and seizures, are less common. Withdrawal can be logically minimized by tapering rather than abruptly discontinuing treatment.

Overdose

Fatal overdose with a benzodiazepine taken alone is rare. The main danger results from an increased depression of the CNS when the agent is combined with other dangerous substances, such as alcohol and/or other sedatives. In general, the coadministration of single doses of benzodiazepines with single doses of alcohol causes a greater CNS depression than that caused by either agent taken alone. This interaction can result in life-threatening, irreversible respiratory and cardiovascular collapse. Death usually results due to respiratory depression and asphyxia.

Effects on the Elderly

Diminished alertness resulting from benzodiazepine therapy in elderly patients may be confused with senility or dementia and thus lead to inappropriate treatment. Benzodiazepines may also cause confusion and severe impairment of mental function. Because the geriatric client is more susceptible to drug effects (such as ataxia or excessive sedation), doses are reduced by 50%. The initial dose should be small, and dosage increments should be made gradually in accordance with the response of the patient.

Clients with Liver Disease

There appears to be a two- to threefold rise in the plasma levels of patients taking long-acting benzodiazepines in association with liver disease. However, short-acting benzodiazepines do not tend to accumulate significantly in these patients and are the agents of choice for relieving anxiety in those with liver disease.

Pregnancy and Children

Increased incidence of cleft lip and palate in the children of women who used benzodiazepines during the first trimester of pregnancy has been reported, although this is being questioned. Most benzodiazepines are in pregnancy category D, though triazolam and temazepam are in category X. In children, only benzodiazepines should be used to manage convulsive disorders.

Benzodiazepine-Receptor Antagonist

Flumazenil (Mazicon), a benzodiazepine-receptor antagonist, is now available to reverse the sedative effects of benzodiazepines after sedation for brief surgical or diagnostic procedures, anesthesia, or benzodiazepine overdose. The drug does not antagonize opioids, nonbenzodiazepine sedatives, or anesthetic drugs. Flumazenil competes with benzodiazepine agonists for receptor sites in the CNS. It has high affinity for receptors but has little intrinsic activity of its own. Benzodiazepine antagonism begins within 1 to 2 minutes after IV injection, reaches a peak in 6 to 10 minutes, and lasts for about 1 hour, when the residual effect of the agonist may return, depending on the doses of the agonist and antagonist. Potential ADEs of flumazenil are nausea, dizziness, headache, blurred vision, increased sweating, and anxiety. It is not effective in treating benzodiazepine-induced respiratory depression, and it can precipitate convulsions in some patients.

Dental Drug Interactions

Potential drug–drug interactions between benzodiazepines and acetaminophen, antifungal agents, disulfiram, and macrolide antibacterial agents have been documented. The mechanism involves a reduction in the hepatic metabolism of benzodiazepines, so continued dosing results in excessive sedation. Corticosteroids may decrease the effect of midazolam by increasing its metabolism. Benzodiazepines may delay the onset of action of naproxen by delaying its rate of absorption. Benzodiazepine effects may be additive with opioid analgesics and result in increased CNS depression.

Dental Considerations

With a reasoned approach to treatment, acute anxiety can be diminished by medications, particularly the benzodiazepines. Fast-acting benzodiazepines that have a short half-life (Table 18-3) are selected for premedication in the anxious or phobic dental client. This allows for the resumption of normal activities soon after the dental appointment. Triazolam has been used with adult clients, and lorazepam or alprazolam have been used in the elderly due to an intermediate onset and short half-life. Midazolam is available in a syrup doseform for children. The parenteral form of midazolam (Versed) is used for adults. When either oral or parenteral benzodiazepines are administered for a dental appointment, the client should be instructed to bring someone to the appointment because the client should not operate a motor vehicle following drug administration. Further instructions should include not signing important papers or operating equipment. Amnesia can persist for up to 45 minutes, so client instructions should be provided in writing.

Barbiturates

Sedative and hypnotic agents depress the CNS. The degree of this reversible depression is dose dependent. Small doses will produce a mild degree of CNS depression described as conscious sedation. *Sedation* is the act of calming or reducing activity or excitement in an individual while allowing consciousness. A larger dose of the same drug will produce a greater CNS depression, resulting in hypnosis. *Hypnosis* is a condition of artificially induced sleep or a trance resembling sleep. The principal effects of the barbiturates are on the CNS, and they depress the transmission of impulses to the cortex with sedative and hypnotic doses. Higher doses appear to act at all levels of the CNS. Barbiturate sedation impairs mental and physical skill to some degree but has *no significant analgesic effects*, so analgesic agents are added when pain relief is needed. Certain barbiturates are also used for their anticonvulsant effects. Selection of a barbiturate is determined in part by the drug's duration of action and the clinical situation. Indications for the use of barbiturates include sedation for anxiety, essential hypertension, hyperthyroidism, and sleep induction in cases of insomnia. The ultra-short-acting barbiturates are important agents in general anesthesia. The long-acting members are of value as antiepileptics. The

Table 18-4	Barbiturates	
Short-Acting	**Oral Adult Dosage**	**Onset of Action**
Pentobarbital (Nembutal)	50 to 100 mg	about 30 min; duration up to 3 h
Secobarbital (Seconal)	50 to 100 mg	about 30 min; duration up to 3 h
Intermediate-Acting		
Amobarbital (Amytal)	100 to 200 mg	40 to 60 min; duration 3 to 6 h
Aprobarbital (Alurate)	40 to 160 mg	40 to 60 min; duration 3 to 6 h
Butabarbital (Butisol)	50 to 100 mg	40 to 60 min; duration 3 to 6 h
Long-Acting		
Phenobarbital (Luminal)	100 to 200 mg	2 to 3 h; duration >6 h
Talbutal (Lotusate)	60 to 120 mg	2 to 3 h; duration >6 h

short- and intermediate-acting agents are used principally as preoperative medications to reduce anxiety. A practical clinical classification of the barbiturates is by duration of action (Table 18-4). Doses are not absolute and must be specific to the individual. Thiopental and methohexital were discussed in Chapter 11.

Adverse Drug Effects

Sedative and hypnotic doses of barbiturates are relatively safe, although they have a narrow safety margin. CNS depression can be exaggerated in elderly and debilitated patients and those with kidney or liver disease. Sedative effects are additive to the sedation produced by alcohol, other CNS depressants, and antihistamines. In the elderly individual, idiosyncratic excitement rather than sedation may result. Because of the potential for acute poisoning, whether intentional or unintentional (automatism), doses must be individualized because death may result from respiratory failure due to overdose. Abrupt withdrawal from barbiturates may cause tremors, restlessness, anxiety, weakness, nausea and vomiting, seizures, delirium, and cardiac arrest.

Dental Drug Interactions

Barbiturates interact with many drugs because they increase the secretion of microsomal enzymes in the liver, thereby increasing the metabolism of many drugs and leading to less-than-adequate therapeutic effects.

Nonbarbiturate Sedatives and Hypnotics

Chloral Hydrate

Chloral derivatives (Table 18-5) are effective general CNS depressants with effects similar to alcohol. *Chloral hydrate*

elixir is commonly used in dentistry as an antianxiety premedication for children. These drugs are orally administered, have a rapid onset (20 to 30 minutes), and have a fairly short duration of action (about 4 hours). The drugs are relatively safe, because therapeutic doses do not produce pronounced respiratory or cardiovascular depression. Exaggerated effects in patients with advanced liver or kidney disease can be anticipated, and large doses or long-term use may produce peripheral vasodilation, hypotension, and some degree of myocardial depression. Gastric irritation with nausea and/or vomiting may be minimized by taking the drug with milk. These agents may be considered for children or the elderly. Liquid preparations are available.

Dental Drug Interactions

Chloral hydrate causes increased CNS depression when used with other CNS depressants, including nitrous oxide.

Antihistamines

Some antihistamines have an effect on the CNS and produce drowsiness. Antihistamines (Table 18-6) are relatively safe compounds, are effective antianxiety agents, and have mild sedative effects. Because of their anticholinergic effects, they have little or no abuse potential, unlike other CNS drugs used for their sedative effects. This benefit makes diphenhydramine (Benadryl) a widely used sedative in pediatric dentistry.

Dental Drug Interactions

Antihistamines decrease the metabolism of many drugs, which increases the potential for toxic accumulation of drugs even when administered in therapeutic doses. This makes use of sedative antihistamines in elderly individuals who take multiple medications risky. There is no effect on the metabolism of local anesthetics or vasoconstrictors.

Table 18-5	Chloral Derivatives
Drugs	**Oral Dose**
Chloral hydrate (Aquachloral Supprettes, Somnote)	500 to 2,000 mg
Triclofos (Triclos)	1,500 mg
Chloral betaine (Beta chlor)	870 to 1,000 mg

Table 18-6	Antihistamines
Drugs	**Oral Dose**
Chlorpheniramine maleate (Chlor-Trimeton)	2 to 4 mg
Diphenhydramine hydrochloride (Benadryl)	25 to 100 mg
Hydroxyzine hydrochloride (Vistaril)	25 to 100 mg

Dental Considerations for Antianxiety Agents

Rules for the dental prescriber include

- knowing the patient well before prescribing;
- being alert for alcohol and drug dependence and concurrent medications being taken;
- providing instructions in writing regarding how to take the medication and warnings for use.

Depression caused by all anxiolytics will add to depression caused by other CNS depressants that the patient may be taking, making it unsafe to perform acts requiring alertness and muscular coordination. The precise quantity of the drug should be calculated according to client characteristics (child, elderly). An exaggerated response may be expected in the young, the elderly, the debilitated, and those with liver or kidney disease. Because anxiolytics do not provide analgesia, their use without adequate pain control may cause patients to become highly excited and act irrationally. Finally, oral health care professionals should never rely exclusively on drugs to provide a calm and cooperative patient; the anxiolytics are not substitutes for patient rapport or for the proper psychologic approach to patient care. These drugs are used for short terms in dentistry, so xerostomia is not long lasting; however, appropriate instructions related to not driving, operating equipment, signing important papers, or performing any task that requires concentration should be provided verbally and in writing.

■ Self-Study Review

1. Review the various reasons for feeling anxiety and consider the impact on the dental hygiene treatment plan.
2. Describe behaviors attributable to psychologic anxiety that characterize dental phobia.
3. Identify classes of drugs used to manage anxiety, and identify examples of agents in each class.
4. List three therapeutic effects of benzodiazepines in dentistry, and describe their mechanisms of action.
5. Identify potential ADEs of benzodiazepines.
6. Describe drug interaction warnings to be given when a benzodiazepine is prescribed.
7. Identify the benzodiazepine antagonist.
8. List dental drugs that may interact with benzodiazepines.
9. Which benzodiazepines are best for the anxious dental patient? Which are best for children?
10. Describe patient instructions when a benzodiazepine is prescribed.
11. Differentiate between *sedation* and *hypnosis*.
12. List the effects of barbiturates (low dose vs. high dose) and their degree of analgesic effect.
13. Describe the mechanism for most barbiturate/drug interactions.
14. Identify nonbarbiturates used for anxiety, and describe when they would be used.

DEPRESSIVE DISORDERS

Depressive disorders can include depression and mania. *Depression* is characterized by changes in mood, activity, behavior, sleep, and neuroendocrine activity. *Mania* can occur as part of a bipolar disorder, which is characterized by recurrent episodes of mania, depression, or both. Because these functions are mediated by neurotransmitters, a logical hypothesis implicates biochemical errors in the CNS as causes of depression. One hypothesis for the cause of depression relates clinical depression to low concentrations of norepinephrine in the brain. Another hypothesis correlates low brain serotonin concentration with depression. An interfacing of the two hypotheses more realistically reflects the complexity of the clinical disease. The diagnosis of depressive disorders is sometimes obscured by anxiety or the multiple complaints that frequently accompany depression. A survey of periodontists revealed respondents were more knowledgeable about the effects of anxiety and stress on pain and wound healing but less knowledgeable about the relationship between depression, medications used for depression, and the impact of depression on periodontal treatment outcomes.[4] Occasionally, severe depression may be secondary to medical illness or previous drug treatment.

Depression

Major depressive disorder (MDD) is a psychiatric illness in which mood, thoughts, and behavioral patterns are impaired for long periods.[1] The condition is characterized by periods of sadness and loss of interest or pleasure in daily activities, and it may be expressed in sleep disturbances, fatigue, and poor concentration abilities. The World Health Organization ranked MDD as the fourth leading cause of disability and premature death in the world. Even when treated, the condition has a recurrence rate of more than 50%. Depression is treated with a combination of counseling and pharmacologic therapy. Because of the high rate of relapse, continued use of the medication is often recommended for up to 1 year following recovery from the initial signs and symptoms. Mild depression is managed with different agents than severe depression. Saint-John's-Wort, an herb, has been shown to be effective for mild depression. It is discussed in more detail in Chapter 20. A variety of antidepressant agents is used for more severe forms of the condition. Table 18-7 lists available agents for management of depressive disorders and includes dental hygiene considerations. Patients beginning antidepressant drug therapy require close monitoring for several weeks. The main causes of treatment failure are inadequate dosage, insufficient duration of treatment, and poor compliance. Low initial doses with gradual increases are recommended for elderly patients who have a higher incidence of ADEs, but they may ultimately require the same doses as younger patients to achieve a therapeutic effect. Therapeutic effects generally begin within a week or two but may take longer to be fully apparent. After dosage has been stabilized, a single evening dose 2 to 3 hours before bedtime is generally as effective as divided doses. These drugs are often taken for extended periods of time, and the chronic xerostomic effects can result in dental caries.

Table 18-7	Antidepressants	
Drug Class	**Examples of Agents**	**Management Considerations**

Atypical	Bupropion (Wellbutrin)
	Nefazodone (Serzone)
	Trazodone (Desyrel)
	Venlafaxine (Effexor)
		Xerostomic effects—salivary
		  lubricants and stimulants; fluoride
		  and xylitol therapy
		Inattention to oral needs—counseling
		  and persuasion techniques
		Orthostatic hypotension (Desyrel)—
		  monitor BP at end of appointment

MAOIs	Isocarboxazid (Marplan)
	Phenelzine (Nardil)
	Tranylcypromine (Parnate)
		Same as above
		Orthostatic hypotension—monitor BP
		  at end of appointment, especially in
		  elderly clients

Serotonin
  reuptake
  inhibitors
	Citalopram (Celexa)
	Escitalopram (Lexapro)
	Fluoxetine (Prozac)
	Fluvoxamine (Luvox)
	Paroxetine (Paxil)
	Sertraline (Zoloft)
		Same as above
		Orthostatic hypotension is uncommon
		  with SSRIs

Tetracyclics	Maprotiline (Ludiomil)
	Mirtazapine (Remeron)
		Xerostomic effects—salivary
		  lubricants and stimulants; fluoride
		  and xylitol therapy
		Inattention to oral needs—counseling
		  and persuasion techniques
		Orthostatic hypotension—monitor BP
		  at end of appointment, especially in
		  elderly clients
		Blood dyscrasias—monitor bleeding,
		  infection

Tricyclics	Amitriptyline (Elavil)
	Amoxapine (Asendin)
	Clomipramine (Anafranil)
	Desipramine (Norpramin)
	Doxepin (Sinequan)
	Imipramine (Tofranil)
	Nortriptyline (Pamelor)
	Protriptyline (Vivactil)
	Trimipramine (Surmontil)
		Same as MAOIs
		Orthostatic hypotension—monitor BP
		  at end of appointment, especially in
		  elderly clients

BP, blood pressure.

Pharmacologic Therapy

Tricyclic Antidepressants

A tricyclic antidepressant (TCA) is generally the first choice for drug treatment of severe depression. All tricyclic drugs are similar in effectiveness. Imipramine (Tofranil and others) and amitriptyline (Elavil and others) are used most extensively. Tricyclics exert their effects by preventing presynaptic neurons from reabsorbing norepinephrine and serotonin from the synaptic space. Thus, the concentration of these two neurotransmitters is elevated, and effects of mood elevation are increased. A new agent has been introduced recently, the tricyclic amoxapine (Asendin). Some TCAs are lethal in overdose situations, and many patients become noncompliant because of unpleasant side effects.

Adverse Drug Effects

The most common ADEs limiting treatment with the TCAs are anticholinergic effects (such as dry mouth, decreased gastrointestinal [GI] motility, mydriasis, cycloplegia, urinary hesitancy or retention, tachycardia and, in high doses, delirium), **dysgeusia** (altered taste sensations), orthostatic hy-

potension (which can cause serious falls, especially in elderly patients), poor concentration, and sedation (which is sometimes welcome).

Elderly patients are more sensitive to the anticholinergic effects of the tricyclic drugs and can develop delirium, especially if the tricyclic is used in combination with antipsychotic drugs, which also have anticholinergic effects. TCAs can slow intraventricular conduction, prolonging the PRS, PR, and QR intervals in the electrocardiogram, and cause complete heart block or ventricular dysrhythmia. Overdose with TCAs can be lethal.

Atypical Antidepressants

The atypical agents (bupropion [Wellbutrin], venlafaxine [Effexor]) exert their effects through varied mechanisms, including selective norepinephrine reuptake inhibition, dopamine reuptake inhibition, and inhibition of monoamine oxidase. The atypical antidepressants (AAs) are as effective as the selective serotonin reuptake inhibitors (SSRIs) and, along with SSRIs, are used as first-line treatments for individuals with mild to moderate depression. Maprotiline has been associated with orthostatic hypotension, electrocardiogram (ECG) changes, tachycardia, and agranulocytosis; mirtazapine has been associated with infrequent reports of agranulocytosis and neutropenia.

Monoamine-Oxidase Inhibitors

Monoamine-oxidase inhibitors (MAOIs), such as phenelzine (Nardil), are older antidepressant agents. They are helpful for some patients who fail to respond to TCAs and may be particularly helpful for those with "atypical depression." They exert an antidepressant effect by nonselective inhibition of monoamine oxidase at the synapse so that norepinephrine and serotonin levels are elevated and neuronal activity is enhanced.

Adverse Drug Effects

The most common side effects include dizziness, drowsiness, orthostatic hypotension, hypertension, dysrhythmias, and anorexia. MAOIs prevent the liver from inactivating tyramine found in aged meats, red wine, beer, and some cheeses, causing norepinephrine blood levels to rise. This can result in fatal hypertensive crisis. Consequently, those taking MAOI agents should avoid these foods, as well as decongestants and drugs containing ephedrine. Xerostomia can occur in some individuals. It is unclear why some drugs can cause opposite effects (orthostatic hypotension and hypertension).

Selective Serotonin Reuptake Inhibitors

The SSRIs are the most common drugs used for depressive disorders, and one is included in the top-20 most commonly prescribed drug list (sertraline [Zoloft]). The SSRIs increase synaptic concentrations of serotonin in the brain by blocking its reuptake into the presynaptic neurons. Thus, the neurotransmitter levels remain free to bind to receptors and cause their mood-stabilizing effect. Paroxetine (Paxil) is approved for a variety of uses, including anxiety, obsessive-compulsive disorder, panic disorder, post-traumatic stress disorder, social anxiety disorder, and major depression.

Adverse Drug Effects

Side effects are different among the wide variety of SSRIs; they have fewer anticholinergic and cardiovascular side effects, although the majority of SSRIs cause xerostomia and dysgeusia. Some agents can cause an increase in bleeding time. Postural hypotension uncommonly occurs with some of the agents. Some agents are reported to cause sialadenitis, gingivitis, and discoloration of the tongue.[1] Individuals with depression are prone to develop periodontitis. Patients taking SSRIs or AAs may develop a movement disorder that includes clenching, grinding of the teeth (bruxism), or both, leading to further destruction of the periodontal attachment.[5] Each drug should be investigated in a drug reference for its specific side effect profile. As a group, these agents have fewer side effects than the other classes of antidepressants.

New Agents

Several new antidepressant agents have recently been introduced, including maprotiline (Ludiomil), a tetracyclic compound, and trazodone (Desyrel), an atypical agent. Clinical experience with these drugs is limited; none has been convincingly shown to be more effective or to act more rapidly than the older tricyclics.

Adverse Drug Effects

The new antidepressant trazodone (Desyrel), which is not structurally related to the tricyclic drugs, causes few, if any, anticholinergic effects, but it can cause orthostatic hypotension and sedation and may cause an increase in ventricular premature contractions in some patients. Maprotiline commonly causes dry mouth, dizziness, orthostatic hypotension, tachycardia, nausea, and blurred vision.

Dental Drug Interactions

Some drugs used in oral health care can interact with antidepressant drugs. Adverse interactions between SSRIs and some medications used in dentistry may occur because these antidepressants inhibit certain metabolic pathways by inhibiting cytochrome P450 enzymes needed to metabolize codeine, benzodiazepines, erythromycin, and carbamazepine. Aspirin should be avoided when SSRIs are taken due to increased bleeding. Barbiturates and benzodiazepines can increase CNS depression in most antidepressants. Clomipramine and maprotiline interact with several drugs used in dentistry. They inhibit the bacteriostatic action of erythromycin, increase the sedative effect of opioid analgesics, and enhance the actions of vasoconstrictors (epinephrine, levonordefrin). Small concentrations of epinephrine (1:100,000) can be used when tricyclic and tetracyclic agents are taken, taking precaution to inject slowly and aspirate to avoid intravascular injection. No more than two cartridges should be used in one appointment, because excessive amounts can result in increased blood pressure. Levonordefrin is contraindicated when tricyclics or tetracyclics are taken due to the possibility of an exaggerated hypertensive response. Acetaminophen should be used in low doses, because higher doses can reduce the metabolic rate of the tetracyclics and tricyclics, leading to toxic levels of the antidepressant. Patients taking MAOIs can receive local anesthetics with vasoconstrictors because the MAOIs do not potentiate the pressor or cardiac effects of direct-acting catecholamines. However, meperidine (Demerol) should be avoided because of a potentially toxic interaction in which severe hyperthermia, hypertension, and tachycardia may develop. The effects of narcotic analgesics may be increased when MAOIs are taken; therefore, narcotics should be prescribed at low doses.

Management Considerations

Some patients may be hesitant to admit they are receiving care for psychiatric reasons because of the stigma associated with mental illness. To overcome such barriers to communication, oral health professionals should have a supportive, nonjudgmental attitude and advise the patient that information will be held confidential.[1] Medical consultation may be necessary if substance abuse is suspected. Patients with a history of alcohol abuse should have liver function test data, a complete blood cell count, and a coagulation profile (international normalized ratio [INR], prothrombin time [PT], partial thromboplastin time [PTT]) if procedures that involve bleeding are planned.

The disease and side effect profile can influence the dental hygiene care plan. The depressive disorder can result in lack of attention to self-care, with resultant periodontal inflammation.[1,2] A 3-month maintenance schedule may be indicated for periodontal care. In other cases toothbrushing and flossing are performed excessively, leading to loss of tooth structure from abrasion. Chronic xerostomic effects as well as a craving for sweets lead to caries and candidiasis. Chronic facial pain, burning sensation of the oral mucosa or tongue, or a TMJ disorder frequently brings the depressed patient for dental care. Profound local anesthesia may be necessary to provide complete treatment and reduce anxiety in the patient. Orthostatic hypotension risk should be considered at the end of the appointment, and the chair should be raised slowly with the patient allowed to sit upright for several minutes before dismissal from the appointment. Allowing the elderly individual to place the feet on the floor and exercise the leg muscles while seated may help the return blood flow to the heart and avoid a hypotensive event. Some authorities recommend measuring the blood pressure in predisposed individuals prior to rising from the dental chair and again after the individual stands. A drug reference to identify the potential for side effects is essential, as well as questioning the client to determine if side effects have occurred in the past.

Mania

Mania can occur as part of a bipolar disorder that is characterized by recurrent episodes of mania, depression, or both. The biologic hypothesis of mania stipulates a functional excess of norepinephrine and serotonin. Conversely, a modified hypothesis proposes a decrease in serotonin secretion in the brain in both depression and mania, with a greater deficit occurring in depression.

Pharmacologic Therapy

Lithium (Eskalith and others) is the drug of choice for patients with mania and for long-term maintenance to prevent both depressive and manic episodes in bipolar disorder. Lithium influences norepinephrine and serotonin levels in the CNS, as well as other neurotransmitters. Lithium may take 2 to 3 weeks to demonstrate a therapeutic effect, and serum concentration levels should be medically monitored. Valproate and carbamazepine, anticonvulsant drugs, are also used to manage mania in those who do not respond to lithium or who cannot take it because of drug complications. During depressive episodes, cautious use of TCAs or MAOIs may also be needed in addition to lithium.

Adverse Drug Effects

Nausea and fatigue can occur in the first weeks of treatment with lithium, even when serum concentrations are in the recommended range. Fine tremors of the hand, edema, and weight gain may persist for the duration of treatment. Lithium-induced tremors can be treated with a beta-adrenergic blocking agent. Confusion is an important toxic effect of lithium that may not be perceived as drug induced.

Hypothyroidism, with swelling of the neck and generalized edema, can result as an ADE of lithium. Oral side effects include increased thirst and dry mouth. Hypotension, hand tremors, and nausea may also affect the dental hygiene treatment plan.

Dental Drug Interactions

Dental drug interactions with lithium include erythromycin and COX-inhibitors. Reduced metabolism of lithium can lead to increased blood levels and toxicity.

■ Self-Study Review

15. Describe the forms of depressive disorders, and identify agents used to manage symptoms of the disorders by class.
16. Long-term therapy can result in what oral problem?
17. Identify ADEs commonly associated with each class relevant to oral health care.
18. List dental drug interactions with the various agents used for depressive disorders.
19. Describe dental hygiene management considerations for the client with a depressive disorder.
20. Identify uses for lithium and ADEs relevant to dental hygiene procedures.

SCHIZOPHRENIA

Schizophrenia is a functional psychosis characterized by major disturbances in thought content, bizarre behavior, a regression in intellectual functioning, inappropriate affective expression, and frequent hallucinations and delusions. The biochemical theory of schizophrenia suggests that abnormal motor and mood states are due to an excess of dopamine, a CNS catecholamine neurotransmitter. Some symptoms of schizophrenia and acute psychoses may improve rapidly after treatment with antipsychotic drugs, but chronic schizophrenia usually requires 3 weeks or more before any benefit is seen, and the full course of improvement may take months. Many patients with chronic schizophrenia require prolonged maintenance drug therapy, but the benefits of antipsychotic drugs are limited for some chronic schizophrenics.

Pharmacologic Therapy

There are three main classes of drugs to manage the condition, including the first-generation phenothiazines and butyrophenones (haloperidol) and second-generation atypical antipsychotic agents. No important differences in effectiveness have been demonstrated among the various phenothiazines or between the phenothiazines and haloperidol (Haldol). These first-generation conventional antipsychotic agents are still used, but atypical second-generation antipsychotic agents,

Table 18-8	Antipsychotic Agents	
Drug Classification	**Agents**	**Management Considerations**
Phenothiazines	Chlorpromazine (Thorazine) Fluphenazine (Prolixin) Mesoridazine (Serentil) Perphenazine (Trilafon) Prochlorperazine (Compazine) Thioridazine (Mellaril) Trifluoperazine (Stelazine)	Tardive dyskinesia—movements of lips, tongue may complicate intraoral procedures Dry mouth—monitor for caries, candidiasis; preventive fluoride therapy and xylitol products Orthostatic hypotension—monitor BP end of appointment
Butyrophenone	Haloperidol (Haldol)	See above
Atypicals	Thiothixene (Navane) Aripiprazole (Abilify) Clozapine (Clozaril) Loxapine (Loxitane) Molindone (Moban) Olanzapine (Zyprexa) Pimozide (Orap) Quetiapine (Seroquel) Risperidone (Risperdal) Ziprasidone (Geodon)	See above

BP, blood pressure.

such as risperidone, are now used more commonly (Table 18-8). Atypical antipsychotic agents have not been shown to offer important advantages in the management of schizophrenia, other than molindone (Moban) which often causes unrelated weight loss, in contrast to the weight gain frequently caused by the phenothiazines and haloperidol. Antipsychotic drugs may have oral and extrapyramidal side effects that can influence the provision of oral health care procedures. Some of the agents in the class are also approved by the Food and Drug Administration (FDA) to manage symptoms of bipolar disorder and Alzheimer disease.

Adverse Drug Effects

Each drug must be investigated for specific associated ADEs, which are numerous. Chlorpromazine (Thorazine and others) causes sedation, postural hypotension, and anticholinergic effects, as well as occasional extrapyramidal (rigidity, **akinesia**, tremor, tardive dyskinesia, and akathisia) effects with long-term therapy. Thioridazine (Mellaril) also sedates and causes hypotension but is less likely to cause extrapyramidal symptoms. Hypotension and sedation are less likely with perphenazine (Trilafon), fluphenazine (Permitil and others), trifluoperazine (Stelazine and others), haloperidol (Haldol), thiothixene (Navane), and molindone (Moban), but all of these drugs tend to cause extrapyramidal symptoms, such as rigidity, akinesia, tremor, and akathisia (motor restlessness). Tardive dyskinesia is one of the most serious ADEs of drugs used to treat schizophrenia; it usually occurs after prolonged therapy and sometimes persists for long periods or for life, even after the drug is discontinued. It can occur, although rarely, less than a year after beginning treatment with antipsychotic drugs. Tardive dyskinesia, which is characterized by involuntary movements (initially of the lips and tongue, but sometimes also of the fingers, toes, or trunk), has also been reported in children. The extrapyramidal symptoms are less frequent with the newer atypical antipsychotics, but they can develop in some individuals. All antipsychotic agents are reported to cause chronic dry mouth.

Dental Drug Interactions

There are no documented drug–drug interactions between agents used to manage schizophrenia and dental therapeutics; however, the absence of evidence is not evidence of safety. Loxapine may produce anxiety and respiratory distress in combination with lorazepam (possible synergism), and their concurrent use should be avoided. Increased orthostatic hypotensive effect of olanzapine with diazepam (decreased metabolism) is possible; here, too, concurrent use should be avoided.

Management Considerations

Tardive dyskinesia can complicate intraoral procedures. Taking care when working in the mouth is essential when sharp instruments are being used. Observe the pattern of tongue movements and try to avoid contact between the instrument tip and the tongue. Panoramic radiography may be the only type of radiograph that can be achieved in this condition. Dry mouth may increase the risk of caries and require an anticaries program (both in-office and at-home fluoride and use of xylitol gum) and professional application of sealants. When a supine position is used, a protocol to prevent orthostatic hypotension should be followed at each appointment.

■ Self-Study Review

21. Identify the agents used for schizophrenia and psychoses (both generic and brand names).

22. Describe ADEs of phenothiazines and management for these effects.

INSOMNIA

The ascending reticular activating system (ARAS), a diffuse collection of neuron cell bodies and neuron fibers in the central brain stem, is the physiologic mechanism for the maintenance of an "awake" cerebral cortex and, conversely, for the transition to an "asleep" cerebral cortex. Input to the ARAS occurs from all sensory modalities, and activity in the ARAS is further influenced by the brain. Using electroencephalographic (EEG) tracings, two states of sleep have been identified: (a) nonrapid eye movement (NREM) and (b) rapid eye movement (REM). The NREM state is further divided into four stages. The sleep cycle begins with stage one, the lightest sleep stage, which is followed by successively deeper stages two, three, and four, with the deepest sleep occurring in stage four. The typical sleep cycle involves a quick passage through stage one and stage two, followed by a moderate period of time in delta sleep, stages three and four. After the four stages of the NREM state, the REM state of sleep associated with dreaming, decreased muscle tone, and high-frequency, low-amplitude EEG waves begins. Approximately 90 minutes after the onset of sleep, a person enters the first REM state, which lasts several minutes. This cycle is repeated four to six times during the night. As the nocturnal sleep period proceeds, NREM sleep consumes less time, and the REM state lengthens and intensifies. The final REM state in a nor-mal sleep cycle usually lasts 30 to 60 minutes. Difficulty in falling asleep, an inability to remain asleep, abbreviated sleep with premature awakening, or a combination of these sleep problems characterizes insomnia.

Pharmacologic Treatment

Sleep disturbances occur in association with many psychiatric and medical disorders. When a major psychiatric or medical illness is present, the primary pharmacologic treatment is directed at the underlying illness. Hypnotic agents may be prescribed for the temporary treatment of insomnia, and when pain causes anxiety and insomnia, analgesics can relieve these symptoms. Insomnia may also occur in otherwise healthy people when they are anxious or incapacitated, and the temporary use of an anxiolytic or hypnotic agent may be appropriate. Benzodiazepines, barbiturates, nonbarbiturate sedatives, and antihistamines are the agents most commonly used (Table 18-9).

Benzodiazepines

Although all benzodiazepines have hypnotic activity, only triazolam, estazolam, lorazepam, temazepam, flurazepam, and quazepam are labeled for the treatment of **insomnia**. The short-acting benzodiazepines are preferred because they are less likely to accumulate with chronic use and produce less daytime sedation. Significant residual effects on driving ability occurring the morning after bedtime administration have been demonstrated with flurazepam; impairment was still detected in the afternoon.

Table 18-9	Agents Used for Insomnia	
Classification	**Drug Names**	**Management Implications**
Barbiturates	Pentobarbital Secobarbital Amobarbital	CNS depression, cardiovascular and respiratory depression
Miscellaneous nonbarbiturates	Chloral hydrate Zolpidem (Ambien) Eszopiclone (Lunesta) Ethchlorvynol (Placidyl) Glutethimide Zaleplon (Sonata) Ramelteon (Rozerem)	Dry mouth—if used on chronic basis, recommend home anticaries products and xylitol. Taste disturbance can occur with eszopiclone. Sugar-free mints and gum can be recommended. Following treatment, monitor for dizziness and assist in balance.
	Meprobamate (Miltown)	An anxiolytic agent, historically used for daytime sedation, is seldom used today because it is highly addicting and is commonly abused.
Benzodiazepines	Estazolam (ProSom) Flurazepam (Dalmane) Lorazepam (Ativan) Quazepam (Doral) Temazepam (Restoril) Triazolam (Halcion)	Dizziness may require monitoring for balance following treatment. Daytime sedation Muscle weakness
Antihistamines	Diphenhydramine hydrochloride (Benadryl)	Dry mouth (chronic use) may require a recommendation of home anticaries products.

Barbiturates

Other drugs used as sedatives or hypnotics (prolonging REM sleep), such as barbiturates, chloral hydrate, and meprobamate (Equanil, Miltown), tend to lose their effectiveness with continued use, can cause severe toxicity with overdose, and at times have been widely abused. Meprobamate was used in the past for daytime sedation due to reduced effects that allow the individual to remain awake but relaxed. This allows an individual to be able to work while taking the medication. Today, the drug is seldom prescribed because of its addicting properties and great abuse potential.

Nonbarbiturate Sedatives

There is a variety of nonbarbiturate sedative hypnotic agents used for insomnia. To facilitate comparison, the products are divided into two groups: Benzodiazepines (discussed above) and miscellaneous nonbarbiturates. The doses prescribed are intended to be hypnotics (agents that produce drowsiness and facilitate sleep). Many of these agents are newly FDA-approved and are increasingly being advertised via the media.

Zolpidem Tartrate

Zolpidem tartrate (Ambien, Ambien CR) is recommended for short-term treatment (7 to 10 days). The controlled release product has two objectives: To decrease the time to produce sleep and to cause extended sleep periods. The drug is taken immediately before bedtime. Elderly or debilitated patients may be sensitive to its effects, requiring an initial dose reduction. Although the chemical structure is unrelated to the benzodiazepines, which nonselectively activate omega-receptor subtypes, zolpidem binds to the omega-receptor preferentially. It is rapidly absorbed from the GI tract and primarily eliminated by renal excretion. Zolpidem should be used with careful surveillance in individuals with a history of drug abuse and addiction.

Adverse Drug Effects

Drowsiness, headache, lightheadedness, nausea, diarrhea, dry mouth, and flulike symptoms are common side effects. Patients should be warned to avoid alcohol and other CNS depressants while taking this drug.

Zaleplon

Zaleplon (Sonata) is recommended for short-term treatment of insomnia. Elderly patients require a dose reduction due to heightened sensitivity to the drug's effects. The chemical structure is unrelated to benzodiazepines, barbiturates, or other drugs with hypnotic properties, and it interacts with the omega-receptor, which is responsible for some properties of benzodiazepines. It is rapidly absorbed in the GI tract, undergoes significant first-pass metabolism, and is excreted primarily by the kidneys. Unlike zolpidem, it has not been shown to increase total sleep time or decrease the number of awakenings. It is to be taken immediately prior to going to bed. Patients should not take the drug with alcohol or use it immediately before engaging in activity requiring complete mental alertness or motor coordination. It should not be taken with drugs that have CNS effects due to increased CNS stimulation.

Adverse Drug Effects

As with all sedative/hypnotic agents, short-term-memory impairment, hallucinations, impaired coordination, dizziness, and lightheadedness can occur. Other side effects were similar between zaleplon and the placebo. Zaleplon has a drug abuse potential similar to that of benzodiazepines. There are no known clinically important interactions with drugs used in dentistry.

Ramelteon

Ramelteon (Rozerem) was FDA approved in 2005 and represents the newest agent for insomnia. This drug is a melatonin-receptor agonist. Melatonin receptors are thought to be involved in the maintenance of the circadian rhythm underlying the normal sleep–wake cycle. It is approved for the treatment of insomnia characterized by difficulty in sleep onset and is taken within 30 minutes of going to bed. Absorption is rapid in the GI tract, with high first-pass metabolism and excretion primarily by the kidneys. It is not to be taken with or immediately after a high-fat meal, because this decreases absorption in the GI tract. No substance abuse potential was observed in clinical trials.

Adverse Drug Effects

The most common ADEs leading to discontinuation of the drug were somnolence, dizziness, nausea, fatigue, headache, and insomnia, but these were all <1%.

Dental Drug Interactions

When administered with azole antifungals (ketoconazole, fluconazole), blood levels of ramelteon were increased due to the inhibition of metabolism.

Eszopiclone

Eszopiclone (Lunesta) was FDA approved in 2004 for treatment of insomnia, improvement of sleep onset, and improvement of sleep maintenance. Its precise mechanism of action is unknown, but it is believed to interact with receptor complexes similar to those of benzodiazepine. It is to be taken immediately before bedtime and should not be taken soon after eating a high-fat meal, due to a decrease in GI absorption and consequent reduction in sleep onset. Doses should be reduced in the elderly.

Adverse Drug Effects

ADEs most commonly observed in placebo-controlled trials included anxiety, confusion, depression, dizziness, headache, respiratory infection, unpleasant taste (34%), and dry mouth (5% to 7%).

Dental Drug Interactions

Eszopiclone should be given in low doses when potent CYP3A4 inhibitors (ketoconazole) are administered at the same time. When administered with azole antifungals (ketoconazole, fluconazole), blood levels were increased due to the inhibition of metabolism.

Antihistamines

Antihistamines, such as diphenhydramine (Benadryl), are also widely used for their sedative side effect and are present in most over-the-counter sleep remedies. Antihistamines cause neither tolerance nor physical dependence, but they are not uniformly effective and may have undesirable ADEs, such as dry mouth.

■ Self-Study Review

23. Describe the NREM and REM stages of sleep.
24. Identify drugs used for insomnia and daytime sedation.

PARKINSON DISEASE OR SYNDROME

In the United States, PD is the fourth-most-common neurodegenerative disorder in the elderly, affecting an estimated half million people. Oral health care providers can expect to be called upon to care for patients with this progressively debilitating disease. To provide competent care to a patient with PD, clinicians must understand the disease, its treatment, and its impact on the patient's ability to undergo and respond to dental care.

PD is considered to be a "striatal dopamine deficiency syndrome." Figure 18-1 illustrates the pathophysiology of the disease. Striatal dopamine deficiency leads to an impaired ability to control the smooth movement of skeletal muscle. The main extrapyramidal symptoms—tremor, **akinesia**, and rigidity—are positively correlated with the degree of the striatal dopamine deficiency. Clinical manifestations of the syndrome are listed in Box 18-1. Orthostatic hypotension, increased salivation and drooling, difficult swallowing, loss of balance and increased tendency to fall, dementia, and parkinsonian motor symptoms (tremors) can affect the provision of dental hygiene services. Tremors associated with parkinsonian symptoms have been referred to as "pill-rolling," "cigarette-rolling," and "to-and-fro" movements. These tremors are present during rest and often disappear on purposeful movement or during sleep. The most common initial symptom is resting tremor of the hands. During stress or anxiety-provoking situations, tremors increase, and initiation of movement becomes increasingly difficult, extremely fatiguing, and inefficient. Akinesia, or **bradykinesia**, is characterized by lack of spontaneous movements and slowness in initiation of movements. Rigidity or increased muscle tone occurs in response to passive movements. It has been noted that tremor and rigidity of the orofacial musculature may induce orofacial pain, TMJ discomfort, cracked teeth, soft tissue trauma, displaced restorations, attrition from rumination, and ptyalism (drooling or lack of salivary control).

Medical Management

In recent years, remarkable advances have occurred in both the pharmacotherapeutic and surgical management of PD.

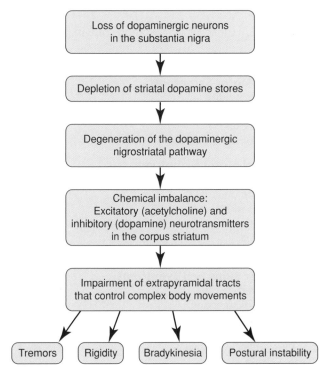

Figure 18-1 The Pathophysiology of Parkinson Disease. (From Dirks SJ, Paunovich ED, Terezhalmy GT, et al. The patient with Parkinson's disease. *Quintessence Int.* 2003;34:379–393, with permission.)

However, no available therapy, including surgery, has been shown to stop the progression of the disease. Medical management is therefore directed at controlling symptoms and maintaining the patient's functional independence for as long as possible. Treatment is individualized and depends on many factors, such as the stage of the disease, the patient's age, the patient's preferences regarding specific risks and benefits, and responses to treatment. The incidence of xerostomia among patients with PD is reported to be as high as 55% (vs. 20% in the general elderly population). Reduced qualitative and quantitative changes in salivary flow are generally related to the parasympatholytic or antimuscarinic effects of the many drugs administered to these patients and not to the pathophysiologic changes of PD itself. Chronic xerostomia may result in painful (burning) oral soft tissue problems and poor tissue adaptation to prostheses. The patient may experience difficulties with mastication, swallowing, and speech. The reduced buffering capacity of the saliva also contributes to an increased incidence of dental caries, exacerbates periodontal disease, and may affect the sensitivity of taste buds, contributing to **dysgeusia**. In addition, xerostomia may predispose to esophageal injury and contribute to nutritional deficiencies and weight loss.

Pharmacologic Treatment

Comprehension of the mechanism of actions of drugs used in PD depends on thorough understanding of the concept that physiologic acetylcholine and dopamine have opposing actions in the CNS. Acetylcholine serves as an excitatory

BOX 18-1. Clinical Manifestations of Parkinson Disease

Cardinal Motor Symptoms
- Muscular rigidity
- Resting tremor
- Bradykinesia
- Loss of postural reflexes

Additional Motor Symptoms
- Masklike face
- Decreased blinking
- Blurred vision
- Dysphagia
- Dysarthria
- Micrographia

Nonmotor Signs and Symptoms
Autonomic
- Bladder dysfunction
- GI problems
- Constipation
- Orthostatic hypotension
- Increased sweating
- Increased salivation
- Sexual dysfunction
- Difficulty swallowing
- Dermatitis
- Olfactory hypofunction
- Sensory disturbances
- Paresthesia
- Pain

Cognitive/Mood Disorders
- Dementia
- Impaired attention
- Impaired cognition
- Depression
- Anxiety
- Sleep disturbances
- Hallucinations

neurotransmitter, while dopamine functions as an inhibitory one. The basic therapeutic problem in PD has been to find suitable compounds that: (a) increase the concentration of dopamine, (b) stimulate the dopamine receptor sites directly, or (c) depress activity at cholinergic receptor sites. Therapeutic classes of agents that increase dopamine are used, as well as anticholinergic agents. The therapeutic agents discussed below are examples of agents that increase dopamine. Table 18-10 illustrates the variety of drugs used to manage the signs and symptoms of PD and ADEs that may influence the dental hygiene treatment plan.

Dopaminergic Agents

Levodopa-Carbidopa

Levodopa is a drug that increases the synthesis of dopamine. It is an inert chemical, but its metabolite, dopamine, is active

pharmacologically. The amount of levodopa to be used depends on the severity of the PD. At the present time, levodopa is combined with carbidopa, a peripheral dopa-decarboxylase inhibitor. The first signs of improvement are usually a subjective feeling of well-being with increased vigor. The symptoms reduce according to the following sequence: Slow disappearance of akinesia, then rigidity, then tremor, which lessens slowly and incompletely. On stopping the drug, the symptoms reappear in reverse order: Tremor, rigidity, and akinesia. The development of involuntary movements may limit the usefulness of levodopa. This dyskinesia is usually manifested in extrapyramidal movements involving the hands, arm, legs, and face. In addition, increased oral activity, with constant chewing, biting, opening and closing of the mouth, and intermittent protrusions of the tongue, is the most frequent oral manifestation. The abnormal involuntary movements ordinarily occur during the time of maximum benefit from levodopa, which is usually 1 to 2 hours after each dose and may last from several minutes up to 1 or 2 hours. To avoid these involuntary movements, it is generally necessary to increase the frequency of drug administration and, at the same time, decrease the dose of levodopa.

Selegiline (L-Deprenyl)

The mechanism of action in the adjunctive treatment of PD is not fully understood. Inhibition of monoamine oxidase type B (MAO-B) activity is of primary importance, although selegiline may act through other mechanisms to increase dopaminergic activity. Clinical evidence indicates that 10 mg of L-deprenyl in combination with levodopa and carbidopa is superior to levodopa with carbidopa in reducing symptoms of PD. The most significant ADEs related to oral health care procedures include tremors, tardive dyskinesia, involuntary movements, and back and leg muscle cramps. Orthostatic hypotension, dry mouth, and nausea are uncommon side effects. This drug should not be administered with the opioid meperidine (Demerol) due to the possibility of a fatal drug interaction.

Bromocriptine

Bromocriptine is a direct dopamine-receptor agonist. As PD progresses, the activity of dopamine substrates may become so low that dopamine cannot be synthesized. In this case, one could stimulate the dopamine receptor sites located postsynaptically with such compounds as bromocriptine. Low-dose bromocriptine has been found to be effective in some, but not all, patients.

Amantadine

Amantadine (Symmetrel) is a drug that blocks the reuptake of dopamine into presynaptic neurons and causes the release of dopamine from neurons. It is used to reverse drug-induced extrapyramidal reactions in parkinsonism. Amantadine is an effective prophylactic agent for the prevention of respiratory infection caused by A_2 influenza (Asian flu) virus strains. Amantadine inhibits the penetration of viruses into cells.

Anticholinergics

In parkinsonian patients, the deficiency of dopamine results in hyperactivity of cholinergic receptors. Therefore,

Table 18-10	Drugs Used to Treat Parkinson Disease	
Drugs	**Mechanism of Action**	**ADEs**
Levodopa-carbidopa (Sinemet, Sinemet CR)	Levodopa is decarboxylated to dopamine in the CNS. Carbidopa prevents the decarboxylation of levodopa in peripheral tissues.	Orthostatic hypotension Arrhythmia Hallucinations Delusions Confusion Dyskinesia
Carbidopa (Lodosyn)	Prevents the decarboxylation of levodopa in peripheral tissues.	No known toxicities when administered alone.
Bromocriptine (Parlodel) Pergolide (Permax) Pramipexole (Mirapex) Ropinirole (Requip)	Dopamine agonists.	Orthostatic hypotension Somnolence Confusion Sudden sleep attacks Dyskinesia Hallucinations Psychosis
Entacapone (Comtan) Tolcapone (Tasmar)	Inhibit catechol-O-methyltransferase (COMT) and prolong the half-life of levodopa.	Nausea Dyskinesia Liver failure
Selegiline (Eldepryl, Carbex)	Irreversibly inhibits monoamine oxidase type B (MAO-B).	Orthostatic hypotension Insomnia Hallucinations
Amantadine (Symmetrel)	Releases dopamine from terminals.	Confusion Hallucinations
Trihexyphenidyl (Artane, Tremin) Benztropine (Cogentin) Procyclidine (Kemadrin) Biperiden (Akineton)	Anticholinergic agents lessen acetylcholine-dopamine imbalance in the striatum.	Xerostomia Sedation Impaired memory Confusion Hallucinations

anticholinergic drugs, trihexyphenidyl (Artane), procyclidine (Kemadrin), biperiden (Akineton), benztropine (Cogentin) may be used to mitigate some of the symptoms. Skeletal muscle relaxants, such as orphenadrine (Norflex), are used to manage motor symptoms. Dry mouth and anticholinergic effects (dizziness or vision problems) are the side effects relevant to dental hygiene care.

Management Considerations

Dental management of the patient with PD requires an awareness of the nature of this neurodegenerative disorder, and physical, cognitive, and behavioral changes (Box 18-2).[6] Short appointments should be scheduled at times near dosing of PD medications. Efforts to minimize stress may decrease its effect on increased tremor activity. A protocol to prevent orthostatic hypotension following treatment must be implemented at each appointment. Functional limitations must be considered prior to dental hygiene procedures and patient instruction. These functional limitations may lead to decreased oral hygiene efficiency and difficulty in controlling oral hygiene devices and retaining dentures. Airway management is essential due to dysfunction in swallowing or using oral rinse preparations. Intraoral procedures may be compromised by involuntary movements of the jaw. Additional oral complications seen as a result of the pharmacologic management of the disease include xerostomia and burning mouth syndrome. When providing oral health care to patients with PD, the goals are to provide effective treatment and prevent

---

BOX 18-2. Management Considerations in Parkinson Disease

1. Be aware of physical, cognitive, and behavioral changes.
2. Schedule short appointments soon after pharmacologic dosing.
3. Minimize stress.
4. Manage orthostatic hypotension.
5. Assess abilities for plaque control and the use of power toothbrushes.
6. Assess ADEs of drug therapy (xerostomia and complications).
7. Perform careful instrumentation to prevent injury.
8. Apply anticaries therapies (fluoride varnish, fluoride in spray bottle, dentifrice).
9. Use chlorhexidine, followed 30 minutes later with fluoride.
10. Discuss oral care needs with the caregiver and train the caregiver in oral physiotherapy methods.

injury during treatment. Oral health education plans should consider the abilities of the individual to effectively use oral hygiene devices and the development of a home fluoride program compatible with the patient's abilities and needs. Topical agents, such as chlorhexidine gluconate and fluoride rinse preparations, are recommended to combat caries, gingivitis, and other periodontal pathoses that result from plaque accumulation. However, these products require the use of a swish and spit technique that may be beyond the capabilities of patients with PD. In such cases, a small spray bottle filled with the therapeutic rinse may be used to gently spray the product on the oral tissues, either by the patient or the caregiver, and the excess suctioned. When the potential for silent aspiration is a concern, gel preparations of these agents may be applied with a toothbrush, a sponge applicator, or a cotton swab. The application of topical fluorides, including a 5% fluoride varnish, should be part of the office-based preventive care. The effectiveness of chemoprevention, using both chlorhexidine and a fluoride, has been demonstrated in patients at high risk for caries and periodontal disease. To maximize therapeutic efficacy of chlorhexidine, it is suggested that the chlorhexidine be used first, followed 30 minutes later by the application of the fluoride gel.[7] The oral health care provider should discuss the patient's oral health care needs and risk factors that may influence preventive and therapeutic strategies with the patient's caregivers and family members. They may offer suggestions on how to manage the patient and facilitate the timing and the sequencing of dental and medical treatment, daily nursing care, and other therapeutic activities. The oral health care provider should also provide the patient's family or caregivers with appropriate training to facilitate the implementation of tasks required to maximize the patient's oral health.

■ Self-Study Review

25. Describe the manifestations of PD and their relevance to oral health care.
26. Identify the etiology of xerostomia in PD.
27. Identify drugs used to manage symptoms of PD and ADEs of each agent.
28. Describe dental hygiene management considerations for the client with PD.

DENTAL HYGIENE APPLICATIONS

A wide variety of conditions are managed with drugs that act on the CNS. In general, the clinician must consider the control of the medical condition for which the drug is used. Drug side effects may have specific management considerations, such as orthostatic hypotension (slowly return the chair to upright, allow the patient to remain seated for several minutes before dismissing), xerostomia (fluoride therapy, xylitol), fine hand tremors (power toothbrushes), and extrapyramidal symptoms of tardive dyskinesia and involuntary movements (may be difficult to complete some oral procedures). Tables within the chapter for the various agents include management considerations specific to those agents. The dental hygienist may be asked to assist in verification of client understanding of dosing instructions and warnings for drugs prescribed by the dentist. For most CNS depressants, instructions should include not signing legally binding documents, making important decisions, or operating equipment. Amnesia caused by benzodiazepines can persist for up to 45 minutes, so client instructions should be provided in writing. A drug reference should be consulted for potential side effects of each specific drug. When nonprescription drugs are recommended, these agents should be investigated to ensure no interaction exists with the CNS agent.

CONCLUSION

Drugs that stimulate the CNS are used for a wide variety of reasons. Anxiety and fear prevents some individuals from seeking dental care. Depression can occur in adults, adolescents, and children. Both the medical condition for which the drugs are used and the drug effects must be considered when planning for dental hygiene care. A concentrated preventive program is important for individuals who experience psychologic disorders, because they may lack proper oral hygiene care and may experience side effects of CNS depressant medications. Many of these agents can result in drug dependence. These various factors must be considered prior to oral care.

References

1. Friedlander AH, Mahler ME. Major depressive disorder: Psychopathology, medical management and dental implications. *J Am Dent Assoc.* 2001;132(5):629–638.
2. Smith TA, Heaton LJ. Fear of dental care: Are we making any progress? *J Am Dent Assoc.* 2003;134(8):1101–1108.
3. Moore R, Brodsgaard I, Mao TK, et al. Fear of injections and report of negative dentist behavior among Caucasians, American and Taiwanese adults from dental school clinics. *Community Dent Oral Epidemiol.* 1996;24:292–295.
4. Kloostra PW, Eber RM, Inglehart MR. Anxiety, stress, depression, and patient's responses to periodontal treatment: Periodontists' knowledge and professional behavior. *J Periodontol.* 2007;78(1):64–71.
5. Gerber PE, Lynd LD. Selective serotonin-reuptake inhibitor-induced movement disorders. *Ann Pharmacother.* 1998;32(6):692–698.
6. Clifford T, Finnerty J. The dental awareness and needs of a Parkinson's disease population. *Gerodontology.* 1995;12:99–103.
7. Ten Cate JM, Parsh PD. Procedures for establishing efficacy of antimicrobial agents for chemotherapeutic caries prevention. *J Dent Res.* 1994;73(3):695–703.

CLINICAL APPLICATION EXERCISES

■ **Exercise 1.** Describe patient instructions when a benzodiazepine is prescribed for a client prior to periodontal therapy.

■ **Exercise 2.** Design a treatment plan for the client taking a drug that has a side effect of tardive dyskinesia.

■ **Exercise 3.** Develop a treatment plan for the patient with PD, identifying considerations for the dental hygiene care plan.

19

Anticonvulsant Drugs

Epilepsy is one of the most common neurologic disorders affecting humans. The term *epilepsy* is synonymous with "seizure disorder." Because the condition is estimated to affect 1% to 3% of the U.S. population, the dental hygienist will likely encounter a client with a seizure disorder at some point.[1] The goal of anticonvulsant medications is to prevent recurrent seizures; therefore, the medical history review must include questioning regarding patient compliance with taking anticonvulsant medications. These drugs do not cure the neurologic disorder and must be taken daily to prevent seizures. Potential adverse drug effects (ADEs) that affect the dental hygiene treatment plan must be considered. This chapter focuses on understanding the disorder, various manifestations and types of seizures, and effects of medications used to control seizures. A description of the acute management of specific seizures that occur during the provision of oral health care services is provided.

SEIZURE DISORDER

Epilepsy is a symptom rather than a disease, and it is characterized by recurrent seizures or convulsions. A *seizure* is a periodic attack of disturbed cerebral function. It can manifest as a motion disturbance, an altered level of consciousness, or a loss of consciousness. It can be an isolated event with an unknown etiology, or it can occur on a recurrent basis. Seizures stem from excessive nerve cell discharges within the brain and are accompanied by sudden disturbances in sensory and/or motor function. The underlying nature of epilepsy is not fully understood, but it is generally believed that in normal brain tissue there is equilibrium between the process of neuronal excitation and inhibition, but in epilepsy the balance is lost in favor of excitation. The imbalance may be localized to one area of the brain (focal), or it may spread to involve the entire brain and spinal cord (generalized), producing a severe convulsion. The underlying disorder of the brain that gives rise to the seizure may be structural, chemical, physiologic, or a combination of all three. Often the etiology is unknown. Some identified causative factors are preventable, such as infections or alcohol-related factors, while others cannot be prevented (Table 19-1). Although the basic mechanism may be the same for all seizures, the triggering mechanism varies from patient to patient. The most common population affected includes children younger than 1 year and individuals older than 75 years.[1] Vascular diseases increase the prevalence of epilepsy in the aging population and represent the

Table 19-1	Causes of Epilepsy	
Preventable/Treatable	**Unpreventable**	
Trauma and asphyxia	Genetic factors	
Infectious diseases, fever	Postvaccination effects	
Complications of pregnancy	Tumors	
Toxicity, alcohol, drugs	Degenerative disorders	
Metabolic, endocrine, and nutritional disorders	Circulatory disturbances	

most common cause of seizures in individuals over 60 years of age.

TYPES OF SEIZURES

Just as there are many causes of epilepsy, so are there many different types of seizures (Table 19-2). Some seizures have signs to signal an oncoming attack (**preictal** signs). Other seizures have no warning signs and are recognized by the events that occur during the seizure. Epilepsy is classified based on the clinical manifestation of the seizure. The two main categories are partial seizures and generalized seizures; seizures that result from a limited or specific area in the brain are described as *simple partial seizures*, and those that involve the entire cerebral cortex are called *generalized seizures*. Some individuals have seizures that evolve from partial into generalized types as the electrical discharges spread from one area of the brain to other areas. In this situation, the simple partial seizure evolves into a complex partial seizure. *Tonic–clonic* (generalized) seizures are the most common form.[2] Some seizures have preictal warning signs (**aura**), and **postictal** confusion occurs with some forms.

Focal or Partial Seizures

Partial seizures are classified into three types: Simple, complex, and partial seizures that evolve to secondary generalized seizures. The types are distinguished by the effects that develop. An affected client may not know the specific type of epilepsy he or she has but may be able to describe its signs and symptoms. The practitioner may be able to predict the necessary treatment modifications based on this information.

Table 19-2	Seizure Classifications
Focal or Partial Seizures	**General Seizures**
Motor	Tonic–clonic convulsion (grand mal)
Sensory	Absence (petit mal)
• Somatic	• Simple
• Visual	• With minor motor accompaniment
• Auditory	• With automatism
• Olfactory	• Continuing or status
Psychomotor	Myoclonic
• Automatism	• Jerks
• Psychical	• Atonic

Simple Partial

Simple partial seizures result from a local discrete spread of excitation that does not become generalized. Jacksonian epilepsy or simple motor seizures often follow physical injury to a brain region, such as that caused by an auto accident. Convulsions in jacksonian seizures are often confined to a single limb or muscle group (jacksonian motor epilepsy) or to specific and localized sensory disturbance (jacksonian sensory epilepsy). In the simple partial seizure, the individual remains conscious but may have a twitching movement, such as a jerking leg or facial twitch. Other signs may include sensory manifestations (such as paresthesia, visual changes, or clenching and smacking of the jaw) or autonomic symptoms (such as tachycardia or dizziness).[2]

Complex Partial

Complex partial seizures result in an altered state of consciousness. They can begin as simple seizures that evolve to affect a greater area of the brain. The typical presentation is a sensory aura followed by impaired consciousness. The patient may be slow to respond or may not respond to commands at all. There may be complex, repetitive motor activity, such as continually tying the shoes. This form of epilepsy is treated with medications or with surgery to remove tissue in the focal area causing the seizure. Surgical treatment often cures the disorder, and the patient becomes seizure free.[2]

Partial Seizure and Secondary Generalized Seizure

The partial seizure and *secondary generalized seizure* can begin as a simple partial or complex partial seizure. Unexplained events allow the electrical discharges to spread and produce asymmetric, tonic–clonic movements. The movements are different from those associated with primary generalized tonic–clonic seizures, which are symmetrical.[2]

■ Self-Study Review

1. Define *epilepsy* and *seizure*. What populations are at increased risk?
2. Differentiate between *generalized* seizure and *focal* seizure characteristics.
3. Describe signs of generalized seizures and partial seizures.
4. Identify the most common seizure types.

Generalized Seizures

Primary generalized seizures involve both hemispheres of the brain and are divided into three common categories, including tonic–clonic, myoclonic, and absence. In contrast to partial seizures, which usually respond to the same anticonvulsant drugs, these types often are treated with drugs specific for the seizure type. Each type has characteristic signs and symptoms that distinguish them from each other. The tonic–clonic form presents the most difficult seizure management in the dental office.

Tonic–Clonic Seizure (Grand Mal)

Unconsciousness and rhythmic, jerking convulsions characterize the *tonic–clonic seizure*. If the individual is standing, loss of consciousness causes a fall to the floor. In the dental chair, the patient can lose consciousness, **nystagmus** can occur, and convulsions can involve the entire body. An *aura* (visual, auditory, epigastric, or psychic) can alert the client of an impending attack, preceding unconsciousness. After the person becomes unconscious, spasm occurs in the diaphragm muscles that explosively forces air out of the lungs, resulting in the epileptic "cry." Generalized motor tonic–clonic seizures follow this high-pitched vocalization. During the tonic component of the seizure, the body stiffens for 10 to 20 seconds, forcing the individual into an arched position when the violent spasm of all body musculature pulls the back muscles. This is followed by convulsions of extremities (clonic phase) for 30 to 40 seconds. In the clonic phase, alternate contraction and relaxation of all muscles occur. Seizures typically last from 2 to 5 minutes. Urinary or fecal control is often lost during a seizure. Postseizure depression of motor and sensory function makes the person sleep for several hours. During this time, the decision would be made for a family member to take the individual home or for emergency medical services (EMS) personnel to be called to transport the person to a hospital facility. Oral signs of this seizure type can include scars involving the lips and tongue and broken or fractured teeth.

Management of Seizure in Dental Office

Preparation for management of the tonic–clonic seizure should include certification in basic life support (BLS) and a protocol for responsibilities of each dental team member in management of the situation (Who calls EMS? Who secures oxygen? Who stays with patient?). At the onset of a seizure, treatment is stopped, instruments and devices are removed from the oral cavity, the situation is assessed, and appropriate management is initiated. If the chair is upright, place the patient in a supine position. Move the bracket tray or equipment that could injure the patient out of the way during the seizure. If the patient alerts the practitioner of an aura (time allowing), the practitioner should move the patient from the dental chair to the floor, away from furniture that could cause injury to the patient. Allow the patient to have the seizure without intervening; nothing should be placed into the patient's mouth.[3] For most seizures, BLS is adequate, and no drugs are used to stop seizure activity. If the seizure lasts over 5 minutes, the EMS system should be activated, and oxygen should be provided by face mask. When EMS arrives, an IV for benzodiazepine administration will be initiated unless the dentist is trained to insert the IV and has already begun emergency treatment.

Myoclonic Seizure

Myoclonic convulsions are generalized seizures that are characterized by rhythmic body jerks without loss of consciousness. The seizure is characterized by sudden, involuntary, excessive movements that last for a few seconds. Movements are similar to sleep jerks or hiccups. The patient is aware of the seizure. This form is often hereditary. The short na-

ture of the episode does not involve a management situation during the dental hygiene appointment.

Absence Seizure (Petit Mal)

The *absence seizure*, another form of generalized seizure, involves neither convulsions nor loss of consciousness. It is characterized by a brief period of impaired consciousness and cessation of activity, often with a motor manifestation, such as twitching of the eyelids. These attacks cause the patient to lose mental awareness of the immediate surroundings and sometimes to simply stare off into space. The affected individual is unaware the seizure is occurring and may describe the signs and symptoms from observations of family members. There is no aura or postictal confusion. This type of seizure, occurring as frequently as several hundred times daily, is most common in the prepubertal years of childhood and often resolves as the child reaches adulthood. Some cases continue into adult life and may be accompanied by generalized tonic–clonic seizures. Patient assessment questioning should involve both the child and parent to determine the risk of seizure and the need for modifications in the treatment plan.

Status Epilepticus

When a seizure does not resolve but instead continues into multiple seizures, an emergency situation that requires immediate intervention can occur. *Status epilepticus* is defined as a seizure that lasts >30 minutes.[2] Any type of seizure can develop into status epilepticus; however, the tonic–clonic seizure that does not resolve is the most dangerous form of this seizure complication, because continuous seizures inhibit respiration to the extent that hypoxia can occur in the brain and cause permanent damage or death. The complication is treated with IV administration of a benzodiazepine (diazepam, lorazepam, or midazolam).[2] The condition may develop in an individual diagnosed with epilepsy or in those who have not been diagnosed. The major cause in children is an infection, resulting in a high fever.[2] Acute causes in adults include stroke, hypoxia, and alcohol intoxication and withdrawal. Airway management is a serious concern, and supplemental oxygen must be provided. Aspiration of oral fluids may complicate management efforts. When the condition develops in the dental office, the EMS system must immediately be activated while oxygen inhalation therapy is started. Individuals who take numerous different anticonvulsant drugs usually have poorly controlled epilepsy and pose an increased risk for status epilepticus.[2]

■ Self-Study Review

5. Identify the seizure type that is most difficult to manage.
6. Describe the events that produce the "epileptic cry."
7. Describe the phases of tonic–clinic seizure.
8. Describe management of the tonic–clonic seizure. When should EMS be summoned?
9. Define and describe *status epilepticus*.

Table 19-3	Treatment of Seizures	
Seizure Disorder	Drugs of Choice	Alternatives
Focal or partial seizures	Phenytoin or carbamazepine	Phenobarbital primidone
Tonic–clonic (grand mal)	Phenytoin, carbamazepine, or valproate	Phenobarbital primidone
Absence (petit mal)	Ethosuximide or valproate	Clonazepam
Myoclonic	Valproate	Clonazepam

Treatment of Epilepsy

The most direct approach one can make toward successful treatment of specific seizure disorders is to determine and resolve, if possible, the primary underlying cause of the attack. Currently, surgical therapy is used in this approach. Another approach that involves recurrent seizure disorder is to control or prevent the seizures by the use of anticonvulsant medications. Medications are supplied as elixirs (which often contain sugar to disguise the taste), tablets, and capsules.

Pharmacologic Management

There is no pharmacologic therapy that cures recurrent epilepsy. Subsequently, signs and symptoms of seizure disorders are managed with a variety of antiseizure medications, with the choice depending on the type of seizure. When recurrent seizure is reported in the individual taking anticonvulsant medications, the most common reason is noncompliance in taking the medication. This illustrates the importance of patient questioning regarding this issue before treatment is initiated. The drugs of choice and alternative drugs for the treatment of the most common types of epileptic seizures are listed in Table 19-3.

Phenytoin

The prototype for the anticonvulsant class of drugs is *phenytoin* (Dilantin). Phenytoin has been approved for the treatment of tonic–clonic and partial seizures. The precise mechanism leading to stabilization of the neuronal membrane by phenytoin is uncertain, but it is believed to (a) limit the development of maximal seizure activity and (b) reduce the spread of seizure process from an epileptic focus. Phenytoin reduces calcium ion transport at the outer nerve membrane by blocking its high-affinity binding sites and prevents the release of norepinephrine, which is necessary for the generation of maximal seizure activity. Phenytoin is absorbed primarily from the duodenum. After absorption, it becomes highly bound to plasma proteins, allowing only a small percentage of the drug to be free for receptor binding. Drugs that may alter the degree of protein binding (such as aspirin) will significantly increase the toxicity of phenytoin and affect the therapeutic usefulness of the drug. Phenytoin is metabolized in the liver to an inactive metabolite and is excreted by the kidneys. Because the membrane-stabilizing effect of phenytoin is not limited to neurons but also works on other excitable tissues,

such as skeletal and heart muscle, it is effective in treating **myotonia** and cardiac arrhythmias.

Adverse Drug Effects

Phenytoin's ADE of interest to oral health care providers is gingival hyperplasia, which occurs in approximately 50% of those who take it (Color Plate 22). It also causes coarsening of the facial features and hirsutism. Serum folic acid and vitamin K concentrations may be depressed, and chronic therapy may cause rickets and osteomalacia due to altered vitamin D metabolism. Phenytoin may cause hypersensitivity reactions characterized by rashes, erythema multiforme (Color Plates 41–43), Stevens-Johnson syndrome, blood dyscrasias, and serum sickness. Long-term therapy can result in loss of bone mineral density. With increasing dosage, phenytoin may cause nystagmus, diplopia, drowsiness, xerostomia, and ataxia. It may interfere with cognitive function in learning situations.

DENTAL HYGIENE MANAGEMENT. Chronic xerostomia is possible because phenytoin is taken on a long-term basis, and at-home fluoride preparations should be recommended to reduce the caries risk.[4] Poor plaque control is a factor in gingival enlargement, and methods to effectively remove plaque biofilm are necessary. This will not eliminate hyperplasia but will reduce the rapidity of enlargement. A 3-month maintenance schedule to manage oral effects is recommended.[2,4]

Carbamazepine

Carbamazepine (Tegretol), another drug in the anticonvulsant class, is structurally related to phenytoin and has similar, but not identical, mechanisms of action. Carbamazepine is recommended for the treatment of generalized tonic–clonic and partial seizures. In addition to its antiepileptic effect, carbamazepine demonstrates sedative, anticholinergic, antidepressant, muscle relaxant, antiarrhythmic, antidiuretic, and neuromuscular transmission inhibitory actions, and it is used for the treatment of trigeminal neuralgia. In therapeutic concentrations, it decreases sodium and potassium conductances and depresses posttetanic potentiation. The oral bioavailability of carbamazepine is relatively high. After absorption, as much as 60% to 70% is bound to plasma proteins. Carbamazepine is metabolized to active derivatives, some of which are excreted unchanged.

Adverse Drug Effects

Carbamazepine commonly causes drowsiness, diplopia, and ataxia, but it has less effect on cognitive function than phenytoin. Blood dyscrasias (thrombocytopenia, leukopenia, aplastic anemia, and agranulocytosis), cardiac toxicity, hepatitis, and Stevens-Johnson syndrome have been reported.

DENTAL HYGIENE MANAGEMENT. The dental hygienist should question the patient about bleeding tendency and recent infection and examine the oral cavity for petechiae or signs of infection to rule out blood dyscrasia. The chewable doseform, frequently prescribed for children, contains sugar to improve the taste. When taken as prescribed (up to four times/day), the risk for caries increases. In this situation, home fluoride therapy and sealants should be recommended.[4]

Dental Drug Interactions

Like phenobarbital, carbamazepine can induce microsomal enzymes in the liver and alter the metabolism of other drugs. This can decrease the effect of doxycycline. The effect of carbamazepine may be increased by erythromycin and propoxyphene. When these drugs are prescribed by the dentist, warnings should be included in patient information.

Phenobarbital

Phenobarbital (Luminal) is a barbiturate that is widely used for the treatment of tonic–clonic and partial seizures, and it is the prototype for this group of anticonvulsant drugs. It is often used in combination with phenytoin. The precise mechanism of action of phenobarbital is not known, but it is believed to inhibit posttetanic potentiation and raise seizure threshold. Phenobarbital is absorbed from the small intestine and becomes bound to protein to the extent of 50%. Phenobarbital is slowly metabolized in the liver, and approximately 20% to 25% of phenobarbital is excreted unchanged in the urine.

Adverse Drug Effects

Compared to phenytoin, phenobarbital is a relatively safe compound. However, in some patients pronounced sedation, reduced activity, and cognitive impairment may be noted. Rare cases of skin reactions, such as Stevens-Johnson syndrome, have been reported.

Primidone

Primidone (Mysoline) is a nonbarbiturate compound that is structurally and functionally related to phenobarbital. Primidone is effective for the same types of seizures as phenobarbital. It is well absorbed from the stomach and does not bind to plasma proteins extensively. Primidone is metabolized to phenobarbital and a related compound, which are both active anticonvulsants.

Adverse Drug Effects

Sedation, vertigo, nausea, and ataxia occur frequently, and primidone can also cause disturbances in behavior, difficulty in concentration, and loss of libido.

Valproate (Valproic Acid)

The term *valproate* is used to refer to this group of drugs, which is not structurally related to other anticonvulsants. The group includes valproic acid, valproate sodium, and divalproex sodium. Valproate is used primarily for the treatment of absence seizures, although it has also been used to prevent tonic–clonic and myoclonic seizures. The mechanism of action of valproate (Depakene) is not fully understood, but it has been postulated to enhance the inhibitory neurotransmitter gamma-aminobutyric acid (GABA). It is rapidly absorbed from the gastrointestinal tract and binds to plasma proteins extensively. Valproate is biotransformed to inactive metabolites, which are eliminated in the kidney.

Adverse Drug Effects

The most common side effects of valproate include nausea, vomiting, and sedation. Valproate inhibits platelet aggregation and can prolong the bleeding time. For procedures where significant bleeding is expected, bleeding time should be determined (20 minutes or less is safe). Because valproate can affect bleeding, other drugs that influence bleeding should be used with caution. Hepatic toxicity, pancreatitis, alopecia, and blood dyscrasias have been noted but are rare.

Clonazepam

Clonazepam (Klonopin), a drug in the benzodiazepine class, interacts with benzodiazepine receptor sites, which in turn enhances postsynaptic GABA transmission. It is used for the treatment of both myoclonic and absence seizures that may be resistant to treatment with other anticonvulsants. ADEs include drowsiness, ataxia, and behavioral disorders.

Ethosuximide

Ethosuximide (Zarontin) is recommended for treatment of uncomplicated absence seizures. The precise mechanism of action of ethosuximide has not been established, but it is believed to enhance inhibitory processes in cortical pathways by augmenting the functions of inhibitory transmitters, such as dopamine and GABA neurotransmitters. Following absorption, ethosuximide does not bind to plasma proteins. It is metabolized in the liver into inactive metabolites. Both the metabolites and the unchanged drug are excreted in the urine.

Adverse Drug Effects

ADEs include nausea, vomiting, headaches, drowsiness, eosinophilia, and leukopenia. Erythema multiforme, Stevens-Johnson syndrome, and a lupuslike syndrome have occasionally been reported.

Gabapentin

Gabapentin is a drug used for adjunctive therapy in the management of partial and generalized seizures. It stabilizes voltage-activated calcium channels in the brain to provide an antiseizure effect, and it is also approved for the treatment of postherpetic neuralgia. Gabapentin is generally well tolerated. Common ADEs include dizziness, somnolence, fatigue, and nystagmus. Severe ADEs include Stevens-Johnson syndrome. No documented drug–drug interactions related to dental therapeutics have been reported.

Felbamate

Felbamate is a drug used for the treatment of refractory partial and tonic–clonic seizures. It stabilizes the inactivated state of voltage-gated Na^+ channels, thereby reducing membrane excitability. Common side effects include photosensitivity, dizziness, abnormal gait, and gastrointestinal irritation. Severe ADEs include aplastic anemia, hepatic failure, and Stevens-Johnson syndrome. No documented drug–drug interactions related to dental therapeutics are reported.

Lamotrigine

Lamotrigine, a drug used in the treatment of refractory complex partial seizures, stabilizes the inactivated state of voltage-gated Na^+ channels, thereby reducing membrane excitability. The drug is also approved for maintenance management in bipolar disorder. The most common ADEs include dizziness, ataxia, somnolence, headache, diplopia, nausea, and vomiting. Life-threatening Stevens-Johnson syndrome and toxic epidermal necrolysis rarely have occurred. No drug–drug interactions related to dental therapeutics are documented.

■ Self-Study Review

10. Identify the drug(s) used for specific seizure types.
11. What is the most common reason for recurrent seizures?
12. Describe ADEs for the various antiseizure drugs.

BOX 19-1. Questions for Epileptic Patients

1. What type of seizure disorder was diagnosed, and when was the condition diagnosed?
2. What drugs are being taken?
3. Has the patient noticed any side effects?
4. How frequently is the medication taken? Has it been taken today?
5. When was the last seizure?
6. Does the patient experience an "aura"? Describe the events of the aura.
7. What occurs during a seizure, and how does it resolve?
8. Has the patient had a seizure during a dental appointment? What caused it?

THE MEDICAL MANAGEMENT OF CHRONIC (NEUROPATHIC) PAIN

The treatment of neuropathic pain disorders with psychotropic pharmacotherapeutic agents is an evolving area of therapy. Unlike patients with acute (nociceptive) pain, patients with chronic pain generally do not respond to conventional analgesic therapy. The anticonvulsants carbamazepine, clonazepam, valproic acid, gabapentin, lamotrigine, topiramate, and phenytoin can relieve neuropathic pain associated with diabetic neuropathy and trigeminal, glossopharyngeal, and postherpetic neuralgia. Other drugs used in treatment include tricyclic antidepressants, such as amitriptyline and imipramine. Although their mechanism of action is unclear, tricyclics can relieve many types of neuropathic pain, including postherpetic neuralgia, burning mouth syndrome, diabetic neuropathy, fibromyalgia, and chronic myofascial pain.

DENTAL HYGIENE APPLICATIONS

During the first appointment with a patient reporting a history of epilepsy, the clinician must obtain a thorough medical history. The dental hygienist begins the assessment by determining if the client had a single seizure or has recurrent seizures. Recurrent seizure disorder has an increased risk for a medical emergency during an appointment. Questioning should include specific questions related to the potential risks in treatment. Box 19-1 includes the most essential questions to gain necessary information. Some authors report that individuals with seizure disorders have poorer oral health than the general population.[5] Factors include the type of seizure (tonic–clonic) and a low socioeconomic status. Recurrent seizures can disable the client and make treatment impossible. As oral health professionals gain a better understanding of the disorder and how it may affect the oral health, the anxiety about providing oral care should be reduced. Regular maintenance for periodontal care should be provided for controlled patients. Uncontrolled disease should be referred for medical intervention, and dental treatment should be resumed as seizure control is obtained. For patients with no history of epilepsy who develop a tonic–clonic seizure, the EMS system should be immediately activated and the seizure should be managed as described earlier.

Relevance of Questioning in Patient Assessment

What Type of Seizure Disorder Was Diagnosed and When?

The well-controlled patient with epilepsy can be treated safely in the dental office. A single seizure from a known cause is unlikely to pose a problem in care. Recurrent seizures are the most risky diagnosis. The possibility of a medical emergency can be identified by asking the patient if seizures are recurring, especially if a tonic–clonic seizure is possible. When diagnosis of epilepsy is recent, the pharmacologic management may not be completely effective. There is a period of drug and dose adjustment to see what therapy prevents the seizures and to determine the dose that can be tolerated by the patient. The determination should be made to see if the drug is preventing seizures for the true treatment risks to be known, particularly if tonic–clonic epilepsy was diagnosed. When dental treatment is likely to involve stressful procedures, it may need to be delayed until the pharmacologic management for seizure control is assured.

What Drug Is Being Taken?

Most patients are controlled with a single antiepileptic drug, but a small group of individuals will require a second anticonvulsant agent. The more anticonvulsant drugs being taken, the greater the risk for status epilepticus. Initially drugs may cause drowsiness, dizziness, or cognitive impairment. These ADEs are usually temporary but may cause noncompliance in taking the medication and missed dental appointments (for example, the patient goes to sleep and does not awake in time to make the appointment or forgets about it altogether).

Some anticonvulsants taken on a long-term basis cause a reduction in bone mineral density, so bisphosphonates may be prescribed to combat the risk for osteoporosis. Follow-up for bisphosphonate education, as described in Chapter 14, should be provided.

Have There Been Any Side Effects?

Potential side effects of agents taken should be investigated. Oral examination for evidence of chronic dry mouth and caries should be completed at each appointment. Bleeding should be monitored during oral débridement when agents that can increase bleeding are taken. Gingival overgrowth occurring with phenytoin therapy can be reduced with strict plaque control. In these individuals, oral health information should include strategies to encourage regular and effective biofilm removal, and the ability to effectively remove plaque with oral devices should be evaluated. Frequent recall visits may be necessary for patients who develop gingival hyperplasia. Caries prevention should be considered for patients taking chewable anticonvulsant agents containing sugar. Drowsiness and lack of attention may influence the oral health education program.

How Often Is the Medication Taken, and Has It Been Taken Today?

The most common reason for uncontrolled seizures is failure to take antiseizure medication as prescribed. Once a patient has been seizure free for 2 years while taking anticonvulsant medications, the physician may reduce the dose or withdraw pharmacologic therapy completely.[2] This is a safe option when the long-term effects of drug therapy are considered. When questioning reveals this history, no alterations to the dental treatment plan are indicated, although the possibility of a seizure during treatment still exists. Most elderly patients will take anticonvulsant drugs for the remainder of their lives.

When Was the Client's Last Seizure?

The goal of anticonvulsant therapy is to keep the individual seizure free. For those affected with recurrent seizures that are uncontrolled by pharmacologic therapy, elective oral health care should be postponed and the patient referred for medical evaluation. Medical consultation will be needed to determine when oral health care procedures can be safely provided. Although seizures can occur in well-controlled patients, they are uncommon. Situations that can lead to a seizure include extreme fatigue, pain, stress, alcohol use, noncompliance in taking anticonvulsant medication, overhead dental lights, use of local anesthetics, and idiopathic causes.

Does the Client Experience an "Aura"? How Would It Be Described?

Information about auras can be used as a strategy to identify an impending seizure during treatment. The patient should be requested to notify the dental hygienist if the aura sensation occurs so that the patient can be moved to a safe area before the seizure develops.

What Occurs During the Seizure, and How Does It Resolve?

Knowing what happens during the seizure helps the practitioner to know what to expect. If the seizure is described as resolving on its own with no need for a summons for the EMS, this guides one to manage the event properly, should it develop. If a tonic–clonic seizure is possible, ensuring the ability to rapidly retrieve oxygen equipment and the location of the emergency medical kit is advisable.

Has the Client Had a Seizure During a Dental Appointment? What Caused It?

Anxiety associated with oral health care has caused seizures. The cause of a previous seizure should be considered and avoided to prevent another seizure during the appointment. Sometimes establishing rapport with the client, explaining treatment procedures, and assuring the client that a break can be taken anytime helps to reduce the anxiety level. Nitrous oxide is an option to relax the client and can be used with anticonvulsant medication. Sudden movements during treatment should be avoided.

■ Self-Study Review

13. Identify follow up questions related to a history of seizure disorder, and explain their use in identifying the need for treatment plan modifications and risks for oral care.

CONCLUSION

Epilepsy affects up to 3% of the U.S. population, and affected patients will present for dental hygiene therapy. A thorough medical assessment will identify most treatment risks and indications. Anticonvulsant therapy is the mainstay to prevent recurrent seizures. These agents are taken chronically, and ADEs are likely to manifest. Management is based on an understanding of the disorder, the pattern of seizures, the risk for a seizure while receiving dental hygiene care, and a determination of preventive therapies for ADEs experienced by the patient. To provide competent care to patients with seizure disorder, clinicians must understand the disease, its treatment, and its impact on the patient's ability to undergo and respond to dental care.

References

1. Wyllie E. *The Treatment of Epilepsy: Principles and Practice.* 2nd ed. Baltimore: Williams & Wilkins; 1997.

CLINICAL APPLICATION EXERCISES

◼ **Exercise 1.** Your 8:00 AM patient arrives late to the appointment. The medical history review reveals a history of tonic–clonic epilepsy. The patient reports taking phenytoin and has not had a seizure in several years. No side effects from the drug are reported, as her dose was lowered recently because she has been seizure free for a prolonged time. What medication effects are relevant to patient assessment, and what are the dental hygiene management considerations?

◼ **Exercise 2.** What topics should be included in the oral health education plan for a patient taking carbamazepine chewable tablets?

◼ **Exercise 3.** WEB ACTIVITY: Do an Internet search for *epilepsy* and identify the official organization for information on the various convulsive disorders. Peruse the site to gain general knowledge on the medical disorder.

2. Bryan RB, Sullivan SM. Management of dental patients with seizure disorders. *Dent Clin North Am.* 2006;50:607–623.
3. Pickett F, Gurenlian J. *The Medical History: Clinical Implications and Emergency Prevention in Dental Settings.* Baltimore: Lippincott Williams & Wilkins; 2005:160.
4. Stoopler ET, Sollecito TP, Greenberg MS. Seizure disorders: Update of medical and dental considerations. *Gen Dent.* 2003; 51(4):361–366.
5. Aragon CE, Burneo JG. Understanding the patient with epilepsy and seizures in the dental practice. *J Can Dent Assoc.* 2007;73(1): 71–76.

Part 4

Drugs Used by Special Populations

20

Herbal and Dietary Supplements

KEY TERMS

Dietary supplement: A natural product used for improved structure and function of the body, including

herbs, vitamins, minerals, and any other product sold as a dietary supplement

KEY ACRONYMS

DSHEA: Dietary Supplement Health and Education Act of 1994
EO: Essential oils, used in many antigingivitis mouth rinses
GMP: Good manufacturing practices
cGMP: Current good manufacturing practices, updated in 2007

SN/AEMS: Special Nutritionals Adverse Event Monitoring System
SJW: Saint-John's-wort, an herb used to treat mild depression

The purported health benefits and aggressive marketing of herbal products and **dietary supplements** have dramatically increased their use during the last decade.[1-3] Because of this popularity, the dental hygienist needs to consider effects of these products as part of the health history review. During this growth period, concerns have been raised about adequate research supporting efficacy claims and lack of uniform product standardizations.[3] Recognition of this trend has prompted increasing concerns about the safety and efficacy of herbal products and other dietary supplements.[4-6] Because they are considered natural products rather than drugs by users, supplements may not be mentioned during the drug interview or listed as medications by patients. The most recent American Dental Association (ADA) health history recognizes the relevance of gathering dietary supplement information, because it includes an item for the reporting of "vitamins, natural or herbal preparations, and/or diet supplements."[7] Reports of adverse drug effects (ADEs) from these products (Box 20-1) that can impact oral health care include postural hypotension (niacin), interaction with drugs used for oral sedation, drowsiness (Saint-John's-wort [SJW], valerian, kava), hypertension and tachycardia (ephedrine), oral ulceration (feverfew leaves,

when chewed), oral mucosal irritation (goldenseal), gastrointestinal (GI) distress (goldenseal, glucosamine, saw palmetto) and increased bleeding (ginkgo, ginseng, garlic, ginger, high doses of Vitamin E).[7-9]

The risk of these potential ADEs should be assessed (client questioning, vital signs, clinical exam) and monitored during dental hygiene treatment.

HERBAL AND NUTRITIONAL SUPPLEMENTS

Over 20,000 herbal (botanical) and other natural products are available in the United States. The term *natural* has been used with herbal products because they are derived from plant sources. The most commonly purchased products include echinacea, feverfew, garlic, ginseng, ginkgo, goldenseal, kava, SJW, saw palmetto, and valerian. Some products are used for health maintenance or for benign, self-limited conditions. Glucosamine and glucosamine/chondroitin have

BOX 20-1. Clinical Considerations for Commonly Used Herbs

Herb	Potential Clinical Effect
Niacin	Postural hypotension
SJW, valerian, kava	Increased sedation with sedative drugs, drowsiness
Ephedrine	Tachycardia, hypertension
Feverfew leaves, goldenseal	Oral ulceration or irritation
Ginkgo, ginseng, garlic, ginger	Increased bleeding
High-dose vitamin E	Increased bleeding
Goldenseal, saw palmetto	GI distress, oral mucosal irritation
Glucosamine	GI distress
Echinacea	Perioral candidiasis

been used successfully to manage symptoms of osteoarthritis. However, others are used to self-treat serious illnesses, such as hawthorn for congestive heart failure, milk thistle for liver disease, and SJW for mild depression.

Herbal products are marketed as dietary supplements in the United States and do not have to comply with the laws for safety and efficacy imposed on drug products. They cannot make claims to cure conditions, but they can make claims to improve structure and function. However, the Food and Drug Administration (FDA) can allow a qualified health claim if scientific evidence supports the claim. For example, soy protein manufacturers are allowed to make the claim that use of their product can reduce the risk for cardiovascular disease when 25 g/day are consumed. When the FDA suggested stricter regulation of the herbal supplement industry, thousands of letters from the general public were sent to Congress to block such regulations. This led to the passage of the Dietary Supplement Health and Education Act of 1994 (DSHEA) to separate supplements from rules on regulated drugs. The act created a new category for herbs, vitamins, minerals, and other products marketed as dietary supplements. Previously, a supplement manufacturer had to prove that its product was safe if challenged by the FDA. Provisions in the 1994 act require the FDA to prove the product was unsafe. Changes in the Federal Food, Drug, and Cosmetic Act in 2006 require the supplement industry to report all serious dietary-supplement-related ADEs to the FDA. In 2007, the FDA drafted regulations requiring manufacturers to test their products for purity, to assure that products do not contain contaminants, and to verify that the contents within the package matches labeling information (*http://www.fda.gov/bbs/topics/NEWS/2007/NEW01657.html*).

During their growth in popularity over the last several years, the promotion of these products has undergone fundamental changes. In the past, herbal products were promoted to consumers primarily by mail-order companies and health food stores. More recently, chain drug stores and grocery stores have aggressively advertised herbal products to con-

sumers in a manner similar to that for nonprescription drug products. The introduction of entire herbal product lines by traditional manufacturers will likely increase this trend. Several national surveys of the U.S. population have reported on the use of nonvitamin or mineral dietary supplements in those age 70 or older, which includes the use of herbal medicines, hormones, oils, and cartilage products.[10,11] There are many reasons for supplement use in older people, such as supplement costs that may be less than for prescription drug products. As well, there is a belief in the efficacy of supplements, their (allegedly) fewer side effects, and their safety compared to prescription drugs.[10,12] While it is well known that many individuals use supplements as part of personal health care, it has been reported that <40% of individuals using these therapies inform their health care providers.[5,10] Conversely, some health care providers may be reluctant to ask patients about alternative medicine use. However, many herbal therapies do have unique pharmacologic actions that can benefit patients. This may be dismissed due to the current paucity of scientific evidence on efficacy and the absence of comprehensive knowledge on the constituents and activities of many herbal and natural products. There are reports of minor to serious complications associated with the use of some natural products.[7] These issues raise concerns among health care providers as to whether some of these therapies pose an excessive public health care risk, or, conversely, does overreactive concern result in delayed use of more effective medical therapies? Given that herbal products are usually complex mixtures of several active ingredients and that they are not subject to the same FDA-regulatory requirements as pharmaceuticals, it is not surprising that little is known about the biological effects of these compounds. Nevertheless, because a substantial portion of the public perceives these products as safe,[10] it is likely that many ADEs associated with herbal medicine and other dietary supplement use have not been recognized or reported.

Safety of Herbal and Nutritional Supplements

Herbal products cannot always be considered as "natural" (and hence, nontoxic) entities, as many consumers believe. Although selected products may have therapeutically beneficial effects, many products cause ADEs and drug interactions similar to those experienced with conventional agents.[9,10] In 1998, 11 poison control centers in the United States recorded 2,332 telephone calls related to ingestion of supplements, with 489 cases strongly associated with supplement use.[12] One third of the events were of greater-than-mild severity, including myocardial infarction (MI), liver failure, bleeding, seizures, and death. Increased symptom severity was associated with the use of several supplements, age, and chronic use. Following reports of cardiovascular events associated with ephedra, in 2004 the FDA issued a regulation prohibiting the sale of dietary supplements containing ephedrine alkaloids and advised consumers to stop using these products (*http://www.cfsan.fda.gov/~lrd/fpephed6.html*). Among the deaths linked to the substance was that of Baltimore Orioles pitching prospect Steve Bechler, "who collapsed and died during spring training

Table 20-1	Selected Adverse Effect with Botanical Products	
Adverse Effect	**Herbal/Supplement**	**Oral Health Care Implications**
Bleeding	Ginkgo, ginseng, garlic, high doses of Vitamin E, angelica, clove, red clover, feverfew	Increased bleeding potential during invasive procedures; monitor clotting
Hepatotoxicity, bleeding	Chaparral, comfrey, kava (oral doseforms)	Reduction in the metabolism of many drugs, increased bleeding potential during invasive procedures; monitor clotting
Postural hypotension	Niacin, yohimbe	Follow protocol to reduce loss of consciousness from postural hypotension
Tachycardia, hypertension	Ephedra (Ma-Huang)	Monitor BP, pulse
Allergic reactions	Coenzyme Q-10, echinacea, milk thistle, pomegranate, wormwood	Watch for skin rash, stomatitis, angioedema, shortness of breath
Oral mucosal irritation, ulceration	Feverfew	Be aware of potential to cause oral ulceration

BP, blood pressure.
(From Therapeutic Research. *Natural Medicines Comprehensive Database.* 7th Ed. Stockton, CA: Therapeutic Research Faculty; 2005, with permission.)

in 2003, supposedly due to taking ephedra-containing supplements to lose weight" (*http://www.washingtonpost.com/wp-dyn/articles/A53586-2005Apr14.html*). A federal judge ruled against the FDA ban on ephedra and in favor of a Utah supplement company that challenged the FDA ban, ruling that ephedra was wrongly being regulated by the FDA as a drug and not a food. Between January 1993 and October 1998, the FDA received 2,621 reports of serious problems involving these products, including 184 deaths.[6] In one study of 386 herb users, 8% had experienced ADEs.[13] Examples of ADEs reported with some botanical products are shown in Table 20-1.

For oral health professionals confronted with inquiries from consumers about the health promotion claims and safety of herbal products, it is important to acknowledge that some of these products have pharmacologically active chemical constituents and, in essence, have drug actions. A large clinical study funded by the National Institute of Health and presented at the June 2007 meeting of the American Society of Clinical Oncology reported that flaxseed slows the growth of tumors in the prostate gland. At the same meeting, another paper was presented that revealed that shark cartilage had no effect on malignant cells.

Drug Interactions

A comprehensive review of known and potential drug–herb interactions shows the interaction potential of herbs with conventional drugs is a critical concern for drugs with narrow therapeutic indexes.[9] For example, many herbal products, such as garlic, ginger, ginseng, ginkgo, and feverfew, possess antiplatelet properties that can be additive when used with drugs known to affect hemostasis, such as warfarin or heparin, albeit through different mechanisms (see Table 20-2 for interactions relevant to dental hygiene care).[14] Recently, significant interactions were identified with hypericum extracts (SJW), including reduced levels of oral contraceptives, cyclosporin, and indinavir. This interaction can lead to birth control failure, rejection of transplanted organs, and treatment failure in HIV disease, respectively.[15] It has been proposed that SJW increases the metabolism of drugs that are affected

by the CYP3A4 mechanism, and because CYP3A4 is involved in the metabolism of >50% of all drugs, SJW is likely to interact with many more drugs than previously had been realized. Some examples of common herb–drug interactions are illustrated in Table 20-2. Herbs can cause coagulation disorders, cardiovascular side effects, water and electrolyte imbalances, endocrine effects, hepatotoxicity, and prolongation of the effects of general anesthetic agents.[16] The American Society of Anesthesiologists recommend that herbal therapy be stopped for 2 weeks prior to surgery involving general anesthesia.

■ Self-Study Review

1. Identify ADEs from various herbal or supplement preparations that can impact oral health care.
2. Identify the federal legislation that allows supplements to be regulated for health claims. What restrictions does the law require for supplements?
3. Review Box 20-1 and Table 20-1 for potential ADEs of botanical products and note their implications in oral health care.
4. Identify potential herb–drug interactions and the specific botanical agents involved.
5. What patient information should be provided when supplements are being consumed and oral surgery is needed?

Standardization of Products

Standardization is the process by which one or more active ingredients of an herb are identified, and all batches of the herb produced by a single manufacturer contain the same amount of active ingredient specified on the label. Consumers expect the component ingredients of their nonprescription and prescription drug products to be standardized to ensure that each dose contains the amount needed to elicit the desired effect. However, consumers may not expect the same level of

Table 20-2 Relevant Herb–Drug Interactions in Oral Health Care

Herb or Dietary Supplement	Interacting Drug/Interaction	Clinical Implications
Garlic, ginger, ginseng, gingko, feverfew, bilberry fruit, bromelain, chamomile, oil of clove, coenzyme Q-10, Cordyceps, evening primrose, guggul, horse chestnut, kava, licorice, tumeric	Warfarin, heparin products, aspirin, clopidogrel, NSAIDs	Increased bleeding; advise patient to stop herb 2 weeks prior to procedures that produce bleeding
SJW	Numerous drug interactions; specifically induces CYP3A4, CYP1A2, and several CYP2 isoenzymes in liver	Increased risk for serotonin syndrome if used with tramadol or meperidine; enhanced sedation theoretically possible with CNS depressants, sedatives; increased potential for photosensitivity when used with tetracyclines: Advise patient to wear sunscreen if exposed to sunlight
Dong quai	Potentiation of antihypertensives, opioids, benzodiazepines, CNS depressants, barbiturates, opioids, antiplatelet drugs (aspirin), warfarin	May increase hypotensive effects leading to postural hypotension following oral care in supine position; increased bleeding
Black cohosh, butterbur, echinacea purpurea	Acetaminophen, NSAIDs, macrolide antibiotics, azole antifungals, dapsone	Additive hepatotoxicity: Avoid use of herb with these drugs
Coleus forskolin, goldenseal, gotu kola, hawthorn, melatonin, nettle root, passion flower, valerian	Benzodiazepines, CNS depressants, barbiturates, opioids	Potential to lower blood pressure, so monitor for orthostatic hypotension; enhanced sedation theoretically possible
Cranberry	Opioids, antidepressants, some antibiotics	Large amounts can reduce urinary pH, theoretically causing increased excretion of drugs
Guar gum	Penicillins	Decreased absorption of penicillin (PEN), use gum 1 hour after PEN dosing
Yohimbe	Indirect-acting sympathomimetics	Due to hypertension side effect, use low doses with aspirating syringe

CNS, central nervous system; NSAIDs, nonsteroidal anti-inflammatory drugs.

standardization for herbal products, either believing that precise formulations are unnecessary or assuming they already are standardized. Herbal medicine advocates may suggest that the therapeutic benefit of herbal products stems from the synergistic action of the variety of natural components in the herb. They argue that some constituents thought to be inactive may play a role in the pharmacokinetics of the active component, and that a standardized extract would diminish or eliminate the beneficial effects of the heterogeneous botanical product. No evidence currently is available to support or refute this argument.

One consequence of the lack of standardization is the variability in the quantity (or the complete absence, in some cases) of the known or supposed active ingredient. Examples include an analysis of 24 ginseng products (from roots of several species of *Panax*, panaxosides), which revealed that 8 (33%) did not contain a detectable panaxoside (which are considered to be the active components), and several products contained less panaxoside content than was stated on the label.[17] In a study of 44 feverfew products, 14 (32%) did not contain the minimum 0.2% parthenolide content that is proposed as the necessary primary active ingredient and concentration. Another 10 products (23%) did not contain any detectable levels of parthenolide.[18]

Good Manufacturing Practice

Good manufacturing practices (GMPs), which are required for foods and drugs, were not required for herbal products or dietary supplements prior to June 2007.[19] GMPs ensure that products meet specific quality standards, are not adulterated or misbranded, and contain the correct ingredients and doses stated on the label. Without GMPs, herbal products were at risk of adulteration and contamination.

The medical literature contains several examples of the adulteration of herbal and natural products with unlabeled ingredients and heavy metals. The FDA has received reports of bradycardia and heart blockage caused by ingesting plantain adulterated with digitalis.[20] This adulteration occurred when an inexperienced harvester mistook the digitalis-containing foxglove for plantain (the two plants are similar in appearance). The product was sold for up to a year by several distributors before the problem was recognized. Melatonin, an herb with sedative properties, in concentrations up to 7.11 μg/g, was found as an adulterant in feverfew, Huang-qin, and SJW products.[21] A 41-year-old woman was reported to have an international normalized ratio (INR) of 11.5 (targeted therapeutic range: 2 to 3.5) after drinking hibiscus tea contaminated with warfarin.[22] One final example of a poor GMP is the practice of incorporating a prescription drug into a supplement product. This trait has been discovered in a variety of products, but one example involved a product promoted for insomnia known as "Sleeping Buddha." This product was found to contain estazolam, a prescription benzodiazepine.[23] These examples illustrate the significant risk to the public for serious adverse health consequences, which could be eliminated by product standardization and requirements for GMPs. In 2003, the FDA drafted "good manufacturing practice requirements" to improve the safety and reliability of supplements, and hearings began in November 2004.[24]

2007 Regulations for Good Manufacturing Practices

On June 22, 2007, the FDA finalized current good manufacturing practices (cGMP) to ensure quality throughout the manufacturing, packaging, labeling, and storing of dietary supplements. The final rule includes requirements for establishing quality control procedures, designing and constructing manufacturing plants, and testing ingredients and the finished product. It also includes requirements for record-keeping and handling consumer product complaints. Regulations requiring manufacturers of dietary supplements to test their products for purity and to provide accurate labeling information help to ensure that consumers will receive the product intended to be purchased and in the quantity established on the label. However, testing is left to the discretion of the companies, and the FDA does not inspect all manufacturing plants to monitor compliance. Companies shown to have unsafe practices in the past are inspected more frequently. If the supplement is found to contain contaminants or to not contain the dietary ingredient represented on the label, the FDA considers the product to be adulterated or misbranded. The final cGMP regulations were effective as of August 24, 2007. Large companies were to comply by June 2008, while firms with fewer than 200 workers had until June 2009 to comply, and small companies with 20 employees or fewer had until June 2010 to comply. After these dates, companies will be compelled to test their products for purity and to verify that the products' strength matches labeling information. Dietary supplement manufacturers, however, will not be required by law to prove the product is safe or effective.

The Federal Trade Commission (FTC) regulates advertising and label claims and has forced some supplement manufacturers to remove advertisements with false or unsubstantiated claims.

Regulatory Issues

From a regulatory perspective, herbal products are classified as dietary supplements. Before 1994, herbs were regulated as foods or drugs, depending on their intended use. Unlike drugs, herbs did not need to be proven safe and effective to be marketed. Dietary supplement manufacturers were given responsibility for determining product safety and verifying that product labeling was not misleading. However, the FDA did not have the authority to intervene unless there was proof that a product was unsafe. When Congress passed the DSHEA in 1994, a separate classification was created for dietary supplements.[23] Under this categorization, herbs were no longer considered to be foods.

Under the FDA rules, a product may make structure, function, and health maintenance claims (e.g., "maintains a healthy prostate") but not disease claims (e.g., "treats benign prostatic hyperplasia") unless FDA approval is gained for the health claim. Products claiming to diagnose, treat, prevent, or cure a disease will be classified as drugs and require proof of safety and efficacy. Manufacturers must be able to provide evidence that a claim is not false or misleading. When manufacturers state that their products affect body structures

or functions, the label must include the following disclaimer: "This statement has not been evaluated by the Food and Drug Administration. This product is not intended to diagnose, treat, cure, or prevent any disease." In addition, companies must notify the FDA that products bear such labels within 30 days after they are on the market.[25]

FDA MedWatch Program

Postmarketing surveillance is an important component of monitoring the safety of herbal products. Reporting ADEs is facilitated through the FDA MedWatch system (Chapter 1). In addition, the FDA developed the Special Nutritionals Adverse Event Monitoring System (SN/AEMS), which is a database of ADEs reported to the FDA that are associated with uses of a special nutritional product: dietary supplements, infant formulas, and medical foods. The SN/AEMS database can be searched online to determine whether a specific dietary supplement is associated with ADEs. The usefulness of this system depends on the extent that ADEs associated with dietary supplements are reported, including herbal products, by health professionals and consumers.

These new FDA measures are important in the regulation of dietary supplements, including herbal products. As these measures are implemented, consumers can place more confidence in the safety, composition, and labeling of herbal products, and health care professionals will be better able to counsel and monitor individuals who take such supplements.

Evidence Base for Dietary Supplements

Table 20-3 provides a bibliographic listing of reliable scientific sources of information on herbal products and alternative medicine. The current direction in medicine is practice-based on reliable scientific evidence. The evaluation of herbal and other natural products as a health care modality should use the evidence-based approach.

In *evidence-based medicine*, product recommendations are determined by the level of evidence available from clinical studies. Box 20-2 illustrates the levels of evidence used in the systematic review process. The levels of evidence range from Level I (trials with the strongest design, such as randomized, controlled trials) to Level V (case reports that provide useful information but no valid evidence for drug effectiveness).[26]

As with any grading system, limitations exist with the levels-of-evidence system. Nonetheless, using such a system can provide an initial approach to objectively evaluate studies of herbal products for study design and determine a grade of recommendation. Herbal products supplied for oral health care have many studies that are Level I status and are discussed below.

Whereas some studies involving herbal products can be graded as having Level I evidence, many published trials have weaker levels of evidence and rank as Level III, IV, or V. Generally, many studies of alternative medicine therapies have flaws in study design, lack evidence of using standardized products, or fail to account for biases. Many of the deficiencies are common to studies of conventional medicine, such as poorly defined exclusion or inclusion criteria and short treatment duration. However, problems such as product quality and standardization are unique to alternative medicine, as

Table 20-3	Reliable Scientific Sources of Information on Supplements

Journals

These journals specifically or regularly address alternative therapies and include original research. The year refers to year of first publication.

English Language, Peer-Reviewed

- *Alternative Medicine Review*, 1996 (academic/scholarly publication)
- *Alternative Therapies in Clinical Practice*, 1994 (academic/scholarly publication)
- *Alternative Therapies in Health and Medicine*, 1995 (academic/scholarly publication)
- *American Journal of Chinese Medicine*, 1973 (abstracting and indexing service, academic/scholarly publication)
- *Focus on Alternative and Complementary Therapies*, 1996 (academic/scholarly publication)
- *HealthInform*, 1995 (newsletter, abstracting and indexing service, academic/scholarly publication)
- *Journal of Alternative and Complementary Medicine: Research on Paradigm, Practice and Policy*, 1993 (academic/scholarly publication)
- *Journal of Herbal Pharmacotherapy*, first issue slated for fall, 2000 (academic/scholarly publication)

Nonpeer-Reviewed or Peer-Review Status Unknown

- *Alternative and Complementary Therapies*, 1994
- *Complementary Therapies in Medicine*,1993 (academic/scholarly publication)
- *Complementary Therapies in Nursing and Midwifery*, 1995 (academic/scholarly publication)
- *HerbalGram*, 1979
- *Phytomedicine*, 1994 (academic/scholarly publication)

Databases

The home page of the Research Council for Complementary Medicine (RCCM) has more details on most of the following. The RCCM's Internet address is provided in the Web site section, below.

- AMED (Alternative and Allied Medicine Database): Produced and updated monthly by the British Library's Medical Information Centre, this database contains 65,000 references from 400 journals on alternative and complementary medicine. Online searches are available through Datastar or MIC-KIBIC. The database is also available on floppy disk and in printed format as the Complementary Medicine Index from the British Library Medical Information Service, Boston Spa, United Kingdom. More details are available from the British Library (01937 546 039).
- CISCOM (Centralized Information Service for Complementary Medicine): This RCCM database of research references and abstracts combines data from MEDLINE, AMED, other specialized European databases, and in-house citation tracking. There is no direct access to the database, but mediated searches can be arranged by calling the RCCM (+44 0207 833 8897). Fees for use of the service start at £15 (UK) and depend on the scale and complexity of the request. Data are provided in printed or electronic format. A special feature of the CISCOM database is a large collection of randomized, controlled trials, including the full registry of the Cochrane Complementary Medicine Field.
- Cochrane Complementary Medicine Field: This section of the Cochrane Library was established to meet the growing need for evidence-based research in alternative medical practices. The primary aim of the database is to compile randomized, controlled trials of alternative medicine interventions, particularly from journals that specialize in this area. The full registry of this database is included in CISCOM (listed above). However, a fee is required for a mediated search of CISCOM. Sometime in the near future, this database will be added to the CCTR of the Cochrane Library. This database is only available to subscribers of the Cochrane Library.
- NAPRALERT (Natural Products Alert): This database contains 125,000 entries on natural products used worldwide, including chemical, pharmacologic, and ethnomedical information, and is updated monthly by Scientific and Technical Information Network. Summary information can be found at http://info.cas.org/ONLINE/DBSS/napralertss.html.
- Natural Medicines Comprehensive Database: This extensive database, maintained by the editors of the *Pharmacist's Letter/Prescriber's Letter*, contains information on over 1,000 herbs and dietary supplements, with an index containing over 7,000 brand names. Each herb/supplement listing includes 15 categories of information that address the most common questions faced by practitioners. The database is well referenced and is available as an electronic version (http://www.naturaldatabase.com) and print version (refer to the references section of this chapter). The Web version is continuously updated and allows more sophisticated searching than does the print version. It also contains a more extensive brand-name index.

Web Sites

- Research Council for Complementary Medicine (RCCM), http://www.rccm.org.uk: The home page contains a comprehensive listing and descriptions of bibliographic databases, indexes, and journals related to alternative medicine. The RCCM is a resource for health care professionals only; they do not serve the lay public. CISCOM is the RCCM's database. Unfortunately, on the completion of existing commitments, the RCCM will cease to operate. At the time of this writing, the home page was still accessible.
- American Botanical Council (ABC), http://www.herbalgram.org: The home page provides access to information on ordering *HerbalGram* (see journals), the *Complete German Commission E Monographs* (see books), and an herb book catalog.
- NIH's National Center for Complementary and Alternative Medicine (NCCAM), http://nccam.nih.gov: The NCCAM facilitates research and evaluation of alternative medical practices and disseminates this information to both health professionals and the public. From the home page, one can access general information on alternative medicine, a listing of program areas, a calendar of events, and the CAM Citation Index. The CAM Citation Index consists of more than 180,000 bibliographic citations from 1963–1998 extracted from the National Library of Medicine MEDLINE database. This database allows one to search or browse the listings, which are organized by CAM system, disease, or method. This database is limited by using MEDLINE, which has only 23 subject headings for alternative medicine and is not as extensive as CISCOM or the Cochrane Library.
- The Cochrane Library, http://www.cochrane.co.uk: This Web site contains information about the Cochrane Library and how to access it. Only abstracts are available free from the Internet. A subscription is required for the other services.
- Center for Food Safety & Applied Nutrition, http://vm.cfsan.fda.gov: This Web site has a section on dietary supplements, including information on the DSHEA and the SN/AEMS.

(Continued)

Table 20-3	*(Continued)*

- International Bibliographic Information on Dietary Supplements (IBIDS), http://dietary-supplements.info.nih.gov/databases/ibids.html: IBIDS is a database of published, international, scientific literature on dietary supplements, including vitamins, minerals, and selected herbal and botanical supplements. It is produced by two government agencies—NIH's Office of Dietary Supplements and the U.S. Department of Agriculture's Food and Nutrition Information Center—and it currently contains 328,000 citations and abstracts.
- Micromedex Internet Healthcare Series, http://www.micromedex.com/products/hcs/ Micromedex is developing a reliable, comprehensive source of information for alternative medicine at this Web site. The AltMedDex System was introduced in February 1999 and will contain more than 50 evidence-based monographs on herbal, vitamin, and other dietary supplements. The clinically focused scientific information also will contain guidelines and recommendations to assist clinicians in making appropriate therapy choices and decisions.
- Office of Dietary Supplements, http://ods.od.nih.gov/databases/ibids.html: This site provides international bibliographic information on dietary supplements and is sponsored by the NIH.
- NIH Clinical Center, http://clinicalcenter.nih.gov: This site is another source for NIH information on supplements.
- University of California, http://nutrition.ucdavis.edu/perspectives: Information source is from the Department of Nutrition Science, UC Davis.
- HerbMed, http://herbmed.org: This site is a free, searchable herbal database operated by the Alternative Medicine Foundation.
- American Herbal Products Association, http://www.ahpa.org: This site is provided by the American Herbal Products Association, publishers of *The Botanical Safety Handbook*.
- Facts & Comparisons, http://www.drugfacts.com: This site is a comprehensive database of potential drug–herb interactions.
- National Center for Complementary and Alternative Medicine, http://nccam.nih.gov: This site contains fact sheets on products and NIH/NCCAM panel reports.
- healthfinder, http://www.healthfinder.gov: This site is a reliable entry point for patients, operated by the U.S. Department of Health and Human Services.

[Adapted from Miller LG, Hume A, Harris IM, et al. White paper on herbal products. *Pharmacotherapy.* 2000;20(7):877–891. Additional source is the Food and Drug Administration Web site (http://www.fda.gov).]

discussed previously. The Agency for Healthcare Research and Quality (formerly the Agency for Health Care Policy and Research), a division of the National Institute of Health, has administered grant applications for well-designed studies of some alternative therapies.[26,27] The Cochrane Library, a group based in Great Britain, has a searchable collection of over 1,500 randomized, controlled trials of alternative medicine interventions.

■ Self-Study Review

6. Explain the process of *standardization* and how it applies to herbal products.
7. Describe issues related to the lack of standardization with botanical products.
8. Explain factors associated with good manufacturing practices. Describe features of the 2007 GMP regulations.
9. Which governmental agency regulates advertising claims for dietary supplements?
10. Identify regulatory issues related to dietary supplements.
11. Identify the system responsible for monitoring ADEs of nutritional supplements.
12. Consider the levels of evidence used in the systematic review process. Which represents strong evidence for the efficacy of a product? Which represents weak evidence?
13. Identify the agency within the National Institute of Health that oversees research on alternative therapies.

BOX 20-2. Levels of Evidence for Systematic Review Process

General Description of Levels of Evidence (LOE)

Level I	Randomized trials or meta-analyses in which lower limits of the confidence interval for the treatment exceed the minimal clinically important benefit
Level II	Randomized trials or meta-analyses in which lower limits of the confidence interval for the treatment overlap the minimal clinically important benefit
Level III	Nonrandomized concurrent cohort studies (studies with one group receiving the treatment and a concurrent group not receiving the treatment)
Level IV	Nonrandomized historic cohort studies (a study in which outcomes from patients receiving a treatment are compared with a historic group with different treatment method)
Level V	Case series without controls

[Based on Oxford Centre for Evidence-based Medicine. Levels of Evidence, 2001, with permission.]

Herbal Products in Dentistry

Herbal products used for oral purposes include essential oil (EO) mouth rinses (thymol, eucalyptol, menthol), xylitol, acemannan, oil of cloves, and triclosan. Sanguinarine, from the bloodroot plant (also called tetter wort), was included in an oral rinse and dentifrice (Viadent products) in the 1980s to reduce gingivitis. Clinical trials were positive, but sanguinaria extract was discovered to have a potential ADE of leukoplakia and was removed from the current Viadent formulation.[28]

Essential Oil Mouth Rinse

The ADA has approved more than 20 mouth rinses that contain the EOs thymol, eucalyptol, and menthol. The proposed mechanism of action of EOs is a bacteriostatic effect. The first manufacturer (Warner/Lambert [now Pfizer Pharmaceutical]) to market the rinse (Listerine) did not promote the scientific evidence base for the combination product to the dental profession. A randomized, controlled trial has demonstrated a statistically significant improvement in gingival bleeding and reduced plaque scores.[29] Communication with the manufacturer (Pfizer) reveals that the Cool Mint Listerine product was used in most of the recent trials. The ADA Seal of Acceptance states that "the product has received the ADA Seal of Acceptance as a safe and effective adjunct to brushing and flossing and regular professional care in helping to reduce supragingival plaque and gingivitis." One EO combination product not yet on the market in the United States has sodium fluoride (100 ppm) in it. It has been shown to be effective in promoting enamel remineralization and fluoride uptake.[30]

Xylitol

Xylitol is a naturally occurring sweetener derived from plants, such as the bark of birch trees. It is comparable in sweetness to sucrose, but xylitol has one fewer carbon and is not fermentable, meaning the xylitol molecule cannot be metabolized by *Streptococcus mutans* to form acids. This property reduces *S. mutans* levels and makes it useful for the antibacterial and cariostatic effects that result. In addition, xylitol has an antibacterial effect in that it inhibits the ability of microbes to adhere and grow in plaque, although there are no xylitol products that claim an antigingivitis effect. It has been demonstrated that if a mother chews xylitol four times a day during the first years of the child's life, the child has much less cariogenic bacterial growth and a decreased risk of caries.[31] Xylitol products are discussed in more detail in Chapter 7.

Acemannan

Acemannan hydrogel is an extract from the aloe vera leaf that has immunomodulating properties. It is marketed as an over-the-counter (OTC) topical patch (Carrington Patch) to reduce the healing time of aphthous ulcerations by causing the ulcerations to heal faster. In a clinical study, acemannan was as effective as a prescription product in healing aphthous ulcerations.[32]

Oil of Cloves (Eugenol)

Oil of cloves, an OTC product, has been used for decades as a topical analgesic for dental pain. School nurses use eugenol as a "toothache medicine" for short-term relief until the child can receive treatment in a dental facility. The product is used empirically in the dental profession, and there are no published studies for efficacy. The proposed mechanism of action is unclear, but it is hypothesized that pulpal nerves are affected in some way to obtund pain.

Triclosan

Triclosan is an herb-based substance that has been shown to produce a statistically significant reduction in plaque and gingivitis when compared to a placebo dentifrice.[33] One triclosan product has the ADA Seal of Acceptance (Colgate Total) for an antigingivitis effect. A recent systematic review of the Cochrane Controlled Trials Register (1986–2003) compared triclosan's effectiveness in reducing plaque accumulation and gingival health with that of fluoride toothpaste.[34] To be included in the systematic review, trials had to be randomized, include adults with plaque and gingivitis, have unsupervised use of the triclosan dentifrice for at least 6 months, and evaluate plaque and gingivitis levels after the 6-month period. Sixteen trials met these criteria at the Level I and Level II evidence levels. The Cochrane group concluded that the triclosan/copolymer dentifrice significantly reduced plaque and gingivitis when compared to fluoride dentifrice alone.

Clinical Studies for Future Products

The efficacy of an herbal-based mouth rinse in conjunction with subgingival irrigation (PikPocket device, Teledyne Corp.) to reduce gingival inflammation was investigated by the Oral Surgery faculty in Mainz, Germany. The mouth rinse contained a mixture of herbal substances (salvia officinalis, metha piperita, menthol, matricaria chamomilla, Commiphora myrrha, carvum carvi, Eugenia caryophyllus, and echinacea purpurea). A double-blind, randomized, 12-week controlled trial with 89 subjects was designed to determine the effect on the plaque index, gingival index, and probe depths. Participants were divided into three groups: Group 1 used the oral irrigator with subgingival tip and an herb mouth rinse mixture, Group 2 used an oral irrigator with subgingival tip and water, and Group 3 used a conventional mouth rinse without subgingival irrigation. Patients were instructed to brush their teeth twice daily for 2 minutes (any technique), and then Groups 1 and 2 applied the specific irrigant within the sulcus using the oral irrigator with subgingival tip twice daily for 5 minutes. Group 3 swished for 1 minute following toothbrushing. There was a statistically significant reduction in bleeding and plaque in Groups 1 and 2, while the plaque and gingival indices in Group 3 were similar to indices at baseline. The authors concluded that subgingival irrigation could be recommended as an adjunctive treatment to reduce gingival inflammation, but it does not reduce probe depths.[35] Results suggest that the addition of the herbal mixture did not provide additional efficacy over the use of the subgingival tip and water in this study. This illustrates the importance of reading the entire study, rather than only the abstract and conclusion.

A small study investigated the effects on healing of the combined extracts from *Centella asiatica* and *Punica granatum* (found in pomegranate rind) incorporated into biodegradable chips and inserted into the sulcus following scaling and root planing in individuals with adult periodontitis.[36] Twenty patients with 260 initial pocket depths of 5 to 8 mm were subjected to periodontal scaling, and then the medicated chips were placed into pockets for the test group following the procedure; they then returned for monthly polishing to remove supragingival plaque. Unmedicated chips were placed into pockets for the control (placebo) group in the same manner and timing as with the test group. The control group received periodontal scaling alone. Pocket-depth probe measurements, attachment level, bleeding on probing, gingival index, and plaque index were recorded at baseline and again at 3 and 6 months. Results showed statistically significant improvements of pocket-depth reduction and attachment levels in the test group patients who received medicated chips when compared to the placebo chip sites at 3 months and at 6 months. The authors reported that the herbal combination extracts incorporated into local delivery chips plus scaling and root planing significantly reduced the clinical signs of chronic periodontitis. This is a small study that needs to be verified by a larger trial, and results cannot be applied to large populations; however, it suggests that herbal extracts may be included in future products for oral health care purposes.

■ Self-Study Review

14. Identify herbal products used for oral care.
15. Which botanical dental product was associated with leukoplakia?
16. Identify oral herbal products with the ADA Seal of Acceptance.
17. Identify the mechanisms of action of herbal products used for oral care.
18. Identify medical and oral health benefits of botanicals discussed in the chapter.

DENTAL HYGIENE APPLICATIONS

All drug histories should include questions about the use of herbal and other natural products. When these products are reported, the potential effects should be investigated in a pharmacologic reference and followed up with the client. Inquiries should address the specific health care purpose for which the patient is using the product. Health care professionals and consumers must be vigilant in detecting and reporting suspected serious ADEs from natural products, as well as prescription drugs and OTC products, to the FDA's MedWatch program. In this manner, consumers are more likely to learn of potential ADEs, with the result of improved safety when they use herbal or natural products, but only if professionals and consumers are proactive in reporting problems.

CONCLUSION

Natural products are marketed as food supplements in the United States, and current law does not require manufacturers to prove safety or effectiveness before selling them. The DSHEA of 1994 was created to separate supplements from being classified and regulated as drugs. Most products are safe if used in the manner described in the labeling instructions; however, due to problems in product quality control,

the product contents identified on the label may not be accurate. The FDA established regulations in 2007 to compel manufacturers to test their products for purity and ensure accuracy of labeling information, but compliance will not be enforced until 2009 and 2010. The dental hygienist must be vigilant to identify potential ADEs that may affect the oral health care treatment plan, and the dentist must consider potential interactions if surgery is planned for the appointment.

References

1. Ervin RB, Wright JD, Reed-Gillette D. Prevalence of leading types of dietary supplements used in the Third National Health and Nutrition Examination Survey, 1988–94. *Adv Data.* 2004; 349:1–7.
2. Radimer K, Bindewald B, Hughes J, et al. Dietary supplement use by U.S. adults: Data from the National Health and Nutrition Examination Survey 1999–2000. *Am J Epidemiol.* 2004; 160:339–349.
3. Eisenberg DM, Kessler RC, Foster C, et al. Unconventional medicine in the United States: Prevalence, costs and patterns of use. *N Engl J Med.* 1993;328:246–252.
4. Eisenberg DM, Davis RB, Ettner SL, et al. Trends in alternative medicine use in the United States, 1990–1997: Results of a follow-up national survey. *JAMA.* 1998;280:1569–1575.
5. Eisenberg DM, Kessler RC, Van Rompay MI, et al. Perceptions about complementary therapies relative to conventional therapies among adults who use both: Results from a national survey. *Ann Intern Med.* 2001;135(5):344–351.
6. Miller LG, Hume A, Harris IM, et al. White paper on herbal products. *Pharmacotherapy.* 2000;20(7):877–891.
7. Pickett F, Gurenlian J. *The Medical History: Clinical Implications and Emergency Prevention in Dental Settings.* Baltimore: Lippincott Williams & Wilkins; 2005:42, 5.
8. Ang-Lee MK, Moss MD, Yuan C. Herbal medicines and perioperative care. *JAMA.* 2001;286:208–216.
9. Miller LG. Herbal medicinals: Selected clinical considerations focusing on known or potential drug–herb interactions. *Arch Intern Med.* 1998;158:2200–2211.
10. Winslow LC, Kroll DJ. Herbs as medicines. *Arch Intern Med.* 1998;158:2192–2199.
11. Astin JA. Why patients use alternative medicine: Results of a national study. *JAMA.* 1998;279:1548–1553.
12. Palmer ME, Haller C, McKinney PE, et al. Adverse events associated with dietary supplements: An observational study. *Lancet.* 2003;361(9352):101–106.
13. Abbot NC, White AR, Ernst E. Complementary medicine. *Nature.* 1996;381:361.
14. Jacobsen PL, Cohan RP, Blumenthal M, et al. Alternative medicine in dentistry. In: Yagiela JA, Dowd FJ, Neidle EA, eds. *Pharmacology and Therapeutics for Dentistry.* 5th ed. St. Louis: Mosby; 2004:880–889.
15. Moore LB, Goodwin B, Jones SA, et al. St. John's wort induces hepatic drug metabolism through activation of the pregnane X receptor. *Proc Natl Acad Sci U S A.* 2000;97(13):7500–7502.
16. Cheng B, Hung CT, Chin W. Herbal medicine and anaesthesia. *Hong Kong Med J.* 2002;8(2):123–130.
17. Liberti LE, DerMarderosian AD. Evaluation of commercial ginseng products. *J Pharm Sci.* 1978;67:1487–1489.
18. Heptinstall S, Awang DVS, Dawson BA, et al. Parthenolide content and bioactivity of feverfew (Tanacetum parthenium (l.) Schultz-Bip.): Estimation of commercial and authenticated feverfew products. *J Pharm Pharmacol.* 1992;44:391–395.
19. Dietary Supplement Health and Education Act (DSHEA), Pub L No. 103-417, 108 Stat 4325 (1994).

CLINICAL APPLICATION EXERCISES

■ **Exercise 1.** A new patient reports for dental hygiene care. Oral examination reveals generalized bleeding and sulcus probe depths of 3 to 4 mm. Questioning reveals the client does not use fluoride products due to a fear of cancer but regularly uses herbal medicines for various maladies. Given the interest in herbal therapies, what oral products could be recommended for an antigingivitis effect?

■ **Exercise 2.** WEB ACTIVITY: The FDA monitors supplements for adulterations. Log on to this URL for an example: http://www.fda.gov:80/bbs/topics/NEWS/2007/NEW01678.html.

■ **Exercise 3.** WEB ACTIVITY: Using Web information in Table 20-3, log on to selected sites to gain knowledge on the extent and reliability of information presented. Scan information relevant to issues in managing oral care when various herbal products are commonly used.

20. Blumenthal M. Industry alert: Plantain adulterated with digitalis. *HerbalGram.* 1997;40:28–29.
21. Murch SJ, Simmons CB, Saxene PK. Melatonin in feverfew and other medicinal plants. *Lancet.* 1997;350:1598–1599.
22. Norcross WA, Ganiats TG, Ralph LP, et al. Accidental poisoning by warfarin-contaminated herbal tea. *West J Med.* 1993;159:80–82.
23. US Food and Drug Administration. FDA warns consumers against taking dietary supplement "Sleeping Buddha." March 10, 1998. Available at: http://www.fda.gov/bbs/topics/news/new00625.html. Accessed May 9, 2008.
24. US Food and Drug Administration. Regulations on statements made for dietary supplements concerning the effect of the product on the structure or function of the body. *Federal Register.* 2000 Jan 6:65:1000–1050.
25. Evidence-Based Medicine Working Group. Evidence-based medicine: A new approach to teaching the practice of medicine. *JAMA.* 1992;268:240–248.
26. Agency for Healthcare Research and Quality. Milk Thistle: Effects on liver disease and cirrhosis and clinical adverse effects, structured abstract. September 2000. Available at: http://www.ahrq.gov/clinic/tp/milkttp.htm. Accessed April 11, 2007.
27. Agency for Healthcare and Quality. Garlic: Effects on cardiovascular risks and disease, protective effects against cancer, and clinical adverse effects, structured abstract. October 2000. Available at: http://www.ahrq.gov/clinic/tp/garlictp.htm. Accessed April 11, 2007.
28. Anderson KM, Stoner GD, Fields HW, et al. Immunohistochemical assessment of Viadent-associated leukoplakia. *Oral Oncol.* 2005;41:200–207.
29. Bauroth K, Charles CH, Mankodi SM, et al. The efficacy of an essential oil antiseptic mouthrinse vs. dental floss in controlling interproximal gingivitis: A comparative study. *J Am Dent Assoc.* 2003;134:359–365.
30. Zero DT, Zhang JZ, Harper DS, et al. The remineralizing effect of an essential oil fluoride mouthrinse in an intraoral caries test. *J Am Dent Assoc.* 2004;135(2):231–237.
31. Featherstone J. Caries update. *Dimen Den Hyg.* 2005;3(2):14.
32. Plemons J. Evaluation of acemannan in the treatment of recurrent aphthous stomatitis. *Wounds.* 1994;6(2):40–45.
33. Triratana T, Rustogi KN, Volpe AR, et al. Clinical effect of a new liquid dentifrice containing triclosan/copolymer on existing plaque and gingivitis. *J Am Dent Assoc.* 2002;133(2):219–225.
34. Davies RM, Ellwood RP, Davies GM. The effectiveness of a toothpaste containing triclosan and polyvinyl-methyl ether maleic acid copolymer in improving plaque control and gingival health: A systematic review. *J Clin Periodontol.* 2004;31:1029–1033.
35. Pistorius A, Willershausen B, Steinmeier E, et al. Efficacy of subgingival irrigation using herbal extracts on gingival inflammation. *J Periodontol.* 2003;74(5):616–622.
36. Sastravaha G, Yotnuengnit P, Booncong P, et al. Adjunctive periodontal treatment with *Centella asiatica* and *Punica granatum* extracts: A preliminary study. *J Int Acad Periodontol.* 2003;5:106–115.

21

Women's Issues: Pregnancy, Lactation, Menopause, and Osteoporosis

This chapter focuses on pharmacologic considerations and clinical management issues relevant to treating women who report pregnancy, lactation, menopause, or bone density changes that lead to osteoporosis. The pregnant or lactating patient presents a number of unique management issues for oral health care providers. Clinicians are responsible for providing safe and effective care for the mother while also considering the safety of the fetus, newborn, infant, or young child. Considerations must include the effects of medications, which may be distributed from the maternal plasma through the placenta to the fetus or to breast milk, exposing the nursing infant to potentially dangerous drug concentrations. In

addition, a number of physiologic and oral changes requiring the attention of oral health care providers may be observed as a consequence of the multiple physiologic changes associated with pregnancy.

Menopause is a physiologic process experienced by women generally after the age of 50. Such symptoms as hot flashes, thinning mucosal tissues, and mood alterations may impact the dental hygiene appointment. Osteoporosis may develop as a complication of loss of estrogen during the aging process. It occurs in both men and women, but women are affected to a greater extent than men.

THE PHYSIOLOGY OF PREGNANCY

Women are normally subject to cyclic hormonal changes related to the menstrual cycle. This cycle is dramatically altered following fertilization of the ovum. Changes include increased production of maternal hormones while placental hormone synthesis begins. Human chorionic gonadotropin prevents normal involution of the corpus luteum after fertilization has occurred. It also stimulates the corpus luteum to secrete large amounts of estrogen and progesterone. Estrogen causes enlargement of the uterus, relaxes the pelvic ligaments in preparation for birth, and prepares the breasts for lactation by increasing growth of the breast ductal structure. In the oral cavity, estrogen provides an energy source to periodontal organisms leading to gingivitis. Progesterone contributes to the preparation of the breasts for lactation and decreases spontaneous contraction of the uterus. Additional hormonal changes during pregnancy include an increased synthesis of growth hormone, insulin, vitamin D, cortisol, aldosterone, and thyroid hormones.

Pregnancy and the Cardiovascular System

The demand on the cardiovascular (CV) system progressively increases during pregnancy. As a result of increased synthesis of estrogen, progesterone, cortisol, and aldosterone associated with pregnancy, water is retained, and the blood volume expands by about 1 to 2 L (30% to 50%). The heart compensates for this volume expansion as cardiac output increases 30% to 50% by the end of the first trimester. As a consequence of these physiologic changes, tachycardia, heart murmur, increased venous blood pressure, and vasomotor instability can develop. Vasomotor instability predisposes patients to postural hypotension and syncope, especially in the first trimester.[1] As venous pressure rises in the later stages of pregnancy, the patient may experience peripheral edema, varicosities, and hemorrhoids.

Pregnancy and the Respiratory System

Expansion of plasma volume also decreases plasma colloid osmotic pressure, which contributes to pulmonary edema during pregnancy. The developing fetus further contributes to reduced respiratory capacity by displacing the diaphragm upward. These events *decrease* residual functional capacity by about 18% at a time when oxygen demand is *increased* by 15% to 20%. Increased cardiac output tends to compensate for the decreased respiratory capacity; however, in the second and third trimesters, exertion or placing the patient in a supine position may precipitate dyspnea. Pregnant patients are also prone to hyperventilation after the first trimester.[2]

Pregnancy and the Renal System

As a result of plasma volume expansion and increased cardiac output during pregnancy, glomerular filtration rate increases by 30 to 50%. The patient may also manifest temporary renal glycosuria secondary to gestational diabetes mellitus (GDM). In the later stages of pregnancy, patients tend to experience increased urinary frequency, urgency, incontinence, and recurrent urinary tract infections.

Pregnancy and the Gastrointestinal System

Nausea, vomiting, and other dyspeptic symptoms, such as increased salivation or heartburn, are common in pregnancy and affect between 50% and 90% of women, although the severity varies. In one study, 83.6% of the mothers reported at least one of these symptoms.[3] Expectant mothers most frequently reported symptoms of morning sickness (51.8%) and heartburn (66.7%). The causes of these symptoms are not clear, but they seem to be related to physiologic and anatomic changes that occur during pregnancy. Progesterone has been implicated in decreasing lower esophageal sphincter tone, which is further compromised by increased intragastric pressure as the stomach is displaced superiorly by the expanding uterus. Nausea and vomiting may lead to inadequate absorption of certain nutrients and minerals (particularly iron). Progesterone also decreases gastrointestinal (GI) motility and alters gastric secretions. As the gastric pH decreases, there is a corresponding increase in acid reflux and a potential for aspiration with serious consequences. Increased appetite and cravings for unusual combinations of foods are common and may lead to a diet that is not nutritionally sound.

Complications of Pregnancy
Preterm Delivery

Preterm delivery, a major contributor to infant death, occurs in 8% of single births to white women and in about 16% of single births to black women. *Preterm delivery* is defined as birth before 37 weeks of gestation. Preterm delivery may be categorized based on clinical presentation as idiopathic, premature rupture of the membranes, and medically indicated. It has been hypothesized that periodontal inflammation is a factor in preterm delivery and low birth weight; however, a large randomized clinical trial (called the Obstetrics and Periodontal Therapy, or OPT, trial) found no causal link between periodontitis and preterm delivery.[4] There were no differences in the rate of preterm birth or in low-birth-weight infants in women who received periodontal treatment when compared to the group who did not receive care.

Pre-Eclampsia and Eclampsia

Pre-eclampsia is a multisystem disorder diagnosed when hypertension associated with proteinuria is found. Hypertension is considered severe if there is sustained systolic elevation ≥ 180 mm Hg and/or sustained diastolic elevation ≥ 110 mm Hg. Blood pressure at these levels is a contraindication to providing elective oral health care. Fetal complications include preterm delivery, fetal growth restriction, hypoxic-neurologic injury, long-term CV morbidity associated with low birth weight, and perinatal death. **Eclampsia** is defined by the onset of convulsions in women with pre-eclampsia. Prevention and treatment of the complications is predicated on prenatal care, timely diagnosis, proper management, and timely delivery.

Gestational Diabetes Mellitus

Glucose intolerance occurs normally during pregnancy, particularly in the third trimester, and GDM is a complicating factor in approximately 7% of all pregnancies. GDM is defined as any degree of glucose intolerance with onset or first recognition developing during pregnancy. Hyperglycemia usually returns to normal following **parturition**. The definition applies whether insulin or diet-only modification is used for treatment, or whether the condition persists after pregnancy. It does not exclude the possibility that unrecognized diabetes mellitus (DM) may have antedated or begun concomitantly with the pregnancy. A fasting plasma glucose level >126 mg/dL or a casual plasma glucose >200 mg/dL meets the threshold for the diagnosis. Women at high risk for GDM are those with marked obesity, previous history of GDM and/or glycosuria, previous birth of a ≥9-pound infant, or a strong family history of DM. High-risk women free of GDM at the initial prenatal screening and average-risk women are retested and tested, respectively, between the 24th and 28th week of gestation. Fasting hyperglycemia in women at risk for GDM is lower than for the nonpregnant individual (>105 mg/dL). This level may be associated with an increased risk of intrauterine fetal death during the last 4 to 8 weeks of gestation. Maternal metabolic surveillance is by daily self-monitoring of blood glucose. Issues related to the dental management of patients with DM were extensively reviewed in a recent publication.[5]

Oral Complications of Pregnancy

The most common oral complication of pregnancy is generalized gingival inflammation, referred to as *pregnancy gingivitis*. Pregnancy gingivitis affects 25% to 100% of pregnant patients and typically occurs during the second to eighth month of pregnancy. Inflammatory changes appear to be in response to poor oral-hygiene-related plaque accumulation exacerbated by increased estrogen, progesterone, and prostaglandin synthesis. These bioactive agents (estrogen, progesterone, prostaglandins) alter gingival vascularity, adversely affect cell-mediated immune function, inhibit collagen synthesis, and modify the subgingival microbial flora.[6] As the flora of subgingival plaque changes, a distinct increase in the proportion of *Prevotella intermedia* contributes to the severity of gingivitis. Women with gingivitis, if left untreated, will continue to have gingival disease following parturition, although the inflammation may be less intense. When the process results in loss of clinical attachment, the condition becomes periodontitis. Occasionally, generalized tooth mobility resulting from inflammatory changes in the gingiva, mineral changes in the lamina dura, and disturbances in the periodontal ligament may be observed. Tooth mobility unrelated to periodontitis appears to resolve following parturition.

Effect of Periodontal Disease on the Fetus

Inflammatory mediators, such as cytokines, interleukin-1, interleukin-6, and TNF-alpha associated with periodontal disease, may adversely affect the placenta and the fetus in ways not clearly defined at this time. They stimulate prostaglandin E_2 synthesis, which affects uterine contraction and increases the likelihood of premature labor.[7] A meta-analysis of periodontal disease in relation to the risk of low birth weight and preterm birth concluded that periodontal disease in pregnant patients significantly increases the risk for low birth weight and preterm birth. However, there is no convincing evidence that treatment of periodontal disease will reduce the risk of low birth weight, or preterm birth.[8] This conclusion was verified in the OPT study, which found that treating periodontal disease in pregnant women improved periodontal health and was safe, but it did not significantly alter rates of preterm delivery, low birth weight, or fetal growth restriction.[4]

Pyogenic Granuloma

Pyogenic granuloma (referred to as pregnancy tumor when observed in a pregnant female) is noted in up to 9.6% of pregnant patients. The neoplasms appear most frequently during the second trimester. These rapidly growing lesions typically arise from the interdental papillae in the maxillary anterior area. They vary in color from bright red to blue, bleed easily, and are usually painless. After parturition, most of these lesions tend to regress, at least partially, but the soft tissue in the affected area may require removal. The mechanisms predisposing to pregnancy tumors are the same as those postulated for pregnancy gingivitis (i.e., increased estrogen and progesterone synthesis in the presence of calculus and poor oral-hygiene-related local factors).

Dental Caries

During the second trimester, fetal calcium and phosphorus requirements increase, but while the fetus does draw calcium from maternal bone, it does not come from dental enamel. The calcium found in enamel is in a stable, crystalline form. Increased maternal absorption and decreased excretion compensates for the increased demand. Although the myth still persists, pregnancy does not cause tooth loss or "soft teeth," and there is no evidence that pregnancy contributes directly to an increased incidence of caries. The clinical impression of increased caries activity may be related to dietary changes, such as an increase in the frequency and amount of carbohydrate-containing food consumed. Gingival tenderness may further contribute to inadequate plaque removal. Two contributing factors for enamel demineralization are demineralization secondary to vomiting associated with morning sickness and that associated with xerostomia. Investigators in one study found that about 44% of the pregnant patients experienced persistent dry mouth attributable to hormonal changes.[9]

Prenatal fluoride administration with the intent to reduce caries risk in the child is controversial. Neither the American Academy of Pediatric Dentistry nor the American Academy of Pediatrics recommends prenatal fluoride supplementation. Of course, in areas where the community water is adequately fluoridated, such supplementation is redundant.

Developmental Effects on Teeth

Rhesus-factor incompatibility may cause intrinsic discoloration of deciduous teeth. Tetracycline-containing products, including doxycycline, are contraindicated during pregnancy due to their potential to discolor the developing dentition of the fetus. Pregnancy-related toxemia, prolonged or difficult delivery, and breach positioning of the fetus have been associated with enamel hypoplasia.[10]

■ Self-Study Review

1. Describe physiologic changes from pregnancy on the following systems: CV, respiratory, renal, and GI. Note the relationships of these changes on the dental hygiene care plan (DHCP).
2. Identify potential complications of pregnancy and describe the relationships on the DHCP.
3. Discuss the effects of periodontal treatment to reduce the physiologic and oral complications, if any.
4. What is the most common oral complication of pregnancy?
5. Describe recommendations for prenatal fluoride supplementation.

Drugs and Pregnancy

During pregnancy, the maternal plasma volume increases, total plasma protein concentrations decrease, total body fat increases, and, therefore, the apparent volume of distribution for many drugs increases. At the same time, drugs excreted by the kidneys may have increased rates of clearance due to increased renal blood flow and glomerular filtration rate. Consequently, when medication is necessary, *increased* dosages of a drug may have to be administered to the mother during critical periods of pregnancy. Most drugs in the maternal bloodstream cross the placenta by simple diffusion along the concentration gradient. During early pregnancy, the placental membrane is relatively thick, which tends to reduce permeability. The thickness decreases and the surface area of the placenta increases in the later trimesters, increasing the passage of drugs to fetal circulation. Each drug has a threshold concentration above which fetal abnormalities can occur and below which no effects are discernible. Whether a drug reaches the threshold concentration in the fetus depends on the chemical nature of the agent (molecular weight, protein binding, lipid solubility, and pKa) and maternal pharmacokinetic factors.

Local Anesthetics Used in the Pregnant Patient

Lidocaine with epinephrine is the local anesthetic of choice in the pregnant client. The addition of the vasoconstrictor reduces entry of the anesthetic into the circulation.

Epinephrine Used in the Pregnant Patient

Epinephrine is used with local anesthetic agents to improve their quality and to prolong the duration of anesthesia. Epinephrine also decreases the peak plasma concentration of the local anesthetic agent and reduces its toxicity. However, there is general concern on the part of many clinicians that epinephrine in local anesthetic agents, by virtue of beta-adrenergic activity, may decrease uterine blood flow. All of the studies investigating this issue concur that the addition of epinephrine to a local anesthetic agent decreases the total dosage of the local anesthetic agent required to provide for adequate pain relief during labor. Investigators using continuous epidural infusion of epinephrine at a rate of up to 0.04 mg/h (similar to concentrations used in dentistry) drew a similar conclusion.[11]

Teratogenic Effects of Drugs

Major malformations are usually the result of exposure to drugs during the critical period of **organogenesis** (first trimester). Exposure during the second and third trimesters usually affects organ function. Any drug in the fetal compartment at the time of birth must also rely on the **neonate's** own metabolic and excretory capabilities, which have not yet fully developed. Consequently, drugs given near term, especially those with long half-lives, may have prolonged actions on the newborn. Finally, drugs that cause maternal addiction are also known to cause fetal addiction. To date, fewer than 30 drugs have proven to be **teratogenic** in humans when used in clinically effective doses, and even fewer are currently in clinical use. Many commonly used drugs, such as acetylsalicylic acid, glucocorticoids, and diazepam, were once thought to be teratogenic. Larger and better controlled studies have subsequently shown these drugs to be safe.[12]

To make an informed decision about prescribing during pregnancy, the clinician must have access to information on which to base that decision. Currently, the pregnancy risk categories devised by the Food and Drug Administration (FDA) are used. The categories described in Box 21-1 are based on the degree to which available information has ruled out risk to the fetus balanced against the drug's potential benefits to the patient. The rate and extent of placental diffusion are determined by plasma protein binding, ionization, and lipid solubility. Placental transfer of drugs from the mother to the fetus is related to the degree of protein binding. Only free, unbound drug is available for placental transfer. Therefore, local anesthetics with the highest protein-binding capacity may have the lowest placental transfer. Lipid-soluble, nonionized agents readily enter fetal blood from the maternal circulation. Table 21-1 shows the protein-binding capacity of local anesthetics used in dentistry. Although lidocaine (pregnancy category B) has a lower protein-binding ratio than several other local anesthetic agents, the other agents are in pregnancy category C. The concentration of a local anesthetic agent is another factor that affects fetal toxicity and, consequently, safety classification. Lidocaine is 2%, whereas mepivacaine is 2% or 3%, and prilocaine and articaine are 4%. Although lidocaine's lipid solubility is high and it has lower protein-binding capacity, it also has the lowest concentration of the drug in its free form because of its pKa. These features and other available evidence make it safest (category B) for use during pregnancy. Pregnancy risk classifications are based on safety studies. See the differences between category B and C in Box 21-1.

Drugs of choice to resolve an emerging dental problem when primary dental care along with the administration or

BOX 21-1. FDA Pregnancy Risk Stratification of Drugs

Category A: Adequate, well-controlled studies in pregnant women have not shown an increased risk of fetal abnormalities.

Category B: Animal studies have revealed no evidence of harm to the fetus; however, there are no adequate and well-controlled studies in pregnant women.

OR

Animal studies have shown an adverse effect, but adequate and well-controlled studies in pregnant women have failed to demonstrate a risk to the fetus.

Category C: Animal studies have shown an adverse effect, and there are no adequate and well-controlled studies in pregnant women.

OR

No animal studies have been conducted, and there are no adequate and well-controlled studies in pregnant women.

Category D: Studies (adequate, well-controlled, or observational) in pregnant women have demonstrated a risk to the fetus. However, the benefit of therapy may outweigh the potential risk.

Category X: Studies (adequate, well-controlled, or observational) in animals or pregnant women have demonstrated positive evidence of fetal abnormalities. The use of the product is contraindicated in women who are or may become pregnant.

Table 21-1 Protein Binding of Local Anesthetic Agents

Local Anesthetic	Systemic Protein Binding (%)
Articaine	60 to 80
Bupivacaine	95.6
Lidocaine	64.3
Mepivacaine	77.5
Prilocaine	55

the aorta). However, with increasing gestational age, the duct closes (usually by birth). *Patent ductus arteriosus* means failure of the duct between the pulmonary artery and the aorta to close by birth. With respect to this discussion, ibuprofen, naproxen, and codeine, if administered during the last trimester of pregnancy, can induce premature closure of the ductus and lead to heart failure in the fetus. This means that the prenatal communication between the left and right sides of the heart closes prematurely in the developing fetus if the mother takes any COX-inhibitor or codeine in the third trimester of pregnancy. Acetaminophen is in pregnancy category B and is safe to use during pregnancy.

Antibacterial Agents

Most antibacterial agents used for oral infections are in pregnancy category B. Clarithromycin, a macrolide, is in category C. Agents in category B are the drugs of choice for the pregnant client.

Drugs During Lactation

With the increasing recognition of the benefits of breast-feeding, consideration must be paid to the benefits versus risks of drug therapy in lactating women. The rate of passage of a drug from plasma to milk is an important determinant of the concentration of the drug in milk. Mechanisms of excretion of drugs in breast milk include both passive diffusion and carrier-mediated transport. The amount of a drug excreted in breast milk depends on the characteristics of the drug, such as the drug's molecular weight, lipid solubility, pK_a, and plasma protein binding. Small, water-soluble nonelectrolytes pass into milk by simple diffusion through aqueous channels in the mammary epithelial membrane that separates plasma from milk. Equilibrium is reached rapidly, and the drug's concentration in milk approximates plasma levels. With larger molecules, only the lipid-soluble, nonionized form passes through the membrane. The pK_a of weak electrolytes is an important determinant of drug concentration in milk, because the pH of milk is generally lower (more acidic) than that of plasma, and milk can act as an "ion trap" for weak bases. At equilibrium, basic drugs may be more concentrated in milk relative to plasma. Conversely, acidic drugs are limited in their ability to enter milk, because they are primarily in their ionized form in plasma. Weak acids that do diffuse into milk will be primarily in the nonionized form, thus causing a net transfer of the drug from milk to plasma. Consequently, at equilibrium, acidic drugs are more concentrated in plasma than in milk.

prescription of such drugs is unavoidable are listed in Table 21-2.[13]

Local Anesthetics

There are two local anesthetics used in dentistry in pregnancy category B. These include lidocaine and prilocaine. Prilocaine has the potential to cause methemoglobinemia in predisposed individuals. There are few adverse drug effects (ADEs) from lidocaine when it is used properly (no more than maximum dose, slow injection, frequent aspiration).

Aspirin and COX-Inhibitors

Aspirin is unsafe in the third trimester of pregnancy only, because it causes premature closure of the patent ductus arteriosus. *Patent* means open, affording free passage, or unobstructed flow of blood in this case. Prior to birth, there is communication between the pulmonary artery and the aorta (that is, a free flow of blood from the pulmonary artery to

| Table 21-2 | Selected Dental Drugs and Use in Pregnancy and Lactation |

Drug	FDA Pregnancy Category	Lactation and Breast-Feeding Considerations
Analgesics		
Acetaminophen	B	Enters breast milk; compatible/safe.
Aspirin	C/D (3rd trimester)	Enters breast milk; avoid use due to potential adverse effects in nursing infants.
Ibuprofen	C/D (3rd trimester)	Not detected in breast milk; use NSAIDs with caution because of potential effects on infant CV system.*
Tramadol	C	Use with caution.*
Hydrocodone# and acetaminophen	C/D (prolonged use or high doses near term)	Acetaminophen is excreted in breast milk. The AAP considers it to be "compatible" with breast-feeding. Information is not available for hydrocodone. The AAP considers codeine to be "compatible" with breast-feeding. The manufacturers recommend discontinuing the medication or to discontinue nursing during therapy.
Hydrocodone# and aspirin	C/D (3rd trimester)	Hydrocodone: No data reported. Aspirin: Avoid use due to potential adverse effects in nursing infants.
Hydrocodone# and ibuprofen	C/D (3rd trimester)	Excretion in breast milk unknown; use with caution.*
Naproxen	C/D (3rd trimester)	Enters breast milk; not recommended.
Oxycodone# and acetaminophen	B/D (prolonged use or high doses near term)	Oxycodone: Excreted in breast milk.* If occasional doses are used during breast-feeding, monitor infant for sedation, GI effects, and changes in feeding pattern. Acetaminophen: May be taken while breast-feeding.
Oxycodone# and aspirin	B/D (3rd trimester)	Oxycodone: Enters breast milk. Aspirin: Avoid in third trimester.
Oxycodone# and ibuprofen	B/D (3rd trimester)	Enters breast milk; use with caution.*
Propoxyphene# and acetaminophen	C/B	Enters breast milk; the AAP considers propoxyphene and acetaminophen to be "compatible" with breast-feeding.
Propoxyphene,# aspirin, caffeine	C/D (3rd trimester)	Enters breast milk; use with caution.* The AAP recommends that aspirin be used with "caution" during breast-feeding; propoxyphene and caffeine (moderate intake) are considered "compatible."
Antianxiety Agents		
Alprazolam	D	Enters breast milk; not recommended (the AAP rates it "of concern"). Symptoms of withdrawal, lethargy, and loss of body weight have been reported in infants exposed to alprazolam and/or other benzodiazepines while nursing. Breast-feeding is not recommended.
Diazepam	D	Enters breast milk; contraindicated (the AAP rates it "of concern"). Avoid. Clinical effects on the infant include sedation.
Midazolam	D	Enters breast milk; contraindicated (the AAP rates it "of concern"). Avoid.
Nitrous oxide	Avoid	Safe; no systemic absorption.
Barbiturates	D	Avoid.
Diphenhydramine	C	Use with caution.*
Antibiotics		
Amoxicillin	B	Enters breast milk; compatible, although sensitization to PEN exists.
Cephalexin	B	Enters breast milk; use caution.* Theoretically, drug absorbed by nursing infant may change bowel flora or cause side effects of CEPH.
Clindamycin	B	Enters breast milk; compatible.

(Continued)

Table 21-2 *(Continued)*

Drug	FDA Pregnancy Category	Lactation and Breast-Feeding Considerations
Doxycycline subantimicrobial (Periostat), doxycycline (Vibramycin), other tetracyclines	D	Tetracyclines enter breast milk. Use of tetracyclines during tooth development may cause permanent discoloration of the teeth and enamel hypoplasia. Avoid use.
Erythromycin	B	Enters breast milk; the AAP considers it "compatible."
Azithromycin	B	Enters breast milk; not recommended (the AAP rates it "of concern").
Clarithromycin	C	Avoid.
Metronidazole	B (may be contraindicated in 1st trimester)	Enters breast milk; not recommended (the AAP rates it "of concern"). It is suggested to stop breast-feeding for 12 to 24 h following a single dose therapy to allow excretion of dose.
Desensitizing Agents/Fluoride Varnishes		
Potassium oxalate (SuperSeal)	Effects on pregnancy are unknown	Effects on nursing are unknown.
Potassium mono-oxalate (Protect)	Effects on pregnancy are unknown	Effects on nursing are unknown.
Potassium nitrate, triclosan (Triclosan)	Effects on pregnancy are unknown	Effects on nursing are unknown.
Sodium fluoride, stannous fluoride (Gel-Kam Dentin Block)	Effects on pregnancy are unknown	Effects on nursing are unknown.
Sodium fluoride (Duraflor, Duraphate)	Effects on pregnancy are unknown	Effects on nursing are unknown.
Strontium chloride, copal resin (Zarosen)	Effects on pregnancy are unknown	Effects on nursing are unknown.
Local Anesthetics: Local Delivery Systems		
Doxycycline hyclate (Atridox)	D	Tetracyclines enter breast milk. Use of tetracyclines during tooth development may cause permanent discoloration of the teeth and enamel hypoplasia.
Chlorhexidine gluconate (Perio-Chip)	C	Safety in nursing unknown.
Minocycline hydrochloride (Arestin)	D	Tetracyclines enter breast milk. Use of tetracyclines during tooth development may cause permanent discoloration of the teeth and enamel hypoplasia.
Lidocaine and prilocaine (Oraqix)	B	Usual dose has not been shown to affect health of nursing infant.
Anesthetic Agents/Vasoconstrictors		
Benzocaine (topical)	C	Excretion in breast milk unknown; low systemic absorption; safe.
Lidocaine and epinephrine	B	Enters breast milk; compatible. Usual dose has not been shown to affect health of nursing infant.
Articaine	C	Usual dose has not been shown to affect health of nursing infant.
Mepivacaine	C	Usual dose has not been shown to affect health of nursing infant.
Mepivacaine and levonordefrin	C	Usual dose has not been shown to affect health of nursing infant.
Prilocaine with epinephrine	B/C	Usual dose has not been shown to affect health of nursing infant.
Prilocaine plain	B	Usual dose has not been shown to affect health of nursing infant.

NSAID, nonsteroidal anti-inflammatory drug; AAP, American Academy of Pediatrics.
* Use in consultation with physician.
# Most opioids appear in breast milk; effects may not be significant.
[Adapted with permission from Sharuga C. Drug administration for the pregnant and nursing patient. *J Prac Hygiene*. 2007;16(2):6–9.]

Local Anesthetics

Safety for use of local anesthetics during lactation has not been established, and, except for bupivacaine, it is unknown if local anesthetics are excreted in breast milk. Excepting bupivacaine, however, all other local anesthetics are considered safe to use in the lactating female.

Antibacterial Agents

Erythromycin is excreted in breast milk, but no ADEs have been reported. Erythromycin and clindamycin are both considered to be compatible with breast-feeding by the American Academy of Pediatrics (AAP). It is unknown if azithromycin or clarithromycin are excreted in breast milk, and both should be used with caution in nursing mothers. Potential problems for the infant include modification of bowel flora and pharmacologic side effects. Most agents are excreted in breast milk in low concentrations and should be used only if the benefit outweighs the risks. An allergic response in the nursing infant who develops hypersensitivity to the drug (such as penicillin, the most allergenic drug) is possible. Because of the potential for causing tumors in studies using mice, the risk/benefit ratio should be considered before administering metronidazole during lactation. Metronidazole is secreted in breast milk in concentrations similar to those found in maternal plasma.

Selecting Drugs During Lactation

Factors that determine the advisability of giving a particular drug to a nursing mother include the potential for acute or long-term, dose-related, and non-dose-related toxicity; dosage and duration of therapy; age of the infant; quantity of milk consumed by the infant; and the drug's effect on lactation. To minimize the infant's exposure to medications in milk, the following strategies are used:

- Delay drug therapy temporarily
- Withhold drug therapy
- Advise the mother to avoid nursing at peak plasma concentrations of the drug
- Time drug administration to the mother before the infant's longest sleep period
- Withhold breast-feeding temporarily (use a bottle)

Dental drugs that are preferred for women who are breast-feeding are listed in Table 21-2. The list, however, is by no means definitive and only contains the drugs commonly prescribed or used in dentistry. The numbers of women and infants studied are small, and very little is known about the long-term effects of these drugs on infants.

Dental Management During Pregnancy and Lactation

The goals of providing dental hygiene care to the pregnant or nursing mother are to develop and implement timely preventive and therapeutic strategies compatible with the patient's physical and emotional ability to undergo and respond to oral health care and to ensure the safety and well-being of the developing fetus, newborn, infant, or young child.

Patient Assessment

Patient assessment should include eliciting a thorough medical history. The history of previous pregnancies should be discussed, including previous miscarriages, history of GDM, hypertension, and pre-eclampsia or eclampsia. It is important to monitor the blood pressure, pulse rate and rhythm, and respiration of the pregnant patient. Hypertension, associated with pre-eclampsia and eclampsia during pregnancy, occurs after the 20th week of gestation. Hypertensive disorders are a leading cause of maternal mortality. Hypotension is often associated with unexplained symptoms, such as fatigue, chronic fatigue syndrome, and recurrent syncope (orthostatic hypotension). Procedures that promote hypotension should be avoided during dental hygiene treatment because it reduces blood flow to the fetus and can result in fetal hypoxia and injury. Hypotension often occurs in supine positioning and is associated with supine hypotensive syndrome.

Supine Hypotensive Syndrome

During the third trimester, the expectant mother may experience increasing fatigue, mild depression, or mood changes, and she may have lower back pain. Difficulty to assume and maintain a comfortable position may be apparent. As the fetal mass grows, it places increasing pressure on the aorta and inferior vena cava, which leads to reduced cardiac output, especially in a supine position. *Supine hypotensive syndrome* (usually seen after the 28th week of gestation) affects up to 8% of expectant mothers and is characterized by lightheadedness, tachycardia, an abrupt fall in blood pressure, and loss of consciousness (syncope). To avoid such episodes, the patient should be placed in a semiupright position; if a supine position is used, the patient should be placed on her left side (left lateral supine position) at an angle of about 15 degrees and allowed to move her legs frequently. This will reposition the fetus away from the inferior vena cava and promote the return blood flow to the heart. A pillow can be placed under the right hip to achieve this position.

Appointment Planning

Dental hygiene services are ideally planned for the second trimester when there is less risk for nausea and the fetal pressure on the vena cava vasculature is minimal. Dental hygiene appointments should be kept relatively short to reduce stress.

Dental Radiography During Pregnancy

The concept of avoiding radiography during pregnancy generally applies to procedures in which the embryo or fetus would be in or near the primary beam. For dental radiography, the primary beam is limited to the head and neck region. Furthermore, standard radiation hygiene practices, such as the use of high-speed film, filtration, collimation, and leaded aprons, greatly reduce fetal exposure. However, if the pregnant patient expresses anxiety about having dental radiography, it is prudent to avoid or minimize the use of diagnostic radiography, especially during the first trimester, the period of organogenesis. An additional consideration involves the pregnant dental health care worker. As long as appropriate radiation safety measures are followed, there is no contraindication to these individuals operating radiographic equipment.[14]

Oral Health Education

Oral health education should begin early in pregnancy. While most dental problems are not directly attributable to pregnancy, the physiologic and behavioral changes that can occur may exacerbate existing dental disease. Although the pregnant patient may be predisposed to developing gingivitis, those who practice good oral hygiene reduce the risk. Therefore, preventive strategies aimed at attaining optimal oral hygiene should be developed and implemented early. Optimal home care should be complemented with recommendations for postdelivery oral care and care of the infant's developing dentition, as well as recommendations for professional intervention. Definitive periodontal maintenance care may be initiated following parturition. Nausea and vomiting are common during the first trimester. The low pH of the vomitus may lead to erosion of the dental enamel. To prevent erosion, brushing should be avoided immediately after vomiting, because the enamel is more vulnerable to erosion following an acid insult. Patients should be advised to rinse thoroughly with a hypertonic sodium bicarbonate solution following each acid challenge.[6] The educational program facilitates oral health care providers to (a) establish a good clinician-patient relationship, (b) reduce the stress and anxiety in treatment, and (c) establish the initiation of a preventive program to ensure a healthy oral environment throughout pregnancy.

■ Self-Study Review

6. Describe alterations in drug administration in the pregnant client.
7. What local anesthetic should be selected for the pregnant client? Discuss vasoconstrictor issues.
8. Describe precautions in local anesthetic administration for the pregnant client.
9. Identify the trimester associated with *teratogenicity*.
10. Identify drugs used in dentistry and their precautions of use during pregnancy.
11. Define the levels A to X in the FDA pregnancy risk stratification.
12. Identify issues of drug use in lactation. Which dental drug has high concentrations in breast milk?
13. Describe dental management recommendations during pregnancy and lactation.

THE MENOPAUSAL PATIENT

Approximately 36 million women in the United States have entered the menopausal stage of life. Menopause follows spontaneous cessation of menses, usually between the ages of 47 and 55. Menopause can also be induced by surgical removal of the ovaries. This procedure usually is performed in conjunction with a hysterectomy as a prophylactic measure to prevent ovarian cancer. In these situations, the production

of estrogen decreases because of an inadequate number of functioning follicles within the ovaries. When estrogen levels decline, the occurrence of menopausal symptoms may develop. These can include hot flashes, night sweats, and vaginal dryness. The risk of developing cardiovascular disease (CVD; myocardial infarction, stroke), and osteoporosis is increased due to estrogen deprivation. It has been suggested that various changes in the body may affect the oral cavity. Hormone replacement therapy (HRT) is sometimes prescribed on a short-term basis to alleviate the uncomfortable symptoms associated with estrogen deficiency.

Hormone Replacement Therapy

HRT has been promoted over the last 40 years to improve quality of life and to reduce the risks of osteoporotic fractures and coronary heart disease (CHD). However, recent clinical trials have reported that HRT is associated with an increased risk for CV events in some individuals, such as myocardial infarction, stroke, peripheral vascular disease, and sudden cardiac death. The U.S. Preventive Services Task Force (USPSTF) recommends against the routine use of unopposed estrogen for the prevention of chronic conditions in postmenopausal women, because good evidence shows that the use of unopposed estrogen results in both benefits and ADEs. The benefits include a reduced risk for fracture (good evidence); ADEs include an increased risk for venous thromboembolism (fair evidence), stroke (fair evidence), dementia (fair evidence), and lower global cognitive functioning (fair evidence). There is fair evidence that unopposed estrogen has no beneficial effect on CHD. The USPSTF concluded that the harmful effects of unopposed estrogen are likely to exceed the chronic disease prevention benefits in most women. The American College of Obstetricians and Gynecologists, American Heart Association, North American Menopause Society, and Canadian Task Force on Preventive Health Care also recommend against use of hormone therapy for the prevention of chronic diseases in postmenopausal women.[15–18]

HRT Schedules

HRT consists of an estrogen and progestin combination product (Prempro) or estrogen alone (Premarin). The progestin is included in the drug regimen to reduce the risk for uterine cancer, a risk when estrogen is taken alone. In women whose uterus has been removed but whose ovaries are still present, unopposed conjugated estrogen is commonly prescribed.

The most common schedule is daily oral administration of tablets containing both estrogen (conjugated estrogen, 0.625 mg) and a progestin (medroxyprogesterone acetate, 2.5 mg). Less common is a regimen using two sets of tablets, one containing estrogen and the other containing estrogen and progestin; the estrogen tablets are taken for the first 14 days of the cycle, and the combination tablets are taken for the last 14 days of the cycle. This schedule of cyclical therapy results in 70% to 90% of women experiencing a regular monthly cycle with normal menstruation.

Estrogen Replacement Therapy

The estrogen replacement therapy (ERT) regimen is an effective method for preventing loss of bone density and fractures in postmenopausal women from **osteopenia** or osteoporosis. *Osteoporosis* is a condition that results from severe thinning and weakening of normal bone. When this occurs, a patient with osteoporosis will have a higher risk of bone fracture. The dominant underlying factor for osteoporosis in postmenopausal women is estrogen deficiency. Many epidemiologic studies have reported that ERT reduced the risk of hip fractures by about 50%. The effect is greatest in long-term users but may be lost after discontinuation of the hormone. A nonhormonal oral bisphosphonate therapy is commonly used to treat or prevent osteoporosis. These drugs (Fosamax, Actonel, Boniva) are discussed in Chapter 14. Raloxifene (Evista), a nonhormonal selective estrogen receptor modulator, is also approved for treatment and prevention of osteoporosis, as well as prevention of breast cancer.

Adverse Drug Effects

Formation of intravascular blood clots is the most likely side effect from HRT and raloxifene therapy. Increased blood pressure is associated with dose levels of hormones in oral contraceptives but is less common with HRT used to relieve menopausal symptoms. Women who smoke while taking supplemental estrogen have an increased risk for formation of intravascular clots leading to stroke. The long-term administration of estrogen/progestin therapy is associated with an increased risk for breast cancer. There is a low risk for the development of osteonecrosis of the jaw with oral bisphosphonates. It appears that taking bisphosphonates for more than 3 years increases the risk. In addition, there is an increased risk for dementia in long-term use of estrogen.

Oral Changes in Menopause

Xerostomia

Studies differ on whether salivation diminishes during menopause. A study assessed salivary flow rates across menopausal status in a cohort of healthy Caucasian women of varying ages. A comparison of salivary flow rates in the parotid and submandibular glands was made between three groups of female individuals according to their menopausal status. The three groups consisted of healthy, dentate, non-medicated women. One group consisted of premenopausal women whose mean age was 39 years. Another group was perimenopausal with a mean age of 48 years. A third group was postmenopausal with a mean age of 69 years. The results showed no significant differences in stimulated or unstimulated parotid salivation between the three groups, but saliva from the submandibular gland decreased in postmenopausal women. There were also no differences in salivary flow rates between those taking estrogen and those who were not medicated. These data suggest that postmenopausal women have decreased unstimulated and stimulated submandibular and sublingual salivary gland flow compared with premenopausal women.[19]

Dental Caries

Dental caries remains one of the top three most common infectious diseases in the world today. Although caries prevalence decreased markedly in children and in adults up to age 40 between 1975 and 2000, the risk for caries in individuals 70 years of age and older has increased. A study evaluated the 5-year incidence of dental caries in a random sample of 60-, 70-, and 80-year-old subjects.[20] Salivary and microbial factors indicated that there is an increased risk of dental caries with age due to unfavorable microbial and xerostomic conditions. The paucity of saliva seen in postmenopausal women may be the most likely factor responsible for the increased prevalence of dental caries. Caries preventive agents, such as fluorides and xylitol gum, should be considered in this situation.

Burning Mouth Syndrome

Burning mouth syndrome (BMS) is an oral disorder presenting as a burning sensation of the tongue and, less frequently, other oral and perioral sites. This condition is probably of multifactorial origin, is often idiopathic, and has an etiology that remains largely obscure. BMS is a disorder typically observed in middle-age and elderly subjects ranging in age from 38 to 78 years. The female-to-male ratio is about 7:1. The term *BMS* clinically describes a variety of chronic oral symptoms that often increase in intensity at the end of each day, and that seldom interfere with sleep. Two specific clinical features define this syndrome: (a) a symptomatic triad, which includes unremitting oral mucosal pain, **dysgeusia**, and xerostomia; and (b) no signs of lesion(s) or other detectable change(s) in the oral mucosa, even in the painful area. This syndrome is commonly observed in specific subgroups of patients, such as peri- or postmenopausal women. Approximately 90% of women who attend health care clinics for their BMS symptoms are peri- or postmenopausal women. They report pain onset ranging from 3 years before to 12 years after menopause. Moreover, 18% to 33% of menopausal women have been reported to exhibit BMS symptoms.

Treatment Options

Various medications have been used to relieve BMS. Patients have shown a good response to long-term therapy with systemic regimens of antidepressants and antianxiety agents. Clonazepam, a benzodiazepine, has been shown to be helpful in reducing the discomfort of BMS. In addition, topical administration of capsaicin within the mouth has provided a partial or even complete remission of the pain. Although a large variety of drugs, medications, and miscellaneous treatments has been proposed to treat BMS, management of this syndrome is still not satisfactory, and there is no definitive cure. BMS remains an enigma.

Taste Alterations

Taste alteration refers to a decrease in the ability to taste foods (hypogeusia) or the presence of a metallic or medicinal taste in the mouth. Other terms for taste alteration are sometimes used: *Dysgeusia* describes changes in how food tastes, and *ageusia* describes the complete loss of the ability to taste foods. Changes in the function of taste buds and neural networks have been noted to occur following the onset of menopause.[21] This effect on taste and neuronal function leads to an adverse alteration in taste sensation and to a reduction of pleasure and comfort from food and presents a risk factor for nutritional deficiencies. Taste alterations are also exacerbated during menopause due to a reduction in saliva production and atrophic gingivitis. There is no treatment to reverse taste alteration.

Periodontal Disease

The deficiency of estrogen in women at menopause is considered a possible risk factor for periodontal attachment loss. One study reported estrogen deficiency was associated with increased frequency of crestal alveolar bone (CAB) density loss in postmenopausal women with periodontal disease.[22] A report of postmenopausal women who did not receive HRT demonstrated that implants placed in the maxilla, but not in the mandible, failed to integrate with bone more often than implants placed in premenopausal women and postmenopausal women receiving HRT.[23] These results suggest that estrogen deficiency and the resultant bony changes associated with menopause may be risk factors for implant failure in the maxilla.

Osteoporosis in the Jaw

Postmenopausal osteoporosis affects the bones of the jaw, as well as other skeletal bones, and may result in tooth loss. Digital periapical dental radiographs have shown that women with osteoporosis of the spine and hip have altered patterns of bone trabeculation in the anterior maxilla and posterior mandible. The relevance of this to predicting periodontal attachment loss is unclear. Conversely, a recent study in healthy postmenopausal women revealed there was not a statistically significant correlation between clinical attachment level and bone mineral density (BMD), so the role of osteoporosis in alveolar bone loss is unclear.[24]

Oral health care professionals have an opportunity to detect osteoporosis based on incidental findings on dental panoramic radiographs. Eroded or thin inferior cortex of the mandible detected on dental panoramic radiographs may be useful for identifying postmenopausal women with low BMD or osteoporosis.[25] For women who have evidence of attachment loss but have low risk factors for it (such as good oral hygiene or regular care), a referral for bone density testing may be appropriate.

Tooth Loss

Estrogen users have been shown to retain more natural teeth than nonusers. Studies also found that the risk of tooth loss was significantly lower in women who used HRT than those who did not.

■ Self-Study Review

14. Describe the effect of menopause on body function and health.
15. Differentiate between indications for *unopposed estrogen* and *estrogen/progesterone* indications. Which hormone is associated with treatment for osteoporosis?
16. Identify risks in taking HRT.
17. Describe oral changes associated with menopause.

Cardiovascular Disease

CVD due to atherosclerosis (coronary artery disease and stroke) is the most common cause of death among postmenopausal women. This increased risk may result from a decrease in estrogen with a consequent increase in atherogenic risk factors, such as increases in total cholesterol and low-density lipoprotein (LDL) serum cholesterol and a decrease in high-density lipoprotein (HDL) serum cholesterol. Panoramic dental radiographs may identify carotid artery atheromas in the neck and may be useful in identifying postmenopausal women at risk of developing strokes.[26] At this time, research has shown an association between periodontal inflammation and formation of atherosclerosis, but there are no studies to demonstrate that periodontal inflammation causes CVD. A recent pilot study (Periodontitis and Vascular Events [PAVE]) investigated whether treatment of periodontal disease reduces the risk for CVD[27] The authors concluded that following 18 months of provision of periodontal treatment to individuals with heart disease there were similar patterns of adverse events between the test group who received periodontal care and the community care group (untreated group). The American Academy of Periodontology (AAP) advises practitioners that oral health education can include telling patients that treatment of periodontal disease "may" help to reduce CVD.[28]

Dental Management

Oral health care practitioners who treat women entering menopause need to consider the oral and systemic changes those patients are experiencing. Dental hygienists should advise women on how to prevent or control oral infections, particularly dental caries and periodontal diseases. Clinical findings of postmenopausal problems during dental examination may include a paucity of saliva, increased dental caries, taste alterations, periodontitis and osteoporosis of the jaws, making the menopausal client unsuitable for conventional prosthetic devices or dental implants. Estrogen deficiency can be considered a possible cause of oral discomfort in some postmenopausal patients, and ERT may improve subjective symptoms.

Medical History

When treating menopausal clients in the oral health care setting, it is recommended that an initial medical history be taken and reviewed with the patient at each appointment. Due to the risk for CVD, blood pressure should be recorded for all new patients at the time of the initial appointment. Conducting medical history reviews and measuring blood pressure are performed primarily to identify contraindications or assess the need for implementing modifications to dental treatment. A second benefit gained by performing these evaluations, however, is the monitoring of underlying medical conditions and being able to inform the client of suspected abnormalities.

Medical Referral

Postmenopausal women younger than 65 years may need to be referred for bone densitometry on the basis of incidental findings on dental panoramic radiographs. Eroded or thin inferior cortex of the mandible detected on dental panoramic radiographs may be useful for identifying postmenopausal women with low BMD or osteoporosis.

Bisphosphonate Therapy

Oral health professionals should be alerted to the possibility that some menopausal women may be taking bisphosphonates for the management of osteoporosis. Although this class of drugs has clear evidence of medical efficacy, there are an increasing number of reports of bisphosphonate-associated osteonecrosis of the jaw that have substantial implications for the patient and for the clinician.[29] Dental professionals should be alerted about this possible complication so patients taking bisphosphonates and those considering elective dental procedures can be properly counseled. A thorough dental examination and necessary tooth extractions with time for healing is recommended before commencing bisphosphonate therapy. For patients already receiving bisphosphonate therapy, close collaboration with the oral surgeon and physician are essential.

Other Therapies

Some menopausal women may be taking raloxifene (Evista) to prevent osteoporosis. Raloxifene is a nonhormonal selective estrogen-receptor modulator that binds to the estrogen receptor, resulting in estrogen-agonist effects on bone and the CV system and estrogen-antagonist effects on endometrial and breast tissue. It is currently approved to prevent and treat osteoporosis in postmenopausal women, and it recently gained approval to prevent breast cancer. There are suggestive data that raloxifene may have favorable effects on the arterial systems in postmenopausal women, thereby lowering the incidence of future adverse CV events. However, other studies have shown that raloxifene did not significantly affect the risk of CVD. The benefits of raloxifene in reducing the risks of invasive breast cancer and vertebral fracture should be weighed against the low risk of venous thromboembolism and fatal stroke.[30]

■ **Self-Study Review**

18. Describe the risk of CVD from estrogen loss. Consider the role of periodontal disease as a causative factor in CVD and AAP guidelines on the issue.
19. Describe dental management for the menopausal client.

DENTAL HYGIENE APPLICATIONS

In view of the dual responsibility that oral health care providers face in treating the pregnant or lactating patient, managing dental hygiene care requires (a) understanding the physiology of pregnancy and that of fetal development; (b)

being aware of potential oral and physiologic complications of pregnancy; (c) appreciating the risk of administering drugs; and (d) anticipating the effects that dental hygiene intervention may have on the woman, fetus, neonate, infant, or young child. Management of the client in menopause has different considerations, mainly including the relevance of osteoporosis and potential implications on periodontal health.

Pregnancy and Lactation

Hormone levels are increased during pregnancy, which can lead to subgingival organism alterations and gingivitis, as well as pyogenic granuloma formation. Oral health education information should include the possibility of these gingival changes and the need for daily, effective biofilm removal to reduce their development. Some women may believe that pregnancy leads to tooth loss and removal of enamel from teeth. This myth should be dispelled, and oral health information on the benefits of xylitol to both the mother and (after delivery of the baby) the child should be included in the education plan. If caries are found, other caries prevention modalities should be recommended (such as in-office fluoride, home fluoride, or sealants). Although elective care during the first two trimesters of pregnancy has been determined to be safe, the second trimester is considered to be the ideal time. Physiologic changes associated with pregnancy should be considered (Box 21-1), and appropriate intervention strategies should be used during dental hygiene care.

Menopause and Osteoporosis

A thorough health history and measurement of vital signs should be investigated, with the goal of identifying uncontrolled conditions and determining the risks in providing oral health care treatment. The oral cavity should be examined for xerostomia, caries (especially root caries), and periodontal disease, and appropriate preventive and therapeutic services should be provided. Radiography may indicate a need to refer the client for bone density levels. For clients taking bisphosphonates, appropriate patient information should be provided (Chapter 14).

CONCLUSION

In order to provide timely and competent care to expectant and breast-feeding patients, clinicians must understand the physiologic processes that occur, as well as the potential complications. The clinician's primary goal should be to provide necessary care for the pregnant patient while minimizing the risk to the fetus or newborn. When questions or complications arise during care, a consultation with the patient's obstetrician is required.

Menopause can result in a variety of changes in the body. The clinician must be aware of these changes and the impact they may have on dental hygiene care. A complete list of medications the patient is taking should be reviewed. Before initiation of an elective procedure, the possible complications associated with the treatment of menopausal patients should be considered. Communication between patient, physician, and the dental team is essential.

CLINICAL APPLICATION EXERCISES

☐ **Exercise 1.** Describe the pharmacologic treatment plan for the patient in the fifth month of pregnancy whose therapy requires periodontal débridement and definitive scaling and root planing.

☐ **Exercise 2.** Describe the pharmacologic treatment plan for the menopausal client when local anesthesia is necessary.

☐ **Exercise 3.** Your pregnant client complains, "Every time I get pregnant, I lose a tooth!" What is the appropriate information to include in the oral health educa-

tion plan for someone who has just learned she is pregnant?

☐ **Exercise 4.** WEB ACTIVITY: Do a search for oral and systemic disease connection. Find the link to the ADA.org A-Z Topic "Oral-systemic health" and read the special October 2006 supplement on the issue (available as a free download at http://jada.ada.org/content/vol137/suppl_2/index.dtl). Follow other links according to your interest. Research published in 2006 disputed the idea that periodontal treatment would reduce low, preterm birth.[4] Search for evidence published in 2007 and 2008. (See *J Den Res.* 2008;84(1):73–78.)

References

1. Clapp JF III, Capeless E. Cardiovascular function before, during, and after the first and subsequent pregnancies. *Am J Cardiol.* 1997;80:1469–1473.
2. Barron WM. The pregnant surgical patient: Medical evaluation and management. *Ann Intern Med.* 1984;101:683–691.
3. Weyerman M, Brenner H, Adler G, et al. *Helicobacter pylori* infection and the occurrence and severity of gastrointestinal symptoms during pregnancy. *Am J Obstet Gynecol.* 2003;189: 526–531.
4. Michalowicz BS, Hodges JS, DiAngelis AJ, et al. Treatment of periodontal disease and the risk of preterm birth. *N Eng J Med.* 2006;355(11):1885–1894.
5. Miley DD, Terezhalmy GT. The patient with diabetes mellitus. *Quintessence Int.* 2005;36(10):779–795.
6. Lee A, McWilliams M, Janchar T. Care of the pregnant patient in the dental office. *Dent Clin North Am.* 1999;43(3):485–494.
7. Offenbacher S, Sieff S, Beck JD. Periodontitis-associated pregnancy complications. *Premat Neonat Med.* 1998;3:82–85.
8. Khader YS, Ta'ani Q. Periodontal diseases and the risk of preterm birth and low birth weight: A meta-analysis. *J Periodontol.* 2005;76:161–165.
9. Steinberg BJ. Women's oral health issues. *J Dent Educ.* 1999; 63:271–275.
10. Casamassimo PS. Maternal oral health. *Dent Clin North Am.* 2001;45:469–478.
11. Okutomi T, Amano K, Morishima HO. Effect of standard diluted epinephrine infusion on epidural anesthesia in labor. *Reg Anesth Pain Med.* 2000;25:529–534.
12. Koren G, Pastuszak A, Ito S. Drugs and pregnancy. *N Engl J Med.* 1998;338:1128–1137.
13. Sharuga C. Drug administration for the pregnant and nursing patient. *J Prac Hyg.* 2007;16(2):6–9.
14. *Radiation Protection in Dentistry.* Bethesda, MD: National Council and Radiation Protection & Measurements; Dec. 31, 2003:30, 67, 81. NCRP Report No. 145.
15. US Preventive Services Task Force. Hormone therapy for the prevention of chronic conditions in postmenopausal women: Recommendations from the U.S. Preventive Services Task Force. *Ann Intern Med.* 2005;142(10):855–860.
16. Mosca L, Appel LJ, Benjamin EJ, et al. Evidence-based guidelines for cardiovascular disease prevention in women. *Circulation.* 2004;109:672–693.
17. North American Menopause Society. Recommendations for estrogen and progestogen use in peri- and postmenopausal

women: October 2004 position statement of the North American Menopause Society. *Menopause.* 2004;11:589–600.
18. Abramson BL. Postmenopausal hormone replacement therapy for primary prevention of cardiovascular and cerebrovascular disease: Recommendation statement from the Canadian Task Force on Preventive Health Care. *CMAJ.* 2004;170:1388–1389.
19. Streckfus CF, Baur U, Brown LJ, et al. Effects of estrogen status and aging on salivary flow rates in healthy Caucasian women. *Gerontology.* 1998;44:32–39.
20. Anusavice KJ. Dental caries: Risk assessment and treatment solutions for an elderly population. *Compend Contin Educ Dent.* 2002;23(10 Suppl):12–20.
21. Friedlander AH. The physiology, medical management and oral implications of menopause. *J Am Dent Assoc.* 2002;133(1):73–81.
22. Payne JB, Zachs NR, Reinhardt RA. The association between estrogen status and alveolar bone density changes in postmenopausal women with a history of periodontitis. *J Periodontol.* 1997;68:24–31.
23. August M, Chung K, Chang Y, et al. Influence of estrogen status on endosseous implant integration. *J Oral Maxillofac Surg.* 2001;59:1285–1289.
24. Pilgram TK, Hildebolt CF, Dotson M, et al. Relationships between clinical attachment level and spine and hip bone mineral density: Data from healthy postmenopausal women. *J Periodontol.* 2002;73:298–301.
25. Taguchi A, Tsuda M, Ohtsuka M, et al. Use of dental panoramic radiographs in identifying younger postmenopausal women with osteoporosis. *Osteoporos Int.* 2006;17(3):387–394.
26. Friedlander AH, Altman L. Carotid artery atheromas in postmenopausal women: Their prevalence on panoramic radiographs and their relationship to atherogenic risk factors. *J Am Dent Assoc.* 2001;132:1130–1136.
27. Beck JD, Couper DJ, Falkner KL, et al. The periodontitis and vascular events (PAVE) pilot study: adverse events. *J Periodontol.* 2008;79:90–96.
28. Khader YS, Albashaireh ZSM, Alomari MA. Periodontal diseases and the risk of coronary heart and cerebrovascular diseases: A meta-analysis. *J Periodontol.* 2004;75:1046–1053.
29. Woo SB, Hellstein JW, Kalmar JR. Systematic review: Bisphosphonates and osteonecrosis of the jaws. *Ann Intern Med.* 2006;144(10):753–761.
30. Barrett-Connor E, Mosca L, Collins P, et al. Raloxifene Use for The Heart (RUTH) trial investigators: Effects of raloxifene on cardiovascular events and breast cancer in postmenopausal women. *N Engl J Med.* 2006;355(2):125–137.

22

Cancer Chemotherapy

The dental hygienist is likely to treat patients who have been treated for various forms of malignancy or who are currently in treatment for cancer. These patients have unique problems that must be addressed. This chapter reviews the pathophysiology of malignancy and the action of chemotherapy to kill or suppress malignant cells. Treatment plan modifications for the disease or drug effects are explained. Oral complications of chemotherapy are reviewed, and recommendations for management of the complications are provided.

PATHOPHYSIOLOGY OF MALIGNANCY

Malignancy may be defined as uncontrolled tissue growth that results from an imbalance between cell division and programmed cell death **(apoptosis)**.[1] Malignant cells arise from normal cells that have undergone transformation related to specific genetic and epigenetic alterations in **oncogenes**, or tumor-suppressor genes. Oncogenes are normal genes that are involved in physiologic processes and whose excessive function (through **amplification**, or mutation) is associated with **carcinogenesis**. Tumor-suppressor genes, like oncogenes, are normal genes that have important functions in cell homeostasis and when suppressed produce changes associated with increased cell multiplication, or neoplasia. Another set of cancer-related genes is represented by genes that affect DNA-repairing enzymes and whose alterations are also associated with malignancy.[2] All three of these mechanisms affect the cell cycle regulatory proteins that govern the initiation, progression, and completion of cell cycle events. A major consequence is cellular abnormalities,

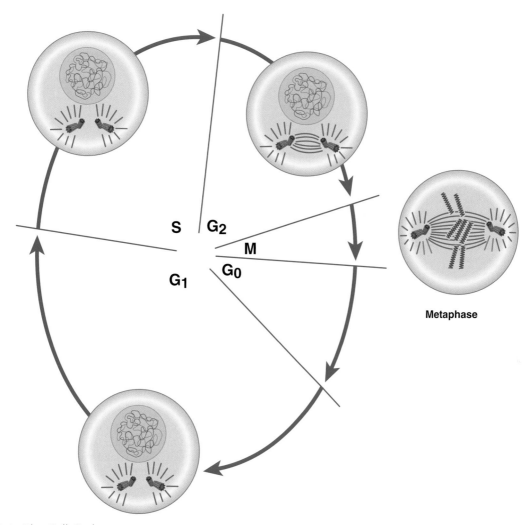

Figure 22-1 The Cell Cycle.

which provide malignant cells with a selective growth advantage.

The Cell Cycle

Understanding the cell cycle lays the foundation for understanding anticancer chemotherapy, because therapy is designed to act at various stages in the cell cycle.[3] The growth of transformed cells into a tumor requires proliferation. Malignant cells, like normal cells, are cycled through the same five physiologic phases: G_0, G_1, S, G_2, and M (Fig. 22-1).[4] The G_0 *phase* is a latent or resting phase during which the cells are preparing to be recruited into the reproductive cycle. The length of time cells spend in this phase is highly variable. Cells recruited from the G_0 phase enter the G_1, or the first active phase, of the reproductive cycle. In the G_1 phase, the cells synthesize ribonucleic acid (RNA), enzymes, and proteins in anticipation of entering subsequent phases of the reproductive cycle. The G_1 phase is followed by the S phase. The predominant event in the *S phase* is the synthesis of deoxyribonucleic acid (DNA). At the end of the S phase, the cells contain twice the original amount of DNA in antici-

pation of cell division. The S phase is followed by the G_2 *phase*, during which a highly specialized DNA that forms the mitotic spindle essential for cell division is created. In the *M (mitotic) phase*, cell division occurs. After creation of a new daughter cell, a cell may resume the cycle at G_1 or move into a resting state in G_0. Malignant cells do not proliferate in isolation. They secrete a variety of chemical mediators to induce the creation of a specialized local environment. Other cells may acquire the capability to move out of the local area, or **metastasize**, and invade tissues throughout the body.

PHARMACOLOGIC BASIS OF ANTICANCER CHEMOTHERAPY

Cell cycle phase-specific chemotherapeutic agents kill cells that are progressing through the active phases of the reproductive cell cycle. Cytotoxic agents kill malignant cells by different mechanisms of action (Fig. 22-2). They may (a) inhibit DNA synthesis and integrity, (b) damage DNA, or (c) inhibit

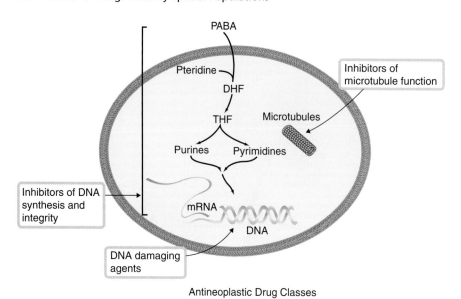

Antineoplastic Drug Classes

Figure 22-2 Mechanisms of Action of Anticancer Chemotherapeutic Agents.

microtubule function. As evident from these mechanisms of action, cytotoxic agents kill cells at different phases of the reproductive cycle, and they may be classified as being either cell cycle phase-specific or cell cycle phase-nonspecific.[3,5] Cell cycle *phase-specific* drugs kill cells which are actively participating in the reproductive cycle. Cell cycle *phase-nonspecific* agents do not depend on cells being in a specific phase and are effective throughout the reproductive cycle.

Pharmacodynamic Considerations

In malignant cells, apoptosis does not occur, and cells continue to grow. Cancer chemotherapy is designed to initiate apoptosis so cells will die.

Inhibitors of DNA Synthesis and Integrity

Table 22-1 illustrates the variety of anticancer agents developed to inhibit DNA synthesis. One can see that the agents inhibit natural mechanisms of cellular function at various stages. Methotrexate, 5-fluorouracil (5-FU), and doxorubicin are commonly used agents.

Analogs of endogenous folates, purines, and pyrimidines are **antimetabolites**. Once incorporated into DNA, the structural differences between these synthetic (or man-made) compounds and their natural counterparts cause a disruption of the structure of DNA, resulting in DNA chain termination, DNA strand breakage, and inhibition of cell growth. These changes initiate apoptosis. Topoisomerase inhibitors prevent DNA from uncoiling and/or "lock" the topoisomerase enzyme in a state that leaves the DNA strand broken. This disruption of DNA structure also initiates apoptosis.

DNA Damaging Agents

Agents that directly damage DNA inhibit development of the precise feature required to maintain a stable genome between generations (Table 22-2). These agents chemically target structural aspects of DNA and disrupt their three-dimensional structure. The disruption of DNA structure initiates apoptosis.

Inhibitors of Microtubule Function

Once a cell has replicated its DNA in the S phase of the cell cycle, it is ready to progress to the G_2 phase and then on to mitosis (M phase). Microtubules, which are critical components of the mitotic spindle, possess an inherent dynamic instability during mitosis and perform critical physiologic functions that culminate in cell division. They locate and attach to the chromosomes, enhance alignment of chromosomes at the equator of the cell, and, finally, separate the diploid pair of chromosomes into each half of the cell. Ultimately, cytokinesis (division of the cytoplasm) occurs, and two daughter cells are formed. In performing their complex

Table 22-1	Chemotherapy Inhibitors of DNA Synthesis
Dihydrofolate reductase inhibitors	Methotrexate
Thymidylate synthase inhibitors	5-Fluorouracil
Inhibitors of purine metabolism	6-Mercaptopurine Pentostatin
Ribonucleotide reductase inhibitors	Hydroxyurea
Purine and pyrimidine analogs	Cladribine Cytarabine Fludarabine Thioguanine

Topoisomerase inhibitors	Amsacrine
	Anthracyclines
	    Daunorubicin
	    Doxorubicin
	    Epirubicin
	Camptothecins
	    Irinotecan
	    Topotecan
	Epipodophyllotoxins
	    Etoposide
	    Teniposide

Table 22-2 Chemotherapeutic Agents That Damage DNA

Agents that directly modify DNA structure	Alkylating agents
	Chlorambucil
	Cyclophosphamide
	Estramustine
	Mechlorethamine
	Melphalan
	Carmustine
	Altretamine
	Lomustine
	Busulfan
	Platinum compounds
	Carboplatin
	Cisplatin
	Oxaliplatin
	Bleomycin

Table 22-3 Inhibitors of Microtubule Function

Agents that inhibit microtubule polymerization	Vinca alkaloids
	Vinblastine
	Vincristine
Agents that inhibit microtubular depolymerization	Taxanes
	Docetaxel
	Paclitaxel

functions, microtubules grow and/or shrink lengthwise. Disruption of microtubule function freezes cells in the M phase, leading eventually to the activation of apoptosis. Table 22-3 lists agents that act by inhibiting microtubule function.

Hormonal Anticancer Drugs

Hormones change the intracellular environment of hormone-dependent cancer cells. They may act either as agonists that activate receptors and inhibit tumor cell growth, or they may act as antagonists that compete with endogenous growth-promoting hormones. Table 22-4 includes various hormones used for cancer chemotherapy. Hormonal therapy may be additive or **ablative** (interfering with cellular functions essential for survival), and, while it influences the course of some cancers, hormonal therapy is primarily palliative and not curative.

Newer Anticancer Agents

Some of the newer anticancer drugs affect signaling mechanisms that drive the cell cycle and act as agonists at receptors to inhibit tumor growth, or they act as antagonists and block growth-promoting endogenous ligands from binding with their receptors.[6] Other therapies for cancer target molecular abnormalities and represent a more specific and less toxic treatment method. These new therapies signal a paradigm shift in the treatment of malignancies. Currently, receptor tyrosine kinases (RTKs), nonreceptor kinases, angiogenic molecules, enzymes involved in extracellular matrix degradation, and enzymes responsible for protein anchorage to cytoplasmic membrane are among the targets against which specific interventions have been developed. Emerging molecular therapies also include targeted gene therapy, which involves the use of nucleic-acid-based molecules. Targeting is achieved through genetically engineered viruses, receptor-ligand interactions, and antibodies. An ingenious antitumor strategy is to deliver the herpes simplex thymidine kinase (HS-TK) gene that selectively metabolizes the antiviral agent ganciclovir to produce a toxic metabolite. This kills the cell expressing the gene. In the management of some malignancies, monoclonal antibodies against the extracellular portion of the RTKs and small-molecule inhibitors of tyrosine kinase activity show promise. An example of this is the use of trastuzumab (Herceptin), a recombinant DNA-derived humanized monoclonal antibody that binds to the herceptin receptor and inhibits the proliferation of some human tumor cells (breast cancer). However, to date, results with gene therapy remain inconclusive.

■ Self-Study Review

1. Describe the genetic influences on carcinogenesis, and define *apoptosis*.

Table 22-4 Hormones Used for Cancer Chemotherapy

Drug Class	Drugs	Mechanisms of Action
Glucocorticosteroids	Prednisone	Cortisol receptor agonists, which inhibit DNA and protein synthesis and interfere with mitosis
Estrogens	Diethylstilbestrol	Estrogen receptor agonist, which overcomes endogenous testosterone
Progestins	Megestrol acetate	Progesterone receptor agonist, which produces an antiluteinizing effect mediated via the pituitary, inhibiting estrogen action
Androgens	Fluoxymesterone	Testosterone receptor agonist, which stimulates RNA polymerase activity, resulting in an increase in protein production
Steroid blockade	Aminoglutethimide	Blocks the enzymatic conversion of cholesterol to delta-5-pregnenolone, which reduces the synthesis of all steroid hormones
Antiandrogens	Flutamide	Inhibits the binding of androgens to receptors in target tissues
Antiestrogens	Tamoxifen	Competitively binds to estrogen receptors in target tissues, produces a nuclear complex that decreases DNA synthesis, and accumulates in the G_0 and G_1 phases
GNRH analog	Leuprolide	Inhibits the secretion of LH and FSH with subsequent decrease in estrogen (females) and testosterone (males) levels

2. What is the role that the cell cycle plays in cancer chemotherapy?
3. Examine Tables 22-1, 22-2, 22-3, and 22-4. Name some of the specific drugs included.
4. Discuss the targeted therapy of newer agents, the use of the herpes gene, and monoclonal antibodies.

Adverse Drug Effects

Cancer chemotherapeutic agents are not selectively tumoricidal. They tend to produce more extensive injury to cancer cells, but they damage normal cells as well. Some side effects may be emotionally and physically distressing, but they are generally not considered dangerous. In contrast, other side effects may be potentially life threatening, and the oncology health care team must focus on monitoring and minimizing these toxicities. In general, most ADEs associated with cancer chemotherapeutic agents are caused by either direct toxic effects on a specific organ or by damage to rapidly dividing normal cell populations (Table 22-5). For example, **alopecia**, or loss of hair, occurs as the hair follicle is damaged and the hair strand is lost. The degree and type of tox-

Table 22-5 ADEs of Cancer Chemotherapeutic Agents

Suppression of bone marrow
Leukopenia
Thrombocytopenia
Anemia
Enhanced susceptibility to infection
Increased incidence of a second malignancy

Gastrointestinal disturbances
Nausea
Vomiting
Diarrhea
Mucositis

Cutaneous manifestations
Erythema
Maculopapular eruptions
Exfoliative dermatitis
Stevens-Johnson syndrome
Alopecia
Hyperpigmentation
Photosensitivity

Cardiotoxicity
Irreversible cardiomyopathy

Pulmonary toxicity

Hepatotoxicity

Renal toxicity

Neurotoxic effects
Pain
Peripheral neuropathies
Convulsions

Inhibition of spermatogenesis, oogenesis, and menstrual cycle

Oral manifestations
Mucositis
Infections (bacterial viral, fungal)
Hemorrhage
Xerostomia
Neurologic complications
Inadequate nutrition

icity depends on the specific agent, dosage, schedule, route of administration, and patient-related predisposing factors.

Oral Manifestations of Adverse Drug Reactions

Mucositis

Mucositis is the most common oral complication, occurring in approximately 40% of patients undergoing standard dose chemotherapy.[7] It is characterized as large ulcerative lesions on the oral epithelium, including the tongue and pharynx, and is very painful (Color Plate 3). With the increasing use of dose-intensified regimens or concomitant chemoradiotherapy regimens, such as may be used for the myeloablative conditioning required for hematopoietic stem cell transplantation (HSCT), the incidence of mucositis approaches 80% to 90%. Consequently, mucositis is recognized as a serious potential dose-limiting toxicity. Of the more than 95 drugs used for the treatment of cancer, fully one third may induce oral toxicity.[5] The drugs most frequently associated with mucositis include bleomycin, doxorubicin, epirubicin, cisplatin, vinblastine, fluorouracil, interferon, methotrexate, and the taxanes. A major concern is that chemotherapy-related mucositis, in addition to being very painful, renders the patient susceptible to systemic infection by odontopathic, periodontopathic, and transient oral microorganisms. In addition to the specific chemotherapeutic agent or agents used, numerous patient-related variables (e.g., age, nutritional status, existing oral flora, oral health status, oral hygiene performance, salivary function, and underlying immunologic status) contribute to the occurrence and severity of mucositis.[8]

Depending on the chemotherapeutic regimen used and other factors discussed above, mucositis develops in about 5 to 10 days following chemotherapy administration. It may progress from erythema to frank ulceration. A "pseudomembrane" consisting of inflammatory cell infiltrates, interstitial exudates, fibrin, and cellular debris is frequently observed. When hydrated by saliva, the lesion appears white or opalescent and may eventually slough, exposing painful ulcerations. These painful ulcerative lesions are noted primarily on nonkeratinized tissues, such as the buccal and labial mucosa (Color Plate 3), the ventrolateral surface of the tongue, and the floor of the mouth. The hard palate, attached gingiva, and dorsal surface of the tongue rarely develop mucositis. Resolution occurs in over 90% of cases within 2 to 3 weeks following cessation of chemotherapy and correlates directly with normalization of the white blood cell count.[8,9]

Fungal Infections

Systemic fungal infections are among the most feared complications of myelosuppressive therapy, and their incidence is rising. *Candida albicans* continues to be the most frequently implicated pathogen, but its incidence is dropping, while the incidence of infection caused by *Aspergillus* species, *C. krusei*, *C. tropicalis*, *C. parapsilosis*, *C. glabrata*, and species of *Mucormycosis* and *Rhizopus* are on the rise. The majority of cases of systemic candidiasis are believed to originate from the oral cavity.[10] Once the organism becomes pathogenic, *C. albicans* may spread to the esophagus or lungs during swallowing or droplet aspiration. Transmission to distant sites is through the hematologic route (bacteremia). The occurrence of noncandidal fungal infections affecting the oral cavity in the immunosuppressed patient is on the rise, and the oral manifestations of such infections may mimic other oral toxicities, making microbiologic determination essential.

Herpes Simplex Virus Infections

As a consequence of their ability to establish long-term latency after primary infection, DNA viruses represent the most frequent cause of viral infection to afflict the immunosuppressed patient. The most relevant of this group are the herpes simplex virus (HSV), the varicella zoster virus (VZV), and the cytomegalovirus (CMV). Clinical images of these infections are shown in Color Plates 18, 19, and 20. Primary HSV infections appear to account for <2% of infections in these patients. The incidence of HSV infection in an unknown mix of seronegative and seropositive patients was reported to be 48%.[11] Data indicate that the optimal period of observation for the detection of recurrent HSV infections is during the 7- to 14-day period following the administration of chemotherapy. The extent and severity of the clinical manifestations of recurrent HSV infection are directly related to the degree of immunosuppression.[12] The lesions of recurrent herpes labialis are quite painful, often demonstrating more extensive clinical involvement than the typical manifestation of vesicles (Color Plate 18), and intraoral recurrent herpes may act to worsen mucositis.

Varicella Zoster Virus Infections

Like HSV, VZV manifests both a primary (chicken pox) and recurrent (shingles) form. Most adults, having experienced their primary disease in childhood, are at risk of recurrence due to immunosuppressive therapy. For reasons not clearly understood, recurrent VZV usually occurs several weeks after the cessation of chemotherapy. Head and neck zoster infection results in painful, unilateral vesicular lesions, which typically follow the distribution of a branch of the trigeminal nerve (Color Plate 19). Intraoral lesions on the palate typically stop at the midline rugae (Color Plate 20). However, severe immunosuppression predisposes to a more widespread atypical distribution pattern. The lesions coalesce into large ulcerations and may linger for weeks before remission occurs.

Hemorrhage

Chemotherapeutic agents may secondarily reduce platelet formation, inducing *thrombocytopenia*, which is the usual cause of intraoral hemorrhage (Color Plate 14). Hemorrhage may occur anywhere in the mouth and may be spontaneous or precipitated by trauma or existing disease. Hemorrhages may present clinically as gingival bleeding or submucosal bleeding with hematoma formation. Profound thrombocytopenia (<20,000 mm³) underlies most of these changes.

Xerostomia

The presence of xerostomia during chemotherapy contributes to the patient's discomfort and risk of infection (Color

Plate 2). Note the dry, shiny texture of the mucosa. Although only a small number of cancer chemotherapeutic agents (i.e., 5-fluorouracil and methotrexate) appear to directly cause xerostomia, dryness of the mucosa can be devastating when it occurs in conjunction with mucositis.[13] Altered salivary flow and salivary histatin levels may be important predisposing factors to oral candidiasis and reduced salivary amylase, and IgA levels may be associated with an increased incidence of oral infections with opportunistic bacterial pathogens. Somewhat paradoxically, there is concern that salivary secretion of toxic agents contributes to the development of mucositis.[13] Chemotherapy-induced mucositis may significantly impair the patient's ability to eat and swallow, leading to significant nutritional problems. The concurrent presence of dry mouth and altered or reduced taste sensation adds to the client's sense of misery.

Neurologic Complications of Pain and Neuropathy

Oral pain may result from mucositis, xerostomia, and infection. Anxiety caused by the diagnosis of cancer may precipitate bruxism and result in temporomandibular joint discomfort. Pain may be associated with acute exacerbations of periodontal disease, root surface sensitivity, or root caries. The sloughing and atrophy of the oral mucosa that occurs because of mucositis cause considerable discomfort. Infections such as pericoronitis or a periodontal or apical abscess can precipitate an acutely painful condition.

Chemotherapy-induced neuropathy (characterized as pain or paresthesia) most often develops after the administration of plant alkaloids (vinblastine, vincristine, etoposide). However, other agents capable of causing neuropathy are altretamine, carboplatin, cisplatin, cladribine, docetaxel, oxaliplatin, paclitaxel, procarbazine, and thalidomide. Often the clinical and radiographic examinations in these cases are unremarkable in that there is no evidence of pain or disease, and the symptoms of neurologic complications may disappear after the chemotherapeutic agent is discontinued.

■ Self-Study Review

5. Examine ADEs in Table 22-5. Which ones are relevant to dental hygiene care?
6. Identify medical issues related to *mucositis*.
7. Describe the oral manifestations of ADEs from chemotherapy.

Complications of Chemotherapy

Oral complications of cancer chemotherapy include mucositis, infection, hemorrhage, xerostomia, neurologic disorders, and nutritional deficiencies. A low neutrophil count is a common ADE of cancer chemotherapy. *Neutrophils* are essential for phagocytosis of bacteria and for the stimulation of the immune system. Filgrastim (Neupogen) and pegfilgrastim (Neulasta) are neutrophil-specific colony-stimulating factors (CSF) administered to patients with neutropenia to combat infection. These drugs enhance the microbicidal activity of neutrophils and mobilize stem cells from the bone marrow into the peripheral circulation. ADEs associated with these drugs include nausea and vomiting, acute respiratory distress syndrome, and splenic rupture.

Recently osteonecrosis of the jaw has been reported with intravenously (IV) administered bisphosphonates that are used to reduce pain and loss of bone from malignant cell proliferation. Bisphosphonate administration by IV is a standard of care when malignancy affects the skeleton. A potential oral ADE of osteonecrosis of the jaw is discussed in Chapter 14. The severity of these conditions may be affected by patient- and therapy-related variables. One of the more important patient-related variables is the patient's oral health status during chemotherapy. Therapy-related variables include the type of agent(s) used and the dosage and frequency of drug administration. It is of paramount importance for clinicians to recognize and anticipate the conditions that predispose patients to complications and include this information in the oral health education program. When oral health is neglected, the oral complications resulting from chemotherapy are more severe and may compromise the treatment and prognosis of the patient.

Management of Oral Complications from Chemotherapy

It has been reported that as many as 40% of patients with cancer may experience acute or chronic oral complications in association with chemotherapy that can adversely affect the oral mucosa, periodontium, pulpal tissues, and salivary glands. The cumulative effects of the oral toxicities described above may be so severe as to require a modification or cessation of the cancer therapy, thus negatively impacting survival. Oral health care providers should, therefore, be an integral part of the multidisciplinary care of cancer chemotherapy patients. When these patients are treated in the oral health care setting, the goals are to develop and implement timely (both short- and long-term), preventive, therapeutic, and palliative/supportive strategies compatible with the patient's physical and emotional ability and desire to receive dental care (Box 22-1).

Preventive Strategies Prior to Chemotherapy

Although acute exacerbations of pre-existing chronic periodontal diseases and acute periapical infections secondary to pulpal necrosis during cancer chemotherapy are rare, odontopathic and periodontopathic organisms have been associated with bacteremia and constitutional symptoms (such as malaise, fever, lymphadenopathy). Consequently, all patients with cancer who receive chemotherapy should have a thorough oral examination, which should include a clinical and radiographic evaluation. Even if therapy has to commence immediately or has already commenced, this examination provides a basis for future comparison and assists in the monitoring and treatment of oral complications. At the least, the patient should be instructed on proper oral hygiene procedures and the importance of avoiding alcohol, tobacco, and caffeine. Some patients become highly motivated to improve their oral health care and minimize oral complications when the importance of this regimen is stressed. Ultimately, however, it is impossible to predict how a given patient will respond to chemotherapy, and close follow-up is mandatory.

Dental Management

If time permits prior to chemotherapy, measures to eradicate potential sources of oral infection should be performed. All patients should receive an oral prophylaxis. Any teeth that are nonrestorable or have severe periodontal involvement should be removed. If an odontogenic abscess is present, the tooth should either be extracted or undergo endodontic therapy. Ideally, all surgical procedures should be completed at least 10 days prior to the onset of neutropenia. Additional therapy should include the restoration of carious teeth, replacement of faulty restorations, smoothing of rough enamel or restored surfaces, and elimination of ill-fitting prostheses. Orthodontic bands should be removed, and the wearing of removable prostheses should be minimized.

Antibiotic Prophylaxis

In all cases, consultation with the managing oncologist is warranted to determine the patient's ability to undergo the anticipated dental therapy. For example, antimicrobial prophylaxis is not recommended for patients with a neutrophil count >2,000/mm^3, while some form of prophylaxis is recommended for counts <2,000/mm^3.[14] The specific antimicrobial regimen should be determined in close consultation with the managing physician, and culturing is recommended when feasible. The drugs included in the American Heart Association regimen of **chemoprophylaxis** are often insufficient to adequately protect the neutropenic patient, and a more aggressive regimen is generally necessary, based on microbiologic culture and sensitivity data.

Mucositis

To date, there are no universally proven and accepted protocols for the prevention and management of mucositis. Universally agreed-upon measures described below are primarily empirical and aimed at improving patient comfort and minimizing infectious complications.

Topical Agents
Palliative care to reduce symptoms includes topical anesthetic agents, such as lidocaine viscous, dyclonine, or diphenhydramine hydrochloride syrup, and a systemic analgesic may be prescribed if necessary. Topical agents are often combined with a coating agent, such as kaolin with pectin (Kaopectate), magnesium hydroxide and/or aluminum hydroxide (Milk of Magnesia, Mylanta, others), in a compounded product referred to as "Miracle Mix." A mucosal covering agent (Rincinol) has been used with some success. However, no comparative studies exist that validate the value of topical anesthetic formulations in treating mucositis. When topical anesthetics are used, the patient should be warned that these agents may initially burn upon application, increase the risk of self-induced trauma, affect taste, and interfere with the pharyngeal phase of swallowing leading to aspiration by depressing the gag reflex. COX-1 inhibitors are contraindicated in patients at risk for hemorrhage, leaving

---

BOX 22-1. Management of Oral Complications of Chemotherapy

Preventive Recommendations

- Prior to the initiation of chemotherapy, all dental and periodontal needs should be treated and resolved. Surgical procedures should precede the onset of neutropenia by 10 days.
- Orthodontic bands should be removed, and wearing of removable prostheses should be minimized.
- Advise the client that neglect of oral health can increase the risk for oral complications during chemotherapy; instruct the patient regarding effective oral hygiene and to avoid alcohol, tobacco, and caffeine to avoid exacerbation of oral complications.

Management Recommendations

- Mucositis: Empirical treatment should be aimed at improving comfort and minimizing the risk for infection. Agents to consider are lidocaine viscous topical anesthetic preparation; diphenhydramine hydrochloride syrup; barrier rinses, such as Miracle Mix, that must be prepared by compounding. Advise that products may burn on application, increase the risk for self-induced trauma, adversely affect taste, interfere with swallowing, and promote gagging. Acetaminophen or opioid analgesics are appropriate. Spicy foods and hard foods should be avoided, and a soft diet is often recommended.
- Infection: When oral complications develop during chemotherapy that require invasive dental treatment (tooth removal, periodontal débridement, and so forth), determine the patient's current neutrophil count from the oncology treatment center. Antibiotic prophylaxis should be considered for neutrophil counts $<2,000/mm^3$. For oral infection, culture and sensitivity tests should be completed prior to determining antimicrobial therapy.
- Hemorrhage: Prevent hemorrhage by repairing sharp restorations, fractured teeth, and so forth. When platelet count is $<20,000/mm^3$, conventional toothbrushing may prove too traumatic. Oral cleansing should be performed every 2 to 4 hours for maximal benefit, but gingival hemorrhage may occur. Advise the patient to use a sponge Toothette device, piece of gauze, or cotton swab soaked in antimicrobial agent (0.12% nonalcoholic chlorhexidine). The oral mucosa should be kept moistened with saline rinses to avoid hemorrhagic complications. Use a nontraumatic flossing technique. Apply pressure to initiate clotting, or use hemostatic agents (absorbable gelatin sponge, aminocaproic acid or tranexamic acid mouth rinses).
- Xerostomia: Advise frequent sipping of water or the use of artificial saliva products. Xylitol gum can be recommended to stimulate salivation. If local measures are insufficient and salivary function is possible, the use of a sialogogue (cevimeline or pilocarpine) oral tablet may be useful.
- Neurologic disorders, pain: Infection should be ruled out or treated. If clenching is practiced, use of an occlusal appliance during sleep may be useful. Opioid analgesics or acetaminophen are often recommended.
- Oral hygiene instruction: Advise use of a nonirritating mouthwash for safe removal of debris, and avoid products containing alcohol, astringents, oils, and antiseptics. Saline mouth rinses with sodium bicarbonate (1/2 tsp each of salt and baking soda in 16 oz water) or saline rinse (1/2 tsp with 8 oz water) are commonly prescribed.
- Osteonecrosis of the jaw: See Chapter 14 for management issues.

---

acetaminophen and opioid-receptor agonists in combination with acetaminophen as the most appropriate systemic analgesics.

Oral Hygiene Instruction

Central to any approach to oral care is the frequent and liberal use of a nonirritating mouthwash for the safe removal of debris. Products containing alcohol, astringents, oils, and antiseptics should be avoided whenever possible. Both saline and sodium bicarbonate (1/2 tsp each of salt and baking soda in 16 oz of water) are commonly prescribed.[15] Sodium bicarbonate reduces oral fluid acidity, dilutes accumulating mucus, and discourages yeast colonization. However, some critics recommend against its use, noting that sodium bicarbonate has an unpleasant taste and contributes to bacterial growth.[16]

This viewpoint leaves saline (1/2 tsp sodium chloride and 8 oz water) as the most neutral and least damaging mouthwash. Patients are further instructed to carefully remove dental plaque, to avoid products irritating to oral soft tissues (such as alcohol and tobacco; hot, spicy, and coarse foods; or fruits and beverages with a high acid content), to refrain from wearing removable prostheses, and to eat a soft diet. Removable prostheses may serve as a source of irritation and bacterial contamination, so they must scrupulously be cleaned or not worn at all. Oral cleansing should be performed frequently (every 2 to 4 hours) in order to maximize benefit. During this time, an appropriate oral hygiene protocol might include a modified mechanical approach consisting of cleaning with a disposable sponge (Toothette device), piece of gauze, or cotton swab soaked in a topical antimicrobial agent (nonalcoholic chlorhexidine 0.12% rinse).

Bacterial Infections

To minimize the potential for acute exacerbation of pre-existing chronic periodontal conditions, a regimen of plaque control consisting of scrupulous oral hygiene should be instituted. There are no universally proven and accepted protocols pertaining to oral hygiene during chemotherapy, and any prescribed regimen must take into account the patient's blood counts, presence of oral ulcerations, and manual dexterity.[17] Acute odontogenic infections may arise during this period, necessitating management. In all cases, consultation with the managing physician is warranted to determine the patient's ability to undergo the anticipated dental therapy.

Fungal Infection

As a consequence of the increased morbidity and mortality associated with fungal septicemia and the difficulty with its diagnosis, evidence of superficial fungal infection in the oropharynx mandates prompt and aggressive therapeutic interventions. Unfortunately, there are few validated recommendations to prevent systemic fungal infection in the myelosuppressed patient, and empirical systemic antifungal therapy remains the standard of care for the febrile chemotherapy patient who does not respond to standard antibacterial therapy. The commonly recommended use of nystatin as a prophylactic or therapeutic agent for oropharyngeal candidiasis in the myelosuppressed patient has not been validated in clinical trials and is no longer encouraged.[8] Fluconazole, in part due to its excellent safety profile and predictable gut absorption, has emerged as the most frequently recommended prophylactic agent to prevent oropharyngeal candidiasis and fungemia in myelosuppressed patients. Parenteral amphotericin B remains the drug of last resort for nonresponsive fungal infections.

Viral Infection

Because of increased susceptibility to HSV, VZV, and CMV infection, and the high incidence of atypical presentations, some investigators recommend prophylactic antiviral agents in the management of severely myelosuppressed patients with evidence of prior viral exposure.[8,18] In the management of patients with milder immunosuppression, oral acyclovir, valacyclovir, or famciclovir may be considered. For resistant cases of HSV or VZV, foscarnet remains the drug of choice. Ganciclovir or foscarnet are the drugs of choice for the pre-emptive treatment and/or treatment of CMV.

Increased Bleeding and Hemorrhage

Prevention is the most effective technique used to avoid hemorrhage. Eliminating potential areas of trauma (sharp restorations, fractured teeth) and pre-existing intraoral disease before chemotherapy minimizes the risk of hemorrhage. When the platelet count is sufficiently low (e.g., <20,000/mm^3), conventional toothbrushing may prove too traumatic. For such cases, swabbing with a sponge soaked in nonalcoholic 0.12% chlorhexidine as described above may be useful. The oral mucosa should be kept moist with saline rinses to avoid friction that may exacerbate a hemorrhagic complication. It has been recommended that conventional toothbrushing two to three times per day and daily flossing be continued during chemotherapy, because the increased risk of infection associated with inadequate oral hygiene may outweigh the theoretical risk of increased bleeding.[8] Accumulated blood should be removed to identify the bleeding site, and then pressure should be applied with moist gauze, periodontal packing, or a mucosal guard. Topical antihemorrhagic agents, such as absorbable gelatin sponges, oxidized cellulose, aminocaproic acid, thrombin, and tranexamic acid, may be applied.[18]

Xerostomia

Dry mouth associated with chemotherapy is usually short lived, returning to normal within a couple months of the cessation of therapy. Patients whose salivary glands can respond to stimulation may benefit from using simple dietary measures, such as frequently sipping water, rinsing frequently with a mouth rinse as described above for mucositis, and chewing sugarless or xylitol-containing gum. Fruit juices and hard, spicy foods should be avoided, and food and drinks should be served cold or tepid. A variety of non-alcohol-containing, non-irritating over-the-counter saliva substitutes, moisturizers, and stimulants are available, but research demonstrating a tangible benefit in their use is lacking. Most currently available saliva substitutes are based upon carboxymethylcellulose, and, while they do provide viscosity, they are a poor substitute for saliva (though one cottonseed oil product [Numoisyn] is reported to be acceptable and closely replicates the feel of saliva). As a consequence, many patients prefer to frequently sip water and not use a saliva substitute. There are few products available for use. For this reason, brand names will be included in the chapter to identify specific products. The use of Biotene oral products (toothpaste, chewing gum, mouthwash) and the oral lubricant Oralbalance may be beneficial and acceptable for some patients. Biotene contains lactoperoxidase, lysozyme, and glucose oxidase. Oralbalance is a hydroxypropyl-methylcellulose-based saliva substitute. Used together, Biotene and Oralbalance are purported to more closely mimic the physiologic actions and texture of saliva than other available agents. If local measures are insufficient, the use of the parasympathomimetic pilocarpine (Salagen) may prove useful. It appears to be effective in patients with residual salivary gland function; however, patients with no salivary reserve require saliva substitutes, such as Numoisyn, Salivart, or Moi-Stir. An oral doseform sialagogue is cevimeline (Evoxac). While this muscarinic agonist is currently only approved for Sjögren-syndrome-induced xerostomia, its use for chemotherapy-induced xerostomia may prove beneficial.

Pain and Neuropathy

A thorough dental examination should be performed to rule out an infectious source of pain, especially when the chemotherapy regimen is capable of inducing neuropathy. Any evidence of infection must be addressed as described above. Pain associated with clenching or bruxism may be eliminated by calling it to the attention of the patient and by the use of an occlusal appliance (bite guard). Patients with mild-to-moderate pain should be treated with a nonopioid analgesic. Patients who present with moderate-to-severe pain or who fail to achieve adequate relief after a trial of a nonopioid analgesic should be treated with a nonopioid in combination with codeine, oxycodone, hydrocodone, or dihydrocodeine.

Nutritional Problems

Measures to control anorexia, nausea, vomiting, and mucositis are important to allow the patient to eat and drink comfortably. Encourage patients to eat frequent, small meals; avoid hot, spicy, acidic, and irritating foods; increase calories and dietary protein; and use nutritional supplements.

■ Self-Study Review

8. Explain the necessity of maintaining oral health during chemotherapy.
9. Describe preventive strategies prior to chemotherapy.
10. Describe dental management of oral complications from chemotherapy.
11. Describe palliative management for mucositis.
12. What products can be recommended in the oral hygiene program?
13. How is pharyngeal candidiasis managed?
14. Describe how to choose the most appropriate tooth-cleaning devices or material when gingival tissues bleed easily.
15. What therapy is recommended for chronic xerostomia?
16. List two oral doseform products used to stimulate salivation.

DENTAL HYGIENE APPLICATIONS

When the patient seeks palliative care for the oral complications of chemotherapy, the dental hygienist may be involved in educating the patient about using the products to resolve the pain and disability involved with the complications. Occasionally, family members will seek information for the patient related to effective products to reduce oral complications. Knowledge of various management procedures and products will allow the dental hygienist to make helpful recommendations. When a patient undergoing cancer chemotherapy presents for dental hygiene treatment, the dental hygienist should question the patient regarding possible oral complications and relay the information to the dentist. Prescriptions would be prepared by the dentist, and the hygienist may be the team member to educate the patient on use of the products. Box 22-1 summarizes management recommendations for oral complications associated with cancer chemotherapy.

CONCLUSION

Oral health professionals must understand the causes of cancer, methods of prevention, management principles, and complications of cancer chemotherapy. They must recognize that patients with cancer require multidisciplinary treatment and coordination of care. The oncologist who manages the patient's care must involve the oral health care provider *before* the initiation of chemotherapy. The oral health care provider must recognize that cancer chemotherapeutic agents are not selective for malignant cells and may produce ADEs. Some side effects may be emotionally and physically distressing to the cancer patient, but they are generally not considered dangerous; in contrast, other side effects may be potentially life threatening, and the health care team must focus on monitoring and minimizing these toxicities. Oral health care providers have the obligation to deliver quality care, in a competent manner before, during, and after cancer chemotherapy.

References

1. Ponder BA. Cancer genetics. *Nature.* 2001;411:336–341.
2. Hoeijmakers JH. Genome maintenance for preventing cancer. *Nature.* 2001;100:57–70.
3. Shapiro GI, Harper JW. Anticancer drug targets: Cell cycle and checkpoint control. *J Clin Invest.* 1999;104(12):1645–1653.
4. Ingwersen KC. Cell cycle kinetics and antineoplastic agents. In: Barton-Burke M, Wilkes G, Ingwersen KC, et al., eds. *Cancer Chemotherapy: A Nursing Process Approach.* 2nd ed. Sudbury, MA: Jones and Bartlett Publishers; 1996:22–42.
5. Abramowicz M., ed. Drugs of choice for cancer. *Treat Guidel Med Lett.* 2003;1(7):41–52.
6. Gibbs JB. Anticancer drug targets: Growth factors and growth factor signaling. *J Clin Invest.* 2000;105(1):9–13.
7. Biron P, Sebban C, Gourmet R, et al. Research controversies in management of oral mucositis. *Support Care Cancer.* 2000; 8:68–71.
8. Epstein JB, Klassen GD. Emerging approaches for prophylaxis and management of oropharyngeal mucositis in cancer therapy. *Exp Opin Emer Drugs.* 2006;11:353–373.
9. Sonis ST. Mucositis as biological process: A new hypothesis for the development of chemotherapy-induced stomatotoxicity. *Oral Oncol.* 1998;34:39–43.
10. National Institutes of Health Consensus Development Panel (1990). Consensus statement: Oral complications of cancer

CLINICAL APPLICATION EXERCISES

☐ **Exercise 1.** Go to a pharmacy and locate products to reduce oral pain. Try to find the Biotene products. Be familiar with the product formulations (gel, mouth rinse, paste) and the instructions for use. This will allow you to provide helpful information should a cancer patient seek your help for oral complications of chemotherapy.

☐ **Exercise 2.** Interview a compounding pharmacist in your area to learn about compounding a coating mouth rinse (often called "Miracle Mix" or "Miracle Mouthrinse") for mucositis. Inquire about the ingredients in the local formulation. In some areas, liquid tetracycline is added to provide an antibacterial effect. Ask the pharmacist for the rationale to support the particular formulation made—for example, "Why is Kaopectate selected over Milk of Magnesia? What liquid antihistamine is used? Is there any possibility for binding the tetracycline molecule with the coating product, rendering it unable to provide a topical antibacterial effect?"

☐ **Exercise 3.** A client presents for oral care with a chief complaint of painful ulcerations associated with recent chemotherapy for breast cancer. She wants to know if there are any products she can use to manage the pain. She reports her oncologist suggested a fluoride gel to use, but it burns her mouth and she is unable to use it. She says her gums bleed when she brushes although she is using a soft toothbrush. She has dry mouth and feels that adds to the burning and pain in her mouth. What will your recommendation be for oral products? Provide rationale for each product.

☐ **Exercise 4.** WEB ACTIVITY: Log on to the Oral Cancer Foundation Web site and read information related to xerostomia suffered by cancer chemotherapy patients (www.oralcancerfoundation.org/dental/xerostomia.htm). This information may be useful to print and supply to patients with xerostomia from chemotherapy.

therapies: Diagnosis, prevention, and treatment. *NCI Monogr.* 9 (whole issue).

11. Montgomery MT, Redding SW, LeMaistre CF. The incidence of oral herpes simplex virus infection in patients undergoing cancer chemotherapy. *Oral Surg Oral Med Oral Pathol.* 1986;61:238–242.

12. National Cancer Institute. Oral complications of chemotherapy and head/neck radiation: Health professional version. 2008: March 13. Available at: http://www.cancer.gov/cancertopics/pdq/supportivecare/oralcomplications/HealthProfessional. Accessed May 30, 2008.

13. Epstein JB, Tsang AHF, Warkentin D, et al. The role of salivary function in modulating chemotherapy-induced oropharyngeal mucositis: A review of the literature. *Oral Surg Oral Med Oral Pathol Oral Radiol Endod.* 2002;94:39–44.

14. Rotea W Jr, Saad ED. Targeted drugs in oncology: New names, new mechanisms, new paradigm. *Am J Health Syst Pharm.* 2003;60(12):1233–1245.

15. Rogers BB. Mucositis in the oncology patient. *Nurs Clin North Am.* 2001;36:745–760.

16. Miller M, Kearney N. Oral care for patients with cancer: A review of the literature. *Cancer Nurs.* 2001;24:241–254.

17. Heimdahl A. Prevention and management of oral infections in cancer patients. *Support Care Cancer.* 1999;7:224–228.

18. Dunn CJ, Goa KL. Tranexamic acid: A review of its use in surgery and other indications. *Drugs.* 1999;57:1005–1032.

23

Substance Abuse

In 2003, an estimated 21.6 million Americans age 12 or older were classified as having substance **dependence** or **addiction**. Oral health care professionals will likely be presented with a patient under the influence of abused substances, some illegal (such as cocaine, methamphetamine [METH], and others) and some legal (such as alcohol or tobacco). In addition to identifying potential drug interacting substances, management issues relevant to dental hygiene practice include offering tobacco cessation information and dealing with the erratic behavior of a client who presents to the dental hygiene appointment while under the influence of illegal drugs or alcohol. In addition, personnel in the dental office may become substance abusers. This presents the practitioner with a dilemma about confronting a staff member regarding suspicions of **drug abuse** and assisting in getting the impaired health care worker to seek treatment. Therefore, the dental hygienist must become aware of drugs of abuse, signs of drug abuse, and dental professional groups that assist in getting individuals into treatment programs.

SUBSTANCE OR DRUG ABUSE

Dentists must be aware of "drug shoppers" who may call the dental office with a complaint of "pain" and request a prescription for a narcotic analgesic. The current health history developed by the American Dental Association includes questions about substance abuse, because some of these drugs interact with drugs used in the provision of oral health care (for example, cocaine and vasoconstrictors). As a secondary strategy to identify those abusing substances, it is important to recognize extraoral and behavioral signs of abusing drugs. **Drug misuse** refers to indiscriminate use of drugs, whereas *drug abuse* refers to chronic self-medication with a drug in excessive quantities, resulting in physical and/or **psychologic dependence**, functional impairment, and behavior that deviates from approved social norms. Psychologic dependence, also referred to as *addiction*, is a behavioral pattern characterized by drug craving, out of control drug usage, overwhelming desire to obtain a drug supply, drug use causing personal and legal problems, denial about the personal drug use, and continuing to use the drug despite personal and legal difficulties. **Physical dependence** is an adaptive state, occurring after prolonged use of a drug, in which discontinuation of the drug causes physical symptoms that are relieved by readministering the same drug or a pharmacologically related drug. Both types of dependence can lead to compulsive patterns of drug use in which the user's lifestyle is focused on taking the drug. Drug abuse is not confined to any particular socioeconomic, cultural, or ethnic group. Drug and alcohol abuse in the workplace is estimated to cost businesses up to $100 billion annually in the United States.[1] In another report, one finds that alcohol is strongly related to assaults, rapes, child abuse, commission of crimes, traffic accidents (nearly 80% of accident fatalities that occur between 8:00 PM and 4:00 AM), suicides, homicides, and unintentional injury fatalities.[2] There are four characteristics of drug abuse (Box 23-1).

BOX 23-1. Characteristics of Drug Abuse

General
Altered state of consciousness
Development of tolerance
Rapid onset of action of desired effects
Abstinence syndrome if the drug is discontinued
　abruptly after an extended period of use

METH Abuse
Inadequate response to local anesthetics
Extensive decay and skin lesions
Paranoia and aggressive behavior
Hypertension and tachyarrhythmia
Nutritional deficiency

BOX 23-2. Stages of Drug Abuse

Experimentation
Regular to risky use
Dependence
Addiction

Stages of Substance Abuse

Experimentation, regular use, risky use, dependence, and addiction are the stages of substance use (Box 23-2). These behaviors can be addressed and treated at any stage, despite the popular myth that people must hit bottom before they can benefit from help.

Experimentation

Substance use starts with a voluntary use of alcohol or other drugs. Often the person is trying to erase another emotional problem, but there are other examples. An older person may self-medicate by drinking alcohol to cope with depression after losing a spouse. A teenager, angry about a parental divorce, may start smoking marijuana or huffing inhalants. Experimentation may even include a husband taking his wife's prescription painkiller to cope with recurring back pain.

Regular-to-Risky Use

The transition from regular to risky use and the reason for its occurrence differs for every individual. While it does not happen to everyone, the National Institute on Alcohol Abuse and Alcoholism (NIAAA) estimates that nearly one third of Americans engage in risky drinking patterns. As a result, what constitutes risky behavior can be difficult to define. If a person's behavior worries close friends and family, the behavior and suspicions should be addressed. The slope from risky behavior to dependence is often hidden, and there are interventions that may reduce or stop the progression to dependence. The Partnership for a Drug-Free America (*http://www.drugfree.org*) has helpful information on dealing with substance abusers. The Partnership for a Drug-Free America also has a comprehensive Web site to educate and provide information for interventions (*http://www.intervenenow.org*). If a family member is a substance abuser, help in understanding and coping with the situation may be needed. Al-Anon is a support group for friends and family members of alcoholics. It provides neutrality and support to persist in helping the impaired individual.

Dependence

Alcohol or drug dependence follows risky behavior. At this stage, alcohol or other drug use may not yet be compulsive and out of control. Many dependent people are able to work, maintain family relationships and friendships, and limit use of alcohol or other drugs to certain time periods, such as weekends or evenings. However it is also difficult for the impaired individual (and for others) to recognize the effect their substance use may be having on themselves, friends, coworkers, and family members. There are appropriate interventions for substance users in this stage and for those close to them. Characteristics of dependence include:

- repeated use of alcohol or other drugs, leading to failure to fulfill major responsibilities related to work, family, school, or other roles;
- repeatedly drinking or using drugs in situations that are physically hazardous, such as driving while intoxicated or using heavy machinery when intoxicated;
- repeated legal problems.

Addiction

Addiction is a medical condition involving serious psychologic and physical changes from repeated heavy use of a substance. Using drugs repeatedly over time changes brain structure and function in ways that can persist after drug use is stopped. The amount of the drug needed to cause this defect is different for everyone, but it is felt that after a certain amount of a drug is consumed, it is as if a switch in the brain is flipped from normal to addicted. The symptoms of addiction are uncontrollable alcohol or other drug craving, seeking, and using that persists even in the face of negative consequences. It is a progressive illness that worsens over time if left untreated. Treatment methods include community resources based on 12-step programs, such as Alcoholics Anonymous, outpatient or residential treatment programs, and various drug treatments, such as methadone treatment of heroin addiction.

Etiologic Factors

The differences in susceptibility to addiction are considered to mainly be related to genetic influences. Very few people are able to return to occasional use after becoming addicted. This does not absolve the addict of responsibility for the behavior, but it explains why an addict cannot stop using by sheer force of will alone. Substance abusers often begin taking the drug to achieve a desirable pharmacologic effect. The drug is used as a coping mechanism to relieve personal problems, and dependence develops. When the individual becomes dependent on the drug for the effects, a genetically associated psychologic mechanism leads to an alteration of the state of mind. This is a feature of central nervous system (CNS) drugs that leads to addiction. In 1990, alcoholism and other chemical dependencies were described by the American Society of Addiction Medicine (ASAM) as primary, chronic, relapsing diseases with genetic, psychosocial, and environmental factors influencing their development and manifestations.[2]

Professional Implications

Prescribing drugs without adequate exploration of the patient's presenting complaint represents drug misuse by a prescriber. Prescribing drugs for prolonged periods of time without medical supervision represents another example. Health care professionals most commonly abuse prescription drugs (benzodiazepines, opioids), alcohol, and tobacco themselves, but the choice of drugs and route of administration typically varies by profession, with dentists abusing nitrous oxide, pharmacists abusing multiple oral drugs, and nurses and physicians abusing injectable drugs.[2] Pressures of the professional work and easy access to narcotic agents place health care professionals at increased risk for drug abuse. Impaired health professionals constitute a hazard to the patient's well-being and to themselves, so they cannot be ignored, overlooked, or left unreported. Health care professionals who own practices must be alert to suspected drug abusers on the staff. Many agencies and most states have mandatory reporting of and active rehabilitation programs for impaired health care professionals. Substance abuse (alcohol and drugs) is considered a "handicap," and such employees may be protected by state and federal employment discrimination laws. The Rehabilitation Act (29 USC §706(7)(B)) states that employers are required to employ these individuals if they can properly perform their job functions and are not a threat to safety or property.[1] Many professional organizations have established assistance programs to help impaired employees and employers with rehabilitation. The goal is to help the impaired individual regain a place in society and the workplace.

■ Self-Study Review

1. Differentiate between drug *misuse* and drug *abuse*.
2. Differentiate between *psychologic* dependence and *physical* dependence.
3. List four characteristics of drug abuse.
4. Describe the five stages of substance abuse.
5. List sources for dealing with issues of substance abuse and what groups they serve.
6. Describe etiologic factors of drug abuse.
7. What are the professional implications of drug abuse?
8. What makes health care professionals at risk for drug abuse?
9. What is the goal of The Rehabilitation Act? Name some features of the act.

Drugs of Abuse

Abused substances are drugs or other materials administered repeatedly in a pattern and amount that may interfere with the health of normal social/occupational functioning of the subject. This definition does not require the development of **tolerance** or dependence, although these often accompany substance abuse. *Tolerance* is characterized by a reduced drug effect following repeated use of the drug and the requirement of higher doses to produce the same effect. *Dependence* is characterized by physiologic and/or behavioral changes that are apparent after discontinuation of a drug, but these withdrawal effects can be reversed by resumption of drug ingestion. **Crosstolerance** means that if a person has become tolerant to the effects of one opioid (heroin, for example), tolerance to other opioids will develop. **Crossdependence** means that a person physically dependent on one drug can

Table 23-1	Substances of Abuse
Opiates/opioids	Morphine
	Heroin
	Codeine
	Oxycodone
	Hydrocodone
	Other narcotic derivatives
Sympathomimetic stimulants	Cocaine
	Amphetamines
	METH
	Methylphenidate
	Nicotine (tobacco)
	Caffeine
Depressants	Barbiturates
	Methaqualone
	Meprobamate
	Ethanol alcohol
Hallucinogens	Mescaline
	LSD
	PCP
Others	Marijuana
	Inhalants (nitrous oxide, amyl nitrite)

switch to another drug in the same class and not have withdrawal symptoms. For example, methadone represents the substitution for heroin or other opioids. Few drugs without CNS effects are abused or misused. The more frequently abused chemically active substances are the xanthines and caffeine, found in coffee, tea, chocolate, and colas. Although these substances are rarely perceived as drugs by the average person, they produce mild stimulant and euphoric effects, and their use can lead to physical dependence. Physical dependence usually occurs only when substances are used over extended times with relatively continuous blood and brain concentrations achieved for days, weeks, or months. Psychologic (or behavioral) dependence usually involves a mindset and intense craving, leading to drug-seeking behavior. Nicotine and ethyl alcohol are the most frequently misused and abused drugs with consequent physical and psychologic dependence. The property of a drug that leads to self-administration is termed *reinforcing efficacy* or *euphorigenic tendency*. Many drugs of abuse, especially the psychomotor stimulants, produce strong **euphoria** and feelings of well-being (Table 23-1). Other CNS drugs, such as anticholinergics, steroids, amphetamines, and levodopa, are examples of agents that may induce altered states of perception, thought, feelings, and drug-induced psychoses as a result of prolonged and concentrated therapeutic use or abuse. The Drug Abuse Warning Network (DAWN) is a federal agency that monitors data on medical and psychologic problems associated with drug use and patterns of drug abuse. Alcohol and cocaine were the number-one and number-two most commonly abused drugs, respectively, that resulted in emergency room visits. This occurred in both males and females. In the 1980s, crack cocaine became popular, and, in the 1990s, cocaine usage increased along with increased transports to emergency rooms. Other drugs in the top categories included heroin/morphine, marijuana/hashish, and amphetamines, including METH/speed and alprazolam (Xanax). In women, acetaminophen was the number-three (number five for men)

most commonly used drug that led to emergency room visitation. This is due to drug misuse (overdose) rather than drug abuse. Drug abuse is a significant public health problem. It has been estimated that over 80% of those in prisons are incarcerated because of drug abuse issues (selling them, committing crimes to get drugs, or taking them). METH use has drastically increased in recent years, and home cooking labs to manufacture METH are a leading cause of law enforcement investigations.

Opiates/Opioids

The most commonly abused opiate is heroin, or diacetyl morphine, synthesized clandestinely from natural morphine. The effects of heroin and morphine are similar, but heroin is about three times more potent and, therefore, contains three times as many "doses" as a corresponding amount of morphine. Other opioid agonists, including hydromorphone (Dilaudid), meperidine (Demerol), and propoxyphene (Darvon), produce similar effects and have similar abuse potential. The opiates act through binding to opioid receptors in the brain.

Heroin

Heroin abusers often begin by smoking or by using subcutaneous (SC) injections (or skin popping) of the drug and progress to intravenous (IV) use (or mainlining). The "rush" that accompanies an IV injection is quite intense. After a few minutes, the rush subsides, and the effects resemble those after oral doseforms. The user feels relaxed and carefree, somewhat dreamy, but able to carry on many normal activities, including normal conversations. The IV administration of illicit drugs often leads to a high incidence of sepsis, hepatitis, infective endocarditis, and bloodborne disease. The individual most commonly at risk for infective endocarditis is the IV drug user.[3,4] Overdose leads to unconsciousness, respiratory depression, and extreme miosis (pinpoint pupils). Opioid antagonists, such as naloxone (Narcan) or naltrexone (ReVia), can immediately reverse these effects. Naltrexone is also used in the treatment of chronic alcohol abuse.

Signs of Withdrawal

The progression to physical dependence occurs gradually for most opiate abusers. The significance of physical dependence to the abuser is the appearance of withdrawal symptoms, called **abstinence syndrome**, about 6 or more hours after the last injection. Many of the signs and symptoms of withdrawal (Table 23-2) are opposite of the effects of acute opiate administration. Unmedicated withdrawal has been termed *cold turkey* because of the appearance of goose bumps accompanying piloerection. Opiates/opioids cross the placental barrier, and if the mother is dependent, the newborn will undergo a withdrawal syndrome beginning 6 to 12 hours after birth. Crossdependence occurs with all full opioid agonists, but not with some partial agonists. Mixed agonist/antagonists and partial agonists, such as pentazocine (Talwin), butorphanol (Stadol), nalbuphine (Nubain), and buprenorphine (Buprenex), have considerably less potential for abuse than full opioid agonists.

Table 23-2	Comparison of Opiate and Depressant Withdrawal

Opiate Withdrawal	Depressant* Withdrawal
Anxiety and dysphoria	Anxiety and dysphoria
Craving and drug-seeking	Craving and drug-seeking
Sleep disturbance	Sleep disturbances
Nausea and vomiting	Nausea and vomiting
Lacrimation	Tremors
Rhinorrhea	Hyperreflexia
Yawning	Hyperpyrexia
Piloerection and gooseflesh	Delirium
Sweating	Seizures
Mydriasis	Possible death
Abdominal cramping	
Hyperpyrexia	
Tachycardia and hypertension	

*Alcohol or barbiturates

Sympathomimetic Stimulants

The most widely known members of the sympathomimetic stimulant class of abused drugs are cocaine, METH, and amphetamine, but various nonamphetamine stimulants, such as methylphenidate (Ritalin, Concerta) and several weight control medications, also have abuse potential. These drugs are centrally acting sympathetic stimulants that enhance catecholaminergic neurotransmission. Cocaine acts in the brain to block the reuptake of dopamine into presynaptic terminal areas, thus enhancing dopamine action. Amphetamines also have dopaminergic actions due to several factors, including an enhanced neurotransmitter release, inhibition of monoamine oxidase enzymatic destruction of amphetamine, reuptake blockade similar to that of codeine, and/or direct postsynaptic receptor activation.

Methamphetamine

METH abuse has increased significantly; the National Survey on Drug Use and Health reports the percentage of METH users who were dependent on the drug increased from 27.5% to 59.3% between 2002 and 2004 (*http://www.oas.samhsa.gov/nhsda.htm*). An estimated 12.3 million Americans over the age of 12 have used the drug at least once, with the majority of users between ages 18 and 34. The drug can be made from inexpensive over-the-counter (OTC) medications and chemicals (lye, muriatic and sulfuric acids) purchased at local retail outlets. Street names include speed, Ice, Chalk, Crank, and Crystal.[5]

METH is a highly addictive synthetic amine that stimulates the release and blocks the reuptake of serotonin, dopamine, and norepinephrine in the brain. The action of these neurotransmitting monoamines is to stimulate the reward centers and give the characteristic high of the substance. Loss of appetite frequently accompanies this effect. The high can last up to 14 hours, during which time the user is impaired, unable to care for children or to prepare meals (Box 23-1).

Long-term use leads to depletion of these neurotransmitters, eliciting depression.[6]

Oral Effects

Oral consequences of using METH are profound, with black to brown areas of extensive decay along the cervical third of teeth, often involving the entire labial surfaces. A METH user may present with the chief complaint, "My teeth are crumbling and falling apart." Frequently teeth cannot be restored and must be extracted. The rapid decay is thought to be due to frequent use of the drug, coupled with drug effects of chronic xerostomia and frequent ingestion of carbonated, sugary beverages. Drug use incites bruxing during the euphoric state, which leads to temporomandibular joint dysfunction, masseter muscle enlargement, and incisal attrition. Fractured teeth that leave retained roots may be found. Oral manifestations of nutritional deficiency may be found, because chronic users have suppressed appetites and do not eat nutritional foods. Periodontal disease can be significant because oral hygiene needs are ignored. The active METH user commonly presents for emergency dental care only, and missed dental appointments or nonpayment for services is common.[6] Pain tolerance may also decrease, resulting in failure of local anesthetic effects.

Central and Physiologic Effects

CNS physiologic changes associated with the use of METH include insomnia, anxiety, paranoia, hallucinations, and aggression. A common paranoic behavior is the perception that the user is being threatened or is in danger. This can lead to violent outbursts and stalking of suspected individuals. Physical symptoms of tachycardia, arrhythmia, and hypertension can develop, leading to stroke.[7] Chronic users have sensations that bugs are crawling under their skin, causing the users to pick and scratch to remove them, which leaves sores on the skin that may become infected. These extraoral signs of METH abuse are discovered during the routine extraoral exam. In addition, the libido increases and can result in risky sexual behavior, leading to contraction of sexually transmitted diseases.[6]

Dental Drug Interactions

Vasoconstrictors found in local anesthetic preparations can lead to increased blood pressure and stroke when METH has been used within the past 24 hours of the local anesthetic/ vasoconstrictor. Pain tolerance may decrease in the METH user, resulting in reduced effects from local anesthesia and presenting a clinical problem. This must be considered before administration of additional local anesthetic doses.

Cocaine

If cocaine is smoked, absorption into the blood is rapid, leading to a quick onset of action similar to that for IV administration. Intranasal and oral administration methods are slower in onset. Cocaine intoxication after IV administration or inhalation generally lasts only about 30 minutes. Users redose frequently in an attempt to maintain the high. In recent years, abuse of freebase cocaine, known as *crack*, has become common. Crack becomes volatile at a lower temperature than does the salt, so crack can be inhaled after heating it in a pipe. Cocaine and other stimulants activate both the central and autonomic sympathetic nervous systems.

Oral Effects

A periodontist reported seeing evidence of cocaine placed within the vestibule as a mode of administration. The vasoconstrictive effects of the drug resulted in loss of attachment in the local area and severe recession of the associated buccal periodontal tissue. When this situation is found in an otherwise healthy periodontal condition, cocaine abuse should be suspected and followed up with the client.

Central and Physiologic Effects

CNS effects include increased alertness, feelings of elation and well-being, increased energy, feelings of competence, and increased sexuality. Athletic performance enhancement has been demonstrated, particularly in sports requiring sustained attention and endurance. Stimulant overdose results in excessive sympathetic nervous system activation, with the resulting tachycardia and hypertension capable of producing myocardial infarction and cerebrovascular hemorrhage. Cocaine can also cause coronary vasospasm and cardiac arrhythmias. Other symptoms include anxiety, feelings of paranoia and impending doom, and restlessness. Patients become unpredictable and sometimes violent. Beta-adrenergic blocking agents, such as propranolol, are effective pharmacologic antagonists, although many patients do not require medication.

Prenatal Use

Cocaine use during pregnancy is associated with complications that include miscarriage, lower gestational age at birth, lower birth weight, and neurobehavioral impairment of the newborn.

Dental Drug Interactions

Researchers reported that cocaine has a high potential to increase the cardiovascular effects of vasoconstrictors (such as tachyarrhythmia and hypertension).[8] There are reports of death (heart attack) when a local anesthetic/vasoconstrictor was given to a patient who had received topical cocaine for nasal surgery. Deaths in dentistry have been reported when the drug combination was used. The authors concluded that vasoconstrictors should be avoided completely in cases of cocaine intoxication. Elective dental treatment is not advised while a patient is using cocaine. One problem in health care is that an individual using cocaine is unlikely to report the practice on the health history. This makes recognition of signs of cocaine abuse essential (see "Oral Effects" and "Central and Physiologic Effects").

Withdrawal Effects

An important component of stimulant intoxication is the letdown that occurs as the drug effects subside. Dysphoria, tiredness, irritability, and mild depression often immediately follow a stimulant intoxication episode. A dangerous pattern of stimulant abuse is that of extended, uninterrupted sequences, referred to as *runs*. Runs result from attempts to maintain a continuous state of intoxication, both to extend the pleasurable feeling and to postpone the postintoxication crash.

■ **Self-Study Review**

10. Differentiate between *tolerance* and *dependence*.
11. Which drugs are most commonly abused? Which drugs are commonly misused?
12. List commonly abused opioids and the signs and symptoms to identify the abuse.
13. What is the relationship of IV drug use and infective endocarditis?
14. Identify the opioid antagonist agents.
15. Describe signs of *abstinence syndrome*.
16. Describe characteristics of METH abuse, including oral changes and physiologic changes that may affect the oral care plan. Describe the potential interaction with vasoconstrictors.
17. Describe oral effects of cocaine abuse.
18. Describe CNS effects of cocaine abuse and any related dental drug interactions.

CNS Depressants

The mechanisms of action of ethanol, barbiturates, and benzodiazepines, the three major therapeutic CNS depressants that are abused, have been described in earlier chapters. Overdose of depressant drugs is characterized by sluggish and miotic pupils, shallow and slow respiration, absence of deep tendon reflexes (or attenuated reflex action), and unresponsive patients. Although benzodiazepines are rarely lethal, they enhance the effects of other depressants—an effect known as dose-dependent CNS depression, including somnolence, impaired coordination, confusion, and coma—especially alcohol, which is often taken concurrently. When the drugs are combined, the usual cause of death is CNS depression leading to respiratory collapse, followed by cardiac arrest.

Repeated use of CNS-depressant drugs produces psychologic and physical dependence. Crossdependence occurs among other barbiturates, nonbarbiturate sedatives, benzodiazepines, and alcohol (dependence on *one* of these drugs results in dependence on *all* of these drugs). Signs and symptoms of depressant withdrawal are often opposite to the acute pharmacologic effects of these drugs. They include dysphoria, anxiety and restlessness, hyper-reflexiveness, insomnia, muscle weakness, and tremor. The occasional appearance of convulsions and delirium make depressant withdrawal a medical emergency.

Ethyl Alcohol

Alcohol abuse is a common problem in the United States. *Alcohol abuse* is defined as the use of alcohol for nonmedical purposes and for altering consciousness. In contrast, *alcohol misuse* means using alcohol in excessive amounts or for longer periods of time than advised. An alcoholic is an alcohol abuser. People who drink excessively on social occasions (binge drinking) or who drink at inappropriate times are misusing alcohol. When used acutely, ethyl alcohol produces inebriation at a blood alcohol concentration >0.15%. The chronic use of alcohol has been shown to cause neuropathy, myopathy, and cerebellar degeneration.

Periodontal Effects

A prospective analysis of the association between alcohol consumption and periodontitis among men who participated in the Health Professionals Follow-up Study (HPFS) suggested that alcohol consumption is an independent modifiable risk factor for periodontitis.[9] The HPFS was a prospective study initiated in 1986 of 51,529 male health professionals (58% dentists, 20% veterinarians, 8% pharmacists, 7% optometrists, 4% osteopathic physicians, and 3% podiatrists), ages 40 to 75 years, who were free from periodontitis at the start of the follow-up period. Alcohol intake was assessed at baseline and updated every 4 years. After adjustment for age, men who drank alcohol were at an 18% to 27% higher risk of periodontal disease compared with nondrinkers. Several plausible biologic explanations exist for a detrimental effect of alcohol on the periodontitis risk. Studies have shown that impaired neutrophil phagocytosis is associated with periodontal disease. Alcohol impairs neutrophil function, contributing to bacterial overgrowth and increased bacterial penetration that may lead to periodontal inflammation. As well, alcohol may have a direct toxic effect on periodontal tissue similar to other tissues of the oropharynx. Finally, high alcohol intake increases monocyte production of inflammatory cytokines, such as tumor necrosis factor-alpha (TNF-α), and interleukins-1 and -6 in the gingival crevice and is associated with periodontitis. Alcohol drinking has been associated with poor oral hygiene in other studies; however, no information was collected on oral hygiene in the HPFS study.

Alcohol Intoxication Therapy

No known antidote for acute alcohol intoxication is available. Disulfiram (Antabuse), a drug used to treat chronic alcoholism, inhibits aldehyde dehydrogenase and should never be used in combination with ethyl alcohol, because it causes severe vomiting. Naltrexone is approved for use in the treatment of chronic alcohol abuse.

Oral Health Care Implications

When alcohol abuse is suspected in the dental patient, management depends on whether the patient is intoxicated, simply shows signs of alcohol abuse (red face, bloodshot eyes, hypertrophy of parotid glands, breath odors of alcohol), or reports substance abuse on the health history. A patient who comes to the appointment in an inebriated state should be rescheduled. The client should be escorted to his or her home by a responsible person, such as a family member, friend, or caregiver. Dental implications for the alcohol abuser include the need for a thorough oral examination due to the increased risk for oral cancer, monitoring of oral self-care (neglect of oral care is common), and questioning about a history of liver disease and subsequent bleeding problems. The diseased liver is unable to store adequate levels of vitamin K, thus reducing the conversion of vitamin K to coagulation factors. Other comorbid conditions include thrombocytopenia, esophageal varices, spontaneous bleeding, and abdominal distension associated with liver failure. Oral complications of alcoholism include glossitis, loss of tongue papillae, and candida infec-

tion (angular cheilitis). Drugs used in dentistry that are metabolized in the liver include amide local anesthetics and benzodiazepines. These drugs may have reduced metabolisms, and blood levels will not fall as rapidly as in the normal patient. Single doses of the drug do not require reduction, but repeated doses may need to be reduced, or the interval between doses prolonged, to prevent excessive blood levels.

A recent review of geriatric alcoholism reported that physiologic changes associated with aging permit the harmful effects of drinking alcohol to become evident at lower levels of consumption than in younger people.[10] Other detrimental effects in this age group include an exacerbation of medical and emotional problems associated with aging and the predisposition to develop adverse drug reactions with psychotherapeutic medications. They suggest the incidence of dental disease in the geriatric population is extensive because of diminished salivary flow and a disinterest in appropriate oral self-care. Many geriatric individuals who drink alcohol also use tobacco products, increasing the risk for oral cancer. Dental hygiene management should include assessment of salivary flow, dental exam for caries and candidiasis, an oral cancer examination, recommendations for anticaries agents, and precaution when advising analgesics that may interact with alcohol or alcohol-related gastrointestinal disease.

Appointment Considerations

Regular visits for oral health services are difficult due to the lifestyle of the addict. Substance abusers frequently miss appointments and may fail to pay for services. Behavior management problems are possible. Medical complications may cause treatment to be delayed in order to complete medical consultations. Vital signs must be measured at every appointment to assess systemic health. Needle tracks may be evident when the blood pressure cuff is placed. Pain tolerance may be decreased, resulting in failure of local analgesic agents to relieve pain. Oral health care providers should require anyone suspected of drug abuse to sign a statement indicating drugs have not been used within the previous 24 hours.[6,9]

Hallucinogens

Abused hallucinogenic (psychedelic) compounds fall into two chemical classes: the amphetamine analogs and the indolamines. Mescaline, or peyote, is the prototypical amphetamine analog **hallucinogen**. Lysergic acid (LSD) is the prototypical indolamine hallucinogen. Other drugs in this group include phencyclidine (PCP), marijuana (cannabis), and others. Nearly all hallucinogens produce varying degrees of sympathomimetic effects, often evident as tachycardia, hypertension, psychomotor stimulation, or euphoria. The most prominent effects are on subjective experience. These effects include (a) lability of mood, (b) altered thought processes, (c) altered visual or auditory perceptions, (d) an experience of having enhanced insights into events and ideas, and (e) impaired judgment. Psychologic dependence can be produced by agents in this group, and tolerance develops early in use. Mood swings can range from profound euphoria to anxiety and terror. Panic states (bad trips) are the symptoms that most commonly lead abusers to seek medical assistance.

Acute Overdose

Although acute overdose is not a common problem with hallucinogenic compounds, a number of other dangers are present. The most significant is the risk of injury caused by impaired judgment. Psychiatric illness may be precipitated by even an occasional encounter with hallucinogenic compounds in subjects with a predisposition to such complications. Another poorly understood aspect of hallucinogen abuse is *flashbacks*, where users re-experience aspects of hallucinogen intoxication despite being drug free.

Lysergic Acid

LSD is the most potent hallucinogen, requiring only micrograms to produce an effect. Overdose of LSD produces widely dilated pupils, hypertension, visual distortions, panic reactions, and paranoia. The user does not lose consciousness during an event, and treatment for acute intoxication is verbal reassurance (talking the user down). Prolonged use leads to mental disturbances, such as panic attacks, depression, flashbacks, and schizophrenic reactions.

Phencyclidine

PCP (or angel dust) was originally developed as an injectable anesthetic in veterinary medicine. Ketamine, a close structural analog of PCP, is currently used during general anesthesia as an anesthetic. PCP inhibits the reuptake of dopamine, serotonin, and norepinephrine. Oral effects include hypersalivation and sweating. CNS stimulation is expressed as a "blank stare"; disorganized thought patterns can lead to bizarre behavior, and muscle twitches and rigidity can occur. Elevated blood pressure and pulse can be found as well.

It was not until smoking became the most common route for PCP administration that the PCP abuse epidemic began. This method of administration allowed users to better titrate the dose. PCP is generally sprinkled onto plant material (e.g., dried parsley or marijuana) and formed into crude cigarettes, sometimes known as *crystal joints* or *killer weed*. Although PCP is the major drug abused in this class, many other analogs of PCP produce similar effects. Ketamine also has PCP-like abuse potential.

The major dangers with PCP abuse are risk-taking behavior and progressive personality changes that culminate in a toxic psychosis. PCP overdose is rarely lethal but may require careful management because of the severe incapacitation of the subject. There is no PCP antagonist available.

Cannabinoids

Marijuana (cannabis) is generally consumed by smoking hand-rolled cigarettes, or *joints*, or by using other smoking paraphernalia. After smoking, the onset of peak intoxication is delayed 15 to 30 minutes. The effects of cannabis generally last from 4 to 6 hours. Except with very high doses, marijuana intoxication is considerably less intense than intoxication with hallucinogens or PCP. Users exhibit mood lability, including euphoria, anxiety, fear, and even panic attacks. Users identify improved experiences of music, movies, sexual behavior, and other activities as strong motivation for their usage. Thought processes, judgment, and time estimation are altered. Marijuana has little direct effect on psychomotor coordination except that altered perception (dreamlike state) and judgment can impair task performance, including driving. Marijuana often produces drowsiness, particularly 1 to 2 hours after smoking. Physiologic effects include tachycardia and conjunctivitis (reddening of sclera). Major dangers of marijuana abuse include preoccupation with marijuana use to the exclusion of other activities (psychologic dependence) and the development of personality changes.

An adverse drug effect of interest to the dental hygienist is the common occurrence of xerostomia in the marijuana user. Other oral effects may include leukoplakia, periodontitis, and heavy smokers of marijuana may have chronic bronchitis.

Medical uses of marijuana (Marinol) include acting as an antiemetic and appetite stimulant in AIDS patients. Recent studies have confirmed that naturally occurring and synthetic cannabinoids are also effective in patients receiving moderately emetogenic chemotherapy. Cannabinoids also increase the appetite, produce euphoria, and have analgesic properties, all of which are useful in patients in terminal stages of cancer.

Inhalants

Many volatile chemicals and gases produce CNS effects and can be subject to abuse. Relatively little is known about the psychopharmacology of these compounds. These chemicals are categorized in the following three broad groups: (a) gases such as nitrous oxide, (b) volatile liquids (gases, glue), and (c) aliphatic nitrites (amyl nitrite).

Nitrous Oxide

Nitrous oxide, a gas used in general anesthesia, produces a short-lived mild intoxication that is characteristic of the early onset of anesthesia. Abuse of nitrous oxide is largely confined to health professionals. When a dental health care worker abuses drugs (nitrous oxide or others), it can present a danger during patient care. It is not uncommon for the individual to be in denial about the addiction or abuse. Because of this denial, confrontation by family members or the office staff may be ineffective. Ultimately, work performance declines and possible mood swings and bizarre behavior (such as throwing instruments) can pose a threat to the staff and to patients. Most state dental associations have "Concerned Committees" to assist those in the dental profession seeking treatment for drug abuse.

Volatile Liquids

Volatile liquids that are abused include anesthetic gases, organic solvents, refrigerants (Freon), and petroleum products. Some of the more popular abused agents are (a) toluene-containing paint thinners, correction fluids, and plastic glues; (b) other alkyl-benzene solvents and cleaners, benzene, and xylene; (c) chlorinated hydrocarbon cleaners and degreasers, such as methyl chloroform and methylene chloride; and (d) general anesthetics. Some of these compounds are suspected carcinogens, some are cardiotoxic or produce ototoxicity, and some produce well-defined neuropathies. When the oral health care professional abuses these agents, neuropathy can result in loss of tactile sensitivity, which can cause impaired ability to hold instruments.

Aliphatic Nitrites

Aliphatic nitrites are volatile liquids. One example is amyl nitrite, which is used medically to treat angina. It is supplied as an ampule, which is broken open so the contents can be inhaled. Nitrites are often abused in conjunction with sexual activity and are popular for their claimed ability to enhance orgasm in men, probably as the result of penile vasodilation. Nitrite use can result in emergencies related to loss of consciousness (syncope).

Nicotine

Tobacco is an addictive product that causes more medical problems than all the other drugs of abuse, except alcohol. Currently, oral health care professionals are encouraged to offer smoking cessation programs in the dental office as a part of the oral health education plan. Tobacco cessation programs are most successful in the individual who desires to stop the smoking habit. Tobacco craving continues in many persons for years after stopping tobacco use. It is well known that tobacco use is a factor in leukoplakia and in squamous cell carcinoma of the oral mucosa, and this information should be included in the program to persuade an individual to stop smoking. As well, smoking is the main etiologic factor in emphysema and other respiratory disorders.

Smoking Cessation Programs

The American Dental Hygienists' Association (ADHA) established guidelines for a smoking cessation program (http://www.askadviserefer.org) within the dental office. This effort is to assist oral health care providers in encouraging patients to stop using tobacco products. In 2000, a National Youth Tobacco Survey (NYTS) was administered anonymously to school-age children. The NYTS was administered to a nationally representative sample of 35,828 students in grades 6 to 12 in 324 schools. A study describing the patterns of *tobacco use counseling* among physicians and dentists (as reported by these adolescents) determined the association between provider advice to quit and cessation activities among current smokers.[11] According to the results, 33% of adolescents who visited a physician or a dentist in the past year reported that a physician counseled them about the dangers of tobacco use, and 20% reported that a dentist provided a similar message. Among students who had smoked in the past year, 16.4% received advice to quit from a physician, and 11.6% received advice to quit from a dentist. Physician or dentist advice to quit was correlated with one or more quit attempts in the past 12 months. Researchers concluded that physician and dentist practice patterns on smoking cessation are well below recommended guidelines and that failure to suggest smoking cessation may represent a missed opportunity to affect adolescent smoking behavior.

Psychologic Effects

Although the psychologic effects of smoked nicotine are fairly subtle, they occur reliably and include mood changes, stress reduction, and some performance enhancement. The nicotine withdrawal syndrome emerges soon after smoking cessation, peaks in 24 to 48 hours, and may last for 10 days or more. The major symptoms of nicotine withdrawal are dysphoria, irritability, anxiety, difficulty concentrating, fatigue, and sleep disturbances. Observable signs include decreased heart rate, increased caloric intake, and weight gain.

Caffeine

Caffeine, together with other methylxanthine stimulants, is present in beverages made from coffee beans or tea leaves. A typical cup of brewed coffee contains 85 to 150 mg of caffeine, and mugs of strong coffee can have upwards of 200 mg per cup. Caffeine is also present in various OTC medications, including analgesic preparations, stimulants, and weight-control products. Excessive consumption of any of these products or combined consumption can result in caffeine intake of well over 1 g/day. Effects are increased alertness, loss of fatigue, and a greater capacity for activities requiring sustained attention. Withdrawal symptoms include headache and irritability.

■ Self-Study Review

19. Identify the usual cause of death from combining alcohol and CNS depressants.
20. Differentiate between alcohol *abuse* and alcohol *misuse*.
21. Describe oral effects of chronic alcohol use.
22. Describe the use of disulfiram and naltrexone in alcohol intoxication.
23. List clinical signs of chronic alcohol abuse.
24. Identify dental implications of alcohol abuse.
25. Identify agents in the hallucinogen classification.
26. Describe behavior changes associated with this class of substances.
27. Identify oral effects of cannabis.
28. Identify the brand-name product for medical cannabis.
29. Describe inhalants used in dentistry that are abused.
30. Describe functional losses that can reduce the ability to effectively practice.
31. Discuss tobacco abuse and its relationship to oral disease.

Substance Abuse Treatment

In addition to stopping drug use, the goal of substance abuse treatment is to return the person to a functional state in the family, workplace, and community. It is clear that no single treatment is appropriate for all individuals and that matching treatment settings, interventions, and services to each individual's specific need is critical to successful treatment. There are three stages of substance abuse treatments:

- Acute care or medical detoxification/stabilization
- Rehabilitation
- Aftercare or continuing care

Acute Care

The purpose of *acute care* is to safely and comfortably remove toxins from the body, to stabilize the patient, and to engage the patient into rehabilitation. It is generally completed within a hospital-type location. Medical detoxification is only the first stage of addiction treatment and by itself does little to change long-term drug use. Medical detoxification safely manages the acute physical symptoms of withdrawal associated with stopping drug use. While detoxification alone is rarely sufficient to help addicts achieve long-term abstinence, some individuals can progress to successful drug addiction treatment.

Medical Treatment

Medications are an important element of treatment for many patients, especially when combined with counseling and other behavioral therapies. Methadone and levo-alpha-acetylmethadol (LAAM) are effective in helping individuals addicted to heroin or other opiates stabilize their lives and reduce illicit drug use. In acute overdose and withdrawal treatment, naloxone (Narcan) is administered for immediate blocking of opioid effects. When the triad of narcotic overdose symptoms (respiratory depression, pinpoint pupils, unconsciousness) is observed, naloxone is the first-line drug used to reverse the acute emergency. For maintenance, naltrexone (ReVia) is used. It has a long (24-hour) duration of action and superior oral bioavailability. Nalmefene (Revex), a new agent administered parenterally, is available for the treatment of acute opioid intoxication (an oral formulation is used for the treatment of alcoholism). Naltrexone is also an effective medication for some opiate addicts and some patients with co-occurring alcohol dependence. Naltrexone is a long-acting synthetic opiate antagonist taken orally (daily or three times a week) that blocks the effects of opiates. It has no potential for abuse and is not addicting. It allows affected individuals to continue working and functioning normally while medicated. Patient noncompliance in taking naltrexone is a common problem, making the treatment most effective for highly motivated people who desire total abstinence, including impaired professionals, parolees, and prisoners in work-release status. Nicotine-containing gum and patches may be used to treat the withdrawal syndrome while patients are participating in a smoking cessation program. For persons addicted to nicotine, these nicotine replacement products or an oral medication (such as bupropion) can be an effective component of treatment. For those with mental disorders, both behavioral treatments and medications may be needed.

Rehabilitation

The purpose of *rehabilitation* is to teach skills necessary to change behavior. A main goal is to reduce threats to progress and engage the patient in the next stage of treatment. Remaining in treatment for an adequate period of time is critical for treatment effectiveness. For most patients, the threshold of significant improvement is reached at about 3 months in treatment. After this threshold is reached, additional treatment can produce further progress toward recovery. Counseling and other behavioral therapies are critical components of ef-

fective treatment for addiction. In therapy, patients address issues of motivation, build skills to resist drug use, replace drug-using activities and peer groups with constructive and rewarding non-drug-using activities and relationships, and improve problem-solving abilities. This therapy is usually provided in a care center where the patient is confined from leaving.

Aftercare

The purpose of *aftercare* is to maintain the behavior change, to support strategies for healthful living, to monitor threats to relapse, and, if relapse occurs, to re-engage the patient to stay in continuing care programs. Possible lapses to drug use during treatment must be monitored continuously. The objective monitoring of a patient's drug and alcohol use, using urinalysis or other tests, can help the patient withstand urges to use drugs. Such monitoring also can provide early evidence of drug use so that the individual's treatment plan can be adjusted. Feedback to patients who test positive for illicit drug use is an important element of monitoring. Recovery from drug addiction can be a long-term process and frequently requires multiple episodes of treatment. As with other chronic illnesses, relapses to drug use can occur during or after successful treatment episodes. Addicted individuals may require prolonged treatment and multiple episodes of treatment to achieve long-term abstinence and fully restored functioning. Participation in self-help programs during and following treatment often is helpful in maintaining abstinence.

■ Self-Study Review

32. Describe the three stages of substance abuse treatment, focusing on elements of each stage.
33. Describe signs of the triad of narcotic overdose.
34. List antagonists used to reverse acute narcotic overdose and the drugs used in maintenance therapy.

DENTAL HYGIENE APPLICATIONS

The dental hygienist must use the medical history information as well as extraoral observation and clinical examination to identify the patient with substance abuse problems. Breath odors may be indicative. Enlarged parotid glands should be investigated for etiologic factors. The practitioner should be aware of the possibility for increased blood pressure and tachyarrhythmia and monitor vital signs each appointment. Awareness of the potential for excessive bleeding when poor liver function is likely and monitoring bleeding during periodontal procedures is necessary. If excessive bleeding is observed, treatment should be stopped and digital pressure applied. Referral for medical evaluation and necessary blood coagulation tests should be requested before treatment progresses. Because alcohol and tobacco use increases the risk for oral cancer, an oral cancer exam should be completed at each maintenance visit. Reduced salivary flow may cause increased caries or candidiasis. Anticaries agents should be recommended if needed, and antifungal therapy should be prescribed by the dentist if indicated. Because opioid abusers develop tolerance to the analgesic effects of opioids, managing dental pain can be difficult. Nonopioid COX-inhibitors may be used. If the patient is in recovery, giving an opioid-containing analgesic can cause the recovery to fail and stimulate the person to begin abusing opiates again. For the alcoholic patient, acidic drugs, such as aspirin and COX-1 inhibitors, should be avoided due to the risk of inducing stomach bleeding. Up to 4 Hg of acetaminophen can be used daily. There is an absolute drug interaction between vasoconstrictors and cocaine that prohibits using the two drugs together. Vasoconstrictors should also be avoided when METH has been used within the past 24 hours. This must be explained to the patient, and the patient must provide assurance that drugs will not be used within 24 hours prior to a dental hygiene appointment at which local anesthesia with a vasoconstrictor is indicated. The vasoconstrictor is needed to reduce periodontal bleeding, and use of a local anesthetic alone may not provide the duration of anesthesia or the degree of hemostasis necessary for the procedure. Nonalcoholic mouth rinse products should be recommended when substance abuse is suspected or for those with a history of alcohol abuse (Box 23-3). Practitioners can advise counseling for drug addiction when the abusing client admits to using drugs. Awareness of the paranoia that accompanies long-term METH use, however, is an indication to not confront the suspected METH user about practitioner suspicions.

BOX 23-4. Web Resources for Substance Abuse

American Society of Addiction Medicine:
    http://www.asam.org
Cocaine Anonymous World Services:
    http://www.ca.org
Drug Abuse Warning Network (DAWN):
    http://dawninfo.samhsa.gov
Drug Enforcement Administration:
    http://www.justthinktwice.com
Narcotics Anonymous World Services:
    http://www.na.org
National Institute on Drug Abuse: http://www.nida.
    nih.gov/infofacts/methamphetamine.html
Substance Abuse & Mental Health Services
    Administration: http://www.samhsa.gov
Substance Abuse Treatment Facility Locator:
    http://www.findtreatment.samhsa.gov
Partnership for a Drug-Free America:
    http://www.drugfree.org

When the oral health care professional suspects a coworker is abusing illicit substances, the suspected drug user must be confronted. Interventions may need to be initiated to assist the individual in getting appropriate treatment. Knowingly permitting someone to treat patients when under the influence of CNS depressants or other illicit drugs will enable the dependence problem to continue as well as put the patient at risk for poor care. In some instances, patient safety may be compromised if the behavior continues.

The results of the 2000 NYTS suggest dentistry is not doing enough to encourage adolescents to stop smoking. Dental hygienists should discuss this issue with adolescents, because the survey indicated many adolescents tried to stop smoking as a result of a physician or dentist recommendation. Smoking cessation programs are available, and every dental hygienist should utilize, or be familiar with, the "askadviserefer" program on the ADHA's Web site. Related Web links for help with substance abuse are included in Box 23-4.

BOX 23-3. Dental Hygiene Management for the Substance-Abusing Patient

Analyze the medical history and extraoral and clinical exam for evidence of drug abuse.
Monitor the patient's vital signs and pulse qualities.
Perform an oral cancer screen, evaluate salivary flow, and recommend anticaries agents as needed.
Provide digital pressure for excessive bleeding and refer the patient for medical evaluation and blood coagulation tests; delay further treatment until medical clearance is supplied.
Acetaminophen (4 Hg/day maximum dose) is the analgesic of choice; avoid aspirin or nonsteroidal anti-inflammatory analgesics for the alcoholic patient, and avoid opioid analgesics for patients in recovery from substance abuse.
Local anesthesia/vasoconstrictor can pose a drug interaction if cocaine or METH is used due to vasoconstrictor–drug interaction. Obtain written assurance from the patient that drugs will not be used within 24 hours of next appointment.
Nonalcoholic rinses should be recommended for assistance in plaque control.

CONCLUSION

Substance and drug misuse and abuse are widespread, despite legislation, enforcement, and educational efforts to curb drug use. Health care professionals must be able to recognize the signs and symptoms of various drugs of abuse. They must also be informed about the proper interventions (pharmacologic and nonpharmacologic) used for treatment of those affected. State professional organizations and boards may have committees to assist impaired oral health care professionals in seeking help for addictions. The impaired oral health care abuser will likely provide less than optimal service, may pose a threat for harm for the patient, and will ultimately

CLINICAL APPLICATION EXERCISES

☐ **Exercise 1.** A patient reports for dental hygiene care with a medical history of alcohol abuse. Vital signs are within normal limits, and the oral exam is noncontributory. The periodontal exam reveals significant attachment loss, heavy calculus deposits, and poor self-care. Describe management implications for this client.

☐ **Exercise 2.** You began working in a dental practice after graduation. The office had never employed a dental hygienist in the past. The other staff included a receptionist and a chairside dental assistant. Everything went well until the second week of working in the office. A patient complained about the recent dental care provided by your employer. The MO posterior restoration had a mesial overhang, the occlusal margins were elevated, and the gingivae apical to the treatment area was abraded. When the dentist came to check the patient following completion of dental hygiene care, a discussion ensued about the client's disapproval of the treatment results. The dentist threw the mirror and explorer across the room, shoved the bracket tray into the wall, and stormed out of the office. What features of the appointment may indicate the dentist has a substance abuse problem?

☐ **Exercise 3.** WEB ACTIVITY: Do an Internet search for "American Dental Association policy on methamphetamine use." This should take you to the URL http://www.ada.org/public/topics/methmouth.asp. Note the overview information and the additional resources to gain full value of information. Aggressive decay is illustrated in the photos contained. Other photos of oral effects can be accessed online by finding this article: Scofield JC. The gravity of methamphetamine addiction. *Dimens Dental Hygiene.* 2007;5(3):16–18. (free access)

☐ **Exercise 4.** WEB ACTIVITY: Find three sources to assist a client who wants to start a smoking cessation program. Evaluate the quality of each Web site for use in a dental office program.

lose the opportunity for professional practice and possibly the license to practice.

References

1. Malatestinic WN, Jorgenson JA. Dealing with substance abuse in the workplace. *Hosp Pharm.* 1991;26(1):102.
2. Baldwin JN, Cook MD. Issues: Psychoactive substance use disorders. In: Young LY, Koda-Kimble MA, eds. *Applied Therapeutics: The Clinical Use of Drugs.* 8th ed. Baltimore: Lippincott, Williams and Wilkins. 2004: 32, 81.
3. Siddiq S, Missri J, Silverman I. Endocarditis in an urban hospital in the 1990s. *Arch Intern Med.* 1996;156:2454–2458.
4. Hoen B. Epidemiology and antibiotic treatment of infective endocarditis: An update. *Heart.* 2006;92:1694–1700.
5. American Dental Association. Methamphetamine use and oral health. *J Am Dent Assoc.* 2005;136:1401.
6. Scofield JC. The gravity of methamphetamine addiction. *Dimens Dental Hygiene.* 2007;5(3):16–18.
7. Ohta K, Mori M, Yoritaka A, et al. Delayed ischemic stroke associated with methamphetamine use. *J Emerg Med.* 2005;28: 165–167.
8. Yagiela JA. Adverse drug interactions in dental practice: Interactions associated with vasoconstrictors. *J Am Dent Assoc.* 1999;139(5):701–709.
9. Pitiphat W, Merchant AT, Rimm EB, Joshipura KJ. Alcohol consumption increases periodontitis risk. *J Dent Res.* 2003;82(7): 509–513.
10. Friedlander, AH, Norman DC. Geriatric alcoholism: Pathophysiology and dental implications. *J Am Dent Assoc.* 2006; 137(3):330–338.
11. Shelly D, Cantrell J, Faulkner D, et al. Physician and dentist tobacco use counseling and adolescent smoking behavior: Results from the 2000 National Youth Tobacco Survey. *Pediatrics.* 2005;115(3):719–725.

24

Joint Disorders: Inflammatory Arthropathies and Gout

There are a variety of joint disorders resulting in pain and inflammation that prompt the individual to seek medical care and pharmacologic relief. These clients may have manifestations in the spinal column, requiring special patient positioning. Some clients may require total joint replacement, necessitating antibiotic prophylaxis prior to oral procedures. The variety of etiologies requires an assortment of differently acting pharmacologic agents. The scope of this chapter is limited to a discussion of pharmacologic strategies in the management of inflammatory **arthropathies** and **gout**. The implications for dental hygiene care are identified.

JOINT DISORDERS

Joint disorders may be infectious, inflammatory (rheumatoid arthritis [RA], juvenile rheumatoid arthritis [JRA], and

spondyloarthropathy), relatively less inflammatory (osteoarthritis [OA] and neurogenic arthropathy), or uric acid crystal induced (gout).

Acute Infectious Arthritis

Acute infectious arthritis is a joint infection that affects **synovial** or **periarticular** tissues and is usually bacterial in origin. Typically, in young adults, the causative organism is *Neisseria gonorrhoeae*, which has spread to a joint via the circulation. Symptoms include rapid onset of pain, effusion, and loss of function, usually within a single joint. Treatment is with intravenous (IV) antibiotics and drainage of purulent exudate from the joint.

Inflammatory Arthropathies

The various inflammatory arthropathies are discussed below. Pharmacologic treatment attempts to relieve symptoms of

Table 24-1	Disease-Modifying Antirheumatic Drugs	
Drug Classes	**Drugs**	**Oral Complications**

DMARDs	TNF inhibitors
	  etanercept
	  infliximab
	  adalimumab
		None

	Immunosuppressants
	  cyclosporine
	  azathioprine
	  methotrexate
		Stomatitis
		  (methotrexate)
		Gingival hyperplasia
		  (cyclosporine)

	Antimalarial agents hydrochloroquine Leflunomide	None

	Gold salts
	  gold sodium
	  thiomalate
	  auranofin
		Stomatitis

	Minocycline	Lupus erythematosus

	Monoclonal antibodies
	  rituximab
		Stevens-Johnson
		  syndrome
		Recurrent herpetic
		  lesions

NSAIDs	See Chapter 8 for additional information	
Corticosteroids	See Chapter 14 for additional information	

inflammation and reduce structural damage to joint tissues. Treatment options include disease-modifying antirheumatic drugs (DMARDs), nonsteroidal anti-inflammatory drugs (NSAIDs/COX inhibitors), and corticosteroids.[1] NSAIDs and corticosteroids are discussed in other chapters. Table 24-1 includes agents classified as DMARDs and their clinical implications for dentistry. A variety of agents are included in this category, including tumor necrosis factor (TNF) blocking agents, gold compounds, antimalarial agents, immunosuppressants, and monoclonal antibodies.

Rheumatoid Arthritis

RA is a chronic autoimmune disease producing damage to joint tissues mediated by inflammatory chemicals, such as cytokines, TNF-alpha, and metalloproteinases. Signs and symptoms include symmetrical inflammation of peripheral joints (e.g., wrists, **metacarpophalangeal** joints), often resulting in progressive destruction of articular surfaces. When the joints of the wrist and fingers are affected, the client may find it difficult to use conventional devices to complete oral hygiene procedures. RA affects about 1% of the general population. Women are affected two to three times more often than men. The classic characteristics are bilateral and symmetric chronic inflammation of the synovial membrane of joints. It may lead to the deterioration and eventual destruction of articular cartilage and bone, resulting in deformities of affected joints.[2] There are extra-articular manifestations of RA as well, including interstitial lung disease, pericardial disease, neutropenia, and xerostomia induced by the development of Sjögren syndrome.[2] Pain management of RA includes the administration of NSAIDs (also referred to as COX inhibitors in Chapter 8). Newer drugs are used to suppress the signs and symptoms of RA. These drugs are generally restricted to rapidly progressing or refractory cases of arthropathies and to patients unable to tolerate standard medications. They are

often referred to as disease-modifying antirheumatic drugs (DMARDs), because they alter the progression of the disease.

Oral Manifestations

Temporomandibular joint (TMJ) pain is a commonly reported complaint among clients with RA.[2] Radiographic findings can include narrow joint spaces, bone erosion, and osteoporosis. Those with longstanding RA may have an increased incidence of periodontal disease, loss of clinical attachment, and tooth loss. It does not appear that inadequate oral hygiene due to functional impairment is a primary factor in the periodontal disease.[3] Those who develop Sjögren syndrome may have excessively dry oral membranes leading to conditions associated with chronic dry mouth (such as caries, candidiasis, or the inability to wear removable prosthetic appliances).

Juvenile Rheumatoid Arthritis

JRA is of unknown etiology, but there appears to be a genetic predisposition and immune-mediated inflammation. The condition usually begins at or before the age of 16. There are three forms of JRA: **polyarticular**, **pauciarticular**, and systemic. The *polyarticular* form (affecting five or more joints) represents approximately 40% of cases. It tends to develop slowly and is similar to adult RA. The *pauciarticular* form (four or fewer joints) is similar in prevalence (40%) and is usually seen in young girls. It manifests as inflammation in the iris of the eye. The *systemic* form (20%) is characterized by fever, rash, splenomegaly, and generalized adenopathy, which usually precedes the development of arthritis. Pharmacologic management of JRA includes the administration of both NSAIDs (to reduce signs and symptoms of inflammation, such as pain and swelling) and DMARDs (to reduce structural damage to joints).

Spondylarthritis

Spondylarthritis (SA) is a systemic disorder that appears to have a genetic basis and probably involves immune-mediated inflammation. This condition usually begins between the ages of 20 and 40 and is characterized by fever, fatigue, anorexia, weight loss, inflammation of the axial skeleton and large peripheral joints, nocturnal back pain, and back stiffness. It is three times more common in men than in women. Pharmacologic management of SA includes the administration of NSAIDs and DMARDs. The client with this type of arthropathy can pose issues related to patient positioning during oral health care procedures if the spine is affected.

Less Inflammatory Arthropathies
Osteoarthritis

OA is a chronic arthropathy characterized by disruption and potential loss of joint cartilage and osteophyte formation. OA is the most common joint disorder, often becoming symptomatic between ages 40 and 50 and being almost universal by age 80. Women are predominately affected from ages 40 to 70, after which men and women are equally affected. This form of arthritis may be primary (idiopathic) or secondary (trauma, related to other disorders that alter the normal structure and function of hyaline cartilage). When the TMJ is affected, the condition is often painless and characterized by **crepitation** when the client chews or opens and closes the mouth. Most OA seen in men below age 40 is the result of trauma. It is characterized by gradual onset, with pain as the earliest symptom. Pain is usually worsened by putting weight on the joint, as in standing and walking, and is relieved by rest. Stiffness follows awakening or inactivity and lessens with movement. Pharmacologic management of OA includes the administration of NSAIDs, glucosamine sulfate, and chondroitin sulfate (supplied as over-the-counter supplements to increase cartilage formation).

Neuropathic Arthritis

Neuropathic arthritis (NA) is a rapidly destructive arthropathy due to impaired pain perception that results from various underlying disorders, most commonly diabetes mellitus and stroke. Pain is a common early manifestation of NA. However, it is often unexpectedly mild because of an impaired ability to sense pain. Other clinical manifestations of NA include joint swelling, deformity from bony overgrowth, and massive synovial effusion leading to instability. Treatment of underlying neurologic disorder may slow progression of the arthropathy.

■ **Self-Study Review**

1. Differentiate between inflammatory joint disorders and less-inflammatory joint disorders.
2. Describe the etiology and clinical features of acute infectious arthritis.
3. Describe the etiology and clinical features of the inflammatory arthropathies, and identify three pharmacologic therapies.
4. Identify an autoimmune disease that is often found in conjunction with RA.
5. Describe forms of JRA.
6. Describe the etiologic and clinical features of the less-inflammatory arthropathies.

Pharmacologic Therapy
Nonsteroidal Anti-Inflammatory Drugs

In the management of arthropathy-associated pain and inflammation, indications for the various NSAIDs are interchangeable, but some patients who do not respond to (or tolerate) one preparation may respond to or tolerate another. The physiologic effects of NSAIDs are due primarily to the inhibition of cyclooxygenase-1 (COX-1) and cyclooxygenase-2 (COX-2) isoenzymes. COX-1 is expressed in most tissues and is responsible for the synthesis of prostaglandins. COX-2 is expressed in various tissues, especially in kidney where it helps to maintain perfusion, and is found at sites of inflammation. Levels of COX-2 and prostaglandins are markedly elevated in the synovial fluid of inflamed joints. NSAIDs

(ibuprofen, naproxen, and others) at therapeutic doses block both COX-1 and COX-2 to varying degrees, while COX-2-selective inhibitors (celecoxib) at therapeutic doses selectively inhibit COX-2. At present, celecoxib (Celebrex) is the only FDA-approved agent of this type on the market. COX-1 and COX-2 inhibitors have analgesic and anti-inflammatory effects, but they have no disease-modifying effects on inflammatory arthropathies. For a more comprehensive discussion of NSAIDs, refer to Chapter 8.

Corticosteroids

Oral corticosteroids (e.g., prednisone) are indicated for rapid relief of symptoms associated with inflammatory joint disease and for control of systemic manifestations, yet most clinicians do not regard corticosteroids as DMARDs or use them as such because of the complications associated with long-term use. Intra-articular injection of a corticosteroid (triamcinolone, methylprednisolone) often can relieve an acutely inflamed arthritic joint with minimal adverse drug effects (ADEs). For a more comprehensive discussion of corticosteroids, refer to Chapter 14.

Disease-Modifying Antirheumatic Drugs

When the diagnosis of an inflammatory joint disease has been established, the general treatment strategy is to start treatment with a DMARD (Table 24-1) for the indication of preventing irreversible damage to joints and then use an NSAID, with or without a corticosteroid, to control symptoms of pain and swelling. When an effective DMARD regimen has been established, the use of NSAIDs and corticosteroids can be minimized. There are several immunomodulating agents that block destructive chemicals involved in the destructive process of chronic inflammation.

Tumor Necrosis Factor Blockers

Recently, immunomodulating agents that block TNF have been introduced with great success. These include etanercept (Enbrel), adalimumab (Humira), infliximab (Remicade), and abatacept (Orencia). They are administered by subcutaneous (SC) injection or by IV administration. Etanercept, the prototypical agent, is discussed here, but the other agents have similar drug effects. This immunomodulating drug is approved for ankylosing **spondylitis**, polyarticular JRA, and RA. The indication is to reduce the signs and symptoms of moderate-to-severe disease in patients who have had an inadequate response to one or more DMARDs. Etanercept can be used alone or in combination with methotrexate. The mechanism of action is that etanercept binds specifically to the cytokine, TNF, and blocks its interaction with TNF receptors, rendering the cytokine biologically inactive. Etanercept can also reduce biologic responses of chemicals induced by TNF, such as interleukins and matrix metalloproteinase. TNF plays a role in various inflammatory conditions, and elevated levels are found in tissues and fluids of patients with RA, SA, and psoriatic conditions. The drug is administered by a single SC injection every other day. It should not be given when sepsis (i.e., infection) or conditions that can metastasize (e.g., tuberculosis) are present or to those patients with conditions that make them at risk for recurrent infection, such as uncontrolled diabetes mellitus. ADEs include gastrointestinal (GI) effects (such as vomiting or abdominal pain), upper respiratory infection, and rare blood dyscrasias, leading to increased infection and bleeding.

Immunosuppressants

Agents in the immunosuppressant category include cyclosporine, azathioprine, and methotrexate. They are administered orally, or in some cases by intramuscular or IV injection, and they are effective in relieving symptoms of RA. Cyclosporine is mainly used to prevent organ rejection following organ transplant, but it can be used to manage signs and symptoms of arthropathy. When NSAID therapy is ineffective, methotrexate is the initial second-line drug. These immunosuppressants have general systemic effects and affect a number of components in the inflammatory response. ADEs are stomatitis, increased infection, blood dyscrasias (thrombocytopenia, bone marrow suppression), GI distress, and **nephrotoxicity**. Cyclosporine is associated with causing gingival hyperplasia. They are used only when NSAID therapy has failed. Methotrexate should not be used concurrently with NSAIDs, because they can displace methotrexate from plasma protein binding sites and the resulting increased blood levels cause toxicity. Cyclosporine is metabolized by CYP3A4 isoenzymes, and inhibitors of this enzyme used in dentistry (erythromycin, clarithromycin, azole antifungals) can cause an increase in cyclosporin blood levels, resulting in toxicity.

Antimalarial Agents

Hydroxychloroquine is an orally administered drug used to prevent malaria. Other pharmacologic immunosuppressive properties make it useful in treating arthropathies, such as RA. It is indicated for treatment of acute or chronic RA patients who have not responded satisfactorily to drugs with less potential for serious side effects. This drug is used for malaria prophylaxis at 300 mg/day, and doses are increased (400 to 600 mg initially) for the antirheumatic effect, leveling off to 200 to 400 mg/day when an adequate response is obtained. There are no drug interactions with agents used in dentistry. The most common ADEs involve vision abnormalities, dizziness, and (rarely) blood dyscrasias.

Leflunomide

Leflunomide is an oral doseform that inhibits an enzyme involved in pyrimidine synthesis. The resulting anti-inflammatory and antiproliferative effects make it useful for RA. The most common ADEs relevant to oral care include abdominal pain, nausea, and cough, although mucosal ulcerations, dry mouth, and taste disturbances are occasionally reported. There are no dental drug interactions.

Gold Salts

Due to their relative toxicity, gold products are now restricted to RA. They are indicated in active cases in which arthritis progresses despite the patient's using NSAIDs, getting adequate rest, and exercising. Gold-related agents used to induce remission of disease are aurothioglucose and auranofin. The mechanism of action for gold-related agents is unknown, but the net effect is a suppression of inflammation and suppression of inflammatory chemicals. These compounds are administered by injection, but there is also an oral doseform of auranofin. Serious ADEs are possible, as are oral ulceration and glossitis. Blood dyscrasias have been reported (leukopenia, agranulocytosis, anemia). These ADEs are dose related and more likely to develop with high-dose therapy. There are no reported interactions with drugs used in dentistry.

Minocycline

Minocycline, a derivative of tetracycline, is used because of its antimatrix metalloproteinase side effect, which is used therapeutically in periodontal inflammation. This inflammatory chemical causes destruction of collagen in the gingival connective tissue and destruction of other collagen-based tissues in the body, such as cartilage. Refer to Chapter 9 for a more detailed discussion of this drug.

Monoclonal Antibodies

Rituximab is a genetically engineered monoclonal antibody approved in 1997 to be used, in combination with methotrexate, to reduce signs and symptoms of moderate-to-severe active RA in adult patients who have had an inadequate response to one or more TNF-antagonist therapies. It is administered as an IV infusion once weekly for four doses (the first course of therapy), and up to eight doses (the second course of therapy if results are inadequate). Corticosteroids are administered by IV prior to each infusion to reduce the incidence and severity of infusion reactions. The mechanism of action is specific binding to a human B lymphocyte antigen that is involved in regulating the early phase of the cell cycle process. Lymphocytic B cells are believed to play a role in the pathogenesis of RA, including activation of the production of rheumatoid factor and other autoantibodies, antigen presentation, T-cell activation, and other proinflammatory cytokine production. The action of rituximab functions to initiate B cell lysis in order to deplete circulating and tissue-based B cells, and it causes significant reductions in IgM and IgG serum antibody levels for up to 6 months postinfusion. The majority of patients showed peripheral B cell depletion for up to 6 months, followed by gradual recovery after that time point. Interleukins and C-reactive protein biologic markers were also reduced. Potential ADEs of interest to dentistry include an increased risk for infection, reactivation of viral diseases (including *herpes simplex*), cardiac arrhythmia and angina, and severe mucocutaneous reactions (Stevens-Johnson syndrome, pemphigus, and others). Monitoring for the development of blood dyscrasia, pulse rate and rhythm, and recent history of angina is recommended.

Clinical Considerations

Individuals with arthropathies may have limited jaw movement, affecting the efficacy of oral hygiene procedures and diminishing the ability to open the mouth enough to accommodate oral procedures. Arthritis may affect the TMJ in the same way as other joints are affected—by causing pain, stiffness, and altered growth (in children). Jaw exercises are recommended to increase the range of opening the mouth. In children if the lower jaw does not develop properly, an overbite may develop, necessitating orthodontic treatment. Some clients may have experienced recent joint replacements that may require prophylactic antibiotics prior to dental hygiene care. Stamina may be affected, necessitating short appointments and use of a mouth prop to relieve muscle fatigue. Side effects (such as poor healing, bleeding, infection, or gingival hyperplasia) for each agent should be investigated and considered during the oral examination. When Sjögren syndrome accompanies RA, xerostomia will require management.

Self-Study Review

7. Identify indications for NSAIDs. What inflammatory chemical is elevated in synovial fluid of inflamed joints?
8. Identify indications for corticosteroids in managing joint arthropathy.
9. Identify the indications to prescribe a DMARD in the pharmacologic therapy that also includes an NSAID.
10. Be able to recognize a DMARD within a list of drugs.
11. Identify the routes of administration of the various pharmacologic therapies for arthropathy.
12. Identify side effects of the various agents that are relevant to oral health care.
13. Identify cyclosporine and methotrexate drug interactions with drugs used in dentistry.
14. How long does the monoclonal antibody effect last?
15. List clinical considerations for a client with joint arthropathy.

GOUT

Gout is arthropathy caused by an imbalance in purine metabolism, resulting in increased uric acid levels that localize in joint spaces. To understand the cause and treatment of gouty arthritis, it is necessary to recall the physiologic principles of nucleotide synthesis. There are five different types of nucleotides found in DNA: Adenine (A), guanine (G), cytosine (C), thymine (T), and uracil (U). Cytosine, thymine, and uracil are pyrimidines. The pyrimidines are readily synthesized, and their metabolic byproducts are easily excreted by the kidneys. Adenine and guanine are purines. Purine synthesis is complex, and the intermediates of purine metabolism are toxic, necessitating tight regulation of purine synthesis and degradation. The final breakdown product of purine metabolism is uric acid, which is barely soluble in blood or urine. If too much uric acid is formed, or too little is excreted in the kidney, uric acid crystals are deposited in joints and surrounding tissues, leading to the development of gout. Urate crystals in the joints and surrounding tissues attract leucocytes, which initiate phagocytosis and the release of chemical mediators of inflammation in the process. Acute attacks often involve the first metatarsophalangeal joint (the big toe). Symptoms include pain, tenderness, warmth, red-

| Table 24-2 | Clinical Features and Pharmacologic Strategies to Treat or Prevent Gout |

Disease Stage	Clinical Features	Pharmacologic Strategies
Hyperuricemia (asymptomatic)	Plasma urate >6 mg/dL in women; >7 mg/dL in men	None
Acute gout	Hyperuricemia Acute arthritis Excruciating pain	NSAIDs Colchicine Glucocorticoids
Chronic gout	Hyperuricemia Development of tophi Recurrent acute attacks	Allopurinol Probenecid Sulfinpyrazone

ness, and swelling. Gout occurs in approximately 0.6% of men and 0.1% of women, primarily after menopause. Drugs from several pharmacologic classes are used to treat and prevent gout (Table 24-2).

Pharmacologic Therapy
Acute Gout

Metabolites of arachidonic acid play an important role in the inflammatory response that enhances the formation of urate crystal deposits in joints. NSAIDs inhibit COX and thereby inhibit prostaglandin and thromboxane synthesis. They affect the inflammatory response to form urate crystals and the associated pain. Clinically, indomethacin is one of the NSAIDs used most often to treat an acute attack of gout. The serious ADEs of NSAIDs include bleeding, salt and water retention, and renal insufficiency.

Colchicine

Colchicine is classified as an antigout agent. In an acutely inflamed joint, colchicine inhibits microtubule formation, which is critical for the alignment and separation of chromosomes during mitosis, and inhibits leukocyte migration and phagocytic activity. In low doses it may be used in the management of chronic gout to inhibit the occurrence of acute attacks. Colchicine inhibits the turnover of epithelial cells in the gastrointestinal tract, and diarrhea is a common complication of therapy. Colchicine has an additional myelosuppressive action.

Glucocorticoids

Glucocorticoids (such as prednisone or methylprednisolone) have powerful anti-inflammatory and immunosuppressive effects and inhibit numerous steps in the inflammatory process during an acute attack of gout. Glucocorticoids have widespread ADEs when administered systemically, so their use is limited for the treatment of acute polyarticular gout or for when there are contraindications, such as renal insufficiency, to other effective therapies. When an acute attack of gout occurs in a single joint and is unresponsive to NSAIDs or colchicine, methylprednisolone can be injected directly into the site of inflammation.

Chronic Gout

Agents That Decrease Uric Acid Synthesis

Allopurinol (Zyloprim) and oxypurinol inhibit xanthine oxidase, an enzyme essential for the conversion of intermediates of purine metabolism to uric acid. The accumulated moderately water-soluble intermediates can be filtered in the kidney. Allopurinol is generally well tolerated. A small number of patients may develop a hypersensitivity reaction characterized by a rash that, in rare instances, can progress to Stevens-Johnson syndrome. For this reason, all patients who develop a cutaneous reaction (rash) to allopurinol should discontinue the drug. The coadministration of amoxicillin and ampicillin may increase the risk of a severe allopurinol-related rash developing. Rarely, allopurinol may cause leukopenia and hepatic necrosis.

Agents That Decrease Uric Acid Excretion

Probenecid and sulfinpyrazone are uricosuric agents that inhibit renal tubule anion exchange and increase the excretion of uric acid. Because probenecid and sulfinpyrazone inhibit the secretion of most anions, they increase the bioavailability of penicillin. Low-dose aspirin may antagonize the action of probenecid. Sulfinpyrazone has an antiplatelet effect; it may cause significant bleeding in patients taking other antiplatelet drugs or anticoagulants.

■ Self-Study Review

16. Describe the etiology and common areas affected by gout.
17. Differentiate between pharmacologic therapy for *acute* gout and *chronic* gout.
18. Which antibiotics should be avoided when allopurinol therapy has produced an associated cutaneous reaction?

DENTAL HYGIENE APPLICATIONS

During planning of the appointment, the following issues should be considered: Can the client open the mouth wide enough to accommodate oral procedures? Should a mouth prop be offered for client comfort? When total joint replacement is reported, is the client in a category that needs antibiotic prophylaxis prior to oral care? Determination of the stamina of the client will affect appointment time scheduling. Patients with longstanding active RA may have increased periodontal destruction. In this condition, it does not appear that inadequate oral hygiene resulting from functional impairment is a primary factor in periodontal disease.[3]

Each drug in the pharmacologic management of arthropathy should be investigated in a drug reference for drug effects that may affect oral health care procedures. Increased infec-

---

> **BOX 24-1.** Dental Hygiene Management of the Client with Arthropathy
>
> Evaluate the limitation of TMJ and consider the use of a mouth prop.
> For a patient with total joint replacement, evaluate the need for antibiotic prophylaxis prior to oral care.
> Determine the need for a short appointment schedule.
> Investigate each agent in pharmacologic therapy for drug effects relevant to the oral care plan.
> Investigate the need to adjust the dental chair to a semisupine position.
> Determine the need for a power toothbrush.
> Include the importance of maintaining oral health and adopting a periodontal maintenance schedule appropriate to oral health in the oral health education discussion.

tion can result from drug therapy. When chronic xerostomia is reported (as in Sjögren syndrome), fluoride therapy may be indicated.[4] Caries may progress despite excellent home care, use of fluoride, and avoidance of cariogenic foods.[2] Chair position may need to be adjusted to a semisupine position, according to the client's comfort level and degree of back pain. If hands are affected, a recommendation of powered devices for effective plaque control can be considered. Oral health education should include the need to avoid oral/periodontal infection, because most agents suppress the inflammatory response. Anti-inflammatory drug effects may indicate a need for a 3- to 4-month maintenance schedule. Box 24-1 summarizes dental hygiene applications.

CONCLUSION

Clients with inflammatory arthropathies can present with situations that may cause changes in the dental hygiene treatment plan, including back pain, disfigured finger joints, and various effects from pharmacologic treatment. Treatment should be provided based on the ability of the individual to receive oral health care.

References

1. Abramowicz M. Treatment guidelines for rheumatoid arthritis. *Treat Guidel Med Lett.* 2005;40(3):83–90.
2. Treister N, Glick M. Rheumatoid arthritis: A review and suggested dental care considerations. *J Am Dent Assoc.* 1999;130(5): 689–698.
3. Kaber UR, Gleissner C, Dehne F, et al. Risk for periodontal disease in patients with longstanding rheumatoid arthritis. *Arthritis Rheum.* 1997;40:2248–2251.
4. Russell SL, Reisine S. Investigation of xerostomia in patients with rheumatoid arthritis. *J Am Dent Assoc.* 1998;129:733–739.

CLINICAL APPLICATION EXERCISES

☐ **Exercise 1.** Investigate the drug etanercept (Enbrel) in a dental drug reference. What are potential drug interactions with drugs used by the dental hygienist? Which ADEs can impact the clinical treatment plan? Describe information to include in the oral health education plan.

☐ **Exercise 2.** WEB ACTIVITY: Log on to the Arthritis Foundation Web site to read their recommendations for treating JRA (http://ww2.arthritis.org/conditions/DiseaseCenter/JRA/treated_eye_dental_diet.asp) and consider related dental care advice.

Appendix

Answers to Clinical Application Exercises

CHAPTER 1

Exercise 1. Example of proper format for drug card on Evista:

Raloxifene (Evista)

- Indication: Bone mineral density (BMD) improvement, prevention of osteoporosis
- Adverse/side effects: Hot flashes, nausea, vomiting, dyspepsia, cough, sinusitis, arthralgia
- Clinical consideration: None of the adverse effects are occurring, but periodontal examination is suggested to determine effects of osteoporosis on oral health.
- Oral health information: Inform the client to notify you if a medication change is made for BMD.

Exercise 2. *Metformin* is taken to control blood glucose levels associated with type II diabetes. It is sold under the brand name Glucophage or Glucophage XR. Dental hygiene treatment plan modifications might include questioning the client to determine the degree of control of diabetes; monitoring for signs of hypoglycemia when other antidiabetic agents are used in combination with metformin; determining if the gastrointestinal (GI) side effects (nausea, abdominal pain) are present and, if so, using a semisupine chair position to provide for comfort during treatment; examining the periodontium for signs of infection and, if disease is found, recommending a more frequent maintenance schedule (3 months, rather than 6 months).

CHAPTER 2

Exercise 1. The antacid medication will influence the pH of the GI tract, so an acidic drug (such as aspirin or other non-steroidal anti-inflammatory drugs [NSAIDs]) will be ionized due to the change in the pH of the stomach and upper small intestines to a more basic pH. This can delay distribution of the drug through biologic membranes. Three options are available: (a) ask the patient to take the aspirin or NSAID an hour before taking the TUMS or 3 hours after taking the TUMS, (b) ask if the TUMS can be stopped for the day of the periodontal débridement, or (c) recommend an analgesic in a weak base form, such as acetaminophen, so the drug molecules will be in a nonionized state. Nonionized drug molecules can cross biologic membranes easily.

Exercise 2. The sublingual formulation of the vasodilating drug will get the drug into the circulation quickly due to the large circulation area of oral tissues and due to the rapid venous return from the sublingual area to the heart and coronary arteries. Nitroglycerin is often prescribed for sublingual administration for chest pain.

Exercise 3. Elderly patients with excess fat should have lower doses of narcotics, because these drugs concentrate in fat and can be released over time, causing a risk of toxicity.

CHAPTER 3

Exercise 1. Questions: "What time did you take the antibiotic today?" "What antibiotic was prescribed?" "What dose did you take?" "Have you noticed any problems since you took the antibiotic?" Treatment record notation: Amoxicillin 2 g taken 1 hour prior to appointment (7:00 AM) for antibiotic prophylaxis, no complications.

Exercise 2. Is the prescription written in ink? Is the prescriber's name, address, and phone identified on the prescription? Is the patient's name, address, and date on the prescription? Is the dentist's DEA number listed? Did the dentist sign the prescription? Is the section "no refills" marked?

Exercise 3. Look at the date of the prescription and the date when it should be refilled. Verify that the expiration date has not passed.

CHAPTER 4

Exercise 1. The effects of the sympathetic branch of the automatic nervous system (ANS) will likely be experienced. Expect tachycardia, elevated levels of blood pressure compared to the normal limits usually experienced by the patient, dry mouth or excessive mucoid salivation, and an increase in blood sugar (hyperglycemia).

Exercise 2. The drugs pilocarpine or cevimeline are often prescribed for xerostomia-related oral problems. These drugs are cholinergic agonists and promote the effects of the parasympathetic nervous system (salivation, lacrimation, urination, defecation). When chronic xerostomia is reported, the teeth should be examined for caries and the mucosa examined for candidiasis. A periodontal exam should be completed.

Exercise 3. The brand name is Pro-Banthine. The drug is an anticholinergic, or muscarinic blocking, agent. Its mechanism of action is to block muscarinic receptors, produce smooth muscle relaxation in the GI tract, and reduce acidity and volume of GI secretions. It is indicated for the treatment of peptic ulcers. Potential adverse effects that may influence the treatment plan include dry mouth, dizziness, tremor, palpitations, bradycardia, nausea, blurred vision, and photophobia. Clinical implications: (a) assess salivation and, if needed, follow protocol for dry mouth (fluoride, xylitol gum); (b) use semisupine chair position if GI pain or acidity is problematic; (c) monitor pulse rate and rhythm; (d) do not shine overhead dental light in eyes; offer dark glasses; (e) frequent recall if oral side effects cause dental disease.

CHAPTER 5

Exercise 1. This exercise is an experience to identify the clinical manifestations of various adverse drug effects. There is no written answer for this exercise.

Exercise 2. The American Academy of Oral Medicine's recommendations for the role of the dental hygienist include explaining to the client that taking a bisphosphonate (BIS) for 3 or more years (oral doseform) or for 6 months (IV doseform) puts the patient at increased risk for osteonecrosis of the jaw. This is a rare side effect associated with drugs in this category. Ways to prevent the condition are unknown at this time, but it is thought that maintaining oral health with regular dental visits and daily home care to remove biofilm is the best method. If the drug is taken to prevent osteoporosis,

the client should be advised to consult with the physician to have a bone density test to determine if the drug still needs to be taken. It is felt that having oral surgery, periodontal surgery involving removal of bone, or any oral surgical procedure is contraindicated until more is known about the risk factors for the development of the condition.

Exercise 3. The client answer should include signs and symptoms of allergy: Rash, itching, erythema, hives. An answer of "nausea, vomiting" would be an adverse effect of codeine, not an allergy.

CHAPTER 6

Exercise 1. When lidocaine is injected apically, the normal tissue pH is approximately 7.3. The drug disassociates to 80% cation form (water soluble), which disperses through connective tissue and reaches the nerve. The other 20% is the base, which is lipid soluble and penetrates the nerve sheath, reaching the axoplasm where the nerve fiber is located. The base disassociates to a 90% cation (24 mg) and 10% base (2.7 mg) due to a 7.0 pH inside the nerve. The cation form binds to receptors in the sodium channels and blocks the nerve impulse.

Inflamed area: The pH changes to a more acidic nature of 6.5. The pH change causes lidocaine to disassociate to 96% cation and only 4% base. This base penetrates the nerve sheath and disassociates to 10.3 mg cation (less than half of the normal concentration) and 1.1 mg base. The low concentration of cation is inadequate to bind to enough receptors to block the impulse conduction effectively.

Exercise 2. Armamentarium: Lidocaine 1:50,000 (one cartridge) for good hemostasis in gingival area; use an aspirating technique to avoid injection into the artery.

Area of injection: Mandibular block for profound anesthesia and to avoid risks associated with acidic pH of gingival area due to inflammation, plus infiltration within attached gingivae of quadrant for hemostasis.

Treatment record entry: Lidocaine 2% (36 mg), EPI 0.018 mg given by infiltration; *or* 1.8 mL lidocaine 2% with 1:100,000 epinephrine, by infiltration.

Exercise 3. Orajel: Benzocaine is the active ingredient; ester local anesthetic. Use: Pain relief when topically applied to oral mucous membranes. Benzocaine is poorly absorbed through mucosa, making it safe in individuals not allergic to esters.

CHAPTER 7

Exercise 1. You will check the list of products accepted by the American Dental Association (ADA) at *http://www.ada.org/ada/seal/category.asp* and search the list for the products in the "toothpaste" and the "mouthrinse" categories. Toothpaste products are listed under the manufacturers which are listed alphabetically. Find the Proctor & Gamble listing and review their approved products. The types of fluoride are not identified in any manufacturer. Access the mouthrinse category. Look at the products under Johnson & Johnson. As of December 2008 only OTC consumer products are eligible for the Seal of Acceptance, and prescription products won't receive Seal approval.

Exercise 2. The rinse is to be used twice a day, preferably at night before going to bed and after breakfast in the morning. Toothbrushing with a dentifrice and the chlorhexidine rinse should be separated by 1 to 2 hours to allow for removal of sodium laurel sulfate from the oral fluids. Side effects may include increased calculus, extrinsic staining, mucosal ulceration, and taste disturbance. Inform the patient that the rinse contains alcohol and to avoid using products that interact with alcohol.

Exercise 3. The answer will correspond to individual findings. The exercise is for personal information.

CHAPTER 8

Exercise 1. A Google search for the Top 200 Drugs in 2007 will bring up several sources (such as *http://www.drugs.com*, *http://www.pharmacytimes.com*).

Exercise 2. From *Dental Drug Reference with Clinical Implications* (LWW 2009), clinical considerations are differentiated from the drug being prescribed by a dentist or being prescribed by medical personnel. The dentist must consider lactation, the age of the patient, the health of the liver, a history of alcoholism, special patient categories (such as elderly, respiratory disease, others), and those with sulfite sensitivity. Potential side effects must be explained and monitored; inquire about other drug therapy being taken by the patient. Oral Health Information: "This prescription contains acetaminophen, the same drug in Tylenol, and if you take more over-the-counter (OTC) acetaminophen or nonaspirin agents for pain, you can get an overdose leading to liver failure. Don't use additional analgesics you have at home. If this drug isn't effective to control your pain, call your physician. Do not wait for pain to start before taking this prescription—get it filled and take it as soon as you get home."

Exercise 3. Aspirin: Arthritis Foundation Pain Reliever, Aspergum, Bayer Children's Aspirin, Bayer Low Adult Strength, Easprin, Ecotrin, Ecotrin Adult Low Strength, Ecotrin Maximum Strength, Empirin, Extended Release Bayer 8-Hour, Extra Strength Bayer, Genprin, Genuine Bayer, 1/2 Halfprin, Halfprin 81, Heartline, Maximum Bayer, Norwich Extra-Strength, St. Joseph Adult Chewable Aspirin, ZORprin.
    CANADA: Alka-Seltzer Flavoured, Asaphen, Asaphen E.C., Entrophen, MSD Enteric Coated ASA, Novasen.
    Acetaminophen: Acephen, Aceta, Acetaminophen Uniserts, Apacet, Anacin Aspirin Free Extra Strength, Aspirin

Free Pain Relief, Children's Dynafed Jr., Children's Fever-All, Children's Genapap, Children's Halenol, Children's Panadol, Children's Silapap, Children's Tylenol, Dapacin, Extra Strength Dynafed E.X., FeverAll, FeverAll Jr. Strength, Genapap, Genapap Extra Strength, Genebs, Genebs X-Tra, Liquiprin, Mapap Children's, Maranox, Meda Cap, Neopap, Oraphen-PD, Panadol, Redutemp, Ridenol, Tapanol, Tempra, Tylenol Arthritis, Tylenol Caplets, Tylenol 8 Hour Extended Relief, Uni-Ace, among others.
    CANADA: Abenol, Apo-Acetaminophen, Atasol, Pediatrix

Exercise 4. The client with a history of asthma may have an allergy to aspirin and aspirin-related medications, such as COX inhibitors. The questions to ask are: "Can you take drugs like ibuprofen?" "When you take an NSAID, do you have symptoms of rhinorrhea (runny nose), urticaria (hives, itching), angioedema (swelling around the mouth, lips), or bronchospasm (difficulty breathing) after taking any pain-relieving medication?"

CHAPTER 9

Exercise 1. Because a penicillin allergy exists, amoxicillin and cephalexin would not be prescribed. Warfarin interacts with the macrolide clarithromycin. The choices are clindamycin or azithromycin.

Exercise 2. When you call to verify the appointment the night before, ask if the antibiotic prescription has been filled, and instruct the patient to take the medication (four 500-mg tablets) 30 minutes to 1 hour prior to the appointment. The day of the appointment, after updating the medical history and vital signs, ask what time the antibiotic tablets were taken (has 30 minutes passed?), how many tablets were taken (four 500-mg tabs for 2 g), and whether any adverse effects have been noticed since the medication was taken. Record all information in the treatment record.

CHAPTER 10

Exercise 1. When nystatin is prescribed by the dentist and the dental hygienist is to instruct the patient on how to take the specific formulation, the directions to the patient are as follows:

- Infant: Tell the parent to give 15 drops to the infant four times daily, on each side of the mouth; clean the dropper after use.
- Child: The frozen nystatin popsicle would be the easiest doseform because it is difficult for the child to hold liquid in mouth for 5 minutes. Allow the frozen pop to dissolve in the mouth, and use five times daily (can be used for adults, also).

- Rinse (suspension): Swish and hold nystatin liquid in mouth approximately 5 minutes, then expectorate; use five times daily.
- Pastille: Place in the mouth and allow to dissolve; use five times daily.
- Cream: Apply cream to denture base that will contact tissue, or apply cream to the area of infection on the palate or other tissue, then place denture; use five times daily.

Exercise 2. Apply Denavir antiviral agent at the first sign of prodrome and reapply every 2 hours (q2h) for 4 days.

CHAPTER 11

Exercise 1. Proper technique of administration should include ensuring that equipment is operational and that the mask has been placed so that the scavenging system is properly functioning, as well as talking with the patient to determine the degree of cognitive function as nitrous oxide is added to gaseous oxygen. The initial administration of 100% oxygen is begun, and nitrous is added slowly. The patient response is monitored to determine when "tingling" is felt. This level is individualized to the patient and may be 30% to 40% nitrous and 70% to 60% oxygen, or approach a 50% to 50% concentration. Vital signs must be monitored every few minutes during the procedure. At the end of the procedure, 100% oxygen must be provided for at least 5 minutes to avoid diffusion hypoxia. Postprocedure instructions should be provided related to potential adverse effects, such as headache. Treatment record entries must include the N_2O concentrations implemented and the length of administration time for the patient.

Exercise 2. Vital signs are indicative of the patient's physical and emotional state, but they do not contraindicate administration of nitrous oxide. Blood pressure values are considered "high normal," the pulse rate is at the upper level of normal, and the respiration is at the upper limits of normal. All indicate a stress response is occurring.

Exercise 3. For a child below the legal age of 18, parental permission is necessary. A consent form signed by the parent or guardian will suffice.

Exercise 4. Chart entry notation: Nitrous oxide administered for 30 minutes at 50% nitrous to 50% oxygen ratio. Vital signs remained in normal range during the procedure.

CHAPTER 12

Exercises 1 and 2 should be completed according to the program's emergency kit contents and oxygen equipment.

Exercise 3. Prior to initiating dental hygiene services, ensure that the patient has brought the personal rescue inhaler to the appointment and has it available for use as needed. Treatment record dialogue: "During treatment the patient began coughing and demonstrated signs of breathing difficulty. It appeared the patient experienced an acute asthma event. Patient was positioned to an upright position and allowed to retrieve bronchodilator inhaler (albuterol). Patient used inhaler twice over a 5-minute period. Oxygen at 10 L/minute with face mask was provided. Signs began to improve. It appeared that fear of the procedure initiated the asthma event. After 10 to 15 minutes, the coughing stopped, breathing improved, and the patient seemed to recover from the asthmatic event. The pulse was still elevated at 102 bpm and respiration was high normal (20 bpm), although still raspy. It was decided to reschedule the appointment and recommend medical assessment for asthma control. Medical consultation will be completed by the dentist regarding the need for an oral anti-anxiety medication prior to dental treatment."

CHAPTER 13

Exercise 1. With a history of painful intraoral conditions that keep the individual from being able to eat, the dentist will likely recommend a topical corticosteroid, such as fluocinonide (Lidex) or clobetasol (Temovate). Application instructions are to apply a dab of the agent with a cotton-tipped applicator to the affected area four to five times per day, as needed. If pain relief is needed to allow the individual to eat, the cream should be applied 30 to 45 minutes before the meal to allow the drug to work and reduce inflammation. Otherwise, the drug is applied after meals, with no rinsing following application, and at bedtime. The agent is used until the ulcer heals, up to 2 weeks.

Exercise 2. The only OTC product approved by the Food and Drug Administration to be used on herpes labialis is docosanol (Abreva). It is applied with a cotton-tipped applicator at the first sign of prodrome or at the earliest stage of the lesion. It can be used five times per day until the lesion heals, and it will reduce the pain associated with a herpes outbreak when applied in the early stages.

CHAPTER 14

Exercise 1. When Fosamax, a BIS, is listed on the health history, one should initially ask how long the drug has been taken. BIS taken for 3 years or longer are associated with the development of osteonecrosis of the jaw. Provide the ADA Patient Information sheet on BIS. Explain that a rare side effect may develop in which bone in the jaw dies. Describe the signs (pain; exposed bone of the jaw, often on the lingual area of the mandible along the mylohyoid ridge; purulent exudate) and tell the patient that the dentist should be notified if these signs develop. Caution that dental disease should be repaired in the early stages before the surrounding bone is affected and that a 3- to 6-month maintenance schedule should identify early dental disease. Provide plaque control skill information as a strategy to assist the individual in maintaining periodontal health.

Exercise 2. When insulin is taken, the individual has type I diabetes. The most common emergency is hypoglycemia, often occurring when insulin is administered and not followed with a meal. Ask the patient when the last dose of insulin was injected and if a meal was consumed after insulin administration. Question the patient about the history of hypoglycemia and how often it occurs to identify the risk during dental hygiene care. After determining how well diabetes is controlled, determine the numbers for the daily blood sugar levels and what value the A1C test revealed. This gives additional information on blood sugar control. Healing problems are possible when blood sugar levels are extremely high (>200). Hypoglycemia is a risk when blood sugar levels are low (<60).

Exercise 3. Use this resource from the American Association of Oral and Maxillofacial Surgeons to investigate information related to BIS-induced osteonecrosis of the jaw.

CHAPTER 15

Exercise 1. Chemical erosion is an oral complication of gastroesophageal reflux disease (GERD), and teeth in this condition can be sensitive. When taken together, Prevacid and clarithromycin (a macrolide) can result in black tongue and glossitis.

Exercise 2. The disease can predispose the patient to regurgitation if placed in the supine position. Questioning the patient to determine the degree of disease control and patient desire related to supine or semisupine chair positioning will be needed. Oral examination will include investigation into chemical erosion from the disease effects. If chemical erosion is found, oral health information will include a warning to rinse with diluted bicarbonate of soda solution and to refrain from brushing the teeth for an hour to prevent removal of enamel. Teeth will be assessed for caries and recommendations made for caries control, as needed. The drugs taken to relieve signs and symptoms of GERD will be investigated for side effects the patient experienced that affect dental hygiene procedures, and alterations in the treatment plan will be made.

Exercise 3. Any acidic drug is contraindicated for peptic ulcer disease. Those analgesics that are acidic include aspirin and COX inhibitors. Acetaminophen would be the indicated analgesic for this medical history.

CHAPTER 16

Exercise 1. The patient must be assessed for infectiousness to the clinician. Measure the temperature to identify a patient with an active, contagious infection. If temperature is within normal limits, assess respiration qualities (sounds apparent?) to determine the need for a semiupright chair position if congestion is present. Monitor possible side effects of current drug therapy (increased blood pressure, tachycardia, xerostomia) by taking vital signs. If xerostomia is possible, recommend home fluoride products.

Exercise 2. The dental hygiene applications in Box 16-2 should be implemented. Drugs are being taken according to the manufacturer recommendations, indicating adequate disease control. Flonase is an inhaled steroid, and a recommendation should be made to rinse the mouth after each use. The oral mucosa should be examined for candidiasis. Maxair is an aerosolized bronchodilator and should be brought to each dental hygiene appointment in case of a bronchoconstriction emergency during the appointment. Aerosolized medications can dry oral tissues and increase plaque and calculus levels. Attention to effective methods for effective oral hygiene may need to be addressed.

Exercise 3. WEB ACTIVITY: This chlorofluorocarbon (CFC) inhaler is thought to be harmful to the ozone layer and is being replaced with the metered-dose inhaler that does not use CFC. This rule establishes December 31, 2008, as the date by which production and sale of single ingredient albuterol CFC metered-dose inhalers (MDIs) must stop, by removing the essential use designation for albuterol MDIs under 2.125.

ODS are substances that deplete stratospheric ozone. They include CFCs. Once released, CFCs rise to the stratosphere. Within the stratosphere, there is a zone about 10 to 25 miles above the Earth's surface in which ozone is relatively highly concentrated. Once in the stratosphere, CFCs are gradually broken down by strong ultraviolet light, and they release chlorine atoms that then deplete stratospheric ozone. Depletion of stratospheric ozone by CFCs and other ODS leads to higher ultraviolet B radiation levels, which in turn has increased skin cancers and cataracts, as well as caused other significant environmental damage. Albuterol MDIs have historically used the CFCs trichlorofluoromethane (CFC-11) and dichlorodifluoromethane (CFC-12) as propellants, both of which are potent and previously common ODS.

CHAPTER 17

Exercise 1. The patient should be asked if he or she has a prescription for nitroglycerin in case of an acute anginal attack. If the answer is "yes," look at the "Refill by [date]" on the label to ensure the drug is still active. To determine if the anginal condition is under control, inquire when the last anginal event occurred and what was done to resolve the pain. Patients who are taking medication to prevent angina, but who are still having episodes, should be referred for medical evaluation before providing stressful dental hygiene treatment. The patient should be instructed to bring the nitroglycerin prescription to the appointment. In the event the prescription is out of date, the patient should secure a new prescription and bring that product to the appointment.

Exercise 2. The patient should be questioned to determine if there was a dose adjustment at the last lab visit. When INR levels are within normal limits and below a level of 3, the patient is told to continue taking the current prescription. When INR levels are increased, the patient is given a prescription for a reduced dose. Inquire about the date of the last lab visit; if it has been a week or longer following the dose adjustment, dental hygiene procedures can be provided. If no change was made to the current prescription, that would indicate INR levels were in an acceptable range. To determine drugs that can affect the INR values, ask the patient if any drugs not usually taken have been recently added. If the patient has started taking a drug that interacts with warfarin, no treatment that could cause bleeding is recommended until after the patient has an INR lab test to determine the risk for hemorrhage.

CHAPTER 18

Exercise 1. Inform the client that the drug will cause sedation and that the patient should have someone bring him or her to the appointment and take him or her home following the appointment. The client should not sign important papers or return to work that requires thought and concentration. Advise against consuming alcohol the day of the appointment. If pain develops, COX inhibitors (ibuprofen or aspirin) can be used, but not acetaminophen. Provide instructions in written form due to amnesia from drug effects.

Exercise 2. Tardive dyskinesia can complicate intraoral procedures. Taking care when working in the mouth is essential when sharp instruments are being used. Observe the pattern of tongue movements and try to avoid contact between the instrument tip and the tongue. Panorex radiography may be the only type of radiograph that can be achieved in this condition.

Exercise 3. Follow the concepts included in Box 18-2.

CHAPTER 19

Exercise 1. Tonic–clonic epilepsy poses a risk for a seizure during oral health care. The past history of control of the seizure disorder with phenytoin reduces the risk. A recent medication change, however, prompts the need for patient monitoring for seizure control during treatment. Stress reduction should be considered, and local anesthesia to reduce pain is appropriate. The oral exam should assess the possibility of gingival hyperplasia and chronic xerostomia. The effects of phenytoin on gingival enlargement and the need for daily, regular plaque removal should be stressed in the oral health education plan. Patient abilities in use of oral hygiene devices should be evaluated. If caries is found, home fluoride products used on a daily basis (such as dentifrice

and mouth rinse) should be recommended. A 3-month maintenance interval should be considered due to the oral side effects of phenytoin and the potential need for periodontal débridement.

Exercise 2. The patient should be informed about the possibility of caries. When chewable carbamazepine is taken, the instruction should include that sugar is in the chewable product, so home fluoride products and xylitol should be used to reduce the risk of dental caries.

Exercise 3. A search should direct the student to the Web site for the Epilepsy Foundation (http://www. epilepsyfoundation.org). Information for individuals affected with the disorder as well as management for seizure activity should be of special interest to the dental hygiene student.

CHAPTER 20

Exercise 1. Both essential oil rinses and the triclosan dentifrice have an established antigingivitis effect. Both products (essential oils and triclosan) are natural products.

Exercise 2,3. Web experience.

CHAPTER 21

Exercise 1. Lidocaine with 1:100,000 epinephrine can be safely used for analgesia during periodontal débridement to reduce bleeding and control pain. Postoperative analgesia can include acetaminophen or ibuprofen.

Exercise 2. There is no contraindication for local anesthesia or any pharmacologic therapy used in oral health care in the menopausal client. This medical history can be treated as one of a healthy patient following established protocol for dental hygiene care.

Exercise 3. The oral health education plan for a pregnant woman should include the need to remove biofilm twice daily to reduce the risk for gingivitis. Information on alveolar bone loss should include that bone (leading to loss of teeth) is not lost significantly around teeth during pregnancy and that control of between-meal eating of sweets and use of fluoride during pregnancy (dentifrice and rinse) should reduce decay, resulting in teeth maintenance. Information on care of the infant's dentition, including advising the patient to use xylitol gum during pregnancy and following birth to help reduce caries in the child, should be provided.

Exercise 4. WEB ACTIVITY: Read the *JADA* October 2006 articles in the special supplement reviewing the literature on the oral/systemic link. Follow links for 2007 and 2008 published evidence, because information changes rapidly on this issue.

CHAPTER 22

Exercise 1. Both cases are activity related and have no specific answers. They will help the practitioner to advise patients and understand the product selection available in the specific geographical area. Instructions for use of products and efficacy to be expected from the products should be learned.

Exercise 2. The aluminum and magnesium in the topical rinses would bind tetracycline and make it unavailable to bind to microbes.

Exercise 3. Determine if the fluoride gel has a neutral pH (pH 5.6), such as in the PreviDent product. Neutral sodium fluoride is the appropriate recommendation during chemotherapy. When gingival bleeding develops, toothbrush bristles, even soft bristles, may irritate gingival tissues. Bleeding may be associated with cellular changes occurring due to chemotherapy and may not be easy to stop. However, a sponge oral cleaning device soaked in a nonalcoholic antiseptic (such as nonalcoholic chlorhexidine or cetylpyridium chloride [Crest Pro-Health] mouth rinse) may be a better product and can be found at most major pharmacies. Numoisyn, a cottonseed oil/glycol product that requires a prescription, may help with xerostomia, as well as other artificial saliva products (Salivart, Moi-Stir). Numoisyn comes in lozenges to stimulate salivation, whereas other products are liquid preparations. Rinsing several times daily with a mild saline solution is also recommended. Chewing xylitol gum will provide an antibacterial effect for caries-causing microorganisms and stimulate salivation.

CHAPTER 23

Exercise 1. A client with a history of alcohol abuse may have increased bleeding during periodontal débridement if significant liver damage has occurred. This issue should be followed up by asking, "Do you bleed for a long time following a cut?" or, "Have you had a lab test to determine your risk for increased bleeding?" If the client response indicates a potential bleeding risk, a medical clearance form and physician consult should be completed to have the appropriate lab test (INR usually) to determine if the vitamin K clotting factor production in the liver is impaired. Acetaminophen can be advised ($\geq$4 g/day, and preferably less, for short-term therapy), as well as a nonalcoholic mouth rinse preparation (nonalcoholic chlorhexidine, nonalcoholic CPC rinse) and an antigingivitis dentifrice. If local anesthesia/vasoconstrictor is to be used, ensure that cocaine has not been consumed in the last 24 hours before the appointment.

Exercise 2. The features of the event that suggest the possibility of substance abuse include client dissatisfaction with dental treatment received and evidence that the work was substandard, followed by abnormal behavior by the dentist in throwing instruments.

CHAPTER 24

Exercise 1. There are no interactions between etanercept and drugs used in dentistry. The client should be questioned about side effects of the drug, such as respiratory symptoms, increased bleeding, and GI symptoms. Questioning related to patient positioning should be included and the chair positioned according to the comfort level of the client. Oral health education should include the need to maintain oral health, because an increased risk for infection is a possible side effect of the drug. This can be accomplished with effective plaque control and regular periodontal maintenance. If the hands and wrists are affected and a manual toothbrush is not effective in biofilm removal, a power toothbrush should be recommended.

Exercise 2. WEB ACTIVITY: Children with juvenile rheumatoid arthritis may have limited jaw movement, affecting the efficacy of oral hygiene procedures and diminishing the ability to open the mouth enough to accommodate oral procedures. Note the various products recommended for use. Also note that some clients may have joint replacements that may require prophylactic antibiotics prior to dental hygiene care. Stamina may be affected, necessitating short appointments.

GLOSSARY

AA: Atypical antidepressant

Ablative: Having to do with the process of interfering with cellular function, causing cell death

Abstinence syndrome: Symptoms experienced by a chemically dependent person who is suddenly deprived of the substance of abuse (also called *withdrawal syndrome*)

ACE: Angiotensin-converting enzyme

Ach: Acetylcholine

ACTH: Adrenocorticotropic hormone

Addiction: Uncontrollable, compulsive drug craving, seeking, and using, even in the face of negative health and social consequences

ADE: Adverse drug effect (or adverse side effect)

ADH: Antidiuretic hormone

Adjuvant: An additional therapy given to enhance or extend the effect of the primary therapy

Adrenergic: A receptor (alpha or beta) or an effect related to the sympathetic nervous system

Adsorbed: A process of pressing a medication onto a chalk tablet, making it available without having to be dissolved

Adverse drug effect: An undesired drug effect that occurs at a normal therapeutic dose

Adverse effects: Unintended responses to a drug, also called "side effects"

Aerobic: An organism that can live only in the presence of oxygen

Afferent: Inflowing; conducting toward an area, such as the CNS

Affinity: The force of attraction of a molecule to a receptor site

Agonist: A drug that has a direct stimulatory effect on a receptor

Akinesia: Absence or loss of the power of voluntary movement

Algogenic substances: Substances liberated by the body during phases of inflammation that can produce pain

Alopecia: Loss of hair, which can be an adverse drug effect from chemotherapy

Alpha receptor: A receptor subtype of the sympathetic nervous system

AMA: American Medical Association

Amplification: The process of making larger

Anaerobic: An organism that can live in the absence of oxygen

Analgesia: Insensibility to pain without loss of consciousness

Analgesics: Agents that relieve pain by inhibiting specific pain pathways

Anaphylactoid response: An allergic response that is not preceded by a prior exposure to the offending drug

ANT: Adrenergic nerve terminal

Antagonist: A drug that interferes with the action of an agonist

Anterograde amnesia: A condition in which no memory extends forward from a particular point in time

Antibacterial: A drug used to kill or suppress the growth of bacteria

Antibiotic: A chemical substance produced by one microorganism (or semisynthetic substances prepared in the laboratory) that is capable of killing or suppressing the growth of other micro-organisms (bacteria, virus, and fungus)

Antibiotic drug resistance: A trait acquired by micro-organisms, either through genetic mutation or by the acquisition of genetic material from other organisms, that allows micro-organisms to resist the action of specific antibiotics

Antimetabolite: A substance bearing a close structural similarity to one required for normal physiologic function that exerts its effect by interfering with the utilization of the essential metabolite

Antipyretic: Capable of reducing fever

Anxiolytic: Having to do with the relief of anxiety

AO: Alveolar osteitis

APAP: Acetaminophen

APF: Acidulated phosphate fluoride

Apnea: Cessation of breathing

Apoptosis: Programmed physiologic cell death

ARAS: Ascending reticular activating system

Arrhythmia: A disturbance in the impulse generation and/or the conduction mechanism of the heart

Arthropathy: Any disease or condition affecting a joint

ASA: Aspirin

ASAM: American Society of Addiction Medicine

Aura: A phenomenon perceived by a patient that is associated with epilepsy and migraine

Autogenous infection: An infection caused by normal flora bacteria

Autonomic nervous system: The involuntary nervous system that includes the parasympathetic and sympathetic divisions; regulates physiologic function of internal organs

Bactericidal: An antibacterial agent capable of killing bacteria

Bacteriostatic: An antibacterial agent capable of suppressing the growth/multiplication of bacteria

Basic life support: Open airway, check breathing, assess evidence of circulation (pulse)

Beta receptor: A receptor subtype of the sympathetic nervous system

Biologic equivalence: The ability of a generic drug to reach blood levels equivalent to those reached by a brandname drug

BIS: Bisphosphonate

BMD: Burning mouth disorder

BMS: Burning mouth syndrome, sometimes occurring in postmenopausal women

Bradykinesia: A decrease in spontaneity of movement

BSA: Body surface area

CAD: Coronary artery disease

Carcinogenesis: Cellular change from normal to malignant cell

Catecholamines: Drugs (agonists) synthesized from tyrosine (dopamine, norepinephrine, epinephrine) that stimulate the sympathetic nervous system

CCB: Calcium channel blocker

Ceiling dose: The dose above which no further beneficial drug effect will occur

Cellular immunity: Immune responses associated with T lymphocytes

Cerebral: Having to do with the brain

Cerebral ischemia: Lack of oxygen in brain tissue

cGMP: Current good manufacturing practices, updated in 2007

Chemoprophylaxis: The prevention of disease by use of chemicals or drugs

Cholinergic: A receptor (muscarinic or nicotinic) or an effect related to the parasympathetic nervous system

CMV: Cytomegalovirus

CNS: Central nervous system

Commensal agents: Agents that live in an environment without causing harm

Compliant patient: A patient who follows the written orders on a prescription as instructed

Conscious sedation: Light sedation to relax the patient who can respond to situations and questions

Contraindication: An inadvisable treatment

COPD: Chronic obstructive pulmonary disease

COX: Cyclooxygenase

COX-I: Cyclooxygenase inhibitors (COX-1, COX-2, COX-3)

CP: Cicatricial pemphigoid

Crepitation: A clicking sound produced by bone to bone or degenerated cartilage surfaces

Crossdependence: Dependence on all drugs in the classification (for example, dependence on heroin will result in dependence on other opioids)

Crosstolerance: Chronic use of a drug produces tolerance to the effects of all drugs in the classification

CVD: Cardiovascular disease

Cytotoxic reaction: A reaction that involves damage to tissue cells; can include overdose

DEA: Drug enforcement administration

Dentinal hyperalgesia: Extreme tooth sensitivity that causes a painful response to stimuli

Dependence: A state in which physiologic and/or behavioral changes and withdrawal symptoms develop when a drug is discontinued, which can be reversed by resumption of drug administration

Depolarization: A relative reduction in polarity of the nerve membrane, allowing for impulse conduction

Dietary supplement: A natural product used for improved structure and function of the body, including herbs, vitamins, minerals, and any other product sold as a dietary supplement

DM: Diabetes mellitus

DMARD: Disease-modifying antirheumatic drug

Doseform: The manner in which the drug formulation is supplied (capsules, tablets, mouth rinse, and so forth)

Drug: A chemical substance used in diagnosis, treatment, or prevention of disease

Drug abuse: Self-administration of a drug, in increasing quantities, resulting in dependence, functional impairment, and deviation from approved social norms

Drug misuse: Indiscriminate or inappropriate use of drugs

DSHEA: Dietary Supplement Health and Education Act of 1994

Dysgeusia: Taste disturbance or perversion

Dysphagia: Impairment of speech sounds

Dysphonia: Altered voice production or voice sounds

Dyspnea: Difficulty breathing; air hunger as a result of hypoxia or too much carbon dioxide in the body

Eclampsia: Onset of convulsions in the individual with preeclampsia

Effector organ: The specific tissue stimulated to act by the postganglionic nerve

Efferent: Outflowing; conducting outward from a given area, such as the CNS

Efficacy: The magnitude of response obtained from optimal receptor site occupancy by a drug

Elixir: A liquid preparation, such as syrup

EM: Erythema multiforme

Emesis: Vomiting

Empirical: The use of experience or statistical probabilities for making drug choices

EMS: Emergency medical services

Endogenous: Originating or produced within the organism or one of its parts

Enteral: The administration of a drug through the GI tract, by mouth

EO: Essential oils, used in many antigingivitis mouth rinses

EPI: Epinephrine

Epistaxis: Nosebleed

Equianalgesic: Equal in the ability for giving pain relief

ERT: Estrogen replacement therapy

Euphoria: A feeling of exaggerated well-being; a pleasure state induced by a drug or substance of abuse

Euthyroid: A normal level of circulating thyroid hormones

Facultative: An organism able to live in either the presence or the absence of oxygen

FDA: Food and Drug Administration

Flatus: Intestinal gas

FSH: Follicle-stimulating hormone

GABA: Gamma-aminobutyric acid

GDM: Gestational diabetes mellitus

General anesthesia: Generalized, reversible depression of the CNS characterized by loss of consciousness, amnesia, and immobility, but not necessarily complete anesthesia

Generic name: The "official" name of a drug listed in a pharmacopeia

GERD: Gastroesophageal reflux disease

Glossodynia: Burning mouth or mucosal tissues

Glycogenolysis: The hydrolysis of glycogen to form glucose

GMP: Good manufacturing practices

Gout: A disorder of blood uric acid levels, resulting in severe, recurrent acute arthritis

Half-life: The time it takes for half the drug to be removed from the body

Hallucinogen: A mind-altering chemical or drug that produces auditory, visual, perceptual, or thought-process disturbances

Hapten: A substance (drug) of low molecular weight that cannot induce antibody formation unless attached to another molecule, usually a protein

HCP: Health care professional

HCTZ: Hydrochlorothiazide

HDL: High-density lipoprotein component of serum cholesterol

Hematopoiesis: The formation of blood or blood cells in the living body (bone marrow)

Hemiparesis: Weakness affecting one side of the body

Hemodynamic: Relating to aspects of blood circulation

HIV: Human immunodeficiency virus

HIVD: Human immunodeficiency viral disease

HPFS: Health Professionals Follow-up Study

HRT: Hormone replacement therapy

HSCT: Hematopoietic stem cell transplantation

HSV: Herpes simplex virus

Humoral substances: Relating to or involving a bodily humor, such as a hormone

Hydrodynamic theory: A theory that the movement of fluid within dentin tubules generates impulse transmission in nerves at the odontoblast connection with dentin

Hyperglycemia: Blood sugar levels >126 mm/mL after a 12-hour fast

Hyper-reactive: A situation in which a smaller than normal dose of a drug produces the intended effect

Hypoglycemia: Low blood glucose level; blood sugar levels <60 mm/mL

Hyporeactive: A situation in which a larger than normal dose of a drug is needed to produce the intended effect

Hypoxia: Inadequate oxygen in body tissues; reduced availability of oxygen to the various cells of the body

Iatrogenic: A result or effect caused inadvertently by a clinician or a clinician's treatment

Ictal: Related to a seizure; *preictal* means prior to a seizure, and *postictal* means following a seizure

Idiosyncrasy: A unique or unexpected drug reaction, often related to genetic variations in the individual

Indication: The intended use for a drug, usually the use approved by the FDA

Infiltration anesthesia: The injection of a local anesthetic solution directly into or adjacent to the tissue to be treated

IM: Intramuscular

Innervate: To supply with nerves

INR: International normalized ratio

International normalized ratio: A test to determine risk of bleeding

Intrinsic activity: The ability to cause an effect or action

Ischemia: Reduction of circulation to an area

IV: Intravenous

JRA: Juvenile rheumatoid arthritis

LA: Local anesthetic

LDL: Low-density lipoprotein component of serum cholesterol

Legend drug: A drug secured by a prescription

LH: Luteinizing hormone

LMWH: Low-molecular-weight heparin

Local anesthesia: A reversible loss of sensation in a defined area associated with the transient inhibition of peripheral nerve conduction

Loading dose: An initial high dose to quickly achieve a therapeutic blood level

LRA: Leukotriene-receptor antagonists

LRT: Lower respiratory tract

MAOI: Monoamine-oxidase inhibitor

MDD: Major depressive disorder

Metabolic equivalent: A measure of functional capacity (MET)

Metacarpophalangeal: Relating to joints of the fingers and the hand

Metastasize: To move a cell from the original tissue to distant sites not normally containing cells of the type

METH: Methamphetamine

MI: Myocardial infarction

MTB: *Mycobacterium tuberculosis*

Muscarinic receptor: A receptor subtype of the parasympathetic nervous system

Mycotic infection: Infection caused by fungi or molds

Myotonia: Delayed relaxation of a muscle after a strong or prolonged contraction

NA: Neuropathic arthritis

NaF: Sodium fluoride

Neonate: A newborn child younger than 1 month of age

Nephrotoxicity: Kidney damage

Nerve block anesthesia: The injection of a local anesthetic agent into or around peripheral nerve trunks or the nerve plexus

Neurotransmitter: A small peptide molecule released by presynaptic cells in response to electrical signals that diffuses across the synaptic cleft and subsequently binds to membrane receptors of postsynaptic cells, producing an excitatory or inhibitory effect

NIAAA: National Institute on Alcohol Abuse and Alcoholism

Nicotinic receptor: A receptor subtype of the parasympathetic nervous system

Nociception: Sensory detection and neuronal transmission of pain stimuli

Nor: Norepinephrine

Noxious: Injurious or harmful

NREM: Nonrapid eye movement

NSAIDs: Nonsteroidal anti-inflammatory drugs

N$_2$O/O$_2$: Nitrous oxide mixed with oxygen

NUG: Necrotizing ulcerative gingivitis

Nystagmus: Involuntary rhythmic oscillation of the eyeballs

NYTS: National Youth Tobacco Survey

OA: Osteoarthritis

OHCW: Oral health care worker

Ointment: A semisolid preparation for external areas of the body

OLP: Oral lichen planus

Oncogenes: Any of a family of genes that normally encode proteins involved in cell growth or regulation but that may foster malignant processes if mutated or activated by contact with retroviruses

ONJ: Osteonecrosis of the jaw

Opioid: Derived from opium; a strong dependence-producing analgesic

Organogenesis: Formation of organs during development of the embryo

Orthopnea: Edema in the lungs as a complication of left-side heart failure

Osteomalacia: Decreased bone mass due to impaired mineralization usually because of severe vitamin D deficiency

Osteopenia: Decreased bone mass, which may be as a result of osteoporosis (decreased bone mass due to increased bone resorption and impaired bone formation) or osteomalacia (decreased bone mass due to impaired mineralization, usually because of severe vitamin D deficiency)

OTC: Over-the-counter (drug)

Palliative care: Methods to provide comfort or reduce the severity of symptoms without curing the condition

Parietal cells: Cells that line the intestines

Parasitism: The evolution from commensal status to causing disease

Parenteral: The administration of a drug bypassing the GI tract, usually through injection into the body in various ways but also including inhalation and topical administration

Paresthesia: Numbness or tingling following return of sensation to an area or following injury to a nerve

Partial agonist: A drug with affinity for the receptor site, but unable to produce a strong effect or action

Parturition: The process of giving birth

Pathognomonic: Specific signs of a given disease, and not associated with other conditions

Pauciarticular: Arthritis affecting only a few joints (four or fewer)

PCP: Phencyclidine (also called *angel dust*)

PD: Parkinson disease

Periarticular: Tissues surrounding a joint

Pharmacodynamics: The mechanisms of drug action involving biochemical and physiologic effects of drugs

Pharmacokinetics: The absorption, distribution, metabolism, and excretion of a drug

Pharmacologic effects: The changes within a body caused by a drug

Pharmacology: The study of drugs and their effects on living tissue

Pharmacopeia: A published source of drug information based on drugs in a given geographical area

Pharmacotherapeutics: The use of pharmacologic agents to diagnose, treat, or prevent disease

Phocomelia: Defective development of the arms or legs, a teratogenic effect

Physical dependence: Dependence related to an altered physiologic state due to increased concentrations of an abused drug

Physiologic status: The state of body functions; could be normal or abnormal

Placebo: A doseform that has no active ingredients; a "sugar pill"

PNS: Parasympathetic nervous system

Polyarticular: Arthritis affecting more than four joints

Positive Nikolsky sign: A clinical sign in which mucosa dislodges from the underlying connective tissue when rubbed

Potency: The concentration at which the drug elicits 50% of its maximal response, related to the drug's affinity for the receptor

Pre-eclampsia: The development of hypertension with proteinuria or edema in pregnancy

Primary oncogenic effect: Malignancy caused by a drug or chemical substance

Proprietary name: The brand name of a drug

Prototype: The first drug in a class of drugs to which all other drugs in the same class are compared

Psychologic dependence: Dependence where the mind controls the craving for a drug

Psychotropic: Capable of affecting the mind, emotions, and behavior

PUD: Peptic ulcer disease

RA: Rheumatoid arthritis

RAS: Recurrent aphthous stomatitis

RDH: Registered dental hygienist

Receptor site: A specialized area on a cell or within a cell where a drug acts to initiate a series of biochemical and physiologic effects

Reflex arc: An automatic motor response to sensory stimuli

REM: Rapid eye movement

RHL: Recurrent herpes labialis

ROA: Route of administration

RTK: Receptor tyrosine kinases, drugs used in chemotherapy

Rx: Latin symbol for "take thou," placed in the body of the prescription

SA: Spondylarthritis

Saprophytic: The ability to live on decaying organic matter

SC: Subcutaneous

Secondary oncogenic effect: Malignancy caused by immune suppression, which allows oncogenic viruses to cause malignant changes in cells

SJS: Stevens-Johnson syndrome

SJW: Saint-John's-wort, an herb used to treat mild depression

SnF: Stannous fluoride

SLUD: Salivation, lacrimation, urination, defecation

SN/AEMS: Special Nutritionals Adverse Event Monitoring System

SNS: Sympathetic nervous system

Somatic nervous system: A part of the peripheral nervous system that controls voluntary skeletal muscle activity and conducts sensory information

Somatic pain: Pain caused by the activation of pain receptors in mucocutaneous and musculoskeletal tissues

Spondylitis: Inflammation of one or more vertebrae

Spondyloarthropathy: Arthritis in the spine

SSRI: Selective serotonin reuptake inhibitor

Status epilepticus: Continuous, uncontrolled seizure

Strong agonist: Drug that produces a significant physiologic response when only a relatively small number of receptors are occupied

Subacute: Disease development without overt clinical signs and symptoms

Substantivity: The ability to produce a prolonged effect, usually through maintaining a bond with receptors

Superinfection: Infection caused by microbes that were not affected by anti-infective therapy, such as a yeast infection following antibiotic therapy

Suprainfection: Opportunistic infection caused by the overgrowth of microorganisms insusceptible to antibacterial therapy

Supraphysiologic: A dose significantly higher than the therapeutic dose

Surfactant: A surface-acting agent, such as an emulsifier or dispersing agent

Synovial: Relating to the membrane of a joint

Tachyphylaxis: The rapid development of tolerance to a drug

TCA: Tricyclic antidepressant

TEN: Toxic epidermal necrolysis

Teratogen: A substance capable of causing fetal deformity

Teratogenic: Capable of causing developmental malformations

Thromboembolic: Having to do with blood clots (thrombus) that enter the circulation (emboli)

Thrombus: A blood clot

TNF: Tumor necrosis factor

Tolerance: A reduced drug effect that results from repeated use, which then necessitates taking higher doses to produce the same effect

Toxicity: Overdose, undesirable effects, or poisoning

TSH: Thyroid-stimulating hormone

Type-A ADE: A predictable adverse drug effect usually associated with the normal dose of a drug, but can include adverse effects of overdose

Type-B ADE: An unpredictable adverse drug effect, not related to the dose

USPSTF: U.S. Preventive Services Task Force

Visceral pain: Pain caused by the activation of pain receptors in internal organs

VZV: Varicella zoster virus

INDEX

Page numbers followed by *b, f* and *t* denote box, figure and table, respectively.